British Pharmacopoeia (Veterinary) 2008

British Pharmacopoeia (Veterinary) 2008

Published on the recommendation of the British Pharmacopoeia Commission pursuant to The Medicines Act 1968 and notified in draft to the European Commission in accordance with Directive 98/34/EEC.

The monographs of the Fifth Edition of the European Pharmacopoeia (2004), as amended by Supplements 5.1 to 5.8 published by the Council of Europe are reproduced either in this edition of the British Pharmacopoeia (Veterinary) or in the associated edition of the British Pharmacopoeia.

see General Notices

Effective date: 1 January 2008

see Notices

London: The Stationery Office

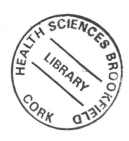

British Pharmacopoeia Commission Office:

Market Towers
1 Nine Elms Lane
London SW8 5NQ
Telephone: +44 (0)20 7084 2561
Fax: +44 (0)20 7084 2566
E-mail: bpcom@mhra.gsi.gov.uk
Web site: www.pharmacopoeia.org.uk

Laboratory:

British Pharmacopoeia Commission Laboratory
Queen's Road
Teddington
Middlesex TW11 0LY
Telephone: +44 (0)20 8943 8960
Fax: +44 (0)20 8943 8962
E-mail: bpcrs@mhra.gsi.gov.uk
Web site: www.bpclab.co.uk

Contents

Notices

Monographs of the European Pharmacopoeia are distinguished by a chaplet of stars against the title. The term European Pharmacopoeia, used without qualification, means the Fifth Edition of the European Pharmacopoeia comprising, unless otherwise stated, the main volume, published in 2004 as amended by any subsequent supplements and revisions.

Patents In this Pharmacopoeia certain drugs and preparations have been included notwithstanding the existence of actual or potential patent rights. In so far as such substances are protected by Letters Patent their inclusion in this Pharmacopoeia neither conveys, nor implies, licence to manufacture.

Effective dates New and revised monographs of national origin enter into force on 1 January 2008. Monographs of the European Pharmacopoeia have previously been published by the Council of Europe and have been brought into effect by means of Notices published in the Belfast, Edinburgh and London Gazettes.

Preface

The British Pharmacopoeia (Veterinary) 2008, a companion volume to the British Pharmacopoeia 2008, is published for Ministers on the recommendation of the British Pharmacopoeia Commission in accordance with Section 99(6) of The Medicines Act 1968.

The British Pharmacopoeia Commission believes that the British Pharmacopoeia (Veterinary) contributes significantly to the overall control of the quality of materials used in the practice of veterinary medicine, by providing an authoritative statement of the quality that a product, material or article is expected to meet at any time during its period of use. The Pharmacopoeial standards, which are publicly available and legally enforceable, are designed to complement and assist the licensing and inspection processes and are part of the system for safeguarding animal and human health.

The British Pharmacopoeia Commission wishes to record its appreciation of the services of all those who have contributed to the preparation of this work.

British Pharmacopoeia Commission

The British Pharmacopoeia Commission is appointed by the NHS Appointments Commission, the body responsible for appointments to all of the Medicines Act 1968 Advisory Bodies.

The duties of the British Pharmacopoeia Commission are as follows:

(a) the preparation under section 99(1) of the Act of any new edition of the British Pharmacopoeia;

(b) the preparation under section 99(1) of the Act, as given effect by section 102(1) thereof, of any amendments of the edition of the British Pharmacopoeia published in 1968 or any new edition of it;

(c) the preparation under section 100 of the Act (which provides for the preparation and publication of lists of names to be used as headings to monographs in the British Pharmacopoeia) of any list of names and the preparation under that section as given effect by section 102(3) of the Act of any amendments of any published list;

(d) the preparation under section 99(6) of the Act, of any compendium, or any new edition thereof, containing information relating to substances and articles which are or may be used in the practice of veterinary medicine or veterinary surgery;

(e) to frame clear and unequivocal technical advice in order to discharge the Commission's responsibilities both for the British Pharmacopoeia, the British Pharmacopoeia (Veterinary) and British Approved Names and as the national pharmacopoeial authority with respect to the European Pharmacopoeia.

Members of the British Pharmacopoeia Commission are appointed for a (renewable) term of 4 years and, under the requirements laid down by the Office of the Commissioner for Public Appointments, can serve for a maximum of 10 years.

Membership of the British Pharmacopoeia Commission

The list below includes those members who served during the period 2006 to 2007.

Chairman **Professor David Woolfson** BSc PhD CChem FRSC MPSNI
Professor of Pharmaceutics, Queens University of Belfast

Vice-Chairman **Mr V'Iain Fenton-May** BPharm MI PharmM FRPharmS
Specialist Quality Controller to the Welsh Hospitals

Dr Anthony H Andrews BVetMed PhD MBIAC DipECBHM FRSM MRCVS
Veterinary Consultant

Professor Graham Buckton BPharm PhD DSc AKC FRPharmS CChem FRSC
Professor of Pharmaceutics; School of Pharmacy, University of London

Professor Donald Cairns BSc PhD MRPharmS CSci CChem MRSC
Associate Head, School of Pharmacy, Robert Gordon University, Aberdeen

Mr Barry Capon CBE (*Lay representative*)
Non-executive Director, Norfolk and Waveney Mental Health Partnership

Professor Alastair Davidson BSc PhD FRPharmS CChem FRSC
Visiting Professor of Pharmaceutical Sciences, University of Strathclyde

Mrs Margaret A Dow MSc PhC
Consultant in the regulation of biological and biotechnological products

Dr Thomas D Duffy BSc PhD FRPharmS CChem MRSC FIQA MRQA
Consultant in quality management systems, quality assurance and training in production, development and QC Laboratories

Mr Christopher Goddard BSc DIS CSci EurChem CChem FRSC
Quality Control Manager, Ashton Pharmaceuticals Limited

Dr Rodney L Horder BPharm PhD MRPharmS
Vice President, Global Pharmaceutical R & D Quality Assurance, Abbott Laboratories

Dr Aileen M T Lee BVMS PhD MRCVS
Member of the Veterinary Medicines Directorate
Specialism: Regulation of Veterinary Immunological Products

Professor Anthony C Moffat BPharm PhD DSc CChem FRSC FRPharmS FFIP
Head, Centre for Pharmaceutical Analysis, The School of Pharmacy, University of London

Membership of Expert Advisory Groups, Panels of Experts and Working Parties

The Commission appointed the following Expert Advisory Groups, Panels of Experts and Working Parties to advise it in carrying out its duties. Membership has changed from time to time; the lists below include all who have served during the period 2006 to 2007.

EXPERT ADVISORY GROUPS

ABS: Antibiotics (formerly Committee E)
R L Horder (*Chairman*), P York (*Vice-Chairman*), A Ambrose, A H Andrews, J F Chissell, J Dolman, P Ellis, S Green, R Harryman, A Livingstone, W Mann, W F H McLean, S Patel, C G Taylor, I R Williams

CX: Excipients (disbanded, 30 June 2006)
G Buckton (*Chairman*), C Mroz (*Vice-Chairman*), E Anno, A C Cartwright, R Cawthorne, M Kearsley, B R Matthews, M I Robertson

HCM: Herbal and Complementary Medicines (formerly Committee G)
A C Moffat (*Chairman*), L A Anderson (*Vice-Chairman*), M Berry, K Chan, T Chapman, A Charvill, K Helliwell, P J Houghton, C Leon, W F H McLean, J D Phillipson, M Pires, J Sumal, E Williamson (*Corresponding member* B P Jackson)

MC1: Medicinal Chemicals (formerly Committee A)
A G Davidson (*Chairman*), D Cairns (*Vice-Chairman*), M Ahmed, L Anderson, J C Berridge, M Broughton, A J Caws, P Fleming, A Hardy, W J Lough, D Malpas

MC2: Medicinal Chemicals (formerly Committee B)
T D Duffy (*Chairman*), C T Goddard (*Vice-Chairman*), D Billington, F Breslin, M Cole, B M Everett, K Goode, A J Hutt, S Jones, M A Lee, J Lim, K McKiernan, B Midcalf, P Murray, M Turgoose

MC3: Medicinal Chemicals (formerly Committee D)
V Fenton-May (*Chairman*), E Williamson (*Vice-Chairman*), S Arkle, J F Chissell, C T Goddard, W J Poling, W K L Pugh, G G Skellern, W H Smith, R Tomlinson, R Torano, I R Williams

NOM: Nomenclature (formerly Panel N)
J K Aronson (*Chairman*), L Tsang (*Vice-Chairman*), M Ahmed, D Cousins, G Gallagher, P W Golightly, D Masieh, A McNaught, H McNulty, G P Moss, R J Taylor, R Thorpe (*Corresponding members* R G Balocco Mattavelli, E M Cortés Montejano, J Robertson)

PCY: Pharmacy (formerly Committee P)
R L Horder (*Chairman*), A D Woolfson (*Vice-Chairman*), M Aulton, E Baker, S Branch, G Buckton, G Davison, G Eccleston, D Elder, R Lowe, B R Matthews, J F McGuire, S C Nichols, R Shaw, M P Summers, K Truman, P Wood

PANELS OF EXPERTS

BIO: Biological and Biotechnological Products (formerly Panel H)
M A Dow (*Chairman*), L Tsang (*Vice-Chairman*), C Booth, A F Bristow, D H Calam, J Cook, T Forsey, R Johnson, J Lawrence, B Mason, A Onadipe, A M Pickett, S Poole, N Randall, D Sesardic, P Sheppard, W J Tarbit, J N A Tettey, A H Thomas, R Thorpe, S Vass

BLP: Blood Products (formerly Panel HB)
B Cuthbertson, A R Hubbard, J Lawrence, T J Snape, R Thorpe, P Varley

IGC: Inorganic and General Chemicals (formerly Panel CI)
C T Goddard (*Chairman*), A C Cartwright, B M Everett, P Henrys, D Malpas, C Mroz, I D Newton

J: Immunological Products (disbanded, 30 June 2006)
M J Corbel, M A Dow, A M Pickett, D Sesardic, A H Thomas

MIC: Microbiology (formerly Panel M)
V Fenton-May (*Chairman*), A H Andrews, R Baird, C Booth, S Denyer, S Gorman, D P Hargreaves, R Johnson, B R Matthews, W F H McLean, P Newby, P Taylor

RAD: Radioactive Materials (formerly Panel R)
S R Hesslewood, D Lui, A M Millar, R D Pickett, S Waters

VIP: Veterinary Immunological Products (formerly Panel JV)
A M T Lee (*Chairman*), A H Andrews, K Redhead, J Salt, P W Wells

WORKING PARTIES

CX: Excipients
G Buckton (*Chairman*), C Mroz (*Vice-Chairman*), E Anno, R Cawthorne, B R Matthews, M I Robertson

UM: Unlicensed Medicines
V Fenton-May (*Chairman*), T D Duffy (*Vice-Chairman*), I Beaumont, C Cable, P Forsey, S Jones, A Lowey, A Nunn, A Pandya, J Smith, D Wallace

Current members of staff of the British Pharmacopoeia Laboratory who have taken part in the production of this edition include:

R Gaur (*Laboratory Manager*), M Azizi, L Fletcher, A Jordan, R Mannan, A Panchal, D Parmar, K Patel, M Patel, N Patel, J Rana, S Rihal

British Pharmacopoeia Staff

Members of staff who have taken part in the production of this edition include:

Secretariat M Vallender (*Editor-in-Chief*)

S Young (*Head of Science*)

A Bentley, M Barrett, A Evans, P Holland, M O'Kane, R A Pask-Hughes, F J Swanson, N Thomas, R L Turner

Administrative M Cumberbatch, B F Delahunty, W Jeffries, L Phillips

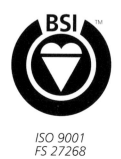

ISO 9001
FS 27268

Introduction

The British Pharmacopoeia (Veterinary) 2008 supersedes the British Pharmacopoeia (Veterinary) 2007. It is published for Ministers on the recommendation of the British Pharmacopoeia Commission in accordance with section 99(6) of the Medicines Act 1968.

This edition is published as a companion volume to the British Pharmacopoeia 2008 and thus contains only those monographs for substances and preparations used exclusively or predominantly in veterinary medicine within the United Kingdom, together with such additional texts as are necessary to support them. It therefore follows that any reference to a monograph, appendix or reagent not contained within this edition is to be construed as a reference to the said monograph, appendix or reagent contained within the British Pharmacopoeia 2008.

This edition, together with the British Pharmacopoeia 2008, contains all the monographs of the 5th edition of the European Pharmacopoeia as amended by Supplements 5.1 to 5.8. Users of the British Pharmacopoeia and British Pharmacopoeia (Veterinary) therefore benefit by finding within these two compendia all current pharmacopoeial standards for veterinary medicines used within the United Kingdom.

Effective Date
The effective date for this edition is 1 January 2008.

Where a monograph which appeared previously in an earlier edition of the British Pharmacopoeia has not been included in this edition, it remains effective in accordance with the Medicines Act 1968.

Expert Advisory Groups and Panels of Experts
A comprehensive review of the membership of the Committees and Panels of Experts was undertaken. The Committees were renamed Expert Advisory Groups (EAGs) and the letter designations for the EAGs and Panels of Experts were changed to reflect more closely the name of the EAG and Panel. The Committee on Excipients was disbanded and its work will now be undertaken by Working Parties of the Pharmacy EAG. The Panel of Experts on Immunological Products was disbanded and the remit of the panel incorporated into that of the Panel of Experts on Biological and Biotechnological Products. The Panel of Experts on Nomenclature was replaced by a new Expert Advisory Group on Nomenclature.

General Notices
Three areas of change have been introduced to the British Pharmacopoeia (Veterinary) General Notices (Part II) as follows.

Definition of terms

A new General Notice has been added to clarify terms such as 'about', 'corresponds' and 'similar' used throughout the publication.
The clarification is intended to facilitate the interpretation of monographs of the British Pharmacopoeia.

Crude Drugs; Traditional Herbal and Complementary; Homoeopathic Medicines

The General Notice on Crude Drugs has been broadened to encompass traditional herbal and complementary medicines. A separate General Notice has also been added to cover Homoeopathic Medicines.

Storage

This General Notice has been amended to clarify the use of the terms 'tamper-evident containers' and 'tamper-proof containers' throughout the Pharmacopoeia.

Additions

A list of monographs included for the first time in the British Pharmacopoeia (Veterinary) 2008 is given at the end of this introduction. It includes a new general monograph of national origin for Veterinary Oral Pastes and 6 new monographs reproduced from Supplements 5.6, 5.7 and 5.8 of the European Pharmacopoeia.

General Monographs

The General Monographs, which are applicable only to veterinary dosage forms, are grouped together within this volume at the beginning of the Formulated Preparations section. They are followed by the individual dosage form monographs arranged in alphabetical order. The General Monographs of the European Pharmacopoeia apply to all individual dosage forms of the type defined rather than only to those preparations for which a specific monograph is described (see the General Notices).

Infrared Reference Spectra

As with the previous edition, the reference spectra are placed in alphabetical order within this edition.

Editorial Changes

Action and use

An extensive review of the Action and use statements has been undertaken. Changes have been made to the monographs included in Volumes I and II of the British Pharmacopoeia 2008. A combined statement is included indicating, where known, the pharmacological action and the therapeutic use of the substance or preparation. For the first time, Action and use statements have been included in relevant monographs for Formulated Preparations.

Stationary phases

A comprehensive review of the terms 'stationary phase A', 'stationary phase B' and 'stationary phase C' has been made and 13 monographs have been amended to refer to the appropriate silica gel for chromatography in this edition.

Dissolution

British Pharmacopoeia monographs have been harmonised with the Ph Eur test method to refer to Apparatus 1 and 2. The 2 veterinary monographs affected have been harmonised.

Chromatographic tests

A new format for chromatographic tests is introduced in this edition to delineate sample preparation, chromatographic conditions, system suitability and acceptance criteria. The format will be harmonised in future editions for all BP monographs.

European Pharmacopoeia

All monographs of the 5th edition of the European Pharmacopoeia, which are used in veterinary practice but not normally in human medicine in the United Kingdom, are reproduced in this edition of the British Pharmacopoeia (Veterinary). Each of these monographs is signified by a European chaplet of stars alongside its title. Additionally, reference to the European Pharmacopoeia monograph number is included immediately below the title in italics in the form 'Ph Eur monograph xxx'. Where the title in the British Pharmacopoeia is different from that in the European Pharmacopoeia, an approved synonym has been created (see Appendix XXI B (Vet)) and the Ph Eur title is included before the monograph number. The entire European Pharmacopoeia text is then bounded by two horizontal lines bearing the symbol 'Ph Eur'.

The European Pharmacopoeia texts have been reproduced in their entirety but, where deemed appropriate, additional statements of relevance to UK usage have been added (e.g. action and use statement, a list of BP (Vet) preparations). It should be noted, however, that in the event of doubt of interpretation in any text of the European Pharmacopoeia, the text published in English under the direction of the Council of Europe should be consulted.

Correspondence between the general methods of the European Pharmacopoeia and the appendices of the British Pharmacopoeia (Veterinary) is indicated in each appendix. A check list is also provided at the beginning of the appendices section. This provides a full listing of the European Pharmacopoeia method texts with their British Pharmacopoeia and British Pharmacopoeia (Veterinary) equivalents.

Pharmacopoeial Requirements

Pharmacopoeial requirements for articles used in veterinary medicine are established on the same basis as those used in human medicine. A proper understanding of the basis upon which these requirements are established is essential for their application and advice is provided within the General Notices of the British Pharmacopoeia (Veterinary) and the Supplementary Chapters to the British Pharmacopoeia. It should be noted that no requirement of the Pharmacopoeia can be taken in isolation. A valid interpretation of any particular requirement depends upon it being read in the context of (i) the monograph as a whole, (ii) the specified method of analysis, (iii) the relevant General Notices and (iv) where appropriate, the relevant general monograph(s).

Where a preparation that is the subject of a monograph in the British Pharmacopoeia is supplied for use in veterinary medicine, the standards of the British Pharmacopoeia apply, unless otherwise justified and authorised. Attention is drawn to the Notice permitting the designation British Pharmacopoeia (Veterinary) [BP (Vet)] to be used in place of the designation British Pharmacopoeia [BP] where a preparation complying with the British Pharmacopoeia is supplied for use in veterinary medicine with the approval of the competent authority.

Innovations

As a new initiative, the British Pharmacopoeia (Veterinary) 2008 will be available as an e-book.

Acknowledgements

The British Pharmacopoeia Commission is greatly indebted to the members of its Expert Advisory Groups and Panels of Experts without whose dedicated enthusiasm and assistance this edition could not have been prepared.

Close co-operation has continued with many organisations at home and overseas. These include the Veterinary Medicines Directorate, the Medicines and Healthcare products Regulatory Agency, the National Institute for Biological Standards and Control, the Royal Pharmaceutical Society of Great Britain, the National Office of Animal Health, the Association of the British Pharmaceutical Industry, the European Pharmacopoeia Commission and the European Directorate for the Quality of Medicines & HealthCare, the Therapeutic Goods Administration (Australia), the Health Protection Branch of the Canadian Department of Health and Welfare, the Committee of Revision of the United States Pharmacopeia, the Essential Drugs and Other Medicines Department of the World Health Organization (WHO) and the WHO Collaborating Centre for Chemical Reference Substances.

The British Pharmacopoeia Commission also acknowledges the advice of the publishing team at The Stationery Office, in particular Mr Phil Halls, Dr Clare Collett and Dr Gill Hodgson, in the production of this edition.

Additions

The following monographs of the British Pharmacopoeia (Veterinary) 2008 were not included in the British Pharmacopoeia (Veterinary) 2007.

Medicinal and Pharmaceutical Substances
Dembrexine Hydrochloride Monohydrate*
Spectinomycin Sulphate Tetrahydrate*

Formulated Preparations: General Monographs
Veterinary Oral Pastes

Immunological Products
Feline Chlamydiosis Vaccine (Inactivated)*
Mycoplasma Gallisepticum Vaccine (Inactivated)*
Salmonella Enteritidis Vaccine (Inactivated) for Chickens*
Salmonella Typhimurium Vaccine (Inactivated) for Chickens*

Omissions

The following monographs of the British Pharmacopoeia (Veterinary) 2007 are not included in the British Pharmacopoeia (Veterinary) 2008.

Formulated Preparations: Specific Monographs
Chloramphenicol Injection

---

* denotes a monograph of the European Pharmacopoeia.

Technical Changes The following monographs in the British Pharmacopoeia (Veterinary) 2008 have been technically amended since the publication of the British Pharmacopoeia (Veterinary) 2007. This list does not include revised monographs of the European Pharmacopoeia. An indication of the nature of the change or the section of the monograph that has been changed is given in *italic type* in the right hand column.

Medicinal and Pharmaceutical Substances
Cefalonium   *Assay*

Changes in Title The following list gives the alterations in the titles of monographs of the British Pharmacopoeia (Veterinary) 2007 that have been retained in the British Pharmacopoeia (Veterinary) 2008.

BRITISH PHARMACOPOEIA (VETERINARY) 2007	BRITISH PHARMACOPOEIA (VETERINARY) 2008
Formulated Preparations: Specific Monographs	
Fenbendazole Veterinary Paste	Fenbendazole Veterinary Oral Paste
Ivermectin Veterinary Paste	Ivermectin Veterinary Oral Paste
Immunological Products	
Veterinary Antisera	Veterinary Immunosera

General Notices

CONTENTS OF THE GENERAL NOTICES

General Notices

Part I

The British Pharmacopoeia (Veterinary) comprises the entire text within this publication. The word 'official' is used in the Pharmacopoeia to signify 'of the Pharmacopoeia'. It applies to any title, substance, preparation, method or statement included in the general notices, monographs and appendices of the Pharmacopoeia. The abbreviation for British Pharmacopoeia (Veterinary) is BP (Vet).

European Pharmacopoeia Monographs of the European Pharmacopoeia are reproduced in this edition of the British Pharmacopoeia (Veterinary) by incorporation of the text published under the direction of the Council of Europe (Partial Agreement) in accordance with the Convention on the Elaboration of a European Pharmacopoeia (Treaty Series No. 32 (1974) CMND 5763) as amended by the Protocol to the Convention (Treaty Series No MISC16 (1990) CMND 1133). They are included for the convenience of users of the British Pharmacopoeia (Veterinary). In cases of doubt or dispute reference should be made to the Council of Europe text.

Monographs of the European Pharmacopoeia are distinguished by a chaplet of stars against the title and by reference to the European Pharmacopoeia monograph number included immediately below the title in italics. The beginning and end of text from the European Pharmacopoeia are denoted by means of horizontal lines with the symbol '*Ph Eur*' ranged left and right, respectively.

The general provisions of the European Pharmacopoeia relating to different types of dosage form are included in the appropriate general monograph in that section of either the British Pharmacopoeia or the British Pharmacopoeia (Veterinary) entitled Monographs: Formulated Preparations. These general provisions apply to all veterinary dosage forms of the type defined, whether an individual monograph is included in the British Pharmacopoeia (Veterinary) or not.

Texts of the European Pharmacopoeia are governed by the General Notices of the European Pharmacopoeia. These are reproduced as Part III of these notices.

Part II

The following general notices apply to the statements made in the monographs of the British Pharmacopoeia (Veterinary) other than those reproduced from the European Pharmacopoeia and to the statements made in the appendices of the British Pharmacopoeia (Veterinary) other than when a method, test or other matter described in an appendix is invoked in a monograph reproduced from the European Pharmacopoeia.

Official Standards   The requirements stated in the monographs of the Pharmacopoeia apply to articles that are intended for veterinary medicinal use but not necessarily to articles that may be sold under the same name for other purposes.
An article intended for veterinary medicinal use that is described by means of an official title must comply with the requirements of the relevant monograph. A formulated preparation must comply throughout its assigned shelf-life (period of validity). The subject of any other monograph must comply throughout its period of use.

A monograph is to be construed in accordance with any general monograph or notice or any appendix, note or other explanatory material that is contained in this edition and that is applicable to that monograph. All statements contained in the monographs, except where a specific general notice indicates otherwise and with the exceptions given below, constitute standards for the official articles. An article is not of Pharmacopoeial quality unless it complies with all of the requirements stated. This does not imply that a manufacturer is obliged to perform all the tests in a monograph in order to assess compliance with the Pharmacopoeia before release of a product. The manufacturer may assure himself that a product is of Pharmacopoeial quality by other means, for example, from data derived from validation studies of the manufacturing process, from in-process controls or from a combination of the two. Parametric release in appropriate circumstances is thus not precluded by the need to comply with the Pharmacopoeia. The general notice on Assays and Tests indicates that analytical methods other than those described in the Pharmacopoeia may be employed for routine purposes.

Requirements in monographs have been framed to provide appropriate limitation of potential impurities rather than to provide against all possible impurities. Material found to contain an impurity not detectable by means of the prescribed tests is not of Pharmacopoeial quality if the nature or amount of the impurity found is incompatible with good pharmaceutical practice.

The status of any statement given under the side-headings Definition, Production, Characteristics, Storage, Labelling or Action and use is defined within the general notice relating to the relevant side-heading. In addition to any exceptions indicated by one of the general notices referred to above, the following parts of a monograph do not constitute standards:
(a) a graphic or molecular formula given at the beginning of a monograph;
(b) a molecular weight; (c) a Chemical Abstracts Service Registry Number;
(d) any information given at the end of a monograph concerning impurities known to be limited by that monograph; (e) information in any annex to a

monograph. Any statement containing the word 'should' constitutes non-mandatory advice or recommendation.

The expression 'unless otherwise justified and authorised' means that the requirement in question has to be met, unless a competent authority authorises a modification or exemption where justified in a particular case. The term 'competent authority' means the national, supranational or international body or organisation vested with the authority for making decisions concerning the issue in question. It may, for example, be a licensing authority or an official control laboratory. For a formulated preparation that is the subject of monograph in the British Pharmacopoeia (Veterinary) any justified and authorised modification to, or exemption from, the requirements of the relevant general monograph of the European Pharmacopoeia is stated in the individual monograph. For example, the general monograph for Tablets requires that Uncoated Tablets, except for chewable tablets, disintegrate within 15 minutes; for Megestrol Tablets a time of 30 minutes is permitted.

Additional statements and requirements applicable to the individual monographs of the British Pharmacopoeia are also included in many of the general monographs of the British Pharmacopoeia for formulated preparations. Such statements and requirements apply also to all monographs for that dosage form included in the British Pharmacopoeia (Veterinary) unless otherwise indicated in either a general monograph or an individual monograph of the British Pharmacopoeia (Veterinary).

Any additions to or modifications of the statements and requirements of the British Pharmacopoeia that are generally applicable to the individual monographs of the British Pharmacopoeia (Veterinary) are provided by means of a supplementary text introduced by a subsidiary heading together with an italicised statement. Thus there is, for example, a supplementary text entitled 'Tablets of the British Pharmacopoeia (Veterinary)' that relates only to the specific monographs for individual tablets that are contained in the British Pharmacopoeia (Veterinary).

Where a monograph on a biological substance or preparation refers to a strain, a test, a method, a substance, *etc.*, using the qualifications 'suitable' or 'appropriate' without further definition in the text, the choice of such strain, test, method, substance, *etc.*, is made in accordance with any international agreements or national regulations affecting the subject concerned.

Definition of Terms Where the term "about" is included in a monograph or test it should be taken to mean approximately (fairly correct or accurate; near to the actual value).

Where the term "corresponds" is included in a monograph or test it should be taken to mean similar or equivalent in character or quantity.

Where the term "similar" is included in a monograph or test it should be taken to mean alike though not necessarily identical.

Further qualifiers (such as numerical acceptance criteria) for the above terms are not included in the BP (Vet). The acceptance criteria for any individual case are set based on the range of results obtained from known reference samples, the level of precision of the equipment or apparatus used and the level of accuracy required for the particular application. The user should determine the variability seen in his/her own laboratory and set in-house acceptance criteria that he/she judges to be appropriate based on the local operating conditions.

Expression of Standards

Where the standard for the content of a substance described in a monograph is expressed in terms of the chemical formula for that substance an upper limit exceeding 100% may be stated. Such an upper limit applies to the result of the assay calculated in terms of the equivalent content of the specified chemical formula. For example, the statement 'contains not less than 99.0% and not more than 101.0% of $C_{20}H_{24}N_2O_2,HCl$' implies that the result of the assay is not less than 99.0% and not more than 101.0%, calculated in terms of the equivalent content of $C_{20}H_{24}N_2O_2,HCl$.

Where the result of an assay or test is required to be calculated with reference to the dried, anhydrous or ignited substance, the substance free from a specified solvent or to the peptide content, the determination of loss on drying, water content, loss on ignition, content of the specified solvent or peptide content is carried out by the method prescribed in the relevant test in the monograph.

Temperature

The Celsius thermometric scale is used in expressing temperatures.

Weights and Measures

The metric system of weights and measures is employed; SI Units have generally been adopted. Metric measures are required to have been graduated at 20° and all measurements involved in the analytical operations of the Pharmacopoeia are intended, unless otherwise stated, to be made at that temperature. Graduated glass apparatus used in analytical operations should comply with Class A requirements of the appropriate International Standard issued by the International Organization for Standardization.

Atomic Weights

The atomic weights adopted are the values given in the Table of Relative Atomic Weights 2001 published by the International Union of Pure and Applied Chemistry (Appendix XXV).

Constant Weight

The term 'constant weight', used in relation to the process of drying or the process of ignition, means that two consecutive weighings do not differ by more than 0.5 milligram, the second weighing being made after an additional period of drying or ignition under the specified conditions appropriate to the nature and quantity of the residue (1 hour is usually suitable).

Expression of Concentrations

The term 'per cent' or more usually the symbol '%' is used with one of four different meanings in the expression of concentrations according to circumstances. In order that the meaning to be attached to the expression in each instance is clear, the following notation is used.

Per cent w/w (% w/w) (percentage weight in weight) expresses the number of grams of solute in 100 g of product.

Per cent w/v (% w/v) (percentage weight in volume) expresses the number of grams of solute in 100 ml of product.

Per cent v/v (% v/v) (percentage volume in volume) expresses the number of millilitres of solute in 100 ml of product.

Per cent v/w (% v/w) (percentage volume in weight) expresses the number of millilitres of solute in 100 g of product.

Usually the strength of solutions of solids in liquids is expressed as percentage weight in volume, of liquids in liquids as percentage volume in volume and of gases in liquids as percentage weight in weight.

When the concentration of a solution is expressed as parts per million (ppm), it means weight in weight, unless otherwise specified.

When the concentration of a solution is expressed as parts of dissolved substance in parts of the solution, it means parts by weight (g) of a solid in parts by volume (ml) of the final solution; or parts by volume (ml) of a liquid in parts by volume (ml) of the final solution; or parts by weight (g) of a gas in parts by weight (g) of the final solution.

When the concentration of a solution is expressed in molarity designated by the symbol M preceded by a number, it denotes the number of moles of the stated solute contained in sufficient Purified Water (unless otherwise stated) to produce 1 litre of solution.

Water Bath   The term 'water bath' means a bath of boiling water, unless water at some other temperature is indicated in the text. An alternative form of heating may be employed providing that the required temperature is approximately maintained but not exceeded.

Reagents   The reagents required for the assays and tests of the Pharmacopoeia are defined in appendices. The descriptions set out in the appendices do not imply that the materials are suitable for use in medicine.

Indicators   Indicators, the colours of which change over approximately the same range of pH, may be substituted for one another but in the event of doubt or dispute as to the equivalence of indicators for a particular purpose, the indicator specified in the text is alone authoritative.

The quantity of an indicator solution appropriate for use in acid—base titrations described in assays or tests is 0.1 ml unless otherwise stated in the text.

Any solvent required in an assay or test in which an indicator is specified is previously neutralised to the indicator, unless a blank test is prescribed.

Caution Statements   A number of materials described in the monographs and some of the reagents specified for use in the assays and tests of the Pharmacopoeia may be injurious to health unless adequate precautions are taken. The principles of good laboratory practice and the provisions of any appropriate regulations such as those issued in the United Kingdom in accordance with the Health and Safety at Work *etc.* Act (1974) should be observed at all times in carrying out the assays and tests of the Pharmacopoeia.

Attention is drawn to particular hazards in certain monographs by means of an italicised statement; the absence of such a statement should not however be taken to mean that no hazard exists.

Titles   Subsidiary titles, where included, have the same significance as the main titles. An abbreviated title constructed in accordance with the directions given in Appendix XXI A has the same significance as the main title.

Titles that are derived by the suitable inversion of words of a main or subsidiary title, with the addition of a preposition if appropriate, are also official titles. Thus, the following are all official titles: Acepromazine Tablets, Tablets of Acepromazine; Catechu Tincture, Tincture of Catechu; Levamisole Injection, Injection of Levamisole.

A title of a formulated preparation that includes the full nonproprietary name of the active ingredient or ingredients, where this is not included in the title of the monograph, is also an official title. For example, the title Acepromazine Maleate Injection has the same significance as Acepromazine

Injection and the title Megestrol Acetate Tablets has the same significance as Megestrol Tablets.

Where the English title at the head of a monograph in the European Pharmacopoeia is different from that at the head of the text incorporated into the British Pharmacopoeia (Veterinary), an Approved Synonym has been declared in accordance with section 65(8) of the Medicines Act 1968. The titles and subsidiary titles, if any, are thus official titles. A cumulative list of such Approved Synonyms is provided in Appendix XXI B (Vet).

Where the names of Pharmacopoeial substances, preparations and other materials occur in the text they are printed with capital initial letters and this indicates that materials of Pharmacopoeial quality must be used. Words in the text that name a reagent or other material, a physical characteristic or a process that is described or defined in an appendix are printed in italic type, for example, *methanol*, *absorbance*, *gas chromatography*, and these imply compliance with the requirements specified in the appropriate appendix.

Chemical Formulae When the chemical composition of an official substance is known or generally accepted, the graphic and molecular formulae, the molecular weight and the Chemical Abstracts Service Registry Number are normally given at the beginning of the monograph for information. This information refers to the chemically pure substance and is not to be regarded as an indication of the purity of the official material. Elsewhere, in statements of standards of purity and strength and in descriptions of processes of assay, it is evident from the context that the formulae denote the chemically pure substances.

Where the absolute stereochemical configuration is specified, the International Union of Pure and Applied Chemistry (IUPAC) *R/S* and *E/Z* systems of designation have been used. If the substance is an enantiomer of unknown absolute stereochemistry the sign of the optical rotation, as determined in the solvent and under the conditions specified in the monograph, has been attached to the systematic name. An indication of sign of rotation has also been given where this is incorporated in a trivial name that appears on an IUPAC preferred list.

All amino acids, except glycine, have the L-configuration unless otherwise indicated. The three-letter and one-letter symbols used for amino acids in peptide and protein sequences are those recommended by the Joint Commission on Biochemical Nomenclature of the International Union of Pure and Applied Chemistry and the International Union of Biochemistry.

In the graphic formulae the following abbreviations are used:

Me	$-CH_3$	Bu^s	$-CH_3(CH_3)CH_2CH_3$
Et	$-CH_2CH_3$	Bu^n	$-CH_2CH_2CH_2CH_3$
Pr^i	$-CH(CH_3)$	Bu^t	$-C(CH_3)_3$
Pr^n	$-CH_2CH_2CH_3$	Ph	$-C_6H_5$
Bu^i	$-CH_2CH(CH_3)_2$	Ac	$-COCH_3$

Definition Statements given under the side-heading Definition constitute an official definition of the substance, preparation or other article that is the subject of the monograph. They constitute instructions or requirements and are mandatory in nature.

Certain medicinal or pharmaceutical substances and other articles are defined by reference to a particular method of manufacture. A statement that a substance or article *is* prepared or obtained by a certain method constitutes part of the official definition and implies that other methods are not permitted. A statement that a substance *may be* prepared or obtained by a certain method, however, indicates that this is one possible method and does not imply that other methods are proscribed.

Additional statements concerning the definition of formulated preparations are given in the general notice on Manufacture of Formulated Preparations.

Production Statements given under the side-heading Production draw attention to particular aspects of the manufacturing process but are not necessarily comprehensive. They constitute mandatory instructions to manufacturers. They may relate, for example, to source materials, to the manufacturing process itself and its validation and control, to in-process testing or to testing that is to be carried out by the manufacturer on the final product (bulk material or dosage form) either on selected batches or on each batch prior to release. These statements cannot necessarily be verified on a sample of the final product by an independent analyst. The competent authority may establish that the instructions have been followed, for example, by examination of data received from the manufacturer, by inspection or by testing appropriate samples.

The absence of a section on Production does not imply that attention to features such as those referred to above is not required. A substance, preparation or article described in a monograph of the Pharmacopoeia is to be manufactured in accordance with the principles of good manufacturing practice and in accordance with relevant international agreements and supranational and national regulations governing medicinal products.

Where in the section under the side-heading Production a monograph on a vaccine defines the characteristics of the vaccine strain to be used, any test methods given for confirming these characteristics are provided as examples of suitable methods. The use of these methods is not mandatory.

Additional statements concerning the production of formulated preparations are given in the general notice on Manufacture of Formulated Preparations.

Manufacture of Formulated Preparations Attention is drawn to the need to observe adequate hygienic precautions in the preparation and dispensing of pharmaceutical formulations. The principles of good pharmaceutical manufacturing practice should be observed.

The Definition in certain monographs for pharmaceutical preparations is given in terms of the principal ingredients only. Any ingredient, other than those included in the Definition, must comply with the general notice on Excipients and the product must conform with the Pharmacopoeial requirements.

The Definition in other monographs for pharmaceutical preparations is presented as a full formula. No deviation from the stated formula is permitted except those allowed by the general notices on Colouring Agents and Antimicrobial Preservatives. Where additionally directions are given under the side-heading Extemporaneous Preparation these are intended for the extemporaneous preparation of relatively small quantities for short-term supply and use. When so prepared, no deviation from the stated directions is permitted. If, however, such a pharmaceutical preparation is manufactured on a larger scale with the intention that it may be stored, deviations from the stated directions are permitted provided that the final product meets the following criteria:

(1) compliance with all of the requirements stated in the monograph;

(2) retention of the essential characteristics of the preparation made strictly in accordance with the directions of the Pharmacopoeia.

Monographs for yet other pharmaceutical preparations include both a Definition in terms of the principal ingredients and, under the side-heading Extemporaneous Preparation, a full formula together with, in some cases, directions for their preparation. Such full formulae and directions are intended for the extemporaneous preparation of relatively small quantities for short-term supply and use. When so prepared, no deviation from the stated formula and directions is permitted. If, however, such a pharmaceutical preparation is manufactured on a larger scale with the intention that it may be stored, deviations from the formula and directions stated under the side-heading Extemporaneous Preparation are permitted provided that any ingredient, other than those included in the Definition, complies with the general notice on Excipients and that the final product meets the following criteria:

(1) accordance with the Definition stated in the monograph;

(2) compliance with all of the requirements stated in the monograph;

(3) retention of the essential characteristics of the preparation made strictly in accordance with the formula and directions of the Pharmacopoeia.

In the manufacture of any official preparation on a large scale with the intention that it should be stored, in addition to following any instruction under the side-heading Production, it is necessary to ascertain that the product is satisfactory with respect to its physical and chemical stability and its state of preservation over the claimed shelf-life. This applies irrespective of whether the formula of the Pharmacopoeia and any instructions given under the side-heading Extemporaneous Preparation are followed precisely or modified. Provided that the preparation has been shown to be stable in other respects, deterioration due to microbial contamination may be inhibited by the incorporation of a suitable antimicrobial preservative. In such circumstances the label states appropriate storage conditions, the date after which the product should not be used and the identity and concentration of the antimicrobial preservative.

Freshly and Recently Prepared The direction, given under the side-heading Extemporaneous Preparation, that a preparation must be freshly prepared indicates that it must be made not more than 24 hours before it is issued for use. The direction that a preparation should be recently prepared indicates that deterioration is likely if the preparation is stored for longer than about 4 weeks at 15° to 25°.

Methods of Sterilisation The methods of sterilisation used in preparing the sterile materials described in the Pharmacopoeia are given in Appendix XVIII. For aqueous preparations, steam sterilisation (heating in an autoclave) is the method of choice wherever it is known to be suitable. Any method of sterilisation must be validated with respect to both the assurance of sterility and the integrity of the product and to ensure that the final product complies with the requirements of the monograph.

Water The term Water used without qualification in formulae for formulated preparations means either potable water freshly drawn direct from the public supply and suitable for drinking or freshly boiled and cooled Purified Water. The latter should be used if the public supply is from a local storage tank or if the potable water is unsuitable for a particular preparation.

Excipients Where an excipient for which there is a Pharmacopoeial monograph is used in preparing an official preparation it shall comply with that monograph. Any substance added in preparing an official preparation shall be innocuous, shall have no adverse influence on the therapeutic efficacy of the active ingredients and shall not interfere with the assays and tests of the Pharmacopoeia. Particular care should be taken to ensure that such substances are free from harmful organisms.

Colouring Agents If in a monograph for a formulated preparation defined by means of a full formula a specific colouring agent or agents is prescribed, suitable alternatives approved in the country concerned may be substituted.

Antimicrobial Preservatives When the term 'suitable antimicrobial preservative' is used it is implied that the preparation concerned will be effectively preserved according to the appropriate criteria applied and interpreted as described in the test for *efficacy of antimicrobial preservation* (Appendix XVI C). In certain monographs for formulated preparations defined by means of a full formula, a specific antimicrobial agent or agents may be prescribed; suitable alternatives may be substituted provided that their identity and concentration are stated on the label.

Characteristics Statements given under the side-heading Characteristics are not to be interpreted in a strict sense and are not to be regarded as official requirements. Statements on taste are provided only in cases where this property is a guide to the acceptability of the material (for example, a material used primarily for flavouring). The status of statements on solubility is given in the general notice on Solubility.

    Solubility Statements on solubility given under the side-heading Characteristics are intended as information on the approximate solubility at a temperature between 15° and 25°, unless otherwise stated, and are not to be considered as official requirements.

    Statements given under side-headings such as Solubility in ethanol express exact requirements and constitute part of the standards for the substances under which they occur.

    The following table indicates the meanings of the terms used in statements of approximate solubilities.

Descriptive term	Approximate volume of solvent in millilitres per gram of solute
very soluble	less than 1
freely soluble	from 1 to 10
soluble	from 10 to 30
sparingly soluble	from 30 to 100
slightly soluble	from 100 to 1000
very slightly soluble	from 1000 to 10,000
practically insoluble	more than 10,000

The term 'partly soluble' is used to describe a mixture of which only some of the components dissolve.

Identification The tests described or referred to under the side-heading Identification are not necessarily sufficient to establish absolute proof of identity. They provide a means of verifying that the identity of the material being examined is in accordance with the label on the container.

Unless otherwise prescribed, identification tests are carried out at a temperature between 15° and 25°.

Reference spectra Where a monograph refers to an infrared reference spectrum, this spectrum is provided in a separate section of the Pharmacopoeia. A sample spectrum is considered to be concordant with a reference spectrum if the transmission minima (absorption maxima) of the principal bands in the sample correspond in position, relative intensities and shape to those of the reference. Instrumentation software may be used to calculate concordance with a previously recorded reference spectrum.

When tests for infrared absorption are applied to material extracted from formulated preparations, strict concordance with the specified reference spectrum may not always be possible, but nevertheless a close resemblance between the spectrum of the extracted material and the specified reference spectrum should be achieved.

Assays and Tests The assays and tests described are the official methods upon which the standards of the Pharmacopoeia depend. The analyst is not precluded from employing alternative methods, including methods of micro-analysis, in any assay or test if it is known that the method used will give a result of equivalent accuracy. Local reference materials may be used for routine analysis, provided that these are calibrated against the official reference materials. In the event of doubt or dispute, the methods of analysis, the reference materials and the reference spectra of the Pharmacopoeia are alone authoritative.

Where the solvent used for a solution is not named, the solvent is Purified Water.

Unless otherwise prescribed, the assays and tests are carried out at a temperature between 15° and 25°.

A temperature in a test for Loss on drying, where no temperature range is given, implies a range of $\pm$ 2° about the stated value.

Visual comparative tests, unless otherwise prescribed, are carried out using identical tubes of colourless, transparent, neutral glass with a flat base and an internal diameter of 16 mm; tubes with a larger internal diameter amy be used but the volume of liquid examined must be increased so that the depth of liquid in the tube is not less than that obtained when the prescribed volume of liquid and tubes 16 mm in internal diameter are used. Equal volumes of the liquids to be compared are examined down the vertical axis of the tubes against a white background or, if necessary, against a black background. The examination is carried out in diffuse light.

Where a direction is given that an analytical operation is to be carried out 'in subdued light', precautions should be taken to avoid exposure to direct sunlight or other strong light. Where a direction is given that an analytical operation is to be carried out 'protected from light', precautions should be taken to exclude actinic light by the use of low-actinic glassware, working in a dark room or similar procedures.

For preparations other than those of fixed strength, the quantity to be taken for an assay or test is usually expressed in terms of the active ingredient. This means that the quantity of the active ingredient expected to be present and the quantity of the preparation to be taken are calculated from the strength stated on the label.

In assays the approximate quantity to be taken for examination is indicated but the quantity actually used must not deviate by more than 10% from that stated. The quantity taken is accurately weighed or measured and the result of the assay is calculated from this exact quantity. Reagents are measured and the procedures are carried out with an accuracy commensurate with the degree of precision implied by the standard stated for the assay.

In tests the stated quantity to be taken for examination must be used unless any divergence can be taken into account in conducting the test and calculating the result. The quantity taken is accurately weighed or measured with the degree of precision implied by the standard or, where the standard is not stated numerically (for example, in tests for Clarity and colour of solution), with the degree of precision implied by the number of significant figures stated. Reagents are measured and the procedures are carried out with an accuracy commensurate with this degree of precision.

The limits stated in monographs are based on data obtained in normal analytical practice; they take account of normal analytical errors, of acceptable variations in manufacture and of deterioration to an extent considered acceptable. No further tolerances are to be applied to the limits prescribed to determine whether the article being examined complies with the requirements of the monograph.

In determining compliance with a numerical limit, the calculated result of a test or assay is first rounded to the number of significant figures stated, unless otherwise prescribed. The last figure is increased by one when the part rejected is equal to or exceeds one half-unit, whereas it is not modified when the part rejected is less than a half-unit.

In certain tests, the concentration of impurity is given in parentheses either as a percentage or in parts per million by weight (ppm). In chromatographic tests such concentrations are stated as a percentage irrespective of the limit. In other tests they are usually stated in ppm unless the limit exceeds 500 ppm. In those chromatographic tests in which a secondary spot or peak in a chromatogram obtained with a solution of the substance being examined is described as corresponding to a named impurity and is compared with a spot or peak in a chromatogram obtained with a reference solution of the same impurity, the percentage given in parentheses indicates the limit for that impurity. In those chromatographic tests in which a spot or peak in a chromatogram obtained with a solution of the substance being examined is described in terms other than as corresponding to a named impurity (commonly, for example, as any (other) *secondary spot* or *peak*) but is compared with a spot or peak in a chromatogram obtained with a reference solution of a named impurity, the percentage given in parentheses indicates an impurity limit expressed in terms of a nominal concentration of the named impurity. In chromatographic tests in which a comparison is made between spots or peaks in chromatograms obtained with solutions of different concentrations of the substance being examined, the percentage given in parentheses indicates an impurity limit expressed in terms of a nominal concentration of the medicinal substance itself. In some monographs, in particular those for certain formulated preparations, the impurity limit is expressed in terms of a nominal concentration of the active moiety rather than of the medicinal substance itself. Where necessary for clarification the terms in which the limit is expressed are stated within the monograph.

In all cases where an impurity limit is given in parentheses, the figures given are approximations for information only; conformity with the requirements is determined on the basis of compliance or otherwise with the stated test.

The use of a proprietary designation to identify a material used in an assay or test does not imply that another equally suitable material may not be used.

Biological Assays and Tests

Methods of assay described as Suggested methods are not obligatory, but when another method is used its precision must be not less than that required for the Suggested method.

For those antibiotics for which the monograph specifies a microbiological assay the potency requirement is expressed in the monograph in International Units (IU) or other Units per milligram. The material is not of pharmacopoeial quality if the upper fiducial limit of error is less than the stated potency. For such antibiotics the required precision of the assay is stated in the monograph in terms of the fiducial limits of error about the estimated potency.

For other substances and preparations for which the monograph specifies a biological assay, unless otherwise stated, the precision of the assay is such that the fiducial limits of error, expressed as a percentage of the estimated potency, are within a range not wider than that obtained by multiplying by a factor of ten the square roots of the limits given in the monograph for the fiducial limits of error about the stated potency.

In all cases fiducial limits of error are based on a probability of 95% ($P = 0.95$).

Where the biological assay is being used to ascertain the purity of the material, the stated potency means the potency stated on the label in terms of International Units (IU) or other Units per gram, per milligram or per millilitre. When no such statement appears on the label, the stated potency means the fixed or minimum potency required in the monograph. This interpretation of stated potency applies in all cases except where the monograph specifically directs otherwise.

Where the biological assay is being used to determine the total activity in the container, the stated potency means the total number of International Units (IU) or other Units stated on the label or, if no such statement appears, the total activity calculated in accordance with the instructions in the monograph.

Wherever possible the primary standard used in an assay or test is the respective International Standard or Reference Preparation established by the World Health Organization for international use and the biological activity is expressed in International Units (IU).

In other cases, where Units are referred to in an assay or test, the Unit for a particular substance or preparation is, for the United Kingdom, the specific biological activity contained in such an amount of the respective primary standard as the appropriate international or national organisation indicates. The necessary information is provided with the primary standard.

Unless otherwise directed, animals used in an assay or a test are healthy animals, drawn from a uniform stock, that have not previously been treated with any material that will interfere with the assay or test. Unless otherwise stated, guinea-pigs weigh not less than 250 g or, when used in systemic toxicity tests, not less than 350 g. When used in skin tests they are white or light coloured. Unless otherwise stated, mice weigh not less than 17 g and not more than 22 g.

Certain of the biological assays and tests of the Pharmacopoeia are such that in the United Kingdom they may be carried out only in accordance with the Animals (Scientific Procedures) Act 1986. Instructions included in such assays and tests in the Pharmacopoeia, with respect to the handling of animals, are therefore confined to those concerned with the accuracy and reproducibility of the assay or test.

Reference Substances and Reference Preparations

Certain monographs require the use of a reference substance, a reference preparation or a reference spectrum. These are chosen with regard to their intended use as prescribed in the monographs of the Pharmacopoeia and are not necessarily suitable in other circumstances.

Any information necessary for proper use of the reference substance or reference preparation is given on the label or in the accompanying leaflet or brochure. Where no drying conditions are stated in the leaflet or on the label, the substance is to be used as received. No certificate of analysis or other data not relevant to the prescribed use of the product are provided. The products are guaranteed to be suitable for use for a period of three months from dispatch when stored under the appropriate conditions. The stability of the contents of opened containers cannot be guaranteed. The current lot is listed in the BP Laboratory website catalogue. Additional information is provided in Supplementary Chapter III E.

Chemical Reference Substances The abbreviation BPCRS indicates a Chemical Reference Substance established by the British Pharmacopoeia Commission. The abbreviation CRS or EPCRS indicates a Chemical Reference Substance established by the European Pharmacopoeia Commission. Some Chemical Reference Substances are used for the microbiological assay of antibiotics and their activity is stated, in International Units, on the label or on the accompanying leaflet and defined in the same manner as for Biological Reference Preparations.

Biological Reference Preparations The majority of the primary biological reference preparations referred to are the appropriate International Standards and Reference Preparations established by the World Health Organisation. Because these reference materials are usually available only in limited quantities, the European Pharmacopoeia has established Biological Reference Preparations (indicated by the abbreviation BRP or EPBRP) where appropriate. Where applicable, the potency of the Biological Reference Preparations is expressed in International Units. For some Biological Reference Preparations, where an international standard or reference preparation does not exist, the potency is expressed in European Pharmacopoeia Units.

Storage

Statements under the side-heading Storage constitute non-mandatory advice. The substances and preparations described in the Pharmacopoeia are to be stored under conditions that prevent contamination and, as far as possible, deterioration. Unless otherwise stated in the monograph, the substances and preparations described in the Pharmacopoeia are kept in well-closed containers and stored at a temperature not exceeding 25°. Precautions that should be taken in relation to the effects of the atmosphere, moisture, heat and light are indicated, where appropriate, in the monographs. Further precautions may be necessary when some materials are stored in tropical climates or under other severe conditions.

The expression 'protected from moisture' means that the product is to be stored in an airtight container. Care is to be taken when the container is opened in a damp atmosphere. A low moisture content may be maintained, if necessary, by the use of a desiccant in the container provided that direct contact with the product is avoided.

The expression 'protected from light' means that the product is to be stored either in a container made of a material that absorbs actinic light sufficiently to protect the contents from change induced by such light or in a container enclosed in an outer cover that provides such protection or stored in a place from which all such light is excluded.

The expression 'tamper-evident container' means a closed container fitted with a device that reveals irreversibly whether the container has been opened, whereas, the expression 'tamper-proof container' means a closed container in which access to the contents is prevented under normal conditions of use. The two terms are considered to be synonymous by the European Pharmacopoeia Commission.

Labelling The labelling requirements of the Pharmacopoeia are not comprehensive and laws governing the statements to be declared on labels of official articles should also be met. In the United Kingdom the provisions of regulations issued in accordance with the Medicines Act 1968, together with those of regulations for the labelling of hazardous materials, should be met.

Only those statements in monographs given under the side-heading Labelling that are necessary to demonstrate compliance or otherwise with the monograph are mandatory. Any other statements are included as recommendations.

Such matters as the exact form of wording to be used and whether a particular item of information should appear on the primary label and additionally, or alternatively, on the package or exceptionally in a leaflet are, in general, outside the scope of the Pharmacopoeia. When the term 'label' is used in Labelling statements of the Pharmacopoeia, decisions as to where the particular statement should appear should therefore be made in accordance with relevant legislation.

The label of every official article states (i) the name at the head of the monograph and (ii) a reference consisting of either figures or letters, or a combination of figures and letters, by which the history of the article may be traced.

The label of every official formulated preparation other than those of fixed strength also states the content of the active ingredient or ingredients expressed in the terms required by the monograph. Where the content of active ingredient is required to be expressed in terms other than the weight of the official medicinal substance used in making the formulation, this is specifically stated under the side-heading Labelling. Thus, where no specific requirement is included under the side-heading Labelling, it is implied that the content of active ingredient is expressed in terms of the weight of the official medicinal substance used in making the formulation. For example, for Diprenorphine Injection, which contains Diprenorphine Hydrochloride but for which the content is expressed in terms of the equivalent amount of diprenorphine, a specific requirement to this effect is included under the

side-heading Labelling. For Megestrol Tablets which contain Megestrol
Acetate and for which the result of the assay is expressed in terms of
megestrol acetate no specific statement is included under the side-heading
Labelling; these Tablets are thus labelled with the nominal weight of
Megestrol Acetate.

These requirements do not necessarily apply to the labelling of articles
supplied in compliance with a prescription.

Action and Use The statements given under this side-heading in monographs are intended
only as information on the principal pharmacological actions or the uses of
the materials in veterinary medicine or pharmacy. It should not be assumed
that the substance has no other action or use. The statements are not
intended to be binding on prescribers or to limit their discretion.

**Antibiotics Intended
for Use in the
Manufacture of
Intramammary
Infusions** Where a monograph for an antibiotic in the British Pharmacopoeia or in the
British Pharmacopoeia (Veterinary) contains specific requirements relating
to sterility or to abnormal toxicity for material intended for use in the
manufacture of a parenteral dosage form, these requirements, together with
any qualification, apply also to any material intended for use in the
manufacture of an intramammary infusion.

**Crude Drugs;
Traditional Herbal
and Complementary
Medicines** *Herbal and complementary medicines are classed as medicines under European
Directive 2001/83/EC as amended. It is emphasised that, although requirements
for the quality of the material are provided in the monograph to assist the
registration scheme by the UK Licensing Authority, the British Pharmacopoeia
Commission has not assessed the safety or efficacy of the material in traditional
use.*

Monograph Title For traditional herbal medicines, the monograph title
is a combination of the established English name together with a description
of use. Monographs for the material that has not been processed (the herbal
drug) and the processed material (the herbal drug preparation) are
published where possible. To distinguish between the two, the word
'Processed' is included in the relevant monograph title. The acronym
'THM' is used in the title to indicate 'Traditional Herbal Medicine'. This
refers to the general use of the material that has not been processed. Where
the acronym 'THMP' is used, this indicates the use of the processed herb
in a 'Traditional Herbal Medicinal Product'.

Definition Under the heading Definition, the botanical name together
with any synonym is given. Where appropriate, for material that has not
been processed, information on the collection/harvesting and/or treatment/
drying of the whole herbal drug may be given. For processed materials,
the method of processing, where appropriate, will normally be given in a
separate section.

Characteristics References to odour are included only where this is
highly characteristic. References to taste are not included.

Control methods Where applicable, the control methods to be used
in monographs are:

(a) macroscopical and microscopical descriptions and chemical/
     chromatographic tests for identification

(b) tests for absence of any related species

(c) microbial test to assure microbial quality

(d) tests for inorganic impurities and non-specific purity tests, including extractive tests, sulphated ash and heavy metals where appropriate

(e) test for Loss on drying or Water

(f) wherever possible, a method for assaying the active constituent(s) or suitable marker constituent(s).

The macroscopical characteristics include those features that can be seen by the unaided eye or by the use of a hand lens. When two species/ subspecies of the same plant are included in the Definition, individual differences between the two are indicated where possible.

The description of the microscopical characteristics of the powdered drug includes information on the dominant or the most specific characters. Where it is considered to be an aid to identification, illustrations of the powdered drug may be provided.

The following aspects are controlled by the general monograph for Herbal Drugs, that is, they are required to be free from moulds, insects, decay, animal matter and animal excreta. Unless otherwise prescribed the amount of foreign matter is not more than 2% w/w. Microbial contamination should be minimal.

In determining the content of the active principle(s) or the suitable marker principle(s) measurements are made with reference to the dried or anhydrous herbal drug. In the tests for Acid-insoluble ash, Ash, Extractive soluble in ethanol, Loss on drying, Sulphated ash, Water, Water-soluble ash and Water-soluble extractive of herbal drugs, the calculations are made with reference to the herbal drug that has not been specifically dried unless otherwise prescribed in the monograph.

Homoeopathic Medicines

Homoeopathic medicines are classed as medicines under European Directive 2001/83/EC as amended. It is emphasised that, although requirements for the quality of the material are provided in the monograph to assist the simplified registration scheme by the UK Licensing Authority, the British Pharmacopoeia Commission has not assessed the safety or efficacy of the material in use.

The statements under Crude Drugs; Traditional Herbal and Complementary Medicines are also applicable to homoeopathic stocks and mother tinctures.

Specific BP monographs for homoeopathic medicines only apply to homoeopathic stocks and mother tinctures. These monographs also include general statements on the methods of preparation of homoeopathic stocks and mother tinctures. Specifications have not been set for final homeopathic products due to the high dilution used in their preparation and the subsequent difficulty in applying analytical methodology.

Identification tests rely predominantly on macroscopical description and thin-layer chromatography. Tests for foreign matter are included when there is the hazard of contamination.

Part III

Monographs and other texts of the European Pharmacopoeia that are incorporated in this edition of the British Pharmacopoeia (Veterinary) are governed by the general notices of the European Pharmacopoeia; these are reproduced below.

GENERAL NOTICES OF THE EUROPEAN PHARMACOPOEIA

1.1. GENERAL STATEMENTS

The General Notices apply to all monographs and other texts of the European Pharmacopoeia.

The official texts of the European Pharmacopoeia are published in English and French. Translations in other languages may be prepared by the signatory States of the European Pharmacopoeia Convention. In case of doubt or dispute, the English and French versions are alone authoritative.

In the texts of the European Pharmacopoeia, the word "Pharmacopoeia" without qualification means the European Pharmacopoeia. The official abbreviation Ph. Eur. may be used to indicate the European Pharmacopoeia.

The use of the title or the subtitle of a monograph implies that the article complies with the requirements of the relevant monograph. Such references to monographs in the texts of the Pharmacopoeia are shown using the monograph title and reference number in *italics*.

A preparation must comply throughout its period of validity; a distinct period of validity and/or specifications for opened or broached containers may be decided by the competent authority. The subject of any other monograph must comply throughout its period of use. The period of validity that is assigned to any given article and the time from which that period is to be calculated are decided by the competent authority in the light of experimental results of stability studies.

Unless otherwise indicated in the General Notices or in the monographs, statements in monographs constitute mandatory requirements. General chapters become mandatory when referred to in a monograph, unless such reference is made in a way that indicates that it is not the intention to make the text referred to mandatory but rather to cite it for information.

The active ingredients (medicinal substances), excipients (auxiliary substances), pharmaceutical preparations and other articles described in the monographs are intended for human and veterinary use (unless explicitly restricted to one of these uses). An article is not of Pharmacopoeia quality unless it complies with all the requirements stated in the monograph. This does not imply that performance of all the tests in a monograph is necessarily a prerequisite for a manufacturer in assessing compliance with the Pharmacopoeia before release of a product. The manufacturer may obtain assurance that a product is of Pharmacopoeia quality from data derived, for example, from validation studies of the manufacturing process and from in-process controls. Parametric release in circumstances deemed appropriate by the competent authority is thus not precluded by the need to comply with the Pharmacopoeia.

The tests and assays described are the official methods upon which the standards of the Pharmacopoeia are based. With the agreement of the competent authority, alternative methods of analysis may be used for control purposes, provided that the methods used enable an unequivocal decision to be made as to whether compliance with the standards of the monographs would be achieved if the official methods were used. In the event of doubt or dispute, the methods of analysis of the Pharmacopoeia are alone authoritative.

Certain materials that are the subject of a pharmacopoeial monograph may exist in different grades suitable for different purposes. Unless otherwise indicated in the monograph, the requirements apply to all grades of the material. In some monographs, particularly those on excipients, a list of functionality-related characteristics that are relevant to the use of the substance may be appended to the monograph for information. Test methods for determination of one or more of these characteristics may be given, also for information.

General Monographs

Substances and preparations that are the subject of an individual monograph are also required to comply with relevant, applicable general monographs. Cross-references to applicable general monographs are not normally given in individual monographs.

General monographs apply to all substances and preparations within the scope of the Definition section of the general monograph, except where a preamble limits the application, for example to substances and preparations that are the subject of a monograph of the Pharmacopoeia.

General monographs on dosage forms apply to all preparations of the type defined. The requirements are not necessarily comprehensive for a given specific preparation and requirements additional to those prescribed in the general monograph may be imposed by the competent authority.

Conventional Terms

The term "competent authority" means the national, supranational or international body or organisation vested with the authority for making decisions concerning the issue in question. It may, for example, be a national pharmacopoeia authority, a licensing authority or an official control laboratory.

The expression "unless otherwise justified and authorised" means that the requirements have to be met, unless the competent authority authorises a modification or an exemption where justified in a particular case.

Statements containing the word "should" are informative or advisory.

In certain monographs or other texts, the terms "suitable" and "appropriate" are used to describe a reagent, micro-organism, test method etc.; if criteria for suitability are not described in the monograph, suitability is demonstrated to the satisfaction of the competent authority.

Interchangeable Methods

Certain general chapters contain a statement that the text in question is harmonised with the corresponding text of the Japanese Pharmacopoeia and/or the United States Pharmacopeia and that these texts are interchangeable. This implies that if a substance or preparation is found to comply with a requirement using an interchangeable method from one of these pharmacopoeias it complies with the requirements of the European Pharmacopoeia. In the event of doubt or dispute, the text of the European Pharmacopoeia is alone authoritative.

1.2. OTHER PROVISIONS APPLYING TO GENERAL CHAPTERS AND MONOGRAPHS

Quantities

In tests with numerical limits and assays, the quantity stated to be taken for examination is approximate. The amount actually used, which may deviate by not more than 10 per cent from that stated, is accurately weighed or measured and the result is calculated from this exact quantity. In tests where the limit is not numerical, but usually depends upon comparison with the behaviour of a reference in the same conditions, the stated quantity is taken for examination. Reagents are used in the prescribed amounts.

Quantities are weighed or measured with an accuracy commensurate with the indicated degree of precision. For weighings, the precision corresponds to plus or minus 5 units after the last figure stated (for example, 0.25 g is to be interpreted as 0.245 g to 0.255 g). For the measurement of volumes, if the figure after the decimal point is a zero or ends in a zero (for example, 10.0 ml or 0.50 ml), the volume is measured using a pipette, a volumetric flask or a burette, as appropriate; otherwise, a graduated measuring cylinder or a graduated pipette may be used. Volumes stated in microlitres are measured using a micropipette or microsyringe.

It is recognised, however, that in certain cases the precision with which quantities are stated does not correspond to the number of significant figures stated in a specified numerical limit. The weighings and measurements are then carried out with a sufficiently improved accuracy.

Apparatus and Procedures

Volumetric glassware complies with Class A requirements of the appropriate International Standard issued by the International Organisation for Standardisation.

Unless otherwise prescribed, analytical procedures are carried out at a temperature between 15 °C and 25 °C.

Unless otherwise prescribed, comparative tests are carried out using identical tubes of colourless, transparent, neutral glass with a flat base; the volumes of liquid prescribed are for use with tubes having an internal diameter of 16 mm, but tubes with a larger internal diameter may be used provided the volume of liquid used is adjusted *(2.1.5)*. Equal volumes of the liquids to be compared are examined down the vertical axis of the tubes against a white background, or if necessary against a black background. The examination is carried out in diffuse light.

Any solvent required in a test or assay in which an indicator is to be used is previously neutralised to the indicator, unless a blank test is prescribed.

Water Bath

The term "water-bath" means a bath of boiling water unless water at another temperature is indicated. Other methods of heating may be substituted provided the temperature is near to but not higher than 100 °C or the indicated temperature.

Drying and Ignition to Constant Mass

The terms "dried to constant mass" and "ignited to constant mass" mean that 2 consecutive weighings do not differ by more than 0.5 mg, the second weighing following an additional period of drying or of ignition respectively appropriate to the nature and quantity of the residue.

Where drying is prescribed using one of the expressions "in a desiccator" or *"in vacuo"*, it is carried out using the conditions described under *2.2.32. Loss on drying.*

Reagents The proper conduct of the analytical procedures described in the Pharmacopoeia and the reliability of the results depend, in part, upon the quality of the reagents used. The reagents are described in general chapter *4*. It is assumed that reagents of analytical grade are used; for some reagents, tests to determine suitability are included in the specifications.

Solvents Where the name of the solvent is not stated, the term "solution" implies a solution in water.

Where the use of water is specified or implied in the analytical procedures described in the Pharmacopoeia or for the preparation of reagents, water complying with the requirements of the monograph on *Purified water (0008)* is used, except that for many purposes the requirements for bacterial endotoxins (*Purified water in bulk*) and microbial contamination (*Purified water in containers*) are not relevant. The term "distilled water" indicates purified water prepared by distillation.

The term "ethanol" without qualification means anhydrous ethanol. The term "alcohol" without qualification means ethanol (96 per cent). Other dilutions of ethanol are indicated by the term "ethanol" or "alcohol" followed by a statement of the percentage by volume of ethanol (C_2H_6O) required.

Expression of Content In defining content, the expression "per cent" is used according to circumstances with one of two meanings:

— per cent *m/m* (percentage, mass in mass) expresses the number of grams of substance in 100 grams of final product;

— per cent *V/V* (percentage, volume in volume) expresses the number of millilitres of substance in 100 millilitres of final product.

The expression "parts per million" (or ppm) refers to mass in mass, unless otherwise specified.

Temperature Where an analytical procedure describes temperature without a figure, the general terms used have the following meaning:

— in a deep-freeze: below − 15 °C;

— in a refrigerator: 2 °C to 8 °C;

— cold or cool: 8 °C to 15 °C;

— room temperature: 15 °C to 25 °C.

1.3. GENERAL CHAPTERS

Containers Materials used for containers are described in general chapter *3.1*. General names used for materials, particularly plastic materials, each cover a range of products varying not only in the properties of the principal constituent but also in the additives used. The test methods and limits for materials depend on the formulation and are therefore applicable only for materials whose formulation is covered by the preamble to the specification. The use of materials with different formulations, and the test methods and limits applied to them, are subject to agreement by the competent authority.

The specifications for containers in general chapter *3.2* have been developed for general application to containers of the stated category, but in view of the wide variety of containers available and possible new developments, the publication of a specification does not exclude the use, in justified circumstances, of containers that comply with other specifications, subject to agreement by the competent authority.

Reference may be made within the monographs of the Pharmacopoeia to the definitions and specifications for containers provided in chapter *3.2. Containers*. The general monographs for pharmaceutical dosage forms may, under the heading Definition/Production, require the use of certain types of container; certain other monographs may, under the heading Storage, indicate the type of container that is recommended for use.

1.4. MONOGRAPHS

Titles Monograph titles are in English and French in the respective versions and there is a Latin subtitle.

Relative Atomic and Molecular Masses The relative atomic mass (A_r) or the relative molecular mass (M_r) is shown, as and where appropriate, at the beginning of each monograph. The relative atomic and molecular masses and the molecular and graphic formulae do not constitute analytical standards for the substances described.

Definition Statements under the heading Definition constitute an official definition of the substance, preparation or other article that is the subject of the monograph.

Limits of content Where limits of content are prescribed, they are those determined by the method described under Assay.

Vegetable drugs In monographs on vegetable drugs, the definition indicates whether the subject of the monograph is, for example, the whole drug or the drug in powdered form. Where a monograph applies to the drug in several states, for example both to the whole drug and the drug in powdered form, the definition states this.

Production Statements under the heading Production draw attention to particular aspects of the manufacturing process but are not necessarily comprehensive. They constitute instructions to manufacturers. They may relate, for example, to source materials; to the manufacturing process itself and its validation and control; to in-process testing; or to testing that is to be carried out by the manufacturer on the final article, either on selected batches or on each batch prior to release. These statements cannot necessarily be verified on a sample of the final article by an independent analyst. The competent authority may establish that the instructions have been followed, for example, by examination of data received from the manufacturer, by inspection of manufacture or by testing appropriate samples.

The absence of a section on Production does not imply that attention to features such as those referred to above is not required. A product described in a monograph of the Pharmacopoeia is manufactured in accordance with a suitable quality system in accordance with relevant international agreements and supranational and national regulations governing medicinal products for human or veterinary use.

Where in the section under the heading Production a monograph on a vaccine defines the characteristics of the vaccine strain to be used, any test methods given for confirming these characteristics are provided for information as examples of suitable methods. Similarly, test methods for choice of vaccine composition are provided for information as examples of suitable methods.

Characters The statements under the heading Characters are not to be interpreted in a strict sense and are not requirements.

SolubilityIn statements of solubility in the section headed Characters, the terms used have the following significance referred to a temperature between 15 °C and 25 °C.

Descriptive term	Approximate volume of solvent in millilitres per gram of solute		
Very soluble	less than	1	
Freely soluble	from	1	to 10
Soluble	from	10	to 30
Sparingly soluble	from	30	to 100
Slightly soluble	from	100	to 1000
Very slightly soluble	from	1000	to 10 000
Practically insoluble	more than		10 000

The term "partly soluble" is used to describe a mixture where only some of the components dissolve. The term "miscible" is used to describe a liquid that is miscible in all proportions with the stated solvent.

Identification The tests given in the identification section are not designed to give a full confirmation of the chemical structure or composition of the product; they are intended to give confirmation, with an acceptable degree of assurance, that the article conforms to the description on the label.

Certain monographs have subdivisions entitled "First identification" and "Second identification". The test or tests that constitute the "First identification" may be used for identification in all circumstances. The test or tests that constitute the "Second identification" may be used for identification provided it can be demonstrated that the substance or preparation is fully traceable to a batch certified to comply with all the other requirements of the monograph.

Tests and Assays **Scope** The requirements are not framed to take account of all possible impurities. It is not to be presumed, for example, that an impurity that is not detectable by means of the prescribed tests is tolerated if common sense and good pharmaceutical practice require that it be absent. See also below under Impurities.

Calculation Where the result of a test or assay is required to be calculated with reference to the dried or anhydrous substance or on some other specified basis, the determination of loss on drying, water content or other property is carried out by the method prescribed in the relevant test in the monograph. The words "dried substance" or "anhydrous substance" etc. appear in parenthesis after the result.

Limits The limits prescribed are based on data obtained in normal analytical practice; they take account of normal analytical errors, of acceptable variations in manufacture and compounding and of deterioration to an extent considered acceptable. No further tolerances are to be applied to the limits prescribed to determine whether the article being examined complies with the requirements of the monograph.

In determining compliance with a numerical limit, the calculated result of a test or assay is first rounded to the number of significant figures stated, unless otherwise prescribed. The last figure is increased by one when the part rejected is equal to or exceeds one half-unit, whereas it is not modified when the part rejected is less than a half-unit.

Indication of permitted limit of impurities For comparative tests, the approximate content of impurity tolerated, or the sum of impurities, may be indicated for information only. Acceptance or rejection is determined on the basis of compliance or non-compliance with the stated test. If the use of a reference substance for the named impurity is not prescribed, this content may be expressed as a nominal concentration of the substance used to prepare the reference solution specified in the monograph, unless otherwise described.

Vegetable drugs For vegetable drugs, the sulphated ash, total ash, water-soluble matter, alcohol-soluble matter, water content, content of essential oil and content of active principle are calculated with reference to the drug that has not been specially dried, unless otherwise prescribed in the monograph.

Equivalents Where an equivalent is given, for the purposes of the Pharmacopoeia only the figures shown are to be used in applying the requirements of the monograph.

Culture media The culture media described in monographs and general chapters have been found to be satisfactory for the intended purpose. However, the components of media, particularly those of biological origin, are of variable quality, and it may be necessary for optimal performance to modulate the concentration of some ingredients, notably:

— peptones and meat or yeast extracts, with respect to their nutritive properties;

— buffering substances;

— bile salts, bile extract, deoxycholate, and colouring matter, depending on their selective properties;

— antibiotics, with respect to their activity.

Storage The information and recommendations given under the heading Storage do not constitute a pharmacopoeial requirement but the competent authority may specify particular storage conditions that must be met.

The articles described in the Pharmacopoeia are stored in such a way as to prevent contamination and, as far as possible, deterioration. Where special conditions of storage are recommended, including the type of container (see 1.3. General chapters) and limits of temperature, they are stated in the monograph.

The following expressions are used in monographs under Storage with the meaning shown.

In an airtight container means that the product is stored in an airtight container *(3.2)*. Care is to be taken when the container is opened in a damp atmosphere. A low moisture content may be maintained, if necessary, by the use of a desiccant in the container provided that direct contact with the product is avoided.

Protected from light means that the product is stored either in a container made of a material that absorbs actinic light sufficiently to protect the contents from change induced by such light, or in a container enclosed in an outer cover that provides such protection, or is stored in a place from which all such light is excluded.

Labelling   In general, labelling of medicines is subject to supranational and national regulation and to international agreements. The statements under the heading Labelling are not therefore comprehensive and, moreover, for the purposes of the Pharmacopoeia only those statements that are necessary to demonstrate compliance or non-compliance with the monograph are mandatory. Any other labelling statements are included as recommendations. When the term "label" is used in the Pharmacopoeia, the labelling statements may appear on the container, the package, a leaflet accompanying the package, or a certificate of analysis accompanying the article, as decided by the competent authority.

Warnings   Materials described in monographs and reagents specified for use in the Pharmacopoeia may be injurious to health unless adequate precautions are taken. The principles of good quality control laboratory practice and the provisions of any appropriate regulations are to be observed at all times. Attention is drawn to particular hazards in certain monographs by means of a warning statement; absence of such a statement is not to be taken to mean that no hazard exists.

Impurities   A list of all known and potential impurities that have been shown to be detected by the tests in a monograph may be given. See also *5.10. Control of impurities in substances for pharmaceutical use.*

Functionality-related Characteristics   A list of functionality-related characteristics that are not the subject of official requirements, but which are nevertheless relevant to the use of a substance, may be appended to a monograph for information (see also *1.1. General statements*, above).

Reference Substances, Reference Preparations and Reference Spectra   Certain monographs require the use of a reference substance, a reference preparation or a reference spectrum. These are chosen with regard to their intended use as prescribed in the monographs of the Pharmacopoeia and are not necessarily suitable in other circumstances. The European Pharmacopoeia Commission does not accept responsibility for any errors arising from use other than as prescribed.

The reference substances, the reference preparations and the reference spectra are established by the European Pharmacopoeia Commission and may be obtained from the Technical Secretariat. They are the official standards to be used in cases of arbitration. A list of reference substances, reference preparations and reference spectra may be obtained from the Technical Secretariat.

Local standards may be used for routine analysis, provided they are calibrated against the standards established by the European Pharmacopoeia Commission.

Any information necessary for proper use of the reference substance or reference preparation is given on the label or in the accompanying leaflet or brochure. Where no drying conditions are stated in the leaflet or on the label, the substance is to be used as received. No certificate of analysis or other data not relevant to the prescribed use of the product are provided. No expiry date is indicated: the products are guaranteed to be suitable for use when dispatched. The stability of the contents of opened containers cannot be guaranteed.

Chemical Reference Substances   The abbreviation CRS indicates a Chemical Reference Substance established by the European Pharmacopoeia

Commission. Some Chemical Reference Substances are used for the microbiological assay of antibiotics and their activity is stated, in International Units, on the label or on the accompanying leaflet and defined in the same manner as for Biological Reference Preparations.

Biological Reference Preparations The majority of the primary biological reference preparations referred to in the European Pharmacopoeia are the appropriate International Standards and Reference Preparations established by the World Health Organisation. Because these reference materials are usually available only in limited quantities, the Commission has established Biological Reference Preparations (indicated by the abbreviation BRP) where appropriate. Where applicable, the potency of the Biological Reference Preparations is expressed in International Units. For some Biological Reference Preparations, where an international standard or reference preparation does not exist, the potency is expressed in European Pharmacopoeia Units.

Reference spectra The reference spectrum is accompanied by information concerning the conditions used for sample preparation and recording the spectrum.

1.5. ABBREVIATIONS AND SYMBOLS

A	Absorbance	n_D^{20}	Refractive index
$A_{1\ cm}^{1\ per\ cent}$	Specific absorbance	Ph. Eur. U.	European Pharmacopoeia Unit
A_r	Relative atomic mass	ppm	Parts per million
$[\alpha]_D^{20}$	Specific optical rotation	R	Substance or solution defined under *4. Reagents*
bp	Boiling point		
BRP	Biological Reference Preparation	R_f	Used in chromatography to indicate the ratio of the distance travelled by a substance to the distance travelled by the solvent front
CRS	Chemical Reference Substance		
d_{20}^{20}	Relative density	R_{st}	Used in chromatography to indicate the ratio of the distance travelled by a substance to the distance travelled by a reference substance
IU	International Unit		
λ	Wavelength		
M	Molarity	RV	Substance used as a primary standard in volumetric analysis (chapter *4.2.1*)
M_r	Relative molecular mass		
mp	Melting point		

Abbreviations used in the monographs on immunoglobulins, immunosera and vaccines

LD_{50}	The statistically determined quantity of a substance that, when administered by the specified route, may be expected to cause the death of 50 per cent of the test animals within a given period	lr/100 dose	The smallest quantity of a toxin that, in the conditions of the test, when mixed with 0.01 IU of antitoxin and injected intracutaneously causes a characteristic reaction at the site of injection within a given period
MLD	Minimum lethal dose		
L+/10 dose	The smallest quantity of a toxin that, in the conditions of the test, when mixed with 0.1 IU of antitoxin and administered by the specified route, causes the death of the test animals within a given period	Lp/10 dose	The smallest quantity of toxin that, in the conditions of the test, when mixed with 0.1 IU of antitoxin and administered by the specified route, causes paralysis in the test animals within a given period
L+ dose	The smallest quantity of a toxin that, in the conditions of the test, when mixed with 1 IU of antitoxin and administered by the specified route, causes the death of the test animals within a given period	Lo/10 dose	The largest quantity of a toxin that, in the conditions of the test, when mixed with 0.1 IU of antitoxin and administered by the specified route, does not cause symptoms of toxicity in the test animals within a given period

Lf dose	The quantity of toxin or toxoid that flocculates in the shortest time with 1 IU of antitoxin
CCID$_{50}$	The statistically determined quantity of virus that may be expected to infect 50 per cent of the cell cultures to which it is added
EID$_{50}$	The statistically determined quantity of virus that may be expected to infect 50 per cent of fertilised eggs into which it is inoculated
ID$_{50}$	The statistically determined quantity of a virus that may be expected to infect 50 per cent of the animals into which it is inoculated

PD$_{50}$	The statistically determined dose of a vaccine that, in the conditions of the tests, may be expected to protect 50 per cent of the animals against a challenge dose of the micro-organisms or toxins against which it is active
ED$_{50}$	The statistically determined dose of a vaccine that, in the conditions of the tests, may be expected to induce specific antibodies in 50 per cent of the animals for the relevant vaccine antigens
PFU	Pock-forming units or plaque-forming units
SPF	Specified-pathogen-free.

Collections of micro-organisms

ATCC	American Type Culture Collection 10801 University Boulevard Manassas, Virginia 20110-2209, USA
C.I.P.	Collection de Bactéries de l'Institut Pasteur B.P. 52, 25 rue du Docteur Roux 75724 Paris Cedex 15, France
IMI	International Mycological Institute Bakeham Lane Surrey TW20 9TY, Great Britain
I.P.	Collection Nationale de Culture de Microorganismes (C.N.C.M.) Institut Pasteur 25, rue du Docteur Roux 75724 Paris Cedex 15, France
NCIMB	National Collection of Industrial and Marine Bacteria Ltd 23 St Machar Drive Aberdeen AB2 1RY, Great Britain

NCPF	National Collection of Pathogenic Fungi London School of Hygiene and Tropical Medicine Keppel Street London WC1E 7HT, Great Britain
NCTC	National Collection of Type Cultures Central Public Health Laboratory Colindale Avenue London NW9 5HT, Great Britain
NCYC	National Collection of Yeast Cultures AFRC Food Research Institute Colney Lane Norwich NR4 7UA, Great Britain
S.S.I.	Statens Serum Institut 80 Amager Boulevard, Copenhagen, Denmark

1.6. UNITS OF THE INTERNATIONAL SYSTEM (SI) USED IN THE PHARMACOPOEIA AND EQUIVALENCE WITH OTHER UNITS

International System Of Units (SI)
The International System of Units comprises 3 classes of units, namely base units, derived units and supplementary units[1]. The base units and their definitions are set out in Table 1.6-1.

The derived units may be formed by combining the base units according to the algebraic relationships linking the corresponding quantities. Some of these derived units have special names and symbols. The SI units used in the European Pharmacopoeia are shown in Table 1.6-2.

Some important and widely used units outside the International System are shown in Table 1.6-3.

The prefixes shown in Table 1.6-4 are used to form the names and symbols of the decimal multiples and submultiples of SI units.

Notes
1. In the Pharmacopoeia, the Celsius temperature is used (symbol t). This is defined by the equation:

$$t = T - T_0$$

where $T_0 = 273.15$ K by definition. The Celsius or centigrade temperature is expressed in degree Celsius (symbol °C). The unit "degree Celsius" is equal to the unit "kelvin".

2. The practical expressions of concentrations used in the Pharmacopoeia are defined in the General Notices.

3. The radian is the plane angle between two radii of a circle which cut off on the circumference an arc equal in length to the radius.

4. In the Pharmacopoeia, conditions of centrifugation are defined by reference to the acceleration due to gravity (g):

$$g = 9.806\,65\ m \cdot s^{-2}$$

5. Certain quantities without dimensions are used in the Pharmacopoeia: *relative density (2.2.5)*, *absorbance (2.2.25)*, *specific absorbance (2.2.25)* and *refractive index (2.2.6)*.

6. The microkatal is defined as the enzymic activity which, under defined conditions, produces the transformation (e.g. hydrolysis) of 1 micromole of the substrate per second.

Table 1.6.-1. – *SI base units*

Quantity		Unit		Definition
Name	Symbol	Name	Symbol	
Length	l	metre	m	The metre is the length of the path travelled by light in a vacuum during a time interval of 1/299 792 458 of a second.
Mass	m	kilogram	kg	The kilogram is equal to the mass of the international prototype of the kilogram.
Time	t	second	s	The second is the duration of 9 192 631 770 periods of the radiation corresponding to the transition between the two hyperfine levels of the ground state of the caesium-133 atom.
Electric current	I	ampere	A	The ampere is that constant current which, maintained in two straight parallel conductors of infinite length, of negligible circular cross-section and placed 1 metre apart in vacuum would produce between these conductors a force equal to 2×10^{-7} newton per metre of length.
Thermodynamic temperature	T	kelvin	K	The kelvin is the fraction 1/273.16 of the thermodynamic temperature of the triple point of water.
Amount of substance	n	mole	mol	The mole is the amount of substance of a system containing as many elementary entities as there are atoms in 0.012 kilogram of carbon-12*.
Luminous intensity	I_v	candela	cd	The candela is the luminous intensity in a given direction of a source emitting monochromatic radiation with a frequency of 540×10^{12} hertz and whose energy intensity in that direction is 1/683 watt per steradian.
* When the mole is used, the elementary entities must be specified and may be atoms, molecules, ions, electrons, other particles or specified groups of such particles.				

Table 1.6.-2. – *SI units used in the European Pharmacopoeia and equivalence with other units*

Quantity		Unit				Conversion of other units into SI units
Name	Symbol	Name	Symbol	Expression in SI base units	Expression in other SI units	
Wave number	ν	one per metre	1/m	m^{-1}		
Wavelength	λ	micrometre	µm	$10^{-6}m$		
		nanometre	nm	$10^{-9}m$		
Area	A, S	square metre	m^2	m^2		
Volume	V	cubic metre	m^3	m^3		$1\ ml = 1\ cm^3 = 10^{-6}\ m^3$
Frequency	ν	hertz	Hz	s^{-1}		
Density	ρ	kilogram per cubic metre	kg/m^3	$kg{\cdot}m^{-3}$		$1\ g/ml = 1\ g/cm^3 = 10^3\ kg{\cdot}m^{-3}$
Velocity	v	metre per second	m/s	$m{\cdot}s^{-1}$		
Force	F	newton	N	$m{\cdot}kg{\cdot}s^{-2}$		$1\ dyne = 1\ g{\cdot}cm{\cdot}s^{-2} = 10^{-5}\ N$ $1\ kp = 9.806\ 65\ N$
Pressure	p	pascal	Pa	$m^{-1}{\cdot}kg{\cdot}s^{-2}$	$N{\cdot}m^{-2}$	$1\ dyne/cm^2 = 10^{-1}\ Pa = 10^{-1}\ N{\cdot}m^{-2}$ $1\ atm = 101\ 325\ Pa = 101.325\ kPa$ $1\ bar = 10^5\ Pa = 0.1\ MPa$ $1\ mm\ Hg = 133.322\ 387\ Pa$ $1\ Torr = 133.322\ 368\ Pa$ $1\ psi = 6.894\ 757\ kPa$
Dynamic viscosity	η	pascal second	Pa·s	$m^{-1}{\cdot}kg{\cdot}s^{-1}$	$N{\cdot}s{\cdot}m^{-2}$	$1\ P = 10^{-1}\ Pa{\cdot}s = 10^{-1}\ N{\cdot}s{\cdot}m^{-2}$ $1\ cP = 1\ mPa{\cdot}s$
Kinematic viscosity	v	square metre per second	m^2/s	$m^2{\cdot}s^{-1}$	$Pa{\cdot}s{\cdot}m^3{\cdot}kg^{-1}$ $N{\cdot}m{\cdot}s{\cdot}kg^{-1}$	$1\ St = 1\ cm^2{\cdot}s^{-1} = 10^{-4}\ m^2{\cdot}s^{-1}$
Energy	W	joule	J	$m^2{\cdot}kg{\cdot}s^{-2}$	$N{\cdot}m$	$1\ erg = 1\ cm^2{\cdot}g{\cdot}s^{-2} =$ $1\ dyne{\cdot}cm = 10^{-7}\ J$ $1\ cal = 4.1868\ J$
Power Radiant flux	P	watt	W	$m^2{\cdot}kg{\cdot}s^{-3}$	$N{\cdot}m{\cdot}s^{-1}$ $J{\cdot}s^{-1}$	$1\ erg/s = 1\ dyne{\cdot}cm{\cdot}s^{-1} =$ $10^{-7}\ W = 10^{-7}\ N{\cdot}m{\cdot}s^{-1} =$ $10^{-7}\ J{\cdot}s^{-1}$
Absorbed dose (of radiant energy)	D	gray	Gy	$m^2{\cdot}s^{-2}$	$J{\cdot}kg^{-1}$	$1\ rad = 10^{-2}\ Gy$
Electric potential, electromotive force	U	volt	V	$m^2{\cdot}kg{\cdot}s^{-3}{\cdot}A^{-1}$	$W{\cdot}A^{-1}$	
Electric resistance	R	ohm	Ω	$m^2{\cdot}kg{\cdot}s^{-3}{\cdot}A^{-2}$	$V{\cdot}A^{-1}$	
Quantity of electricity	Q	coulomb	C	$A{\cdot}s$		
Activity of a radionuclide	A	becquerel	Bq	s^{-1}		$1\ Ci = 37{\cdot}10^9\ Bq = 37{\cdot}10^9\ s^{-1}$
Concentration (of amount of substance), molar concentration	c	mole per cubic metre	mol/m^3	$mol{\cdot}m^{-3}$		$1\ mol/l = 1M = 1\ mol/dm^3 = 10^3\ mol{\cdot}m^{-3}$
Mass concentration	ρ	kilogram per cubic metre	kg/m^3	$kg{\cdot}m^{-3}$		$1\ g/l = 1\ g/dm^3 = 1\ kg{\cdot}m^{-3}$

Table 1.6.-3. – *Units used with the International System*

Quantity	Unit		Value in SI units
	Time	Symbol	
Time	minute	min	1 min = 60 s
	hour	h	1 h = 60 min = 3600 s
	day	d	1 d = 24 h = 86 400 s
Plan angle	degree	°	$1° = (\pi/180)$ rad
Volume	litre	l	$1 l = 1 dm^3 = 10^{-3} m^3$
Mass	tonne	t	$1 t = 10^3$ kg
Rotational frequency	revolution per minute	r/min	$1 r/min = (1/60) s^{-1}$

Table 1.6.-4. – *Decimal multiples and sub-multiples of units*

Factor	Prefix	Symbol	Factor	Prefix	Symbol
10^{18}	exa	E	10^{-1}	deci	d
10^{15}	peta	P	10^{-2}	centi	c
10^{12}	tera	T	10^{-3}	milli	m
10^9	giga	G	10^{-6}	micro	μ
10^6	mega	M	10^{-9}	nano	n
10^3	kilo	k	10^{-12}	pico	p
10^2	hecto	h	10^{-15}	femto	f
10^1	deca	da	10^{-18}	atto	a

Monographs

Medicinal and Pharmaceutical Substances

MEDICINAL AND PHARMACEUTICAL SUBSTANCES

Acepromazine Maleate

$C_{19}H_{22}N_2OS,C_4H_4O_4$ 442.5   *3598-37-6*

Action and use
Dopamine receptor antagonist; neuroleptic.

Preparations
Acepromazine Injection

Acepromazine Tablets

DEFINITION
Acepromazine Maleate is 2-acetyl-10-(3-dimethylaminopropyl) phenothiazine hydrogen maleate. It contains not less than 98.5% and not more than 101.0% of $C_{19}H_{22}N_2OS,C_4H_4O_4$, calculated with reference to the dried substance.

CHARACTERISTICS
A yellow, crystalline powder.

Soluble in *water*; freely soluble in *chloroform*; soluble in *ethanol (96%)*; slightly soluble in *ether*.

IDENTIFICATION
A. Dissolve 20 mg in 2 ml of *water*, add 3 ml of 2M *sodium hydroxide*, extract with 5 ml of *cyclohexane* and evaporate to dryness under reduced pressure. The *infrared absorption spectrum* of the residue, Appendix II A, is concordant with the *reference spectrum* of acepromazine *(RSV 01)*.

B. Complies with the test for *identification of phenothiazines*, Appendix III A, applying to the plate 1 µl of each solution and using *acepromazine maleate BPCRS* for the preparation of solution (2).

C. Dissolve 0.2 g in a mixture of 3 ml of *water* and 2 ml of 5M *sodium hydroxide* and shake with three 3-ml quantities of *ether*. Add to the aqueous solution 2 ml of *bromine solution*, warm in a water bath for 10 minutes, heat to boiling, cool and add 0.25 ml to a solution of 10 mg of *resorcinol* in 3 ml of *sulphuric acid*. A bluish black colour develops on heating for 15 minutes in a water bath.

TESTS
Acidity
pH of a 1.0% w/v solution, 4.0 to 4.5, Appendix V L.

Melting point
136° to 139°, Appendix V A.

Related substances
Complies with the test for *related substances in phenothiazines*, Appendix III A, but using a mixture of 75 volumes of n-*hexane*, 17 volumes of *butan-2-one* and 8 volumes of *diethylamine* as the mobile phase.

Loss on drying
When dried to constant weight at 105°, loses not more than 1.0% of its weight. Use 1 g.

Sulphated ash
Not more than 0.2%, Appendix IX A.

ASSAY
Dissolve 0.4 g in 50 ml of *acetic anhydride* and carry out Method I for *non-aqueous titration*, Appendix VIII A, using *crystal violet solution* as indicator. Each ml of 0.1M *perchloric acid VS* is equivalent to 44.25 mg of $C_{19}H_{22}N_2OS,C_4H_4O_4$.

Alfadolone Acetate

$C_{23}H_{34}O_5$ 390.5   *23930-37-2*

Action and use
Intravenous general anaesthetic.

DEFINITION
Alfadolone Acetate is 3α-hydroxy-11,20-dioxo-5α-pregnan-21-yl acetate. It contains not less than 96.0% and not more than 103.0% of $C_{23}H_{34}O_5$, calculated with reference to the dried substance.

CHARACTERISTICS
A white to creamy white powder.

Practically insoluble in *water*; freely soluble in *chloroform*; soluble in *ethanol (96%)*; practically insoluble in *petroleum spirit (boiling range, 60° to 80°)*.

IDENTIFICATION
A. The *infrared absorption spectrum*, Appendix II A, is concordant with the *reference spectrum* of alfadolone acetate *(RSV 02)*.

B. The *light absorption*, Appendix II B, in the range 230 to 350 nm of a 0.4% w/v solution in *ethanol (96%)* exhibits a maximum only at 290 nm. The *absorbance* at 290 nm is about 0.7.

C. Complies with the test for *identification of steroids*, Appendix III A, using *impregnating solvent II* and *mobile phase D*.

TESTS
Light absorption
Absorbance of a 0.20% w/v solution in *ethanol (96%)* at 235 nm, not more than 0.60, calculated with reference to the dried substance, Appendix II B.

Related substances
Carry out the method for *thin-layer chromatography*, Appendix III A, using *silica gel G* as the coating substance and a mixture of equal volumes of *ethyl acetate* and *toluene* as the mobile phase. Apply separately to the plate 10 µl of each of three solutions of the substance being examined in a

mixture of equal volumes of *chloroform* and *methanol* containing (1) 5.0% w/v, (2) 0.15% w/v and (3) 0.050% w/v. After removal of the plate, dry it in a current of air until the solvent has evaporated, spray with a saturated solution of *cerium (IV) sulphate* in *sulphuric acid (50%)* and heat at 110° for 1 hour. Any *secondary spot* in the chromatogram obtained with solution (1) is not more intense than the spot in the chromatogram obtained with solution (2) (3%) and not more than one such spot is more intense than the spot in the chromatogram obtained with solution (3) (1%).

Loss on drying
When dried to constant weight at 105°, loses not more than 1.0% of its weight. Use 1 g.

Sulphated ash
Not more than 0.1%, Appendix IX A.

ASSAY
Carry out the *tetrazolium assay of steroids*, Appendix VIII J, allowing the reaction to proceed at 35° for 2 hours. Calculate the content of $C_{23}H_{34}O_5$ from the *absorbance* obtained by repeating the operation using *alfadolone acetate BPCRS* in place of the substance being examined.

Alfaxalone

$C_{21}H_{32}O_3$ 332.5   *23930-19-0*

Action and use
Intravenous general anaesthetic.

DEFINITION
Alfaxalone is 3α-hydroxy-5α-pregnane-11, 20-dione. It contains not less than 95.0% and not more than 103.0% of $C_{21}H_{32}O_3$, calculated with reference to the dried substance.

CHARACTERISTICS
A white to creamy white powder.

Practically insoluble in *water*; freely soluble in *chloroform*; soluble in *ethanol (96%)*; practically insoluble in *petroleum spirit (boiling range, 60° to 80°)*.

IDENTIFICATION
A. The *infrared absorption spectrum*, Appendix II A, is concordant with the *reference spectrum* of alfaxalone *(RSV 03)*.

B. Complies with the test for *identification of steroids*, Appendix III A, using *impregnating solvent II* and *mobile phase D*.

C. In the Assay, the chromatogram obtained with solution (2) shows a peak having the same retention time as the peak due to *alfaxalone BPCRS* in the chromatogram obtained with solution (1).

TESTS
Light absorption
Absorbance of a 0.20% w/v solution in *ethanol (96%)* at 235 nm, not more than 0.20, calculated with reference to the dried substance, Appendix II B.

Related substances
Carry out the method for *thin-layer chromatography*, Appendix III A, using *silica gel G* as the coating substance and a mixture of equal volumes of *ethyl acetate* and *toluene* as the mobile phase. Apply separately to the plate 10 μl of each of three solutions of the substance being examined in a mixture of equal volumes of *chloroform* and *methanol* containing (1) 5.0% w/v, (2) 0.15% w/v and (3) 0.050% w/v. After removal of the plate, dry it in a current of air until the solvent has evaporated, spray with a saturated solution of *cerium (IV) sulphate* in *sulphuric acid (50%)* and heat at 110° for 1 hour. Any *secondary spot* in the chromatogram obtained with solution (1) is not more intense than the spot in the chromatogram obtained with solution (2) (3%) and not more than one such spot is more intense than the spot in the chromatogram obtained with solution (3) (1%).

Loss on drying
When dried to constant weight at 105°, loses not more than 1.0% of its weight. Use 1 g.

Sulphated ash
Not more than 0.1%, Appendix IX A.

ASSAY
Carry out the method for *liquid chromatography*, Appendix III D, using the following solutions. For solution (1) dilute 25 ml of a solution in *propan-2-ol R1* containing 0.2% w/v of *alfaxalone BPCRS*, 0.01% w/v of *alfadolone acetate BPCRS* and 0.03% w/v of *betamethasone EPCRS* (internal standard) to 100 ml with *carbon dioxide-free water*. For solution (2) dilute 25 ml of a solution in *propan-2-ol R1* containing 0.2% w/v of the substance being examined to 100 ml with *carbon dioxide-free water*. For solution (3) dilute 25 ml of a solution in *propan-2-ol R1* containing 0.2% w/v of the substance being examined and 0.03% w/v of the internal standard to 100 ml with *carbon dioxide-free water*.

The chromatographic procedure may be carried out using (a) a stainless steel column (10 cm × 5 mm) packed with *octadecylsilyl silica gel for chromatography* (5 μm) (Spherisorb ODS 1 is suitable) and maintained at 60°, (b) as the mobile phase with a flow rate of 1 ml per minute a mixture of *propan-2-ol R1* and *carbon dioxide-free water* adjusted so that the *resolution factor* between the peaks due to alfadolone acetate (retention time about 5 minutes) and alfaxalone (retention time about 6 minutes) is more than 1.0 (a mixture of 25 volumes of *propan-2-ol R1* and 75 volumes of *carbon dioxide-free water* is usually suitable) and (c) a detection wavelength of 205 nm.

Calculate the content of $C_{21}H_{32}O_3$ in the substance being examined using the declared content of $C_{21}H_{32}O_3$ in *alfaxalone BPCRS*; peak areas or peak heights may be used irrespective of the symmetry factor.

Amitraz

$C_{19}H_{23}N_3$ 293.4   *33089-61-1*

Action and use
Topical parasiticide; acaricide.

Preparations
Amitraz Dip Concentrate (Liquid)
Amitraz Dip Concentrate (Powder)
Amitraz Pour-on

DEFINITION
Amitraz is *N*-methylbis (2,4-xylyliminomethyl) amine.
It contains not less than 97.0% and not more than 101.0%
of $C_{19}H_{23}N_3$, calculated with reference to the anhydrous
substance.

CHARACTERISTICS
A white to buff powder.

Practically insoluble in *water*; decomposes slowly in *ethanol
(96%)*; freely soluble in *acetone*.

IDENTIFICATION
The *infrared absorption spectrum*, Appendix II A, is concordant
with the *reference spectrum* of amitraz *(RSV 04)*.

TESTS
Related substances
Prepare a solution containing 0.010% w/v of *2,4-
dimethylaniline*, 0.20% w/v of *form-2',4'-xylidide BPCRS* and
0.20% w/v of *N,N'-bis(2,4-xylyl)formamidine BPCRS* in
methyl acetate (solution A). Disperse 30 mg of *N-methyl-N'-
(2,4-xylyl)formamidine hydrochloride BPCRS* in 5 ml of *methyl
acetate*, add about 32 mg of *triethylamine*, mix with the aid of
ultrasound for 2 minutes, filter, wash the filter with a small
amount of *methyl acetate* and add sufficient *methyl acetate* to
the combined filtrate and washings to produce 25 ml
(solution B) (about 0.1% w/v of *N-methyl-N'-(2,4-
xylyl)formamidine*). Carry out the method for *gas
chromatography*, Appendix III B, using the following
solutions. Solution (1) is a 5.0% w/v solution of the
substance being examined in *methyl acetate*. Solution (2) is a
mixture of equal volumes of solution A and solution B.

The chromatographic procedure may be carried out using *a
fused silica capillary column* (10 m × 0.53 mm) bonded with a
film (5 μm) of *poly [methyl(95)phenyl(5)]siloxane* (Chrompack
CP-SIL 8 CB is suitable) at an initial temperature of 125°,
maintained at 125° for 5 minutes, increasing linearly to 270°
at a rate of 5° per minute and maintained at 270° for
15 minutes with the inlet port at 230° and the detector at
300° and a flow rate of 12 ml per minute for the carrier gas.
Inject 1 μl of each of solutions (1) and (2).

In the chromatogram obtained with solution (2) the peaks
following the solvent peak, in order of emergence, are due to
2,4-dimethylaniline, form-2',4'-xylidide, N-methyl-N'-(2,4-
xylyl)formamidine and N,N'-bis(2,4-xylyl)formamidine.

In the chromatogram obtained with solution (1), the area of
any peak corresponding to 2,4-dimethylaniline, form-2',4'-
xylidide, N-methyl-N'-(2,4-xylyl)formamidine and
N,N'-bis(2,4-xylyl)formamidine is not greater than the area
of the corresponding peak in the chromatogram obtained
with solution (2) (0.1%, 2%, 1% and 2% respectively) and
the area of any other secondary peak is not greater than the
area of the peak due to 2,4-dimethylaniline in the
chromatogram obtained with solution (2) (0.1%).

Water
Not more than 0.1% w/w, Appendix IX C, Method IA.
Use 5 g and a mixture of equal volumes of *chloroform* and
2-chloroethanol in place of *anhydrous methanol*.

Sulphated ash
Not more than 0.2%, Appendix IX A.

ASSAY
Prepare a 2% v/v solution of *squalane* (internal standard) in
methyl acetate (solution C) and carry out the method for *gas
chromatography*, Appendix III B, using the following
solutions. For solution (1) dissolve 0.15 g of the substance
being examined in sufficient *methyl acetate* to produce 30 ml.
For solution (2) dissolve 0.15 g of the substance being
examined in 10 ml of solution C and add sufficient *methyl
acetate* to produce 30 ml. For solution (3) prepare a
1.50% w/v solution of *amitraz BPCRS* in solution C and
dilute 1 volume of this solution to 3 volumes with *methyl
acetate*.

The chromatographic procedure may be carried out using a
fused silica capillary column (15 m × 0.53 mm) coated with
a 1.5 μm film of methyl silicone gum (Chrompack CP-Sil
5 CB is suitable) and maintained at 220° with the inlet port
at 230° and the detector at 300° and a flow rate of 12 ml per
minute for the carrier gas. Inject 1 μl of each solution.

The assay is not valid unless, in the chromatogram obtained
with solution (3), the *resolution factor* between the peaks
corresponding to squalane and amitraz is at least 3.0.

Calculate the content of $C_{19}H_{23}N_3$ from the chromatograms
obtained using the declared content of $C_{19}H_{23}N_3$ in
amitraz BPCRS.

STORAGE
Amitraz should be kept in a well-closed container, which may
contain paraformaldehyde, packed in separate sachets as a
stabiliser.

IMPURITIES

A. 2,4-dimethylaniline (2,4-xylidine),

B. form-2',4'-xylidide,

C. *N*-methyl-*N'*-(2,4-xylyl)formamidine,

D. *N,N'*-bis(2,4-xylyl)formamidine.

Amprolium Hydrochloride

$C_{14}H_{19}ClN_4,HCl$ 315.3   *137-88-2*

Action and use
Antiprotozoal; prevention and treatment of coccidiosis
(veterinary).

DEFINITION
Amprolium Hydrochloride is 1-(4-amino-2-propylpyrimidin-
5-ylmethyl)-2-methylpyridinium chloride hydrochloride.
It contains not less than 97.5% and not more than 101.0%
of $C_{14}H_{19}ClN_4,HCl$, calculated with reference to the dried
substance.

CHARACTERISTICS
A white or almost white powder; odourless or almost
odourless.

Freely soluble in *water*; slightly soluble in *ethanol (96%)*; very
slightly soluble in *ether*; practically insoluble in *chloroform*.

IDENTIFICATION
A. The *infrared absorption spectrum*, Appendix II A, is
concordant with the *reference spectrum* of amprolium
hydrochloride *(RSV 07)*.

B. The *light absorption*, Appendix II B, in the range 230 to
350 nm of a 0.002% w/v solution in 0.1M *hydrochloric acid*
exhibits two maxima, at 246 nm and 262 nm. The
absorbances at the maxima are about 0.84 and about 0.80,
respectively.

C. To 1 mg add 5 ml of *naphthalenediol reagent solution*;
a deep violet colour is produced.

D. Yields the reactions characteristic of *chlorides*,
Appendix VI.

TESTS
Picoline
Dissolve 1.5 g in 30 ml of *water* in a distillation flask, add
20 ml of a saturated solution of *potassium carbonate*

sesquihydrate, connect the flask to a coarse-fritted aerator
extending to the bottom of a 100-ml graduated cylinder
containing 50 ml of 0.05M *hydrochloric acid*, and pass air,
which has previously been passed through *sulphuric acid* and
glass wool, through the system for 60 minutes. To 5 ml of
the hydrochloric acid solution add sufficient
0.05M *hydrochloric acid* to produce 200 ml. The *absorbance* of
the resulting solution at 262 nm is not greater than 0.52,
Appendix II B.

Loss on drying
When dried to constant weight at 100° at a pressure not
exceeding 0.7 kPa, loses not more than 1.0% of its weight.
Use 1 g.

Sulphated ash
Not more than 0.1%, Appendix IX A.

ASSAY
Carry out Method I for *non-aqueous titration*,
Appendix VIII A, using 0.3 g and *1-naphtholbenzein solution*
as indicator. Each ml of 0.1M *perchloric acid VS* is equivalent
to 15.77 mg of $C_{14}H_{19}ClN_4,HCl$.

Apramycin Sulphate

,2½H$_2$SO$_4$

$C_{21}H_{41}N_5O_{11},2\frac{1}{2}H_2SO_4$ 784.8   *41194-16-5*

Action and use
Aminoglycoside antibacterial.
Preparations
Apramycin Veterinary Oral Powder
Apramycin Premix

DEFINITION
Apramycin Sulphate is the sulphate of 4-*O*-
[(2*R*,3*R*,4a*S*,6*R*,7*S*,8*R*,8a*R*)-3-amino-6-(4-amino-
4-deoxy-α- D-glucopyranosyloxy)-8-hydroxy-7-
methylaminoperhydropyrano[3,2-*b*]pyran-2-yl]-2-
deoxystreptamine. It is produced by the growth of certain
strains of *Streptomyces tenebrarius* or obtained by any other
means. The potency is not less than 430 Units per mg,
calculated with reference to the anhydrous substance.

CHARACTERISTICS
A light brown powder or granular material; hygroscopic.

Freely soluble in *water*; practically insoluble in *acetone*,
in *ethanol (96%)*, in *ether* and in *methanol*.

IDENTIFICATION
A. Carry out the method for *thin-layer chromatography*,
Appendix III A, using a silica gel F_{254} precoated plate
(Merck silica gel 60 F_{254} plates are suitable) and as the
mobile phase a mixture of 20 volumes of *chloroform*,
40 volumes of 13.5M *ammonia* and 60 volumes of *methanol*,
equilibrated for 1 hour before use. Allow the solvent front to

ascend 10 cm above the line of application. Apply separately to the plate 5 µl of each of three solutions in *water* containing (1) 0.1% w/v of the substance being examined, (2) 0.07% w/v of *apramycin BPCRS* and (3) 0.07% w/v each of *apramycin BPCRS* and *tobramycin EPCRS*. After removal of the plate, allow it to dry in a current of warm air, spray with a mixture of equal volumes of a 46% w/v solution of *sulphuric acid* and a 0.2% w/v solution of *naphthalene-1,3-diol* in *ethanol (96%)* and heat at 150° for 5 to 10 minutes. The principal spot in the chromatogram obtained with solution (1) corresponds in colour and position to that in the chromatogram obtained with solution (2). The test is not valid unless the chromatogram obtained with solution (3) shows two clearly separated principal spots.

B. In the test for Related substances, the retention time of the principal peak in the chromatogram obtained with solution (1) corresponds to that of the principal peak in the chromatogram obtained with solution (2).

C. Yields reaction A characteristic of *sulphates*, Appendix VI.

TESTS

Sulphate

25.0 to 30.0% of SO_4, calculated with reference to the anhydrous substance, when determined by the following method. Dissolve 0.25 g in 100 ml of *water*, adjust to pH 11 with 13.5M *ammonia* and add 10 ml of 0.1M *barium chloride VS*. Titrate with 0.1M *disodium edetate VS* using 0.5 mg of *phthalein purple* as indicator; add 50 ml of *ethanol (96%)* when the colour of the solution begins to change and continue the titration until the violet-blue colour disappears. Each ml of 0.1M *barium chloride VS* is equivalent to 9.606 mg of SO_4.

Caerulomycin and dipyridyl derivatives

Dissolve 0.5 g in *water* in a 100 ml graduated flask, add 10 ml of *methanol* and dilute to 100 ml with *water*. Place 5 ml in a 25 ml graduated flask and add 5 ml of an acetate buffer prepared by dissolving 8.3 g of *anhydrous sodium acetate* in 25 ml of *water*, adding 12 ml of *glacial acetic acid* and diluting to 100 ml with *water*. Mix, add 1 ml of a 10% w/v solution of *hydroxylamine hydrochloride* in *water* and mix again. Add 5 ml of a 1% w/v solution of *ammonium iron(II) sulphate* and dilute to 25 ml with *water*. Measure the *absorbance* of the resulting solution at 520 nm, Appendix II B, using in the reference cell a solution obtained by carrying out the same procedure without the substance being examined. The *absorbance* is not greater than that obtained by repeating the test using 5 mg of *2,2'-dipyridyl* dissolved in 10 ml of *methanol* and diluted to 100 ml with *water* and beginning at the words 'Place 5 ml in a 25-ml graduated flask...' (1%).

Related substances

Carry out the method for *liquid chromatography*, Appendix III D, using the following solutions. Solution (1) is a 0.50% w/v of the substance being examined in *water*. Solution (2) is a 0.35% w/v of *apramycin BPCRS* in *water*. For solution (3) dilute 1 volume of solution (1) to 20 volumes with *water*.

The chromatographic procedure may be carried out using a column (25 cm × 4 mm) packed with fast cation-exchange polymeric beads (13 µm) with sulphonic acid functional groups (Dionex Fast Cation-1R is suitable) and a stainless steel post-column reaction coil (380 cm × 0.4 mm) with internal baffles, maintained at 130°. Use in the reaction coil *ninhydrin reagent I* at a flow rate approximately the same as that for the mobile phase. For mobile phase A use a solution containing 1.961% w/v of *sodium citrate*, 0.08% v/v

of *liquefied phenol* and 0.5% v/v of *thiodiglycol*, adjusted to pH 4.25 using *hydrochloric acid*. Mobile phase B is a solution containing 4.09% w/v of *sodium chloride* and 3.922% w/v of *sodium citrate* with 0.08% v/v of *liquefied phenol*, adjusted to pH 7.4 with *hydrochloric acid*. Degas both mobile phases using *helium* and use a flow rate of 0.8 ml per minute. Equilibrate the column using a mixture containing 75% of mobile phase A and 25% of mobile phase B. After each injection elute for 3 minutes using the same mixture and then carry out a linear gradient elution for 6 minutes to 100% of mobile phase B. Elute for a further 21 minutes using 100% of mobile phase B, then step-wise, re-equilibrate to a mixture of 75% of mobile phase A and 25% of mobile phase B and elute for at least 10 minutes. Use a detection wavelength of 568 nm.

The test is not valid unless, in the chromatogram obtained with solution (2), the *resolution factor* between compound A and 3-hydroxyapramycin, identified as indicated in the reference chromatogram supplied with *apramycin BPCRS*, is at least 0.8.

In the chromatogram obtained with solution (1) the areas of any peaks corresponding to 3-hydroxyapramycin, lividamine/2-deoxystreptamine (combined), compound A and compound B (identified as indicated in the reference chromatogram supplied with *apramycin BPCRS*) are not greater than 2.8, 2.0, 0.8 and 0.8 times respectively the area of the principal peak in the chromatogram obtained with solution (3) (7%, 5%, 2% and 2% respectively), the area of any other *secondary peak* is not greater than 0.8 times the area of the principal peak in the chromatogram obtained with solution (3) (2%) and the sum of the areas of all the *secondary peaks* is not greater than 6 times the area of the principal peak in the chromatogram obtained with solution (3) (15%). Disregard any peak with an area less than 0.04 times the area of the principal peak in the chromatogram obtained with solution (3) (0.1%).

Sulphated ash

Not more than 1.0%, Appendix IX A, Method II. Use 1 g.

Water

Not more than 10.0% w/w, Appendix IX C. Use 0.25 g.

ASSAY

Carry out the *biological assay of antibiotics*, Appendix XIV A, Method B. The precision of the assay is such that the fiducial limits of error are not less than 95% and not more than 105% of the estimated potency.

LABELLING

The label states (1) the number of Units per mg; (2) the date after which the material is not intended to be used; (3) the conditions under which it should be stored.

Apramycin Sulphate intended for use in the manufacture of a parenteral dosage form is decolourised and complies with the above requirements with the following modifications.

Preparation Apramycin Injection

DEFINITION

The potency is not less than 550 Units per mg, calculated with reference to the anhydrous substance.

Related substances

Carry out the method as described above.

In the chromatogram obtained with solution (1) the areas of any peaks corresponding to 3-hydroxyapramycin, lividamine/2-deoxystreptamine (combined) and compound A (identified as indicated in the reference chromatogram supplied with *apramycin BPCRS*) are not greater than twice the area of the principal peak in the chromatogram obtained with solution (3) (5% each), the area of any peak corresponding to compound B is not greater than 0.8 times the area of the principal peak in the chromatogram obtained with solution (3) (2%), the area of any other *secondary peak* is not greater than 0.8 times the area of the principal peak in the chromatogram obtained with solution (3) (2%) and the sum of the areas of all the *secondary peaks* is not greater than 4.8 times the area of the principal peak in the chromatogram obtained with solution (3) (12%). Disregard any peak with an area less than 0.04 times the area of the principal peak in the chromatogram obtained with solution (3) (0.1%).

STORAGE

If the substance is sterile, the container should be sterile, tamper-evident and sealed so as to exclude micro-organisms.

LABELLING

The label states, in addition, (1) that the material is suitable for parenteral use; (2) where applicable, that it is sterile.

Apramycin Sulphate intended for use in the manufacture of a parenteral dosage form without a further appropriate sterilisation procedure complies with the following additional requirement.

Sterility

Complies with the *test for sterility*, Appendix XVI A.

IMPURITIES

A. caerulomycin,

B. lividamine,

C. 2-deoxystreptamine,

D. 3-hydroxyapramaycin; *R* = OH,

E. 'compound A',

F. 'compound B'.

Azaperone

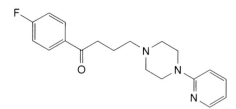

(*Azaperone for Veterinary Use,
Ph Eur monograph 1708*)

$C_{19}H_{22}FN_3O$ 327.4   1649-18-9

Action and use

Dopamine receptor antagonist; neuroleptic (veterinary).

Preparation

Azaperone Injection

Ph Eur

DEFINITION

1-(4-Fluorophenyl)-4-[4-(pyridin-2-yl)piperazin-1-yl]butan-1-one.

Content

99.0 per cent to 101.0 per cent (dried substance).

CHARACTERS

Appearance

White or almost white powder.

Solubility

Practically insoluble in water, freely soluble in acetone and in methylene chloride, soluble in alcohol.

It shows polymorphism.

IDENTIFICATION

Infrared absorption spectrophotometry (*2.2.24*)

Preparation Discs.

Comparison azaperone CRS.

If the spectra obtained show differences, dissolve the substance to be examined and the reference substance separately in *acetone R*, evaporate to dryness and record new spectra using the residues.

TESTS

Appearance of solution

The solution is clear (*2.2.1*) and not more intensely coloured than reference solution Y_6 (*2.2.2, Method II*).

Dissolve 1.0 g in 25 ml of a 14 g/l solution of *tartaric acid R*.

Related substances

Liquid chromatography (*2.2.29*).

Test solution Dissolve 0.100 g of the substance to be examined in *methanol R* and dilute to 10.0 ml with the same solvent.

Reference solution (a) Dissolve 5.0 mg of *azaperone CRS* and 6.0 mg of benperidol CRS in *methanol R* and dilute to 200.0 ml with the same solvent.

Reference solution (b) Dilute 1.0 ml of the test solution to 100.0 ml with *methanol R*. Dilute 5.0 ml of the solution to 20.0 ml with *methanol R*.

Column:

— *size: l* = 0.10 m, Ø = 4.6 mm,
— *stationary phase: base-deactivated octadecylsilyl silica gel for chromatography R* (3 μm),
— *temperature*: 25 °C.

Mobile phase:
— *mobile phase A*: dissolve 1.4 g of *anhydrous sodium sulphate R* in 900 ml of *water R*, add 16.0 ml of *0.01 M sulphuric acid* and dilute to 1000 ml with *water R*,
— *mobile phase B*: *methanol R*.

Time (min)	Mobile phase A (per cent *V/V*)	Mobile phase B (per cent *V/V*)
0 - 15	95 → 20	5 → 80
15 - 20	20	80
20 - 21	20 → 95	80 → 5

Flow rate 1.5 ml/min.

Detection Spectrophotometer at 230 nm.

Equilibration At least 4 min with the mobile phase at the initial composition.

Injection 10 µl.

Relative retention with reference to azaperone (retention time = about 9 min): impurity A = about 0.9; impurity B = about 1.1; impurity C = about 1.15.

System suitability Reference solution (a):
— *resolution*: minimum 8.0 between the peaks due to azaperone and to benperidol.

Limits:
— *impurity A*: not more than the area of the principal peak in the chromatogram obtained with reference solution (b) (0.25 per cent),
— *total of impurities B and C*: not more than 3 times the area of the principal peak in the chromatogram obtained with reference solution (b) (0.75 per cent),
— *total*: not more than 4 times the area of the principal peak in the chromatogram obtained with reference solution (b) (1.0 per cent),
— *disregard limit*: 0.2 times the area of the principal peak in the chromatogram obtained with reference solution (b) (0.05 per cent).

Loss on drying (*2.2.32*)
Maximum 0.5 per cent, determined on 1.000 g by drying *in vacuo* at 60 °C for 4 h.

Sulphated ash (*2.4.14*)
Maximum 0.1 per cent, determined on 1.0 g.

ASSAY
Dissolve 0.130 g in 70 ml of a mixture of 1 volume of *anhydrous acetic acid R* and 7 volumes of *methyl ethyl ketone R*. Titrate with *0.1 M perchloric acid*, using 0.2 ml of *naphtholbenzein solution R* as indicator.

1 ml of *0.1 M perchloric acid* is equivalent to 16.37 mg of $C_{19}H_{22}FN_3O$.

STORAGE
Protected from light.

IMPURITIES

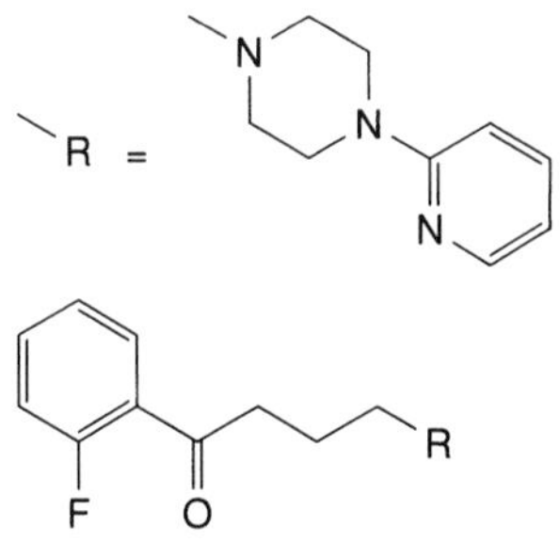

A. 1-(2-fluorophenyl)-4-[4-(pyridin-2-yl)piperazin-1-yl]butan-1-one,

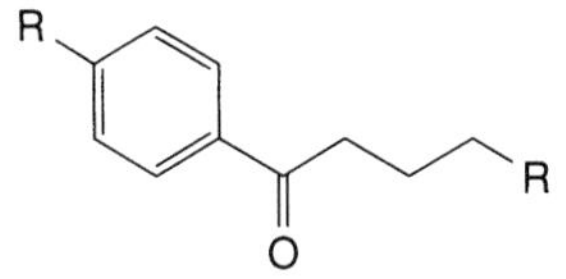

B. 4-[4-(pyridin-2-yl)piperazin-1-yl]-1-[4-[4-(pyridin-2-yl)piperazin-1-yl]phenyl]butan-1-one,

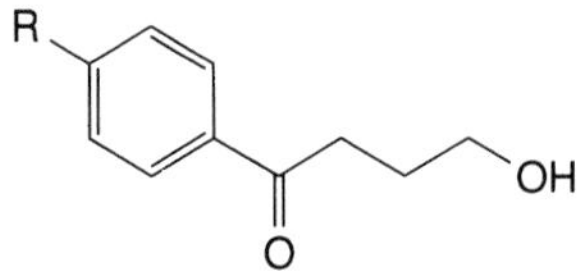

C. 4-hydroxy-1-[4-[4-(pyridin-2-yl)piperazin-1-yl]phenyl]butan-1-one.

_____ *Ph Eur*

Calcium Copperedetate

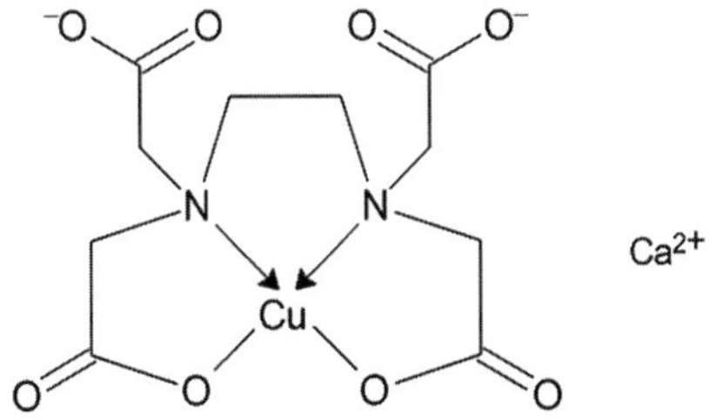

$C_{10}H_{12}CaCuN_2O_8,2H_2O$ 427.6

Action and use
Used in the treatment of copper deficiency.

Preparation
Calcium Copperedetate Injection

DEFINITION
Calcium Copperedetate is the dihydrate of calcium [ethylenediaminetetra-acetato(4-)-*N*,*N'*,*O*,*O'*]copper(II). It contains not less than 9.1% and not more than 9.7% of calcium, Ca, and not less than 14.4% and not more than 15.3% of copper, Cu, both calculated with reference to the dried substance.

CHARACTERISTICS
A blue, crystalline powder.

Freely soluble in *water*, the solution gradually precipitating the tetrahydrate; practically insoluble in *ethanol (96%)*.

IDENTIFICATION

A. Dissolve 0.2 g in 5 ml of *water* and add 1 ml of 6M *acetic acid* and 2 ml of *dilute potassium iodide solution*. The solution remains clear and deep blue.

B. Ignite 0.2 g, dissolve the residue in 3 ml of 2M *hydrochloric acid*, neutralise the solution with 5M *ammonia* and add 1 ml of 6M *acetic acid* and 2 ml of *dilute potassium iodide solution*. A white precipitate is produced and iodine is liberated, colouring the supernatant liquid brown.

C. Dissolve 0.5 g in 10 ml of *water*, acidify with 2M *hydrochloric acid*, add 25 ml of a 10% v/v solution of *mercaptoacetic acid* and filter. Make the filtrate alkaline with 5M *ammonia* and add 5 ml of a 2.5% w/v solution of *ammonium oxalate*. A white precipitate is produced which is soluble in *hydrochloric acid* but only sparingly soluble in 6M *acetic acid*.

TESTS

Lead

Not more than 25 ppm of Pb when determined by the following method. Dissolve 1.25 g in 10 ml of *hydrochloric acid*, dilute to 25 ml with *water* and determine by *atomic absorption spectrophotometry*, Appendix II D, measuring at 283.3 nm and using a lead hollow-cathode lamp as the radiation source and *lead standard solution (100 ppm Pb)*, diluted if necessary with *water*, to prepare the standard solutions.

Zinc

Not more than 200 ppm of Zn when determined by the following method. Dissolve 1.0 g in 20 ml of *hydrochloric acid*, dilute to 200 ml with *water* and determine by *atomic absorption spectrophotometry*, Appendix II D, measuring at 213.9 nm and using a zinc hollow-cathode lamp as the radiation source and *zinc standard solution (5 mg/ml Zn)* diluted if necessary with *water*, to prepare the standard solutions.

Loss on drying

When dried to constant weight at 105°, loses not more than 2.0% of its weight. Use 1 g.

ASSAY

For copper

Ignite 4 g at 600° to 700°, cool and heat the residue with 12 ml of a mixture of equal volumes of *hydrochloric acid* and *water* on a water bath for 15 minutes. Add 10 ml of *water*, filter and dilute the filtrate to 100 ml with *water* (solution A); reserve a portion for the Assay for calcium. To 25 ml of solution A add 25 ml of *water* and 10 ml of *bromine solution*, boil to remove the bromine, cool and add *dilute sodium carbonate solution* until a faint permanent precipitate is produced. Add 3 g of *potassium iodide* and 5 ml of 6M *acetic acid* and titrate the liberated iodine with 0.1M *sodium thiosulphate VS*, using *starch mucilage* as indicator, until only a faint blue colour remains; add 2 g of *potassium thiocyanate* and continue the titration until the blue colour disappears. Each ml of 0.1M *sodium thiosulphate VS* is equivalent to 6.354 mg of Cu.

For calcium

To 5 ml of solution A add 10 ml of *water* and 10 ml of a 10% v/v solution of *mercaptoacetic acid*, allow to stand until the precipitate has coagulated, dilute to 100 ml with *water*, add 5 ml of 5M *sodium hydroxide* and titrate with 0.05M *disodium edetate VS*, using *methyl thymol blue mixture* as indicator, until the solution becomes a full purple colour,

adding the titrant slowly as the end point is approached. Each ml of 0.05M *disodium edetate VS* is equivalent to 2.004 mg of Ca.

Catechu

Pale Catechu

Action and use
Intestinal astringent.

Preparation
Catechu Tincture

When Powdered Catechu is prescribed or demanded, material complying with the appropriate requirements below shall be dispensed or supplied.

DEFINITION

Catechu is a dried aqueous extract prepared from the leaves and young shoots of *Uncaria gambier* (Hunter) Roxb.

CHARACTERISTICS

Odourless or almost odourless.

Macroscopical Catechu usually occurs as cubes, which are sometimes more or less agglutinated and mixed with fragments of broken cubes; the cubes are friable and porous and measure about 2.5 cm in each direction; larger cubes and brick-shaped pieces, up to 4 cm long, also occur and are sometimes broken. Their colour is dull, pale greyish brown to dark reddish brown externally and pale brown internally.

Microscopical The diagnostic characters are: the abundant yellowish brown masses of acicular catechin crystals, soluble in hot *water*; varying amounts of fragments from the leaves and flowering shoots of the plant including: unicellular covering trichomes, 250 to 540 μm long with lignified walls, pitted at the base, some with one or two thin transverse septa; fewer smaller trichomes, 25 to 45 μm long, conical, with warty, unlignified walls, epidermal cells of the leaves thin-walled with a finely striated cuticle and *paracytic* stomata, Appendix XI H, on the lower epidermis only; reddish brown corolla segments with numerous covering trichomes and characteristic pitted and lignified cicatrices in the epidermis; parenchymatous cells containing calcium oxalate as cluster crystals and crystal sand; subspherical pollen grains, 11 to 18 μm in diameter with three pores, three furrows and a minutely pitted exine; occasional fragments of cork.

IDENTIFICATION

Warm 0.3 g with 2 ml of *ethanol (96%)*, cool and filter. Add 2 ml of 5M *sodium hydroxide* to the filtrate, shake, add 2 ml of *petroleum spirit (boiling range, 40° to 60°)*, shake and allow to separate. A brilliant greenish fluorescence is produced in the upper layer.

TESTS

Matter insoluble in ethanol (96%)

Not more than 34.0%, calculated with reference to the dried material, when determined by the following method. Macerate 5 g, in *coarse powder*, with 100 ml of *ethanol (96%)*, allow to stand for 6 hours shaking frequently and allow to stand for a further 18 hours. Filter, wash the residue with *ethanol (96%)* and dry to constant weight at 100°.

Starch

The residue obtained in the test for Matter insoluble in ethanol (96%) contains not more than an occasional starch granule.

Water-insoluble matter
Not more than 33.0%, calculated with reference to the dried material, when determined by the method for Matter insoluble in ethanol (96%), but using *water* in place of the *ethanol (96%)*.

Loss on drying
When dried to constant weight at 105°, loses not more than 15.0% of its weight. Use 1 g.

Ash
Not more than 8.0%, Appendix XI J.

Cefalonium

$C_{20}H_{18}N_4O_5S_2,2H_2O$ 494.5   *5575-21-3 (anhydrous)*

Action and use
Cephalosporin antibacterial.

Preparations
Cefalonium Eye Ointment
Cefalonium Intramammary Infusion (Dry Cow)

DEFINITION
Cefalonium is 3-(4-carbamoyl-1-pyridiniomethyl)-7-[(2-thienyl)acetamido]-3-cephem-4-carboxylate dihydrate. It contains not less than 95.0% and not more than 103.5% of $C_{20}H_{18}N_4O_5S_2$, calculated with reference to the anhydrous substance.

CHARACTERISTICS
A white or almost white crystalline powder.

Very slightly soluble in *water* and in *methanol*; soluble in *dimethyl sulphoxide*; insoluble in *dichloromethane*, in *ethanol (96%)* and in *ether*. It dissolves in dilute acids and in alkaline solutions.

IDENTIFICATION
A. The *infrared absorption spectrum*, Appendix II A, is concordant with the *reference spectrum* of cefalonium *(RSV 09)*.

B. The *light absorption*, Appendix II B, in the range 220 to 350 nm of a 0.002% w/v solution in *water* exhibits two maxima, at 235 nm and at 262 nm. The *absorbance* at 235 nm is about 0.76 and at 262 nm is about 0.62.

TESTS
Specific optical rotation
Dissolve 0.25 g with the aid of gentle heat in sufficient *dimethyl sulphoxide* to produce 50 ml. Allow the solution to stand for 30 minutes before measurement of the optical rotation. The *specific optical rotation* in the resulting solution is -50 to -56, calculated with reference to the anhydrous substance, Appendix V F.

Related substances
Carry out the method for *thin-layer chromatography*, Appendix III A, using *silica gel F_{254}* as the coating substance

and a mixture of 10 volumes of *glacial acetic acid*, 10 volumes of 1M *sodium acetate* and 30 volumes of *propan-2-ol* as the mobile phase but allowing the solvent front to ascend 12 cm above the line of application. Apply separately to the plate 4 µl of each of the following solutions in 8.3M *acetic acid* containing (1) 2.5% w/v of the substance being examined, (2) 0.05% w/v of the substance being examined, (3) 0.025% w/v of the substance being examined, (4) 0.005% w/v of the substance being examined and (5) 0.05% w/v of each of *cefalotin sodium EPCRS* and *isonicotinamide*. After removal of the plate, allow it to dry in air and examine under *ultraviolet light (254 nm)*. Any *secondary spot* in the chromatogram obtained with solution (1) is not more intense than the spot in the chromatogram obtained with solution (2) (2%), not more than one such spot is more intense than the spot in the chromatogram obtained with solution (3) (1%) and not more than three such spots are more intense than the spot in the chromatogram obtained with solution (4) (0.2% each). The test is not valid unless the chromatogram obtained with solution (5) shows two clearly separated spots.

Sulphated ash
Not more than 0.2%, Appendix IX A.

Water
6.5 to 8.5% w/w, Appendix IX C. Use 0.5 g.

ASSAY
Measure the *absorbance* of a 0.002% w/v solution at the maximum at 262 nm, Appendix II B. Calculate the content of $C_{20}H_{18}N_4O_5S_2$ from the *absorbance* obtained using a 0.002% w/v solution of *cefalonium BPCRS* and from the declared content of $C_{20}H_{18}N_4O_5S_2$ in *cefalonium BPCRS*.

STORAGE
Cefalonium should be protected from light and stored at a temperature not exceeding 30°.

Cefalonium intended for use in the manufacture of either a parenteral dosage form or an intramammary infusion without a further appropriate sterilisation procedure complies with the following additional requirement.

Sterility
Complies with the *test for sterility*, Appendix XVI A.

IMPURITIES

A. cefalotin,

B. 3-hydroxymethyl-7β-(2-thienylacetamido)-3-cephem-4-carboxylic acid,

C. 3-hydroxymethyl-7β-(2-thienylacetamido)-3-cephem-4-carboxylic acid lactone,

D. isonicotinamide.

Clazuril

(Clazuril for Veterinary Use, Ph Eur monograph 1714)

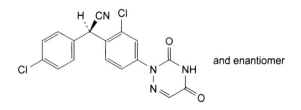

C₁₇H₁₀Cl₂N₄O₂   373.2   *101831-36-1*

$C_{17}H_{10}Cl_2N_4O_2$ 373.2   *101831-36-1*

Action and use

Treatment of coccidiosis; antiprotozoal (veterinary).

Ph Eur

DEFINITION

(2RS)-[2-Chloro-4-(3,5-dioxo-4,5-dihydro-1,2,4-triazin-2(3H)-yl)phenyl](4-chlorophenyl)acetonitrile.

Content

99.0 per cent to 101.0 per cent (dried substance).

CHARACTERS

Appearance

White or light yellow powder.

Solubility

Practically insoluble in water, freely soluble in dimethylformamide, slightly soluble in alcohol and in methylene chloride.

IDENTIFICATION

A. Melting point *(2.2.14)*: 199 °C to 203 °C.

B. Infrared absorption spectrophotometry *(2.2.24)*.

Comparison   Ph. Eur. reference spectrum of clazuril.

TESTS

Related substances

Liquid chromatography *(2.2.29)*.

Test solution   Dissolve 20.0 mg of the substance to be examined in a mixture of equal volumes of *tetrahydrofuran R* and *water R* and dilute to 20.0 ml with the same mixture of solvents.

Reference solution (a)   Dissolve 5 mg of *clazuril for system suitability CRS* in a mixture of equal volumes of

tetrahydrofuran R and water R and dilute to 5.0 ml with the same mixture of solvents.

Reference solution (b)   Dilute 1.0 ml of the test solution to 100.0 ml with a mixture of equal volumes of *tetrahydrofuran R* and *water R*. Dilute 2.0 ml of this solution to 10.0 ml with a mixture of equal volumes of *tetrahydrofuran R* and *water R*.

Column:

— *size*: $l = 0.10$ m, $\varnothing = 4.6$ mm,

— *stationary phase*: octadecylsilyl silica gel for chromatography R (3 μm),

— *temperature*: 35 °C.

Mobile phase:

— *mobile phase A*: mix 100 volumes of a 7.7 g/l solution of *ammonium acetate R* adjusted to pH 6.2 with a 10 per cent *V/V* solution of *anhydrous formic acid R*, 150 volumes of *acetonitrile R* and 750 volumes of *water R*,

— *mobile phase B*: mix 100 volumes of a 7.7 g/l solution of *ammonium acetate R* adjusted to pH 6.2 with a 10 per cent *V/V* solution of *anhydrous formic acid R*, 850 volumes of *acetonitrile R* and 50 volumes of *water R*,

Time (min)	Mobile phase A (per cent V/V)	Mobile phase B (per cent V/V)
0 - 20	100 → 0	0 → 100
20 - 25	0	100
25 - 30	0 → 100	100 → 0
30 - 40	100	0

Flow rate   1.0 ml/min.

Detection   Spectrophotometer at 230 nm.

Injection   5 μl.

System suitability   Reference solution (a):

— *peak-to-valley ratio*: minimum 1.5, where H_p = height above the baseline of the peak due to impurity G and H_v = height above the baseline of the lowest point of the curve separating this peak from the peak due to clazuril,

— the chromatogram obtained is concordant with the chromatogram supplied with *clazuril for system suitability CRS*.

Limits:

— *correction factors*: for the calculation of contents, multiply the peak areas of the following impurities by the corresponding correction factor: impurity G = 1.4; impurity H = 0.8;

— *any impurity*: not more than the area of the principal peak in the chromatogram obtained with reference solution (b) (0.2 per cent);

— *total*: not more than 3 times the area of the principal peak in the chromatogram obtained with reference solution (b) (0.6 per cent);

— *disregard limit*: 0.25 times the area of the principal peak in the chromatogram obtained with reference solution (b) (0.05 per cent); disregard the peaks due to the solvents.

Loss on drying *(2.2.32)*

Maximum 0.5 per cent, determined on 1.000 g by drying in an oven at 100-105 °C for 4 h.

Sulphated ash *(2.4.14)*

Maximum 0.1 per cent, determined on 1.0 g.

ASSAY

Dissolve about 0.260 g in 35 ml of *tetrahydrofuran R* and add 35 ml of *water R*. Titrate with *0.1 M sodium hydroxide*, determining the end-point potentiometrically (*2.2.20*). Carry out a blank titration.

1 ml of *0.1 M sodium hydroxide* is equivalent to 37.32 mg of $C_{17}H_{10}Cl_2N_4O_2$.

STORAGE

Protected from light.

IMPURITIES

A. R = OH: (*2RS*)-[2-chloro-4-(3,5-dioxo-4,5-dihydro-1,2,4-triazin-2(*3H*)-yl)phenyl](4-chlorophenyl)acetic acid,

C. R = NH₂: (*2RS*)-2-[2-chloro-4-(3,5-dioxo-1,2,4-triazin-2(*3H*)-yl)phenyl]-2-(4-chlorophenyl)acetamide,

B. R = NH₂: 2-[3-chloro-4-[(*RS*)-(4-chlorophenyl)cyanomethyl]phenyl]-3,5-dioxo-2,3,4,5-tetrahydro-1,2,4-triazine-6-carboxamide,

D. R = N(CH₃)₂: 2-[3-chloro-4-[(*RS*)-(4-chlorophenyl)cyanomethyl]phenyl]-*N,N*-dimethyl-3,5-dioxo-2,3,4,5-tetrahydro-1,2,4-triazine-6-carboxamide,

E. R = OCH₃: methyl 2-[3-chloro-4-[(*RS*)-(4-chlorophenyl)cyanomethyl]phenyl]-3,5-dioxo-2,3,4,5-tetrahydro-1,2,4-triazine-6-carboxylate,

F. R = OC₂H₅: ethyl 2-[3-chloro-4-[(*RS*)-(4-chlorophenyl)cyanomethyl]phenyl]-3,5-dioxo-2,3,4,5-tetrahydro-1,2,4-triazine-6-carboxylate,

G. 2-[3-chloro-4-(4-chlorobenzoyl)phenyl]-1,2,4-triazine-3,5(*2H,4H*)-dione,

H. [2-chloro-4-(3,5-dioxo-4,5-dihydro-1,2,4-triazin-2(*3H*)-yl)phenyl][4-[[2-chloro-4-(3,5-dioxo-4,5-dihydro-1,2,4-triazin-2(*3H*)-yl)phenyl]cyanomethyl]phenyl](4-chlorophenyl)acetonitrile,

I. (*Z*)-2-[[3-chloro-4-[(*RS*)-(4-chlorophenyl)cyanomethyl]phenyl]diazanylidene]acetamide.

Ph Eur

Cloprostenol Sodium

$C_{22}H_{28}ClNaO_6$ 446.9   *55028-72-3*

Action and use
Prostaglandin (PGF$_{2\alpha}$) analogue.

Preparation
Cloprostenol Injection

DEFINITION

Cloprostenol Sodium is (±)-(5*Z*)-7-(1*R*,3*R*,5*S*)-2-[(1*E*,3*R*)-4-(3-chlorophenoxy)-3-hydroxybut-1-enyl]-3,5-dihydroxycyclopentylhept-5-enoate. It contains not less than 97.5% and not more than 102.5% of $C_{22}H_{28}ClNaO_6$, calculated with reference to the anhydrous substance.

CAUTION *Cloprostenol Sodium is extremely potent and extraordinary care should be taken in any procedure in which it is used.*

CHARACTERISTICS

A white or almost white, amorphous powder; hygroscopic.

Freely soluble in *water*, in *ethanol (96%)* and in *methanol*; practically insoluble in *acetone*.

IDENTIFICATION

A. The *infrared absorption spectrum*, Appendix II A, is concordant with the *reference spectrum* of cloprostenol sodium *(RSV 11)*.

B. Yields reaction A characteristic of *sodium salts*, Appendix VI.

TESTS

Related substances

Carry out the method for *liquid chromatography*, Appendix III D, using two solutions of the substance being examined in *absolute ethanol* containing (1) 2.0% w/v and (2) 0.050% w/v.

The chromatographic procedure may be carried out using (a) a stainless steel column (25 cm × 4.6 mm) packed with *silica gel for chromatography* (5 µm) (Partisil is suitable), (b) a mixture of 1 volume of *glacial acetic acid*, 70 volumes of *absolute ethanol* and 930 volumes of *hexane* as the mobile phase with a flow rate of 1.8 ml per minute and (c) a detection wavelength of 220 nm.

Inject 5 µl of each solution. Using solution (2) adjust the attenuation to obtain a principal peak with a height corresponding to at least 50% of full-scale deflection of the recorder. Allow the chromatography to proceed for twice the retention time of the peak due to Cloprostenol.

In the chromatogram obtained with solution (1) the sum of the areas of any *secondary peaks* is not greater than the area of the principal peak in the chromatogram obtained with solution (2) (2.5%).

Water

Not more than 3.0% w/w, Appendix IX C. Use 50 mg dissolved in 1 ml of *absolute ethanol*.

ASSAY

Carry out the method for *liquid chromatography*, Appendix III D, using two solutions in *absolute ethanol* containing (1) 0.08% w/v of the substance being examined and (2) 0.08% w/v of *cloprostenol sodium BPCRS*.

The chromatographic procedure may be carried out using (a) a stainless steel column (25 cm × 4.6 mm) packed with *silica gel for chromatography* (5 µm) (Partisil is suitable), (b) a mixture of 1 volume of *glacial acetic acid*, 100 volumes of *absolute ethanol* and 900 volumes of *hexane* as the mobile phase with a flow rate of 1.8 ml per minute and (c) a detection wavelength of 220 nm.

Inject 5 µl of each solution. Calculate the content of $C_{22}H_{28}ClNaO_6$ from the chromatograms obtained and using the declared content of $C_{22}H_{28}ClNaO_6$ in *cloprostenol sodium BPCRS*.

STORAGE

Cloprostenol Sodium should be protected from light and moisture.

IMPURITIES

A. (±)-(5*Z*)-7-(1*R*,3*R*,5*S*)-2-[(1*E*,3 *S*)-4-(3-chlorophenoxy)-3-hydroxybut-1-enyl]-3,5-dihydroxycyclopentylhept-5-enoate *(epimer)*,

B. (±)-(5*E*)-7-(1*R*,3*R*,5*S*)-2-[(1*E*,3 *R*)-4-(3-chlorophenoxy)-3-hydroxybut-1-enyl]-3,5-dihydroxycyclopentylhept-5-enoate *(trans-isomer)*.

Closantel Sodium Dihydrate

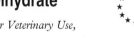

(Closantel Sodium Dihydrate for Veterinary Use, Ph Eur monograph 1716)

and enantiomer

$C_{22}H_{13}Cl_2I_2N_2NaO_2,2H_2O$ 721   *61438-64-0*

Action and use
Antihelminthic.

Ph Eur _____

DEFINITION

N-[5-Chloro-4-[(*RS*)-(4-chlorophenyl)cyanomethyl]-2-methylphenyl]-2-hydroxy-3,5-diiodobenzamide sodium salt dihydrate.

Content
98.5 per cent to 101.5 per cent (anhydrous substance).

CHARACTERS

Appearance
Yellow powder, slightly hygroscopic.

Solubility
Very slightly soluble in water, freely soluble in ethanol (96 per cent), soluble in methanol.

It shows polymorphism.

IDENTIFICATION

A. Infrared absorption spectrophotometry *(2.2.24)*.

Preparation   Discs without recrystallisation.

Comparison   *closantel sodium dihydrate CRS*.

B. Dissolve 0.1 g in 2 ml of *ethanol (96 per cent) R*. The solution gives reaction (a) of sodium *(2.3.1)*.

TESTS

Appearance of solution
The solution is clear *(2.2.1)* and not more intensely coloured than reference solution GY_4 *(2.2.2, Method II)*.

Dissolve 0.50 g in *ethanol (96 per cent) R* and dilute to 50 ml with the same solvent.

Related substances
Liquid chromatography *(2.2.29)*.

Prepare the solutions immediately before use and protect from light.

Test solution Dissolve 0.100 g of the substance to be examined in *methanol R* and dilute to 10.0 ml with the same solvent.

Reference solution (a) Dissolve 10 mg of *closantel for system suitability CRS* (containing impurities A to J) in *methanol R* and dilute to 1.0 ml with the same solvent.

Reference solution (b) Dilute 1.0 ml of the test solution to 100.0 ml with *methanol R*. Dilute 5.0 ml of this solution to 25.0 ml with *methanol R*.

Column:
— *size*: l = 0.10 m, Ø = 4.6 mm,
— *stationary phase*: base-deactivated octadecylsilyl silica gel for chromatography R (3 μm),
— *temperature*: 35 °C.

Mobile phase:
— *mobile phase A*: to 100 ml of a 7.7 g/l solution of ammonium acetate R previously adjusted to pH 4.3 with acetic acid R, add 50 ml of acetonitrile R and 850 ml of water R;
— *mobile phase B*: to 100 ml of a 7.7 g/l solution of ammonium acetate R previously adjusted to pH 4.3 with acetic acid R, add 50 ml of water R and 850 ml of acetonitrile R;

Time (min)	Mobile phase A (per cent *V/V*)	Mobile phase B (per cent *V/V*)
0 - 2	50	50
2 - 22	50 → 20	50 → 80
22 - 27	20	80
27 - 28	20 → 50	80 → 50
28 - 32	50	50

Flow rate 1.5 ml/min.

Detection Spectrophotometer at 240 nm.

Injection 10 μl.

Relative retention With reference to closantel (retention time = about 16 min): impurity A = about 0.07; impurity B = about 0.48; impurity C = about 0.62; impurity D = about 0.65; impurity E = about 0.82; impurity F = about 0.89; impurity G = about 0.93; impurity H = about 1.13; impurity I = about 1.16; impurity J = about 1.55.

System suitability Reference solution (a):
— *resolution*: baseline separation between the peaks due to impurity G and closantel,
— the chromatogram obtained is similar to the chromatogram supplied with *closantel for system suitability CRS*.

Limits:
— *correction factors*: for the calculation of contents, multiply the peak areas of the following impurities by the corresponding correction factor: impurity A = 1.5; impurity B = 1.3;
— *impurity G*: not more than 2.5 times the area of the principal peak in the chromatogram obtained with reference solution (b) (0.5 per cent);
— *impurities F, H, I*: for each impurity, not more than 1.5 times the area of the principal peak in the chromatogram obtained with reference solution (b) (0.3 per cent);
— *impurities A, B, C, D, E, J*: for each impurity, not more than the area of the principal peak in the chromatogram obtained with reference solution (b) (0.2 per cent);

— *any other impurity*: for each impurity, not more than the area of the principal peak in the chromatogram obtained with reference solution (b) (0.2 per cent);
— *total*: not more than 7.5 times the area of the principal peak in the chromatogram obtained with reference solution (b) (1.5 per cent);
— *disregard limit*: 0.25 times the area of the principal peak in the chromatogram obtained with reference solution (b) (0.05 per cent).

Water *(2.5.12)*
4.8 per cent to 5.8 per cent, determined on 0.250 g.
Use a mixture of 1 volume of *dimethylformamide R* and 4 volumes of *methanol R* as the solvent.

ASSAY
Dissolve 0.500 g in 50 ml of a mixture of 1 volume of *anhydrous acetic acid R* and 7 volumes of *methyl ethyl ketone R*. Titrate with *0.1 M perchloric acid*, determining the end-point potentiometrically *(2.2.20)*.

1 ml of *0.1 M perchloric acid* is equivalent to 68.5 mg of $C_{22}H_{13}Cl_2I_2N_2NaO_2$.

STORAGE
In an airtight container, protected from light.

IMPURITIES
Specified impurities A, B, C, D, E, F, G, H, I, J.

A. 2-hydroxy-3,5-diiodobenzoic acid,

and enantiomer

B. (2*RS*)-(4-amino-2-chloro-5-methylphenyl)(4-chlorophenyl)ethanenitrile,

and enantiomer

C. R1 = H, R2 = CO_2H, R3 = I: (2*RS*)-[2-chloro-4-[(2-hydroxy-3,5-diiodobenzoyl)amino]-5-methylphenyl](4-chlorophenyl)acetic acid,

D. R1 = H, R2 = $CONH_2$, R3 = I: *N*-[4-[(1*RS*)-2-amino-1-(4-chlorophenyl)-2-oxoethyl]-5-chloro-2-methylphenyl]-2-hydroxy-3,5-diiodobenzamide,

E. R1 = H, R2 = CN, R3 = Cl: 3-chloro-*N*-[5-chloro-4-[(*RS*)-(4-chlorophenyl)cyanomethyl]-2-methylphenyl]-2-hydroxy-5-iodobenzamide,

F. R1 + R2 = O, R3 = I: *N*-[5-chloro-4-(4-chlorobenzoyl)-2-methylphenyl]-2-hydroxy-3,5-diiodobenzamide,

G. R1 = H, R2 = C(=NH)OCH₃, R3 = I: methyl (2RS)-2-[2-chloro-4-[(2-hydroxy-3,5-diiodobenzoyl)amino]-5-methylphenyl]-2-(4-chlorophenyl)acetimidate,

H. R1 = H, R2 = CO-OCH₃, R3 = I: methyl (2RS)-[2-chloro-4-[(2-hydroxy-3,5-diiodobenzoyl)amino]-5-methylphenyl](4-chlorophenyl)acetate,

I. R1 = R3 = H, R2 = CN: N-[5-chloro-4-[(RS)-(4-chlorophenyl)cyanomethyl]-2-methylphenyl]-2-hydroxy-5-iodobenzamide,

J. N-[5-chloro-4-[[4-[[2-chloro-4-[(2-hydroxy-3,5-diiodobenzoyl)amino]-5-methylphenyl]cyanomethyl]phenyl](4-chlorophenyl)cyanomethyl]-2-methylphenyl]-2-hydroxy-3,5-diiodobenzamide.

_____ Ph Eur

Cloxacillin Benzathine

C₁₆H₂₀N₂,(C₁₉H₁₈ClN₃O₅S)₂   1112.1   32222-55-2

Action and use
Penicillin antibacterial.

Preparations
Cloxacillin Benzathine Intramammary Infusion (Dry Cow)

Ampicillin Trihydrate and Cloxacillin Benzathine Intramammary Infusion (Dry Cow)

DEFINITION
Cloxacillin Benzathine is N,N'-dibenzylethylenediammonium bis[(6R)-6-(3-o-chlorophenyl-5-methylisoxazole-4-carboxamido)penicillanate]. It contains not less than 92.0% of C₁₆H₂₀N₂,(C₁₉H₁₈ClN₃O₅S)₂ and not less than 20.0% and not more than 22.0% of benzathine, C₁₆H₂₀N₂, each calculated with reference to the anhydrous substance.

CHARACTERISTICS
A white or almost white powder.

Slightly soluble in water; freely soluble in methanol; slightly soluble in ethanol (96%) and in propan-2-ol.

IDENTIFICATION
A. The infrared absorption spectrum, Appendix II A, is concordant with the reference spectrum of cloxacillin benzathine (RSV 12).

B. Shake 0.1 g with 1 ml of 1M sodium hydroxide for 2 minutes, add 2 ml of ether, shake for 1 minute and allow to separate. Evaporate 1 ml of the ether layer to dryness, dissolve the residue in 2 ml of glacial acetic acid and add 1 ml of dilute potassium dichromate solution. A golden yellow precipitate is produced.

C. Shake 50 mg with 10 ml of water and filter. To 5 ml of the filtrate add a few drops of silver nitrate solution. No precipitate is produced. Heat 50 mg with 2 ml of alcoholic potassium hydroxide solution on a water bath for 15 minutes, add 15 mg of activated charcoal, shake and filter. Acidify the filtrate with 2M nitric acid. The solution yields reaction A characteristic of chlorides, Appendix VI.

TESTS
Water
Not more than 5.0% w/w, Appendix IX C. Use 0.5 g.

ASSAY
For cloxacillin benzathine
To 60 mg add 40 ml of methanol, shake to dissolve, add 25 ml of 1M sodium hydroxide and allow to stand for 30 minutes. Add 27.5 ml of 1M hydrochloric acid and sufficient water to produce 100 ml, mix, transfer 20 ml of the solution to a stoppered flask, add 30 ml of 0.01M iodine VS, close the flask with a wet stopper and allow to stand for 15 minutes protected from light. Titrate the excess of iodine with 0.02M sodium thiosulphate VS, using starch mucilage, added towards the end of the titration, as indicator. Add a further 12 mg of the substance being examined to 10 ml of water, swirl to disperse, add 30 ml of 0.01M iodine VS and titrate immediately with 0.02M sodium thiosulphate VS, using starch mucilage, added towards the end of the titration, as indicator. The difference between the titrations represents the volume of 0.01M iodine VS equivalent to the total penicillins present. Calculate the content of C₁₆H₂₀N₂,(C₁₉H₁₈ClN₃O₅S)₂ from the difference obtained by carrying out the assay simultaneously using cloxacillin benzathine BPCRS and from the declared content of C₁₆H₂₀N₂,(C₁₉H₁₈ClN₃O₅S)₂ in cloxacillin benzathine BPCRS.

For benzathine
To 1 g add 30 ml of a saturated solution of sodium chloride and 10 ml of 5M sodium hydroxide, shake well, and extract with four 50 ml quantities of ether. Wash the combined extracts with three 10 ml quantities of water, extract the combined washings with 25 ml of ether and add the extract to the main ether solution. Evaporate the ether solution to low bulk, add 2 ml of absolute ethanol and evaporate to dryness. To the residue add 50 ml of anhydrous acetic acid and titrate with 0.1M perchloric acid VS, using 0.1 ml of 1-naphtholbenzein solution as indicator. Repeat the operation without the substance being examined. The difference between the titrations represents the amount of perchloric acid required to neutralise the liberated base. Each ml of 0.1M perchloric acid VS is equivalent to 12.02 mg of C₁₆H₂₀N₂.

STORAGE
Cloxacillin Benzathine should be kept in an airtight container. If the material is sterile, the container should be sterile, tamper-evident and sealed so as to exclude micro-organisms.

LABELLING

The label states, where applicable, that the material is sterile.

Cloxacillin Benzathine intended for use in the manufacturer of either a parenteral dosage form or an intramammary infusion without a further appropriate sterilisation procedure complies with the following additional requirement.

Sterility

Complies with the *test for sterility*, Appendix XVI A.

Cobalt Oxide

Co$_3$O$_4$ 240.8   *1307-96-9*

Action and use

Used in the prevention of cobalt deficiency in ruminants.

Preparation

Cobalt Depot-tablets

DEFINITION

Cobalt Oxide consists of cobalt(II,III) oxide (tricobalt tetraoxide) with a small proportion of cobalt(III) oxide (dicobalt trioxide). It contains not less than 70.0% and not more than 75.0% of Co, calculated with reference to the substance ignited at about 600°.

CHARACTERISTICS

A black powder.

Practically insoluble in *water*. It dissolves in mineral acids and in solutions of the alkali hydroxides.

IDENTIFICATION

A. Dissolve 50 mg, with warming, in 5 ml of *hydrochloric acid* and add 10 ml of *water*. To 2 ml of the solution add 1 ml of 5M *sodium hydroxide*. A blue precipitate which becomes pink on warming is produced. Reserve the remainder of the solution for use in test B.

B. Neutralise 10 ml of the solution reserved in test A with 5M *sodium hydroxide* and add 0.5 ml of 6M *acetic acid* and 10 ml of a 10% w/v solution of *potassium nitrite*. A yellow crystalline precipitate is produced.

Loss on ignition

When ignited at about 600°, loses not more than 1.0% of its weight. Use 1 g.

ASSAY

Dissolve 0.1 g in 20 ml of *hydrochloric acid*, by repeated evaporation if necessary. Add 300 ml of *water*, 4 g of *hydroxylamine hydrochloride* and 25 ml of 13.5M *ammonia*. Warm to 80° and titrate with 0.05M *disodium edetate VS*, using *methyl thymol blue mixture* as indicator, until the colour changes from blue to purple. Each ml of 0.05M *disodium edetate VS* is equivalent to 2.946 mg of Co.

Decoquinate

C$_{24}$H$_{35}$NO$_5$ 417.6   *18507-89-6*

Action and use

Antiprotozoal (veterinary).

Preparation

Decoquinate Premix

DEFINITION

Decoquinate is ethyl 6-decyloxy-7-ethoxy-4-hydroxyquinoline-3-carboxylate. It contains not less than 99.0% and not more than 101.0% of C$_{24}$H$_{35}$NO$_5$, calculated with reference to the dried substance.

CHARACTERISTICS

A cream to buff-coloured, microcrystalline powder; odourless or almost odourless.

Insoluble in *water*; very slightly soluble in *chloroform* and in *ether*; practically insoluble in *ethanol (96%)*.

IDENTIFICATION

A. The *infrared absorption spectrum*, Appendix II A, is concordant with the *reference spectrum* of decoquinate *(RSV 14)*.

B. The *light absorption*, Appendix II B, in the range 230 to 350 nm of the solution used in the test for Light absorption exhibits a well-defined maximum only at 265 nm.

TESTS

Light absorption

Dissolve 40 mg in 10 ml of hot *chloroform* and, keeping the solution warm, dilute slowly with 70 ml of *absolute ethanol*. Cool and dilute to 100 ml with *absolute ethanol*. Immediately dilute 10 ml to 100 ml with *absolute ethanol*. To 10 ml of the solution add 10 ml of 0.1M *hydrochloric acid* and dilute to 100 ml with *absolute ethanol*. The *absorbance* of the resulting solution at the maximum at 265 nm is 0.38 to 0.42, calculated with reference to the dried substance, Appendix II B.

Related substances

Carry out the method for *thin-layer chromatography*, Appendix III A, using a silica gel F$_{254}$ precoated plate (Merck silica gel 60 F$_{254}$ plates are suitable) and a mixture of 5 volumes of *anhydrous formic acid*, 10 volumes of *absolute ethanol* and 85 volumes of *chloroform* as the mobile phase. Apply separately to the plate 10 µl of each of three solutions in *chloroform* containing (1) 1.0% w/v of the substance being examined, prepared with the aid of heat, (2) 0.0050% w/v of *diethyl 4-decyloxy-3-ethoxyanilinomethylenemalonate BPCRS* and (3) 0.010% w/v of the substance being examined. After removal of the plate, allow it to dry in air and examine under *ultraviolet light (254 nm)*. In the chromatogram obtained with solution (1) any spot corresponding to diethyl 4-decyloxy-3-ethoxyanilinomethylenemalonate is not more intense than the spot in the chromatogram obtained with solution (2) (0.5%) and any other *secondary spot* is not more intense than the spot in the chromatogram obtained with solution (3) (1%).

Loss on drying

When dried to constant weight at 105°, loses not more than 0.5% of its weight. Use 1 g.

Sulphated ash

Not more than 0.1%, Appendix IX A.

ASSAY

Dissolve 1 g in a mixture of 50 ml of *chloroform* and 50 ml of *anhydrous acetic acid* and carry out Method I for *non-aqueous titration*, Appendix VIII A, using *crystal violet solution* as indicator. Each ml of 0.1M *perchloric acid VS* is equivalent to 41.76 mg of $C_{24}H_{35}NO_5$.

Deltamethrin

$C_{22}H_{19}Br_2NO_3$ 505.2   *52918-63-5*

Action and use

Insecticide (veterinary).

Preparation

Deltamethrin Pour-on

DEFINITION

Deltamethrin is (*S*)-α-cyano-3-phenoxybenzyl-(1*R*,3*R*)-3-(2,2-dibromovinyl)-2,2-dimethylcyclopropane carboxylate. It contains not less than 97.0% and not more than 101.0% of $C_{22}H_{19}Br_2NO_3$.

CHARACTERISTICS

A white to buff-coloured, crystalline powder.

Insoluble in *water*; soluble in *ethanol (96%)* and in *acetone*.

IDENTIFICATION

A. The *infrared absorption spectrum*, Appendix II A, is concordant with the *reference spectrum* of deltamethrin (*RSV 47*).

B. In the test for Related substances the principal spot in the chromatogram obtained with solution (2) corresponds to that in the chromatogram obtained with solution (5).

TESTS

Specific optical rotation

In a 4% w/v solution in *toluene*, +55.5 to +58.5, Appendix V F.

Becisthemic acid chloride

Not more than 0.2% when determined by the following method. Dissolve 2 g in 100 ml of *methanol* with moderate heating, if necessary, and cool. Titrate with 0.02M *potassium hydroxide VS* using a solution containing 0.8% w/v of *dimethyl yellow* and 0.08% w/v of *methylene blue* in *methanol* as indicator to a green end point. Each ml of 0.02M *potassium hydroxide VS* is equivalent to 6.329 mg of becisthemic acid chloride, $C_8H_9Br_2ClO$.

Becisthemic acid and becisthemic anhydride

Not more than 1% in total when determined by the following methods.

Becisthemic acid

Dissolve 2 g in 100 ml of *ethanol (96%)* with moderate heating. Cool in an ice-bath and immediately titrate with 0.02M *sodium hydroxide VS* using a 1% w/v solution of *1-naphtholbenzein* in *ethanol (96%)* solution as indicator to a green end point. Correct the volume of titrant for any contribution due to the becisthemic acid chloride content using the following expression:

$$V \times P_2/P_1$$

where V = titration volume obtained in the becisthemic acid chloride test,

      P_1 = weight of sample used in the becisthemic chloride test,

      P_2 = weight of sample used in this test.

Each ml of 0.02M *sodium hydroxide VS* is equivalent to 5.959 mg of becisthemic acid, $C_8H_{10}Br_2O_2$.

Becisthemic anhydride

To 1.0 g add 10 ml of 0.01M *aniline* in *cyclohexane* and 10 ml of *glacial acetic acid*. Stopper the flask and allow to stand at room temperature for 1 hour. Titrate with 0.01M *perchloric acid VS* using *crystal violet solution* as indicator. Repeat the procedure omitting the substance being examined. Correct the volume of titrant for any contribution due to twice the becisthemic acid chloride content calculated using the above formula. Each ml of 0.01M *perchloric acid VS* is equivalent to 5.779 mg of becisthemic anhydride, $C_{16}H_{18}Br_4O_3$.

Related substances

Carry out the method for *thin-layer chromatography*, Appendix III A, using a silica gel F_{254} precoated plate (Merck silica gel 60 F_{254} plates are suitable) and as the mobile phase a mixture of 20 volumes of *di-isopropyl ether* and 80 volumes of *hexane*. Apply separately to the plate 10 μl of each of five solutions in *toluene* containing (1) 2.0% w/v of the substance being examined, (2) 0.5% w/v of the substance being examined, (3) 0.020% w/v of the substance being examined, (4) 0.010% w/v of the substance being examined and (5) 0.5% w/v of *deltamethrin BPCRS*. After removal of the plate, allow it to dry in air and examine under *ultraviolet light (254 nm)*. Any *secondary spot* in the chromatogram obtained with solution (1) is not more intense than the spot in the chromatogram obtained with solution (3) (1%) and not more than two such spots are more intense than the spot in the chromatogram obtained with solution (4) (0.5%).

ASSAY

Carry out the method for *liquid chromatography*, Appendix III D, using solutions in the mobile phase containing (1) 0.1% w/v of *deltamethrin BPCRS*, (2) 0.1% w/v of the substance being examined and (3) 0.1% w/v of *deltamethrin impurity standard BPCRS*.

The chromatographic procedure may be carried out using (a) a stainless steel column (25 cm × 4.6 mm) packed with *silica gel for chromatography* (5 μm) (Zorbax Sil is suitable), (b) as the mobile phase with a flow rate of 1.3 ml per minute a mixture of 0.04 volume of *propan-2-ol*, 2 volumes of *acetonitrile*, 10 volumes of *dichloromethane* and 100 volumes of *hexane* and (c) a detection wavelength of 278 nm.

The test is not valid unless, in the chromatogram obtained with solution (3), a peak due to (*R*)-deltamethrin appears immediately before the principal peak, as indicated in the reference chromatogram supplied with *deltamethrin impurity standard BPCRS*.

Calculate the content of $C_{22}H_{19}Br_2NO_3$ using the declared content of $C_{22}H_{19}Br_2NO_3$ in *deltamethrin BPCRS*.

IMPURITIES

The impurities limited by the requirements of this monograph include:
— Becisthemic acid,
— Becisthemic anhydride,
— Becisthemic acid chloride.

Dembrexine Hydrochloride Monohydrate

(*Dembrexine Hydrochloride Monohydrate for Veterinary Use, Ph Eur monograph 2169*)

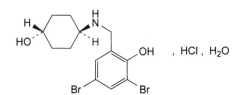

$C_{13}H_{17}Br_2NO_2$, HCl, H_2O 433.6   *83200-09-3*

Ph Eur

DEFINITION

trans-4-[(3,5-Dibromo-2-hydroxybenzyl)amino]cyclohexanol hydrochloride monohydrate.

Content

98.0 per cent to 101.0 per cent (anhydrous substance).

CHARACTERS

Appearance

White or almost white, crystalline powder.

Solubility

Slightly soluble in water, freely soluble in methanol, slightly soluble in anhydrous ethanol.

IDENTIFICATION

A. Infrared absorption spectrophotometry (*2.2.24*).

Comparison   dembrexine hydrochloride monohydrate CRS.

B. It gives reaction (a) of chlorides (*2.3.1*).

TESTS

Related substances

Liquid chromatography (*2.2.29*). *Prepare the solutions immediately before use.*

Test solution   Dissolve 25.0 mg of the substance to be examined in *methanol R* and dilute to 10.0 ml with the same solvent.

Reference solution (a)   Dilute 1.0 ml of the test solution to 50.0 ml with *methanol R*. Dilute 1.0 ml of this solution to 10.0 ml with *methanol R*.

Reference solution (b)   Dissolve 2.5 mg of *tribromophenol R* (impurity E) in *methanol R* and dilute to 50.0 ml with the same solvent. To 1.0 ml of this solution add 1.0 ml of the test solution and dilute to 10.0 ml with *methanol R*.

Blank solution   Methanol R.

Column:
— *size*: l = 0.15 m, Ø = 4.0 mm;
— *stationary phase*: endcapped octadecylsilyl silica gel for chromatography R (5 µm);
— *temperature*: 40 °C.

Mobile phase:
— mobile phase A: dissolve 1.0 g of *potassium dihydrogen phosphate R* in 900 ml of *water R*, adjust to pH 7.4 with *0.5 M potassium hydroxide* and dilute to 1000 ml with *water R*; mix 80 volumes of this solution with 20 volumes of *methanol R*;
— mobile phase B: methanol R, acetonitrile R (20:80 *V/V*);

Time (min)	Mobile phase A (per cent *V/V*)	Mobile phase B (per cent *V/V*)
0 - 7	75	25
7 - 15	75 → 50	25 → 50
15 - 20	50	50
20 - 25	50 → 75	50 → 25
25 - 30	75	25

Flow rate   1.0 ml/min.

Detection   Spectrophotometer at 250 nm.

Injection   10 µl.

Relative retention   With reference to dembrexine (retention time = about 6 min): impurity A = about 2.3; impurity B = about 1.3.

System suitability   Reference solution (b):
— *resolution*: minimum 2 between the peaks due to dembrexine and impurity E.

Limits:
— *impurities A, B*: for each impurity, not more than the area of the principal peak in the chromatogram obtained with reference solution (a) (0.2 per cent);
— *unspecified impurities*: for each impurity, not more than the area of the principal peak in the chromatogram obtained with reference solution (a) (0.2 per cent);
— *total*: not more than 2.5 times the area of the principal peak in the chromatogram obtained with reference solution (a) (0.5 per cent);
— *disregard limit*: 0.5 times the area of the principal peak in the chromatogram obtained with reference solution (a) (0.1 per cent); disregard any peak due to the blank.

Water (*2.5.12*)

3.5 per cent to 5.0 per cent, determined on 0.500 g.

Sulphated ash (*2.4.14*)

Maximum 0.1 per cent, determined on 1.0 g.

ASSAY

Dissolve 0.350 g in 40 ml of *methanol R*. Add 40 ml of *acetone R* and 1 ml of *0.1 M hydrochloric acid*. Carry out a potentiometric titration (*2.2.20*) using *0.1 M sodium hydroxide*. Read the volume added between the 2 points of inflexion.

1 ml of *0.1 M sodium hydroxide* is equivalent to 41.56 mg of $C_{13}H_{18}Br_2ClNO_2$.

IMPURITIES

Specified impurities   A, B.

Other detectable impurities   (The following substances would, if present at a sufficient level, be detected by one or other of the tests in the monograph. They are limited by the general acceptance criterion for other/unspecified impurities and/or by the general monograph *Substances for pharmaceutical use* (*2034*). It is therefore not necessary to identify these impurities for demonstration of compliance. See also *5.10. Control of impurities in substances for pharmaceutical use*): C, D, E.

A. *trans*-4-[(3,5-dibromo-2-hydroxybenzylidene)amino]cyclohexanol,

B. *cis*-4-[(3,5-dibromo-2-hydroxybenzyl)amino]cyclohexanol,

C. R1 = CHO, R2 = R3 = Br:
3,5-dibromo-2-hydroxybenzaldehyde,

D. R1 = CHO, R2 = R3 = H: 2-hydroxybenzaldehyde
(salicylaldehyde),

E. R1 = R2 = R3 = Br: 2,4,6-tribromophenol.

Ph Eur

Detomidine Hydrochloride

(*Detomidine Hydrochloride for Veterinary Use,
Ph Eur monograph 1414*)

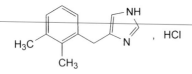

$C_{12}H_{15}ClN_2$ 222.7   90038-01-0

Action and use
Alpha$_2$-adrenoceptor agonist.

Ph Eur

DEFINITION
Detomidine hydrochloride for veterinary use contains not less than 98.5 per cent and not more than the equivalent of 101.5 per cent of 4-(2,3-dimethylbenzyl)-1*H*-imidazole hydrochloride, calculated with reference to the dried substance.

CHARACTERS
A white or almost white, hygroscopic, crystalline powder, soluble in water, freely soluble in alcohol, very slightly soluble in methylene chloride, practically insoluble in acetone.

It melts at about 160 °C.

IDENTIFICATION
A. Examine by infrared absorption spectrophotometry (*2.2.24*), comparing with the spectrum obtained with *detomidine hydrochloride CRS*. Examine the substances prepared as discs. If the spectra obtained show differences, dry the substance to be examined and the reference substance in an oven at 100 °C to 105 °C and record new spectra.

B. It gives reaction (a) of chlorides (*2.3.1*).

TESTS
Appearance of solution
Dissolve 0.25 g in *water R* and dilute to 25 ml with the same solvent. The solution is clear (*2.2.1*) and colourless (*2.2.2, Method II*).

Related substances
Examine by liquid chromatography (*2.2.29*).

Test solution   Dissolve 25.0 mg of the substance to be examined in 20 ml of the mobile phase and dilute to 50.0 ml with the mobile phase.

Reference solution (a)   Dilute 0.20 ml of the test solution to 100.0 ml with the mobile phase.

Reference solution (b)   Dissolve 1 mg of *detomidine impurity B CRS* in the mobile phase and dilute to 100 ml with the mobile phase. Dilute 1 ml of the solution to 10 ml with reference solution (a).

The chromatographic procedure may be carried out using:
— a stainless steel column 0.15 m long and 4.6 mm in internal diameter packed with *octylsilyl silica gel for chromatography R* (5 µm),
— as mobile phase at a flow rate of 1 ml/min a mixture of 35 volumes of *acetonitrile R* and 65 volumes of a 2.64 g/l solution of *ammonium phosphate R*,
— as detector a spectrophotometer set at 220 nm.

When the chromatograms are recorded in the prescribed conditions, the retention time of detomidine is about 7 min and the relative retention times of impurities A, B and C with respect to detomidine are about 0.4, 2.0 and 3.0, respectively. Inject 20 µl of reference solution (a). Adjust the sensitivity of the system so that the height of the principal peak in the chromatogram obtained is at least 50 per cent of the full scale of the recorder. Inject 20 µl of reference solution (b). The test is not valid unless: the resolution between the peaks corresponding to detomidine and to impurity B is at least 5.

Inject 20 µl of the test solution. Continue the chromatography for four times the retention time of the principal peak. Multiply the area of any peak (corresponding to the impurity C and its diastereoisomer) eluting with a relative retention time of about 3, by the correction factor 2.7. The sum of the areas of such peaks is not greater than 2.5 times the area of the principal peak in the chromatogram obtained with reference solution (a) (0.5 per cent); the area of any other peak apart from the principal peak and the peak corresponding to the impurity C is not greater than the area of the principal peak in the chromatogram obtained with reference solution (a) (0.2 per cent); the sum of the areas of all the peaks apart from the principal peak is not greater than five times the area of the principal peak in the chromatogram obtained with reference solution (a) (1 per cent). Disregard any peak with an area less than 0.25 times the area of the principal peak in the chromatogram obtained with reference solution (a).

Loss on drying (*2.2.32*)
Not more than 0.5 per cent, determined on 1.000 g by drying in oven at 100 °C to 105 °C.

Sulphated ash *(2.4.14)*
Not more than 0.1 per cent, determined on 1.0 g.

ASSAY
Dissolve 0.170 g in 50 ml of *alcohol R*. Add 5.0 ml of *0.01 M hydrochloric acid*. Carry out a potentiometric titration *(2.2.20)*, using *0.1 M sodium hydroxide*. Read the volume added between the two points of inflection.

1 ml of *0.1 M sodium hydroxide* corresponds to 22.27 mg of $C_{12}H_{15}ClN_2$.

STORAGE
Store in an airtight container.

IMPURITIES

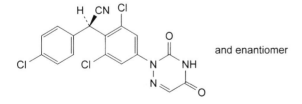

A. (*RS*)-(2,3-dimethylphenyl)(1*H*-imidazol-4-yl)methanol,

B. (*RS*)-(1-benzyl-1*H*-imidazol-5-yl)(2,3-dimethylphenyl)methanol,

C. 4-[(2,3-dimethylcyclohexyl)methyl]-1*H*-imidazole.

_____ Ph Eur

Diclazuril

(Diclazuril for Veterinary Use,
Ph Eur monograph 1718)

$C_{17}H_9Cl_3N_4O_2$ 407.6   *101831-37-2*

Action and use
Antiprotozoal (veterinary); coccidiosis.

Ph Eur _____

DEFINITION
(*RS*)-(4-Chlorophenyl)[2,6-dichloro-4-(3,5-dioxo-4,5-dihydro-1,2,4-triazin-2(3*H*)-yl)phenyl]acetonitrile.

Content
99.0 per cent to 101.0 per cent (dried substance).

CHARACTERS
Appearance
White or light yellow powder.

Solubility
Practically insoluble in water, sparingly soluble in dimethylformamide, practically insoluble in alcohol and methylene chloride.

IDENTIFICATION
Infrared absorption spectrophotometry *(2.2.24)*.

Comparison   Ph. Eur. reference spectrum of diclazuril.

TESTS
Related substances
Liquid chromatography *(2.2.29)*.

Test solution   Dissolve 20.0 mg of the substance to be examined in *dimethylformamide R* and dilute to 20.0 ml with the same solvent.

Reference solution (a)   Dissolve 5 mg of *diclazuril for system suitability CRS* in *dimethylformamide R* and dilute to 5.0 ml with the same solvent.

Reference solution (b)   Dilute 1.0 ml of the test solution to 100.0 ml with *dimethylformamide R*. Dilute 5.0 ml of the solution to 20.0 ml with *dimethylformamide R*.

Column:
— *size*: *l* = 0.10 m, Ø = 4.6 mm,
— *stationary phase*: *base-deactivated octadecylsilyl silica gel for chromatography R* (3 μm),
— *temperature*: 35 °C.

Mobile phase:
— *mobile phase A*: mix 10 volumes of a 6.3 g/l solution of *ammonium formate R* adjusted to pH 4.0 with *anhydrous formic acid R*, 15 volumes of *acetonitrile R* and 75 volumes of *water R*,
— *mobile phase B*: mix 10 volumes of a 6.3 g/l solution of *ammonium formate R* adjusted to pH 4.0 with *anhydrous formic acid R*, 85 volumes of *acetonitrile R* and 5 volumes of *water R*,

Time (min)	Mobile phase A (per cent *V/V*)	Mobile phase B (per cent *V/V*)
0 - 20	100 → 0	0 → 100
20 - 25	0	100
25 - 26	0 → 100	100 → 0
26 - 36	100	0

Flow rate   1.0 ml/min.

Detection   Spectrophotometer at 230 nm.

Injection   5 μl.

System suitability   Reference solution (a):
— *peak-to-valley ratio*: minimum of 1.5, where H_p = height above the baseline of the peak due to impurity D and H_v = height above the baseline of the lowest point of the curve separating this peak from the peak due to diclazuril.

Limits:
— *correction factors*: for the calculation of contents, multiply the peak areas of the following impurities by the corresponding correction factor: impurity D = 1.9; impurity H = 1.4,

— *impurity D*: not more than 0.4 times the area of the principal peak in the chromatogram obtained with reference solution (b) (0.1 per cent),

— *any other impurity*: not more than the area of the principal peak in the chromatogram obtained with reference solution (b) (0.25 per cent),

— *total*: not more than 4 times the area of the principal peak in the chromatogram obtained with reference solution (b) (1.0 per cent),

— *disregard limit*: 0.2 times the area of the principal peak in the chromatogram obtained with reference solution (b) (0.05 per cent).

Loss on drying (*2.2.32*)
Maximum 0.5 per cent, determined on 1.000 g by drying in an oven at 100-105 °C for 4 h.

Sulphated ash (*2.4.14*)
Maximum 0.1 per cent, determined on 1.0 g.

ASSAY
Dissolve 0.150 g in 75 ml of *dimethylformamide R*. Carry out a potentiometric titration (*2.2.20*), using *0.1 M tetrabutylammonium hydroxide*. Read the volume added at the second inflexion point. Carry out a blank titration.

1 ml of *0.1 M tetrabutylammonium hydroxide* is equivalent to 20.38 mg of $C_{17}H_9Cl_3N_4O_2$.

STORAGE
Protected from light.

IMPURITIES
Specified impurities   A, B, C, D, E, F, G, H, I.

and enantiomer

A. R = Cl, R′ = CO₂H: 2-[3,5-dichloro-4-[(RS)-(4-chlorophenyl)cyanomethyl]phenyl]-3,5-dioxo-2,3,4,5-tetrahydro-1,2,4-triazine-6-carboxylic acid,

B. R = OH, R′ = H: (RS)-[2,6-dichloro-4-(3,5-dioxo-4,5-dihydro-1,2,4-triazin-2(3H)-yl)phenyl](4-hydroxyphenyl)acetonitrile,

C. R = Cl, R′ = CONH₂: 2-[3,5-dichloro-4-[(RS)-(4-chlorophenyl)cyanomethyl]phenyl]-3,5-dioxo-2,3,4,5-tetrahydro-1,2,4-triazine-6-carboxamide,

G. R = Cl, R′ = CO-O-[CH₂]₃-CH₃: butyl 2-[3,5-dichloro-4-[(RS)-(4-chlorophenyl)cyanomethyl]phenyl]-3,5-dioxo-2,3,4,5-tetrahydro-1,2,4-triazine-6-carboxylate,

D. X = O: 2-[3,5-dichloro-4-(4-chlorobenzoyl)phenyl]-1,2,4-triazine-3,5(2H,4H)-dione,

F. X = H₂: 2-[3,5-dichloro-4-(4-chlorobenzyl)phenyl]-1,2,4-triazine-3,5(2H,4H)-dione,

and enantiomer

E. R = NH₂: (RS)-(4-amino-2,6-dichlorophenyl)(4-chlorophenyl)acetonitrile,

H. R = H: (RS)-(4-chlorophenyl)(2,6-dichlorophenyl)acetonitrile,

I. N,2-bis[3,5-dichloro-4-[(4-chlorophenyl)cyanomethyl]phenyl]-3,5-dioxo-2,3,4,5-tetrahydro-1,2,4-triazine-6-carboxamide.

Ph Eur

Dihydrostreptomycin Sulphate

(*Dihydrostreptomycin Sulphate for Veterinary Use, Ph Eur monograph 0485*)

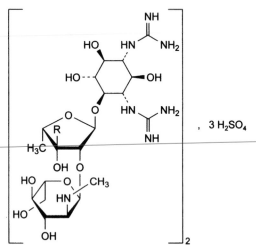

, 3 H₂SO₄

Compound	R	Molec. Formula	M_r
dihydrostreptomycin sulphate	CH₂OH	$C_{42}H_{88}N_{14}O_{36}S_3$	1461
streptomycin sulphate	CHO	$C_{42}H_{84}N_{14}O_{36}S_3$	1457

Action and use
Aminoglycoside antibacterial.

Ph Eur

DEFINITION
Main compound
bis[N,N′′′-[(1R,2R,3S,4R,5R,6S)-4-[[5-deoxy-2-O-[2-deoxy-2-(methylamino)-α-L-glucopyranosyl]-3-C-(hydroxymethyl)-α-

L-lyxofuranosyl]oxy]-2,5,6-trihydroxycyclohexane-1,3-diyl]diguanidine] trisulphate.

Sulphate of a substance obtained by catalytic hydrogenation of streptomycin or by any other means. Semi-synthetic product derived from a fermentation product.

Stabilisers may be added.

Content:
— *sum of dihydrostreptomycin sulphate and streptomycin sulphate*: 95.0 per cent to 102.0 per cent (dried substance);
— *streptomycin sulphate*: maximum 2.0 per cent (dried substance).

PRODUCTION
The method of manufacture is validated to demonstrate that the product, if tested, would comply with the following test.

Abnormal toxicity (*2.6.9*)
Inject into each mouse 1 mg dissolved in 0.5 ml of *water for injections R*.

CHARACTERS
Appearance
White or almost white, hygroscopic powder.

Solubility
Freely soluble in water, practically insoluble in acetone, in ethanol (96 per cent) and in methanol.

IDENTIFICATION
First identification A, E.

Second identification B, C, D, E.

A. Examine the chromatograms obtained in the assay.

Results The principal peak in the chromatogram obtained with the test solution is similar in retention time and size to the principal peak in the chromatogram obtained with reference solution (a).

B. Thin-layer chromatography (*2.2.27*).

Test solution Dissolve 10 mg of the substance to be examined in *water R* and dilute to 10 ml with the same solvent.

Reference solution (a) Dissolve the contents of a vial of *dihydrostreptomycin sulphate CRS* in 5.0 ml of *water R*. Dilute 1.0 ml of this solution to 5.0 ml with *water R*.

Reference solution (b) Dissolve the contents of a vial of *dihydrostreptomycin sulphate CRS* in 5.0 ml of *water R*.

Reference solution (c) Dissolve 10 mg of *kanamycin monosulphate CRS* and 10 mg of *neomycin sulphate CRS* in *water R*, add 2.0 ml of reference solution (b), mix thoroughly and dilute to 10 ml with *water R*.

Plate *TLC silica gel plate R*.

Mobile phase 70 g/l solution of *potassium dihydrogen phosphate R*.

Application 10 μl.

Development Over 2/3 of the plate.

Drying In a current of warm air.

Detection Spray with a mixture of equal volumes of a 2 g/l solution of *1,3-dihydroxynaphthalene R* in *ethanol (96 per cent) R* and a 460 g/l solution of *sulphuric acid R*; heat at 150 °C for 5-10 min.

System suitability Reference solution (c):
— the chromatogram shows 3 clearly separated spots.

Results The principal spot in the chromatogram obtained with the test solution is similar in position, colour and size to the principal spot in the chromatogram obtained with reference solution (a).

C. Dissolve 0.1 g in 2 ml of *water R* and add 1 ml of α-*naphthol solution R* and 2 ml of a mixture of equal volumes of *strong sodium hypochlorite solution R* and *water R*. A red colour develops.

D. Dissolve 10 mg in 5 ml of *water R* and add 1 ml of *1 M hydrochloric acid*. Heat in a water-bath for 2 min. Add 2 ml of a 5 g/l solution of α-*naphthol R* in *1 M sodium hydroxide* and heat in a water-bath for 1 min. A violet-pink colour is produced.

E. It gives reaction (a) of sulphates (*2.3.1*).

TESTS
Solution S
Dissolve 2.5 g in *carbon dioxide-free water R* and dilute to 10 ml with the same solvent.

Appearance of solution
Solution S is not more intensely coloured than intensity 5 of the range of reference solutions of the most appropriate colour (*2.2.2, Method II*). Allow to stand protected from light at about 20 °C for 24 h; solution S is not more opalescent than reference suspension II (*2.2.1*).

pH (*2.2.3*)
5.0 to 7.0 for solution S.

Specific optical rotation (*2.2.7*)
− 83.0 to − 91.0 (dried substance).

Dissolve 0.200 g in *water R* and dilute to 10.0 ml with the same solvent.

Related substances
Liquid chromatography (*2.2.29*).

Test solution Dissolve 50.0 mg of the substance to be examined in *water R* and dilute to 10.0 ml with the same solvent.

Reference solution (a) Dissolve the contents of a vial of *dihydrostreptomycin sulphate CRS* (containing impurities A, B and C) in 5.0 ml of *water R*.

Reference solution (b) Dilute 1.0 ml of the test solution to 100.0 ml with *water R*.

Reference solution (c) Dilute 5.0 ml of reference solution (b) to 50.0 ml with *water R*.

Reference solution (d) Dissolve 10 mg of *streptomycin sulphate CRS* in *water R*, add 2 ml of the test solution and dilute to 20 ml with *water R*.

Column:
— *size*: *l* = 0.25 m, Ø = 4.6 mm;
— *stationary phase*: *octadecylsilyl silica gel for chromatography R* (5 μm);
— *temperature*: 45 °C.

Mobile phase Solution in water R containing 4.6 g/l of *anhydrous sodium sulphate R*, 1.5 g/l of *sodium octanesulphonate R*, 120 ml/l of *acetonitrile R1* and 50 ml/l of a 27.2 g/l solution of *potassium dihydrogen phosphate R* adjusted to pH 3.0 with a 22.5 g/l solution of *phosphoric acid R*.

Flow rate 1.0 ml/min.

Detection Spectrophotometer at 205 nm.

Injection 20 μl.

Run time 1.5 times the retention time of dihydrostreptomycin.

Identification of impurities Use the chromatogram supplied with *dihydrostreptomycin sulphate CRS* and the chromatogram obtained with reference solution (a) to identify the peaks due to streptomycin and impurities A, B and C.

Relative retention With reference to dihydrostreptomycin (retention time = about 57 min): impurity A = about 0.2; impurity B = about 0.8; streptomycin = about 0.9; impurity C = about 0.95.

System suitability:
— *resolution:* minimum 2.5 between the peaks due to streptomycin and dihydrostreptomycin in the chromatogram obtained with reference solution (d); if necessary, adjust the amount of sodium sulphate in the mobile phase;
— the chromatogram obtained with reference solution (a) is similar to the chromatogram supplied with *dihydrostreptomycin sulphate CRS*.

Limits:
— *correction factor:* for the calculation of content, multiply the peak area of impurity A by 0.5;
— *impurities A, B:* for each impurity, not more than the area of the principal peak in the chromatogram obtained with reference solution (b) (1.0 per cent);
— *impurity C:* not more than twice the area of the principal peak in the chromatogram obtained with reference solution (b) (2.0 per cent);
— *any other impurity:* for each impurity, not more than the area of the principal peak in the chromatogram obtained with reference solution (b) (1.0 per cent);
— *total:* not more than 5 times the area of the principal peak in the chromatogram obtained with reference solution (b) (5.0 per cent);
— *disregard limit:* the area of the principal peak in the chromatogram obtained with reference solution (c) (0.1 per cent); disregard the peak due to streptomycin.

Heavy metals (*2.4.8*)
20 ppm.

1.0 g complies with test C. Prepare the reference solution using 2 ml *of lead standard solution (10 ppm Pb) R*.

Loss on drying (*2.2.32*)
Maximum 5.0 per cent, determined on 1.000 g by drying under high vacuum at 60 °C for 4 h.

Sulphated ash (*2.4.14*)
Maximum 1.0 per cent, determined on 1.0 g.

Bacterial endotoxins (*2.6.14*)
Less than 0.50 IU/mg, if intended for use in the manufacture of parenteral dosage forms without a further appropriate procedure for removal of bacterial endotoxins.

ASSAY

Liquid chromatography (*2.2.29*) as described in the test for related substances with the following modification.

Injection Test solution and reference solution (a).

Calculate the percentage content of $C_{42}H_{88}N_{14}O_{36}S_3$ and of $C_{42}H_{84}N_{14}O_{36}S_3$ using the chromatogram obtained with reference solution (a) and the declared contents of *dihydrostreptomycin sulphate CRS*. Calculate the sum of these percentage contents.

STORAGE

In an airtight container, protected from light. If the substance is sterile, store in a sterile, airtight, tamper-proof container.

LABELLING

The label states, where applicable, the name and quantity of any added stabiliser.

IMPURITIES

Specified impurities *A, B, C.*

Other detectable impurities (The following substances would, if present at a sufficient level, be detected by one or other of the tests in the monograph. They are limited by the general acceptance criterion for other/unspecified impurities and/or by the general monograph *Substances for pharmaceutical use (2034)*. It is therefore not necessary to identify these impurities for demonstration of compliance. See also *5.10. Control of impurities in substances for pharmaceutical use*): D.

A. *N,N'''-[(1R,2s,3S,4R,5r,6S)-2,4,5,6-tetrahydroxycyclohexane-1,3-diyl]diguanidine* (streptidine),

B. *N,N'''-[(1S,2R,3R,4S,5R,6R)-2,4,5-trihydroxy-6-[[β-D-mannopyranosyl-(1→4)-2-deoxy-2-(methylamino)-α-L-glucopyranosyl-(1→2)-5-deoxy-3-C-(hydroxymethyl)-α-L-lyxofuranosyl]oxy]cyclohexane-1,3-diyl]diguanidine* (dihydrostreptomycin B),

C. unknown structure,

D. *N,N'''*-[(1*R*,2*R*,3*S*,4*R*,5*R*,6*S*)-4-[[3,5-dideoxy-2-*O*-[2-deoxy-2-(methylamino)-α-L-glucopyranosyl]-3-(hydroxymethyl)-α-L-arabinofuranosyl]oxy]-2,5,6-trihydroxycyclohexane-1,3-diyl]diguanidine (deoxydihydrostreptomycin).

Ph Eur

Dimetridazole

C₅H₇N₃O₂   141.1   *551-92-8*

Action and use
Antiprotozoal (veterinary).

Preparations
Dimetridazole Premix
Dimetridazole Veterinary Oral Powder

DEFINITION
Dimetridazole is 1,2-dimethyl-5-nitroimidazole. It contains not less than 98.0% and not more than 101.0% of C₅H₇N₃O₂, calculated with reference to the anhydrous substance.

CHARACTERISTIC
An almost white to brownish yellow powder which darkens on exposure to light; odourless or almost odourless.

Slightly soluble in *water*; freely soluble in *chloroform*; sparingly soluble in *ethanol (96%)*; slightly soluble in *ether*.

IDENTIFICATION
A. The *infrared absorption spectrum*, Appendix II A, is concordant with the *reference spectrum* of dimetridazole *(RSV 16)*.

B. The *light absorption*, Appendix II B, in the range 230 to 350 nm, of a 0.002% w/v solution in *methanol* exhibits a well-defined maximum only at 309 nm. The *absorbance* at the maximum at 309 nm is about 1.3.

C. Dissolve 0.1 g in 20 ml of *ether*, add 10 ml of a 1% w/v solution of *picric acid* in *ether*, induce crystallisation and allow to stand. A precipitate is produced which after washing with

ether and drying at 105° has a *melting point* of about 160°, Appendix V A.

TESTS
Melting point
138° to 141°, Appendix V A.

2-Methyl-5-nitroimidazole
Carry out the method for *thin-layer chromatography*, Appendix III A, protected from light, using *silica gel GF₂₅₄* as the coating substance and a mixture of 1 volume of *propan-2-ol* and 9 volumes of *chloroform* as the mobile phase. Apply separately to the plate 5 μl of each of two solutions in *chloroform* containing (1) 2.0% w/v of the substance being examined and (2) 0.010% w/v of *2-methyl-5-nitroimidazole BPCRS*. After removal of the plate allow it to dry in air and examine under *ultraviolet light (254 nm)*. Any spot in the chromatogram obtained with solution (1) corresponding to 2-methyl-5-nitroimidazole is not more intense than the spot in the chromatogram obtained with solution (2) (0.5%).

Water
Not more than 1.0% w/w, Appendix IX C. Use 1.0 g.

Sulphated ash
Not more than 0.1%, Appendix IX A.

ASSAY
Carry out Method I for *non-aqueous titration*, Appendix VIII A, using 0.3 g and *crystal violet solution* as indicator. Each ml of 0.1M *perchloric acid VS* is equivalent to 14.11 mg of C₅H₇N₃O₂.

STORAGE
Dimetridazole should be protected from light.

Dimpylate

C₁₂H₂₁N₂O₃PS   304.4   *333-41-5*

Action and use
Insecticide.

DEFINITION
Dimpylate is *O,O*-diethyl *O*-(2-isopropyl-6-methylpyrimidin-4-yl)phosphorothioate. It contains not less than 95.0% and not more than 101.0% of C₁₂H₂₁N₂O₃PS, calculated with reference to the anhydrous substance.

CHARACTERISTICS
A clear, yellowish brown, slightly viscous liquid.

Practically insoluble in *water*; miscible with *ethanol (96%)*, with *ether* and with most organic solvents.

IDENTIFICATION
A. The *infrared absorption spectrum*, Appendix II A, is concordant with the *reference spectrum* of dimpylate *(RSV 49)*.

B. In the Assay, the chromatogram obtained with solution (1) shows a peak with the same retention time as the peak due to dimpylate in the chromatogram obtained with solution (3).

TESTS

Toluene

Not more than 1% v/v when determined by the test for *residual solvents*, Appendix VIII L.

Related substances

Carry out the method for *gas chromatography*, Appendix III B, using the following solutions. Solution (1) contains 0.5% w/v of the substance being examined in *dichloromethane*. Solution (2) contains 0.5% w/v of the substance being examined and 0.025% w/v of *diethyl phthalate* (internal standard) in *dichloromethane*. Solution (3) contains 0.0020% w/v of the substance being examined and 0.025% w/v of *diethyl phthalate* in *dichloromethane*. Solution (4) contains 0.5% w/v of *dimpylate for chromatography BPCRS* and 0.025% w/v of *diethyl phthalate* in *dichloromethane*. Solution (5) contains 0.012% v/v of *toluene* in *dichloromethane*.

The chromatographic procedure may be carried out using (a) a fused silica capillary column (15 m × 0.32 mm) coated with a 1 μm film of dimethyl silicone gum (SE-54 is suitable) fitted with a precolumn (0.2 m × 0.53 mm) coated with a 1 μm film of dimethyl silicone gum, the temperature programme described below with the inlet port at room temperature and the detector at 280° and (b) *hydrogen* as the carrier gas at a flow rate of 40 ml per minute and *nitrogen* as the make up gas with a flow rate of 50 ml per minute.

Time (minute)	Temperature	Comments
0 → 1	35°	Isothermal
1 → 15.5	35° → 180°	Linear increase 10°/minute
15.5 → 23.5	180°	Isothermal
23.5 → 30.5	180° → 250°	Linear increase 10°/minute
30.5 → 40.5	250°	Isothermal

In the chromatogram obtained with solution (3) the retention time of the internal standard is about 18.5 minutes and of dimpylate, about 23 minutes. The test is not valid unless the chromatogram obtained with solution (4) closely resembles that supplied with *dimpylate for chromatography BPCRS*.

In the chromatogram obtained with solution (2) identify any peaks corresponding to 4-ethoxy-2-isopropyl-6-methylpyrimidine, *O,O,S*-triethyl phosphorothioate, 3-ethyl-2-isopropyl-6-methyl-4-oxo-3,4-dihydropyrimidine, tetraethyl thionopyrophosphate, tetraethyl dithionopyrophosphate and *O,O*-diethyl *O*-(2-isopropyl-6-methylpyrimidin-4-yl)phosphate from the chromatogram supplied with *dimpylate for chromatography BPCRS*. The area of any peak corresponding to 4-ethoxy-2-isopropyl-6-methylpyrimidine or 3-ethyl-2-isopropyl-6-methyl-4-oxo-3,4-dihydropyrimidine is not greater than 2.5 times the area of the peak due to dimpylate in the chromatogram obtained with solution (3) (1% of each), the area of any peak corresponding to *O,O,S*-triethyl phosphorothioate is not greater than 1.25 times the area of the peak due to dimpylate in the chromatogram obtained with solution (3) (0.5%), the area of any peak corresponding to tetraethyl thionopyrophosphate is not greater than 0.02 times the area of the peak due to dimpylate in the chromatogram obtained with solution (3) (0.02%, assuming a response factor of 0.4), the area of any peak

corresponding to tetraethyl dithionopyrophosphate is not greater than 0.25 times the area of the peak due to dimpylate in the chromatogram obtained with solution (3) (0.2%, assuming a response factor of 0.5), the area of any peak corresponding to *O,O*-diethyl *O*-(2-isopropyl-6-methylpyrimidin-4-yl)phosphate is not greater than 0.75 times the area of the peak due to dimpylate in the chromatogram obtained with solution (3) (0.3%) and the area of any other *secondary peak* is not greater than 0.5 times the area of the peak due to dimpylate in the chromatogram obtained with solution (3) (0.2%). Disregard any peak corresponding to toluene.

Water

Not more than 0.1% w/w, Appendix IX C. Use 2 g.

ASSAY

Carry out the method for *gas chromatography*, Appendix III B, using solutions in *4-methylpentan-2-one* containing (1) 0.2% w/v of the substance being examined, (2) 0.2% w/v of the substance being examined and 0.15% w/v of *diethyl phthalate* (internal standard) and (3) 0.2% w/v of *dimpylate BPCRS* and 0.15% w/v of *diethyl phthalate*.

The chromatographic procedure may be carried out using (a) a fused silica capillary column (15 m × 0.53 mm) coated with a 1.5 μm film of dimethyl silicone gum (SE-54 from J & W Scientific is suitable) at a temperature of 110° increasing linearly at a rate of 6° per minute to 215° with the inlet port at 250° and the detector at 250° and (b) *helium* as the carrier gas at a flow rate of 20 ml per minute with *nitrogen* as the make up gas with a flow rate of 10 ml per minute.

The assay is not valid unless, in the chromatogram obtained with solution (3), the *resolution factor* between the peaks due to dimpylate and the internal standard is at least 2.

Calculate the content of $C_{12}H_{21}N_2O_3PS$ from the chromatograms obtained and using the declared content of $C_{12}H_{21}N_2O_3PS$ in *dimpylate BPCRS*.

IMPURITIES

The impurities limited by the requirements of this monograph include:

A. Diethyl disulphide,

B. *O,O*-Diethyl chlorophosphorothioate,

C. 4-Ethoxy-2-isopropyl-6-methylpyrimidine,

D. *O,O,O*-Triethyl phosphorothioate,

E. *O,O,S*-Triethyl phosphorothioate,

F. 3-Ethyl-2-isopropyl-6-methyl-4-oxo-3,4-
dihydropyrimidine,

G. 4-Hydroxy-2-isopropyl-6-methylpyrimidine,

H. Tetraethyl thionopyrophosphate,

I. Tetraethyl dithionopyrophosphate,

J. *O,O*-Diethyl *O*-(2-isopropyl-6-methylpyrimidin-4-
yl)phosphate,

K. *O,O*-Diethyl *S*-(2-isopropyl-6-methylpyrimidin-4-
yl)phosphorothiophate,

L. *O,S*-Diethyl *O*-(2-isopropyl-6-methylpyrimidin-4-
yl)phosphorothiophate,

M. Bis(2-isopropyl-6-methylpyrimidin-4-yl) sulphide,

N. *O*-ethyl *O,O*-(2-isopropyl-6-methylpyrimidin-4-
yl)phosphorothiophate.

Dinitolmide

$C_8H_7N_3O_5$ 225.1 *148-01-6*

Action and use
Antiprotozoal (veterinary).

DEFINITION
Dinitolmide is 3,5-dinitro-*o*-toluamide. It contains not less
than 98.0% and not more than 100.5% of $C_8H_7N_3O_5$,
calculated with reference to the dried substance.

CHARACTERISTICS
A cream to light tan powder.

Practically insoluble in *water*; soluble in *acetone*; slightly
soluble in *chloroform*, in *ethanol (96%)* and in *ether*.

IDENTIFICATION
A. The *infrared absorption spectrum*, Appendix II A, is
concordant with the *reference spectrum* of dinitolmide
(RSV 17).

B. Heat 1 g with 20 ml of 9M *sulphuric acid* under a reflux
condenser for 1 hour, cool, add 50 ml of *water* and filter.
The *melting point* of the residue, after washing with *water*
and drying at 105°, is about 205°, Appendix V A.

TESTS
Acid value
Not more than 5.0, Appendix X B, using 0.5 g and 50 ml
of *ethanol (96%)* as the solvent.

Melting point
177° to 181°, Appendix V A.

Related substances
Carry out the method for *thin-layer chromatography*,
Appendix III A, using a silica gel F$_{254}$ precoated plate
(Merck plates are suitable) and a mixture of 5 volumes of

glacial acetic acid, 10 volumes of *methanol* and 85 volumes of *chloroform* as the mobile phase. Apply separately to the plate 10 μl of each of three solutions in *acetone* containing (1) 2.5% w/v of the substance being examined, (2) 0.0125% w/v of the substance being examined and (3) 0.0125% w/v of *o-toluic acid*. After removal of the plate allow it to dry in air and examine under *ultraviolet light (254 nm)*. Spray with *titanium(III) chloride solution* diluted 1 to 5 with *water*, heat at 100° for 5 minutes and spray with *alcoholic dimethylaminobenzaldehyde solution*. When examined under ultraviolet light the spot in the chromatogram obtained with solution (3) is more intense than any corresponding spot in the chromatogram obtained with solution (1) (0.5%). By each method of visualisation any *secondary spot* in the chromatogram obtained with solution (1) is not more intense than the spot in the chromatogram obtained with solution (2) (0.5%).

Loss on drying
When dried to constant weight at 105°, loses not more than 1.0% of its weight. Use 1 g.

ASSAY
Dissolve 0.15 g in *acetone* and dilute to 50 ml. To 10 ml of this solution add 10 ml of *glacial acetic acid* and 15 ml of a 40% w/v solution of *sodium acetate*. Maintain a stream of *carbon dioxide* through the flask throughout the determination. Add 25 ml of 0.1M *titanium(III) chloride VS* and allow to stand for 5 minutes. Add 10 ml of *hydrochloric acid*, 10 ml of *water*, and 1 ml of a 10% w/v solution of *potassium thiocyanate*. Titrate with 0.1M *ammonium iron(III) sulphate VS* until the solution becomes colourless and then orange. Repeat the operation without the substance being examined. The difference between the titrations represents the amount of titanium(III) chloride required to reduce the dinitolmide. Each ml of 0.1M *titanium(III) chloride VS* is equivalent to 1.876 mg of $C_8H_7N_3O_5$.

Diprenorphine Hydrochloride

$C_{26}H_{35}NO_4,HCl$ 462.1   *16808-86-9*

Action and use
Opioid receptor antagonist.

Preparation
Diprenorphine Injection

DEFINITION
Diprenorphine Hydrochloride is *N*-cyclopropylmethyl-7,8-dihydro-7α-(1-hydroxy-1-methylethyl)-6-*O*-methyl-6α,14α-ethanonormorphine hydrochloride. It contains not less than

98.5% and not more than 101.0% of $C_{26}H_{35}NO_4,HCl$, calculated with reference to the dried substance.

CHARACTERISTICS
A white or almost white, crystalline powder.

Sparingly soluble in *water*; slightly soluble in *ethanol (96%)*; very slightly soluble in *chloroform*; practically insoluble in *ether*.

IDENTIFICATION
A. The *infrared absorption spectrum*, Appendix II A, is concordant with the *reference spectrum* of diprenorphine hydrochloride *(RSV 18)*.

B. The *light absorption*, Appendix II B, in the range 230 to 350 nm of a 0.02% w/v solution in 0.1M *hydrochloric acid* exhibits a maximum only at 287 nm. The *absorbance* at the maximum is about 0.70.

C. The *light absorption*, Appendix II B, in the range 230 to 350 nm of a 0.02% w/v solution in 0.1M *sodium hydroxide* exhibits a maximum only at 301 nm. The *absorbance* at the maximum is about 1.1.

D. Yields reaction A characteristic of *chlorides*, Appendix VI.

TESTS
Acidity
pH of a 2.0% w/v solution, 4.5 to 6.0, Appendix V L.

Specific optical rotation
In a solution prepared by dissolving 0.5 g in sufficient *methanol* to produce 25 ml, -97.0 to -107.0, calculated with reference to the dried substance, Appendix V F.

Related substances
Carry out the method for *thin-layer chromatography*, Appendix III A, using *silica gel G* as the coating substance and a mixture of 1 volume of *water*, 5 volumes of *methanol*, 30 volumes of *butan-2-one*, 80 volumes of *acetone* and 100 volumes of *cyclohexane* as the mobile phase. Apply separately to the plate 20 μl of each of two solutions of the substance being examined in *methanol* containing (1) 2.0% w/v and (2) 0.020% w/v. Add at each point of application 10 μl of a mixture of 4 volumes of *methanol* and 1 volume of 13.5M *ammonia*. After removal of the plate, allow it to dry in air and spray with a 1% w/v solution of *iodine* in *methanol*. Any *secondary spot* in the chromatogram obtained with solution (1) is not more intense than the spot in the chromatogram obtained with solution (2) (1%).

Loss on drying
When dried to constant weight at 105°, loses not more than 2.0% of its weight. Use 1 g.

Sulphated ash
Not more than 0.1%, Appendix IX A.

ASSAY
Carry out Method I for *non-aqueous titration*, Appendix VIII A, using 0.5 g, adding 7 ml of *mercury(II) acetate solution* and using *crystal violet solution* as indicator. Each ml of 0.1M *perchloric acid VS* is equivalent to 46.21 mg $C_{26}H_{35}NO_4,HCl$.

STORAGE
Diprenorphine Hydrochloride should be protected from light.

Enilconazole

(Enilconazole for Veterinary Use,
Ph Eur monograph 1720)

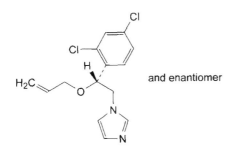

and enantiomer

$C_{14}H_{14}Cl_2N_2O$ 297.2   *73790-28-0*

Action and use
Antifungal.

Ph Eur

DEFINITION
1-[(2*RS*)-2-(2,4-Dichlorophenyl)-2-(prop-2-enyloxy)ethyl]-
1*H*-imidazole.

Content
98.5 per cent to 101.5 per cent (dried substance).

CHARACTERS
Appearance
Clear, yellowish, oily liquid or solid mass.

Solubility
Very slightly soluble in water, freely soluble in alcohol,
in methanol and in toluene.

IDENTIFICATION
Infrared absorption spectrophotometry (*2.2.24*).

Comparison   enilconazole CRS.

TESTS
Optical rotation (*2.2.7*)
− 0.10° to + 0.10°.

Dissolve 0.1 g in *methanol R* and dilute to 10 ml with the
same solvent.

Related substances
Gas chromatography (*2.2.28*). *Prepare the solutions immediately*
before use and protect from light.

Test solution   Dissolve 0.100 g of the substance to be
examined in *toluene R* and dilute to 100.0 ml with the same
solvent.

Reference solution (a)   Dissolve 10.0 mg of *enilconazole CRS*
and 10.0 mg of *enilconazole impurity E CRS* in *toluene R* and
dilute to 100.0 ml with the same solvent.

Reference solution (b)   Dilute 5.0 ml of the test solution to
100.0 ml with *toluene R*. Dilute 1.0 ml of this solution to
10.0 ml with *toluene R*.

Column:
— *material*: fused silica,
— *size*: *l* = 25 m, Ø = 0.32 mm,
— *stationary phase*: chemically bonded
   poly(dimethyl)(diphenyl)siloxane R (film thickness
   0.52 μm).

Carrier gas   *helium for chromatography R.*

Flow rate   1.3 ml/min.

Split ratio   1:38.

Temperature:

	Time (min)	Temperature (°C)
Column	0 - 6.4	100 → 260
	6.4 - 14	260
Injection port	-	250
Detector	-	300

Detection   Flame ionisation.

Injection   2 μl.

Relative retentions with reference to enilconazole (retention
time = about 10 min): impurity A = about 0.6;
impurity B = about 0.7; impurity C = about 0.8;
impurity D = about 0.9; impurity F = about 1.1.

System suitability   Reference solution (a):
— *resolution*: minimum 2.5 between the peaks due to
   enilconazole and impurity E.

Limits:
— *any impurity*: not more than twice the area of the principal
   peak in the chromatogram obtained with reference
   solution (b) (1.0 per cent), and not more than one such
   peak has an area greater than the area of the principal
   peak in the chromatogram obtained with reference
   solution (b) (0.5 per cent),
— *total*: not more than 4 times the area of the principal peak
   in the chromatogram obtained with reference solution (b)
   (2.0 per cent),
— *disregard limit*: 0.1 times the area of the principal peak in
   the chromatogram obtained with reference solution (b)
   (0.05 per cent).

Loss on drying (*2.2.32*)
Maximum 0.5 per cent, determined on 1.000 g by drying
in vacuo at 40 °C for 4 h.

Sulphated ash (*2.4.14*)
Maximum 0.1 per cent, determined on 1.0 g.

ASSAY
Dissolve 0.230 g in 50 ml of a mixture of 1 volume of
anhydrous acetic acid R and 7 volumes of *methyl ethyl ketone R*.
Titrate with *0.1 M perchloric acid* using 0.2 ml of
naphtholbenzein solution R as indicator.

1 ml of *0.1 M perchloric acid* is equivalent to 29.72 mg of
$C_{14}H_{14}Cl_2N_2O$.

STORAGE
In an airtight container, protected from light.

IMPURITIES

Cl

Cl

H

H_2C

O

N

R2   R1

and enantiomer

A. R1 = R2 = H: (2*RS*)-2-(2,4-dichlorophenyl)-2-(prop-2-
enyloxy)ethanamine,

B. R1 = H, R2 = CH₂-CH=CH₂: *N*-[(2*RS*)-2-(2,4-
dichlorophenyl)-2-(prop-2-enyloxy)ethyl]prop-2-en-1-amine,

C. R1 = CHO, R2 = H: *N*-[(2*RS*)-2-(2,4-dichlorophenyl)-2-(prop-2-enyloxy)ethyl]formamide,

D. R1 = CHO, R2 = CH₂-CH=CH₂: *N*-[(2*RS*)-2-(2,4-dichlorophenyl)-2-(prop-2-enyloxy)ethyl]-*N*-(prop-2-enyl)formamide,

and enantiomer

E. (1*RS*)-1-(2,4-dichlorophenyl)-2-(-1*H*-imidazol-1-yl)ethanol,

and enantiomer

F. 1-[(2*RS*)-2-(3,4-dichlorophenyl)-2-(prop-2-enyloxy)ethyl]-1*H*-imidazole.

_____ *Ph Eur*

Etamiphylline Camsilate

C₁₃H₂₁N₅O₂,C₁₀H₁₆O₄S   511.6   *19326-29-5*

Action and use
Non-selective phosphodiesterase inhibitor (xanthine); treatment of reversible airways obstruction.

Preparations
Etamiphylline Injection
Etamiphylline Tablets
Etamiphylline Veterinary Oral Powder

DEFINITION
Etamiphylline Camsilate is
7-(2-diethylaminoethyl)theophylline camphorsulphonate.
It contains not less than 98.0% and not more than 102.0%
of C₁₃H₂₁N₅O₂,C₁₀H₁₆O₄S, calculated with reference to
the dried substance, when determined by both methods
described under the Assay.

CHARACTERISTICS
A white or almost white powder.

Very soluble in *water*; soluble in *chloroform* and in *ethanol (96%)*; very slightly soluble in *ether*.

IDENTIFICATION
A. The *light absorption*, Appendix II B, in the range 230 to 350 nm of a 0.004% w/v solution exhibits a maximum only at 274 nm. The *absorbance* at 274 nm is about 0.70.

B. The *infrared absorption spectrum*, Appendix II A, is concordant with the *reference spectrum* of etamiphylline camsilate *(RSV 51)*.

C. Fuse 0.1 g with a pellet of *sodium hydroxide*, dissolve in *water* and neutralise with *hydrochloric acid*. The resulting solution yields reaction A characteristic of *sulphates*, Appendix VI.

TESTS
Melting point
202° to 206°, Appendix V A.

Acidity
pH of a 10% w/v solution, 3.9 to 5.4, Appendix V L.

Free etamiphylline
Not more than 2.0% w/w when determined by Method I for *non-aqueous titration*, Appendix VIII A, using 2 g dissolved in 75 ml of *acetic anhydride* and determining the end point potentiometrically. Each ml of 0.1M *perchloric acid VS* is equivalent to 27.93 mg of free etamiphylline.

Related substances
Carry out the method for *thin-layer chromatography*, Appendix III A, using *silica gel HF₂₅₄* as the coating substance and a mixture of 80 volumes of *chloroform*, 20 volumes of *ethanol (96%)* and 1 volume of 13.5M *ammonia* as the mobile phase. Apply separately to the plate 10 μl of each of two solutions of the substance being examined in *water* containing (1) 4.0% w/v and (2) 0.0080% w/v. After removal of the plate, allow it to dry in air and examine under *ultraviolet light (254 nm)*. Any *secondary spot* in the chromatogram obtained with solution (1) is not more intense than the spot in the chromatogram obtained with solution (2) (0.2%).

Loss on drying
When dried to constant weight at 105°, loses not more than 0.5% of its weight. Use 1 g.

Sulphated ash
Not more than 0.2%, Appendix IX A.

ASSAY
For camphorsulphonic acid
Dissolve 1 g in 25 ml of *methanol*, previously neutralised with 1M *sodium hydroxide VS*, and titrate with 0.1M *sodium hydroxide VS* using *thymol blue solution* as indicator. Each ml of 0.1M *sodium hydroxide VS* is equivalent to 51.16 mg of C₁₃H₂₁N₅O₂,C₁₀H₁₆O₄S.

For etamiphylline
Dissolve 0.15 g in 20 ml of 2M *hydrochloric acid*, add 12 ml of a 5% w/v solution of *silicotungstic acid* and allow to stand for 5 hours. Filter, wash the residue with 2M *hydrochloric acid* until the filtrate yields no precipitate with a 1% w/v solution of *quinine hydrochloride* and dry at 110°. Each g of residue is equivalent to 0.2830 g of C₁₃H₂₁N₅O₂,C₁₀H₁₆O₄S.

Ethopabate

C$_{12}$H$_{15}$NO$_4$ 237.3   *59-06-3*

Action and use
Antiprotozoal.

DEFINITION
Ethopabate is methyl 4-acetamido-2-ethoxybenzoate.
It contains not less than 96.0% and not more than 101.0%
of C$_{12}$H$_{15}$NO$_4$, calculated with reference to the dried
substance.

CHARACTERISTICS
A white or pinkish white powder. It melts at about 148°.

Very slightly soluble in *water*; soluble in *chloroform* and in
methanol; sparingly soluble in *ethanol (96%)*; slightly soluble
in *ether*.

IDENTIFICATION
A. The *infrared absorption spectrum*, Appendix II A, is
concordant with the *reference spectrum* of ethopabate
(RSV 20).

B. In the Assay, the retention time of the principal peak in
the chromatogram obtained with solution (1) is the same as
that of the principal peak in the chromatogram obtained with
solution (2).

TESTS
Related substances
Carry out the method for *liquid chromatography*,
Appendix III D, using the following solutions in a mixture of
equal volumes of *methanol* and *water*. Solution (1) contains
0.040% w/v of the substance being examined.
For solution (2) dilute 1 volume of solution (1) to
100 volumes. Solution (3) contains 0.040% w/v of
ethopabate BPCRS and 0.010% w/v of *methyl 4-acetamido-
2-hydroxybenzoate BPCRS*.

The chromatographic procedure may be carried out using
(a) a stainless steel column (30 cm × 3.9 mm) packed with
particles of silica the surface of which has been modified by
chemically-bonded phenyl groups (10 µm) (Waters
µBondapak phenyl is suitable), (b) 30 volumes of *acetonitrile*,
150 volumes of *methanol* and 450 volumes of 0.15M *sodium
hexanesulphonate*, adjusted to pH 2.5 with *orthophosphoric acid*,
as the mobile phase with a flow rate of 1 ml per minute and
(c) a detection wavelength of 268 nm. Maintain the
temperature of the column at 45°.

The test is not valid unless, in the chromatogram obtained
with solution (3), the *resolution factor* between the peaks due
to ethopabate and methyl 4-acetamido-2-hydroxybenzoate is
at least 1.2.

In the chromatogram obtained with solution (1) the area of
any peak eluting before the peak corresponding to methyl
4-acetamido-2-hydroxybenzoate (identified by the peak in the
chromatogram obtained with solution (3)) is not greater than
0.1 times the area of the principal peak in the chromatogram
obtained with solution (2) (0.1%); the area of any other
secondary peak is not greater than the area of the principal
peak in the chromatogram obtained with solution (2) (1%)
and the sum of the areas of all the *secondary peaks* is not
greater than twice the area of the principal peak in the
chromatogram obtained with solution (2) (2%).

Loss on drying
When dried at 60° at a pressure of 2 kPa for 2 hours,
loses not more than 1.0% of its weight. Use 1 g.

Sulphated ash
Not more than 0.1%, Appendix IX A.

ASSAY
Carry out the method for *liquid chromatography*,
Appendix III D, using the following solutions in a mixture of
equal volumes of *methanol* and *water*. Solution (1) contains
0.002% w/v of the substance being examined. Solution (2)
contains 0.002% w/v of *ethopabate BPCRS*. Solution (3)
contains 0.002% w/v of *ethopabate BPCRS* and 0.010% w/v
of *methyl 4-acetamido-2-hydroxybenzoate BPCRS*.

The chromatographic conditions described under Related
substances may be used.

The test is not valid unless, in the chromatogram obtained
with solution (3), the *resolution factor* between the peaks due
to ethopabate and methyl 4-acetamido-2-hydroxybenzoate is
at least 1.2.

Calculate the content of C$_{12}$H$_{15}$NO$_4$ in the substance being
examined using the declared content of C$_{12}$H$_{15}$NO$_4$ in
ethopabate BPCRS.

IMPURITIES

A. 4-aminosalicylic acid,

B. methyl 2-ethoxy-4-aminobenzoate,

C. methyl 2-hydroxy-4-aminobenzoate,

D. methyl 4-acetamido-2-hydroxybenzoate,

E. ethyl 4-acetamido-2-ethoxybenzoate.

Etorphine Hydrochloride

$C_{25}H_{33}NO_4,HCl$ 448.0   13764-49-3

Action and use
Opioid receptor agonist; analgesic.

Preparations
Etorphine and Acepromazine Injection

Etorphine and Levomepromazine Injection

DEFINITION
Etorphine Hydrochloride is $(6R,7R,14R)$-7,8-dihydro-7-[(1R)-1-hydroxy-1-methylbutyl]-6-O-methyl-6,14-ethenomorphine hydrochloride. It contains not less than 98.0% and not more than of 101.0% of $C_{25}H_{33}NO_4,HCl$, calculated with reference to the dried substance.

CAUTION *Etorphine Hydrochloride is extremely potent and extraordinary care should be taken in any procedure in which it is used. Any spillage on the skin should be washed off at once. In the case of accidental injection or absorption through broken skin or mucous membrane, a reversing agent should be injected immediately.*

CHARACTERISTICS
A white or almost white, microcrystalline powder.

Sparingly soluble in *water* and in *ethanol (96%)*; very slightly soluble in *chloroform*; practically insoluble in *ether*.

IDENTIFICATION
A. The light absorption, Appendix II B, in the range 230 to 350 nm of a 0.02% w/v solution in 0.1M *hydrochloric acid* exhibits a maximum only at 289 nm. The *absorbance* at the maximum is about 0.68.

B. The *light absorption*, Appendix II B, in the range 230 to 350 nm of a 0.02% w/v solution in 0.1M *sodium hydroxide* exhibits a maximum only at 302 nm. The *absorbance* at the maximum is about 1.2.

C. Carry out the method for *thin-layer chromatography*, Appendix III A, in subdued light using *silica gel GF$_{254}$* as the coating substance and a mixture of 10 volumes of *diethylamine*, 20 volumes of *ethyl acetate* and 70 volumes of *toluene* as the mobile phase. Apply separately to each half of

the plate 1 μl of each of two solutions in *methanol* containing (1) 2.0% w/v of the substance being examined and (2) 1.8% w/v of *diprenorphine BPCRS*. Add at each point of application 10 μl of a mixture of 4 volumes of *methanol* and 1 volume of 13.5M *ammonia*. After removal of the plate, allow it to dry in air and examine under *ultraviolet light (254 nm)*. Spray one half of the plate with a mixture of 5 volumes of *chloroplatinic acid solution*, 35 volumes of *dilute potassium iodide solution* and 60 volumes of *acetone*. Spray the other half of the plate with a mixture of 1 volume of *iron(III) chloride solution R1* and 1 volume of *dilute potassium hexacyanoferrate(III) solution*. The principal spot in the chromatogram obtained with solution (1) has an Rf value of about 1.15 relative to that of the spot in the chromatogram obtained with solution (2), absorbs ultraviolet light and yields a reddish violet colour with the iodoplatinate spray reagent and a blue colour with the iron—hexacyanoferrate spray reagent.

D. Yields reaction A characteristic of *chlorides*, Appendix VI.

TESTS
Acidity
pH of a 2.0% w/v solution, 4.0 to 5.5, Appendix V L.

Specific optical rotation
In a solution prepared by dissolving 0.5 g in sufficient *methanol* to produce 25 ml, -122 to -132, calculated with reference to the dried substance, Appendix V F.

Related substances
Carry out in subdued light the method for *thin-layer chromatography*, Appendix III A, using *silica gel G* as the coating substance and a mixture of 10 volumes of *diethylamine*, 20 volumes of *ethyl acetate* and 70 volumes of *toluene* as the mobile phase. Apply separately to the plate 20 μl of each of two solutions of the substance being examined in *methanol* containing (1) 2.0% w/v and (2) 0.020% w/v. Add at each point of application 10 μl of a mixture of 4 volumes of *methanol* and 1 volume of 13.5M *ammonia*. After removal of the plate, allow it to dry in air and spray with a 1% w/v solution of *iodine* in *methanol*. Any *secondary spot* in the chromatogram obtained with solution (1) is not more intense than the spot in the chromatogram obtained with solution (2) (1%).

Loss on drying
When dried to constant weight at 105°, loses not more than 4.0% of its weight. Use 1 g.

Sulphated ash
Not more than 0.1%, Appendix IX A.

ASSAY
Carry out Method I for *non-aqueous titration*, Appendix VIII A, using 0.5 g, adding 7 ml of *mercury(II) acetate solution* and using *crystal violet solution* as indicator. Each ml of 0.1M *perchloric acid VS* is equivalent to 44.80 mg of $C_{25}H_{33}NO_4,HCl$.

STORAGE
Etorphine Hydrochloride should be protected from light.

Febantel

(Febantel for Veterinary Use, Ph Eur monograph 2176)

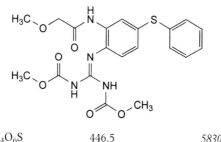

C$_{20}$H$_{22}$N$_4$O$_6$S   446.5   *58306-30-28*

Action and use
Anthelmintic.

Ph Eur

DEFINITION
Dimethyl *N,N′*-[[[2-[(methoxyacetyl)amino]-4-(phenylsulphanyl)phenyl]imino]methylene]dicarbamate.

Content
97.5 per cent to 102.0 per cent (dried substance).

CHARACTERS
Appearance
White or almost white, crystalline powder.

Solubility
Practically insoluble in water, soluble in acetone, slightly soluble in anhydrous ethanol.

It shows polymorphism.

IDENTIFICATION
Infrared absorption spectrophotometry *(2.2.24)*.

Comparison   febantel CRS.

If the spectra obtained in the solid state show differences, dissolve the substance to be examined and the reference substance separately in *acetone R*, evaporate to dryness and record new spectra using the residues.

TESTS
Related substances
Liquid chromatography *(2.2.29)*.

Solvent mixture   acetonitrile R, tetrahydrofuran R (50:50 V/V).

Test solution (a)   Dissolve 0.100 g of the substance to be examined in the solvent mixture and dilute to 10.0 ml with the solvent mixture.

Test solution (b)   Dilute 5.0 ml of test solution (a) to 100.0 ml with the solvent mixture.

Reference solution (a)   Dilute 1.0 ml of test solution (a) to 100.0 ml with the solvent mixture. Dilute 1.0 ml of this solution to 10.0 ml with the solvent mixture.

Reference solution (b)   Dissolve 50.0 mg of *febantel CRS* in the solvent mixture and dilute to 10.0 ml with the solvent mixture. Dilute 5.0 ml of this solution to 50.0 ml with the solvent mixture.

Reference solution (c)   Dissolve 5 mg of *febantel for system suitability CRS* (containing impurities A, B and C) in 1.0 ml of the solvent mixture.

Column:
— *size: l* = 0.15 m, Ø = 4.0 mm;
— *stationary phase: spherical end-capped octadecylsilyl silica gel for chromatography R1 (5 μm).*

Mobile phase   Dissolve 6.8 g of *potassium dihydrogen phosphate R* in 1000 ml of *water for chromatography R*. Mix 350 ml of *acetonitrile R* with 650 ml of this solution.

Flow rate   1.0 ml/min.

Detection   Spectrophotometer at 280 nm.

Injection   10 μl of test solution (a) and reference solutions (a) and (c).

Run time   1.5 times the retention time of febantel.

Elution order   impurity A, impurity B, impurity C, febantel.

Retention time   febantel = about 32 min.

System suitability   Reference solution (c):
— *resolution*: minimum 3.0 between the peaks due to impurities A and B and minimum 4.0 between the peaks due to impurities B and C.

Limits:
— *impurities A, B, C*: for each impurity, not more than the area of the principal peak in the chromatogram obtained with reference solution (a) (0.1 per cent);
— *unspecified impurities*: for each impurity, not more than twice the area of the principal peak in the chromatogram obtained with reference solution (a) (0.20 per cent);
— *total*: not more than 5 times the area of the principal peak in the chromatogram obtained with reference solution (a) (0.5 per cent);
— *disregard limit*: 0.5 times the area of the principal peak in the chromatogram obtained with reference solution (a) (0.05 per cent).

Heavy metals *(2.4.8)*
Maximum 20 ppm.

1.0 g complies with test F. Prepare the reference solution using 2 ml of *lead standard solution (10 ppm Pb) R*.

Loss on drying *(2.2.32)*
Maximum 0.5 per cent, determined on 1.000 g by drying in an oven at 100-105 °C for 2 h.

Sulphated ash *(2.4.14)*
Maximum 0.1 per cent, determined on 1.0 g.

ASSAY
Liquid chromatography *(2.2.29)* as described in the test for related substances with the following modification.

Injection   Test solution (b) and reference solution (b).

Calculate the percentage content of C$_{20}$H$_{22}$N$_4$O$_6$S from the declared content of *febantel CRS*.

IMPURITIES
Specified impurities   A, B, C.

A. methyl [[2-[(methoxyacetyl)amino]-4-(phenylsulphanyl)phenyl]carbamimidoyl]carbamate,

B. R = CH$_2$-OCH$_3$: 2-(methoxymethyl)-5-(phenylsulphanyl)-1*H*-benzimidazole,

C. R = NH-CO-OCH$_3$: methyl [5-(phenylsulphanyl)-1*H*-benzimidazol-2-yl]carbamate (fenbendazole).

Ph Eur

Fenbendazole

*(Fenbendazole for Veterinary Use,
Ph Eur monograph 1208)*

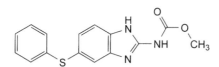

$C_{15}H_{13}N_3O_2S$ 299.4   *43210-67-9*

Action and use
Antihelminthic.

Preparations
Fenbendazole Granules

Fenbendazole Veterinary Oral Paste

Fenbendazole Veterinary Oral Powder

Fenbendazole Veterinary Oral Suspension

Ph Eur

DEFINITION
Fenbendazole for veterinary use contains not less than
98.0 per cent and not more than the equivalent of
101.0 per cent of methyl [5-(phenylsulphanyl)-1*H*-
benzimidazol-2-yl]carbamate, calculated with reference
to the dried substance.

CHARACTERS
A white or almost white powder, practically insoluble in
water, sparingly soluble in dimethylformamide, very slightly
soluble in methanol.

IDENTIFICATION
Examine by infrared absorption spectrophotometry *(2.2.24)*,
comparing with the spectrum obtained with
fenbendazole CRS. Examine the substances prepared as discs.

TESTS
Related substances
Examine by liquid chromatography *(2.2.29)*.

Test solution   Dissolve 50.0 mg of the substance to be
examined in 10.0 ml of *hydrochloric methanol R.*

Reference solution (a)   Dissolve 50.0 mg of *fenbendazole CRS*
in 10.0 ml of *hydrochloric methanol R*. Dilute 1.0 ml of this
solution to 200.0 ml with *methanol R*. Dilute 5.0 ml of this
second solution to 10.0 ml with *hydrochloric methanol R.*

Reference solution (b)   Dissolve 10.0 mg of *fenbendazole
impurity A CRS* in 100.0 ml of *methanol R*. Dilute 1.0 ml of
this solution to 10.0 ml with *hydrochloric methanol R.*

Reference solution (c)   Dissolve 10.0 mg of *fenbendazole
impurity B CRS* in 100.0 ml of *methanol R*. Dilute 1.0 ml of
this solution to 10.0 ml with *hydrochloric methanol R.*

Reference solution (d)   Dissolve 10.0 mg of *fenbendazole CRS*
and 10.0 mg of *mebendazole CRS* in 100.0 ml of *methanol R*.
Dilute 1.0 ml of this solution to 10.0 ml with *hydrochloric
methanol R.*

The chromatographic procedure may be carried out using:
— a stainless steel column 0.25 m long and 4.6 mm in
   internal diameter packed with *octadecylsilyl silica gel for
   chromatography R* (5 μm),
— as mobile phase at a flow rate of 1 ml/min:

Mobile phase A   Mix 1 volume of *anhydrous acetic acid R*,
30 volumes of *methanol R* and 70 volumes of *water R*,

Mobile phase B   Mix 1 volume of *anhydrous acetic acid R*,
30 volumes of *water R* and 70 volumes of *methanol R*,

Time (min)	Mobile phase A (per cent *V/V*)	Mobile phase B (per cent *V/V*)	Comment
0 - 10	100 → 0	0 → 100	linear gradient
10 - 40	0	100	isocratic
40 - 50	0 → 100	100 → 0	re-equilibration

— as detector a spectrophotometer set at 280 nm.

When the chromatograms are recorded in the prescribed
conditions, the retention time for fenbendazole is about
19 min. Inject separately 10 μl of each solution. The test is
not valid unless, in the chromatogram obtained with
reference solution (d), the resolution between the peaks
corresponding to fenbendazole and mebendazole is at
least 1.5.

In the chromatogram obtained with the test solution: the area
of the peaks corresponding to impurity A and impurity B is
not greater than 2.5 times the area of the corresponding peak
in the chromatograms obtained with reference solution (b)
and reference solution (c) (0.5 per cent); the area of any
peak, apart from the principal peak and the peaks
corresponding to impurity A and impurity B respectively, is
not greater than twice the area of the principal peak in the
chromatogram obtained with reference solution (a)
(0.5 per cent); the sum of the areas of all the peaks, apart
from the principal peak, is not greater than 4 times the area
of the principal peak in the chromatogram obtained with
reference solution (a) (1 per cent). Disregard any peak with
an area less than 0.2 times that of the principal peak in the
chromatogram obtained with reference solution (a).

Heavy metals *(2.4.8)*
1.0 g complies with limit test C for heavy metals (20 ppm).
Prepare the standard using 2 ml of *lead standard
solution (10 ppm Pb) R.*

Loss on drying *(2.2.32)*
Not more than 1.0 per cent, determined on 1.000 g by
drying in an oven at 100-105 °C for 3 h.

Sulphated ash *(2.4.14)*
Not more than 0.3 per cent, determined on 1.0 g.

ASSAY
Dissolve 0.200 g in 30 ml of *anhydrous acetic acid R*, warming
gently if necessary. Cool and titrate with *0.1 M perchloric acid*,
determining the end-point potentiometrically *(2.2.20)*.

1 ml of *0.1 M perchloric acid* is equivalent to 29.94 mg of
$C_{15}H_{13}N_3O_2S$.

STORAGE
Protected from light.

IMPURITIES

A. R = H: methyl (1*H*-benzimidazol-2-yl)carbamate,

B. R = Cl: methyl (5-chloro-1*H*-benzimidazol-2-
yl)carbamate.

Fenthion

C$_{10}$H$_{15}$O$_3$PS$_2$ 278.3   55-38-9

Action and use
Insecticide.

DEFINITION
Fenthion is O,O-dimethyl O-4-methylthio-*m*-tolylphosphorothioate. It contains not less than 90.0% and not more than 100.5% of C$_{10}$H$_{15}$O$_3$PS$_2$.

CHARACTERISTICS
A yellowish brown, oily substance.

Immiscible with *water*; miscible with *chloroform* and with *ethanol (96%)*.

IDENTIFICATION
A. The *infrared absorption spectrum*, Appendix II A, is concordant with the *reference spectrum* of fenthion *(RSV 21)*.

B. Carry out the method for *thin-layer chromatography*, Appendix III A, using *silica gel GF$_{254}$* as the coating substance and a mixture of 1 volume of *acetone* and 4 volumes of *hexane* as the mobile phase. Apply separately to the plate 2 μl of each of two solutions in *chloroform* containing (1) 0.5% w/v of the substance being examined and (2) 0.5% w/v of *fenthion BPCRS*. After removal of the plate, allow it to dry in air and examine under *ultraviolet light (254 nm)*. The spot in the chromatogram obtained with solution (1) corresponds to that in the chromatogram obtained with solution (2).

C. To 0.15 ml add 3 ml of *propan-2-ol* and 0.2 g of *potassium hydroxide* and heat on a water bath for 15 minutes. Add 5 ml of *water*, heat for a further 5 minutes, cool, dilute to 50 ml with *water* and add 3 ml of *iodinated potassium iodide solution*. A green colour is produced which gradually fades.

Related substances
Carry out the method for *thin-layer chromatography*, Appendix III A, using a silica gel F$_{254}$ precoated plate (Merck silica gel 60 F$_{254}$ plates are suitable) and a mixture of 1 volume of *acetone* and 4 volumes of *hexane* as the mobile phase. Apply separately to the plate 10 μl of each of three solutions of the substance being examined in *methanol* containing (1) 2.0% w/v, (2) 0.12% w/v and (3) 0.040% w/v. After removal of the plate, allow it to dry in air and examine under *ultraviolet light (254 nm)*. Any spot in the chromatogram obtained with solution (1) with an Rf value of about 0.36 relative to that of the principal spot is not more intense than the spot in the chromatogram obtained with solution (2) (6%) and any other *secondary spot* is not more intense than the spot in the chromatogram obtained with solution (3) (2%).

ASSAY
Carry out the method for *gas chromatography*, Appendix III B, using solutions in *chloroform* containing (1) 0.4% w/v of *fenthion BPCRS* and 0.2% w/v of *dibutyl phthalate* (internal standard), (2) 0.4% w/v of the substance being examined and (3) 0.4% w/v of the substance being examined and 0.2% w/v of the internal standard.

The chromatographic procedure may be carried out using (a) a glass column (1.5 m × 4 mm) packed with *acid-washed, silanised diatomaceous support* (80 to 100 mesh) coated with 3% w/w of phenyl methyl silicone fluid (OV 17 is suitable) and maintained at 225°.

Calculate the content of C$_{10}$H$_{15}$O$_3$PS$_2$ using the declared content of C$_{10}$H$_{15}$O$_3$PS$_2$ in *fenthion BPCRS*.

Fluanisone

C$_{21}$H$_{25}$FN$_2$O$_2$ 356.4   1480-19-9

Action and use
Dopamine receptor antagonist; neuroleptic.

DEFINITION
Fluanisone is 4'-fluoro-4-[4-(2-methoxyphenyl)piperazin-1-yl]-butyrophenone. It contains not less than 98.0% and not more than 101.0% of C$_{21}$H$_{25}$FN$_2$O$_2$, calculated with reference to the dried substance.

CHARACTERISTICS
White or almost white to buff-coloured crystals or powder; odourless or almost odourless. It exhibits polymorphism.

Practically insoluble in *water*; freely soluble in *chloroform*, in *ethanol (96%)*, in *ether* and in dilute solutions of organic acids.

IDENTIFICATION
A. The *infrared absorption spectrum*, Appendix II A, is concordant with the *reference spectrum* of fluanisone *(RSV 22)*. If the spectra are not concordant, dissolve 0.1 g of the substance being examined in 3 ml of *dichloromethane* and evaporate the solvent at room temperature, scratching the side of the container occasionally with a glass rod and prepare a new spectrum of the residue.

B. The *light absorption*, Appendix II B, in the range 230 to 350 nm of a 0.002% w/v solution in a mixture of 9 volumes of *propan-2-ol* and 1 volume of 0.1M *hydrochloric acid* exhibits a well-defined maximum only at 243 nm. The *absorbance* at 243 nm is about 1.1.

C. Heat 0.5 ml of *chromic-sulphuric acid mixture* in a small test tube in a water bath for 5 minutes; the solution wets the side of the tube readily and there is no greasiness. Add 2 to 3 mg of the substance being examined and again heat in a water bath for 5 minutes; the solution does not wet the side of the tube and does not pour easily from the tube.

TESTS
Melting point
72° to 76°, Appendix V A.

Related substances
Carry out the method for *thin-layer chromatography*, Appendix III A, using a silica gel GF$_{254}$ precoated plate

(Merck silica gel 60 plates are suitable) and a mixture of 10 volumes of *ethanol (96%)* and 90 volumes of *chloroform* as the mobile phase. Apply separately to the plate 10 μl of each of four solutions in *chloroform* containing (1) 2.0% w/v of the substance being examined, (2) 0.010% w/v of the substance being examined, (3) 0.020% w/v of *4'-fluoro-4-chlorobutyrophenone BPCRS* and (4) 0.010% w/v of *1-(2-methoxyphenyl)piperazine BPCRS*. After removal of the plate, allow it to dry in air and expose to iodine vapour for 15 minutes. Any spots in the chromatogram obtained with solution (1) corresponding to 4'-fluoro-4-chlorobutyrophenone and 1-(2-methoxyphenyl)piperazine are not more intense than the spots in the chromatograms obtained with solutions (3) and (4) respectively (1% and 0.5%, respectively); and any other *secondary spot* in the chromatogram obtained with solution (1) is not more intense than the spot in the chromatogram obtained with solution (2) (0.5%).

Loss on drying
When dried to constant weight at 40° at a pressure not exceeding 0.7 kPa, loses not more than 0.5% of its weight. Use 1 g.

Sulphated ash
Not more than 0.1%, Appendix IX A.

ASSAY
Carry out Method I for *non-aqueous titration*, Appendix VIII A, using 0.15 g and *crystal violet solution* as indicator. Each ml of 0.1M *perchloric acid VS* is equivalent to 17.82 mg of $C_{21}H_{25}FN_2O_2$.

STORAGE
Fluanisone should be protected from light.

Flunixin Meglumine

(*Flunixin Meglumine for Veterinary Use,*
Ph Eur monograph 1696)

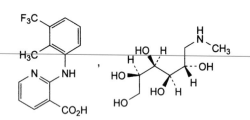

$C_{21}H_{28}F_3N_3O_7$ 491.5   *42461-84-7*

Action and use
Cyclo-oxygenase inhibitor; analgesic; anti-inflammatory.

Ph Eur

DEFINITION
2-[[2-Methyl-3-(trifluoromethyl)phenyl]amino]pyridine-3-carboxylic acid, 1-deoxy-1-(methylamino)-D-glucitol.

Content
99.0 per cent to 101.0 per cent (dried substance).

CHARACTERS
Appearance
White or almost white, crystalline powder.

Solubility
Freely soluble in water and in methanol, practically insoluble in acetone.

IDENTIFICATION
A. Specific optical rotation (*2.2.7*): − 9.0 to − 12.0 (dried substance), determined on solution S (see Tests).
B. Infrared absorption spectrophotometry (*2.2.24*).
Comparison flunixin meglumine CRS.

TESTS
Solution S
Dissolve 2.50 g in *carbon dioxide-free water R* and dilute to 50.0 ml with the same solvent.

Appearance of solution
Solution S is clear (*2.2.1*) and not more intensely coloured than reference solution Y_7 (*2.2.2, Method II*).

pH (*2.2.3*)
7.0 to 9.0 for solution S.

Related substances
Liquid chromatography (*2.2.29*).

Test solution Dissolve 50.0 mg of the substance to be examined in the mobile phase and dilute to 10.0 ml with the mobile phase.

Reference solution (a) Dissolve 5.0 mg of *flunixin impurity B CRS* in 1.0 ml of the test solution and dilute to 50.0 ml with the mobile phase.

Reference solution (b) Dissolve 5.0 mg of *2-chloronicotinic acid R* (impurity A) in the mobile phase and dilute to 50.0 ml with the mobile phase. To 2.0 ml of this solution add 2.0 ml of reference solution (a) and dilute to 20.0 ml with the mobile phase.

Reference solution (c) Dissolve 50 mg of *flunixin impurity C CRS* in the mobile phase and dilute to 100 ml with the mobile phase.

Column:
— *size*: $l = 0.125$ m, Ø = 4.0 mm,
— *stationary phase*: octadecylsilyl silica gel for chromatography R (5 μm).

Mobile phase Mix 300 volumes of *water R* and 700 volumes of *acetonitrile R*, and add 0.25 volumes of *phosphoric acid R*.

Flow rate 1.0 ml/min.

Detection Spectrophotometer at 254 nm.

Injection 10 μl.

Run time 5 times the retention time of flunixin.

Relative retention With reference to flunixin (retention time = about 3.1 min): impurity A = about 0.4; impurity C = about 0.6; impurity B = about 0.7; impurity D = about 4.2.

System suitability Reference solution (a):
— *resolution*: minimum 3.5 between the peaks due to impurity B and flunixin.

Limits:
— *correction factor*: for the calculation of content, multiply the peak area of impurity C by 1.9,
— *impurity A*: not more than the area of the corresponding peak in the chromatogram obtained with reference solution (b) (0.2 per cent),
— *impurity B*: not more than the area of the corresponding peak in the chromatogram obtained with reference solution (b) (0.2 per cent),
— *impurities C, D*: for each impurity, not more than the area of the peak due to flunixin in the chromatogram obtained with reference solution (b) (0.2 per cent),

— *any other impurity*: for each impurity, not more than the area of the peak due to flunixin in the chromatogram obtained with reference solution (b) (0.2 per cent),

— *total*: not more than 2.5 times the area of the peak due to flunixin in the chromatogram obtained with reference solution (b) (0.5 per cent),

— *disregard limit*: 0.25 times the area of the peak due to flunixin in the chromatogram obtained with reference solution (b) (0.05 per cent).

Loss on drying (*2.2.32*)
Maximum 0.5 per cent, determined on 1.000 g by drying in an oven at 100-105 °C for 4 h.

Sulphated ash (*2.4.14*)
Maximum 0.1 per cent, determined on 1.0 g.

ASSAY
Dissolve 0.175 g in 50 ml of *anhydrous acetic acid R*. Titrate with *0.1 M perchloric acid*, determining the end-point potentiometrically (*2.2.20*).

1 ml of *0.1 M perchloric acid* is equivalent to 24.57 mg of $C_{21}H_{28}F_3N_3O_7$.

IMPURITIES
Specified impurities   A, B, C, D.

A. R = H: 2-chloropyridine-3-carboxylic acid,

C. R = C_2H_5: ethyl 2-chloropyridine-3-carboxylate,

B. 2-methyl-3-(trifluoromethyl)aniline,

D. ethyl 2-[[2-methyl-3-(trifluoromethyl)phenyl]amino]pyridine-3-carboxylate.

Ph Eur

Serum Gonadotrophin

(Equine Serum Gonadotrophin for Veterinary Use, Ph Eur monograph 0719)

Action and use
Equine serum gonadotrophin.

Preparation
Serum Gonadotrophin Injection

Ph Eur

DEFINITION
Equine serum gonadotrophin for veterinary use is a dry preparation of a glycoprotein fraction obtained from the serum or plasma of pregnant mares. It has follicle-stimulating and luteinising activities. The potency is not less than 1000 IU of gonadotrophin activity per milligram, calculated with reference to the anhydrous substance.

PRODUCTION
Equine serum gonadotrophin may be prepared by precipitation with alcohol (70 per cent *V/V*) and further purification by a suitable form of chromatography. It is prepared in conditions designed to minimise microbial contamination.

CHARACTERS
Appearance
White or pale grey, amorphous powder.

Solubility
Soluble in water.

IDENTIFICATION
When administered as prescribed in the assay it causes an increase in the mass of the ovaries of immature female rats.

TESTS
Water (*2.5.12*)
Maximum 10.0 per cent, determined on 80 mg.

Bacterial endotoxins (*2.6.14, method C*)
Less than 0.035 IU per IU of equine serum gonadotrophin, if intended for use in the manufacture of parenteral dosage forms without a further appropriate procedure for the removal of bacterial endotoxins.

ASSAY
The potency of equine serum gonadotrophin is estimated by comparing under given conditions its effect of increasing the mass of the ovaries of immature female rats with the same effect of the International Standard of equine serum gonadotrophin or of a reference preparation calibrated in International Units.

The International Unit is the activity contained in a stated amount of the International Standard, which consists of a mixture of a freeze-dried extract of equine serum gonadotrophin from the serum of pregnant mares with lactose. The equivalence in International Units of the International Standard is stated by the World Health Organisation.

Use immature female rats of the same strain, 21 to 28 days old, differing in age by not more than 3 days and having masses such that the difference between the heaviest and the lightest rat is not more than 10 g. Assign the rats at random to 6 equal groups of not fewer than 5 animals. If sets of 6 litter mates are available, assign one litter mate from each set to each group and mark according to litter.

Choose 3 doses of the reference preparation and 3 doses of the preparation to be examined such that the smallest dose is sufficient to produce a positive response in some of the rats and the largest dose does not produce a maximal response in all the rats. Use doses in geometric progression: as an initial approximation total doses of 8 IU, 12 IU and 18 IU may be tried, although the dose will depend on the sensitivity of the animals used and may vary widely.

Dissolve separately the total quantities of the preparation to be examined and of the reference preparation corresponding to the doses to be used in sufficient of a sterile 9 g/l solution of *sodium chloride R* containing 1 mg/ml of *bovine albumin R* such that each single dose is administered in a volume of about 0.2 ml. Store the solutions at 5 ± 3 °C.

Inject subcutaneously into each rat the dose allocated to its group. Repeat the injections 18 h, 21 h, 24 h, 42 h and 48 h after the first injection. Not less than 40 h and not more than 72 h after the last injection, kill the rats and remove the ovaries. Remove any extraneous fluid and tissue and weigh the 2 ovaries immediately. Calculate the results by the usual statistical methods, using the combined mass of the 2 ovaries of each animal as the response.

The estimated potency is not less than 80 per cent and not more than 125 per cent of the stated potency. The confidence limits ($P = 0.95$) of the estimated potency are not less than 64 per cent and not more than 156 per cent of the stated potency.

STORAGE

In an airtight container, protected from light, at a temperature not exceeding 8 °C. If the substance is sterile, store in a sterile, airtight, tamper-proof container.

LABELLING

The label states:
— the potency in International Units per milligram,
— where applicable, that the substance is free from bacterial endotoxins.

Ph Eur

Levamisole

(*Levamisole for Veterinary Use,*
Ph Eur monograph 1728)

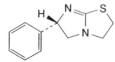

C₁₁H₂₂N₂S $\qquad$ 204.3 $\qquad$ *14769-73-4*

Action and use
Immunostimulant; antihelminthic.

Ph Eur

DEFINITION
(6*S*)-6-Phenyl-2,3,5,6-tetrahydroimidazo[2,1-*b*]thiazole.

Content
98.5 per cent to 101.5 per cent (anhydrous substance).

CHARACTERS
Appearance
White or almost white powder.

Solubility
Slightly soluble in water, freely soluble in alcohol and in methanol.

It shows polymorphism.

IDENTIFICATION
A. It complies with the test for specific optical rotation (see Tests).

B. Infrared absorption spectrophotometry (*2.2.24*).

Comparison   Ph. Eur. reference spectrum of levamisole.

If the spectra show differences, dissolve the substance to be examined in *methylene chloride R*, evaporate to dryness and record a new spectrum using the residue.

TESTS
Solution S
Dissolve 2.50 g in *ethanol R* and dilute to 50.0 ml with the same solvent.

Appearance of solution
Solution S is clear (*2.2.1*) and not more intensely coloured than reference solution BY₆ (*2.2.2, Method II*).

Specific optical rotation (*2.2.7*)
− 85 to − 89 (anhydrous substance), determined on solution S.

Related substances
Liquid chromatography (*2.2.29*). *Prepare the solutions immediately before use, protect from light and keep below 25 °C.*

Test solution   Dissolve 0.100 g of the substance to be examined in methanol R and dilute to 10.0 ml with the same solvent.

Reference solution (a)   Dissolve 50 mg of levamisole hydrochloride for system suitability CRS in methanol R, add 0.5 ml of concentrated ammonia R and dilute to 5.0 ml with methanol R.

Reference solution (b)   Dilute 1.0 ml of the test solution to 100.0 ml with methanol R. Dilute 5.0 ml of the solution to 25.0 ml with methanol R.

Column:
— *size*: l = 0.10 m, Ø = 4.6 mm,
— *stationary phase: base-deactivated octadecylsilyl silica gel for chromatography R (3 µm).*

Mobile phase:
— *mobile phase A: dissolve 0.5 g of ammonium dihydrogen phosphate R in 90 ml of water R; adjust to pH 6.5 with a 40 g/l solution of sodium hydroxide R and dilute to 100 ml with water R,*
— *mobile phase B: acetonitrile R.*

Time (min)	Mobile phase A (per cent *V/V*)	Mobile phase B (per cent *V/V*)
0 - 8	90 → 30	10 → 70
8 - 10	30	70
10 - 11	30 → 90	70 → 10

Flow rate   1.5 ml/min.

Detection   Spectrophotometer at 215 nm.

Equilibration   At least 4 min with the mobile phase at the initial composition.

Injection   10 µl.

Relative retention with reference to levamisole (retention time = about 3 min): impurity A = about 0.9;

impurity B = about 1.4; impurity C = about 1.5; impurity D = about 1.6; impurity E = about 2.0.

System suitability Reference solution (a):
— the chromatogram obtained is similar to the chromatogram supplied with *levamisole hydrochloride for system suitability CRS*.

Limits:
— *correction factors*: for the calculation of content, multiply the peak areas of the following impurities by the corresponding correction factor: impurity A = 2.0; impurity B = 1.7; impurity C = 2.9; impurity D = 1.3; impurity E = 2.7;
— *impurities A, B, C, D, E*: for each impurity, not more than the area of the principal peak in the chromatogram obtained with reference solution (b) (0.2 per cent);
— *any other impurity*: not more than half the area of the principal peak in the chromatogram obtained with reference solution (b) (0.1 per cent);
— *total*: not more than 1.5 times the area of the principal peak in the chromatogram obtained with reference solution (b) (0.3 per cent);
— *disregard limit*: 0.25 times the area of the principal peak in the chromatogram obtained with reference solution (b) (0.05 per cent).

Water (2.5.12)
Maximum 0.5 per cent, determined on 1.00 g.

Sulphated ash (2.4.14)
Maximum 0.1 per cent, determined on 1.0 g.

ASSAY
Dissolve 0.150 g in 50 ml of a mixture of 1 volume of *anhydrous acetic acid R* and 7 volumes of *methyl ethyl ketone R*. Titrate with *0.1 M perchloric acid*, using 0.2 ml of *naphtholbenzein solution R* as indicator.

1 ml of *0.1 M perchloric acid* is equivalent to 20.43 mg of $C_{11}H_{12}N_2S$.

STORAGE
In an airtight container, protected from light.

IMPURITIES

A. 3-[(2RS)-2-amino-2-phenylethyl]thiazolidin-2-one,

B. 3-[(E)-2-phenylethenyl]thiazolidin-2-imine,

C. (4RS)-4-phenyl-1-(2-sulphanylethyl)imidazolidin-2-one,

D. 6-phenyl-2,3-dihydroimidazo[2,1-b]thiazole,

E. 1,1′-[(disulphane-1,2-diyl)bis(ethylene)]bis[(4RS)-4-phenylimidazolidin-2-one].

Ph Eur

Levomepromazine

and enantiomer

$C_{19}H_{24}N_2OS$ 328.5   *60-99-1*

Action and use
Dopamine receptor antagonist; neuroleptic.

Preparation
Etorphine and Levomepromazine Injection

DEFINITION
Levomepromazine is (R)-3-(2-methoxyphenothiazin-10-yl)-2-methylpropyldimethylamine. It contains not less than 99.0% and not more than 101.0% of $C_{19}H_{24}N_2OS$, calculated with reference to the dried substance.

CHARACTERISTICS
A white or slightly cream-coloured, crystalline powder.

Practically insoluble in *water*; slightly soluble in *ethanol (96%)*; freely soluble in *ether*.

IDENTIFICATION
A. The *infrared absorption spectrum*, Appendix II A, is concordant with the *reference spectrum* of levomepromazine (RSV 25).

B. The *light absorption*, Appendix II B, in the range 230 to 350 nm of a 0.001% w/v solution in 0.1M *hydrochloric acid* exhibits a maximum at 250 nm and a less well-defined maximum at 300 nm. The *absorbance* at 250 nm is about 0.75. Protect the solution from light.

C. Complies with the test for *identification of phenothiazines*, Appendix III A, using *levomepromazine BPCRS* to prepare solution (2).

D. Dissolve about 5 mg in 2 ml of *sulphuric acid* and allow to stand for 5 minutes. A deep purple colour is produced.

TESTS

Melting point

124° to 127°, Appendix V A.

Specific optical rotation

In a 5% w/v solution in *chloroform*, -15 to -18, calculated with reference to the dried substance, Appendix V F.

Related substances

Complies with the test for *related substances in phenothiazines*, Appendix III A, using *mobile phase C*.

Loss on drying

When dried to constant weight at 105°, loses not more than 0.5% of its weight. Use 1 g.

Sulphated ash

Not more than 0.1%, Appendix IX A.

ASSAY

Dissolve 1 g in 200 ml of *acetone* and carry out Method I for *non-aqueous titration*, Appendix VIII A, using 3 ml of a saturated solution of *methyl orange* in *acetone* as indicator. Each ml of 0.1M *perchloric acid VS* is equivalent to 32.85 mg of $C_{19}H_{24}N_2OS$.

STORAGE

Levomepromazine should be protected from light.

Meclofenamic Acid

$C_{14}H_{11}Cl_2NO_2$ 296.2   *644-62-2*

Action and use

Cyclo-oxygenase inhibitor; analgesic; anti-inflammatory.

Preparation

Meclofenamic Acid Granules

DEFINITION

Meclofenamic Acid is *N*-(2,6-dichloro-*m*-tolyl)anthranilic acid. It contains not less than 98.5% and not more than 100.5% of $C_{14}H_{11}Cl_2NO_2$, calculated with reference to the dried substance.

CHARACTERISTICS

A white or almost white, crystalline powder.

Practically insoluble in *water*; soluble in *dimethylformamide* and in 1M *sodium hydroxide*; sparingly soluble in *ether*; slightly soluble in *chloroform* and in *ethanol (96%)*.

IDENTIFICATION

A. The *infrared absorption spectrum*, Appendix II A, is concordant with the *reference spectrum* of meclofenamic acid (RSV 26).

B. The *light absorption*, Appendix II B, in the range 230 to 350 nm of a 0.002% w/v solution in 0.1M *sodium hydroxide* exhibits two maxima, at 279 nm and 317 nm. The *absorbances* at the maxima are about 0.45 and about 0.33, respectively.

C. Dissolve about 25 mg in 15 ml of *chloroform*. The solution exhibits a strong blue fluorescence when examined under ultraviolet light.

D. Dissolve about 1 mg in 2 ml of *sulphuric acid* and add 0.05 ml of 0.02M *potassium dichromate*. An intense purple colour is produced, which rapidly fades to purplish brown.

TESTS

Clarity and colour of solution

A 5.0% w/v solution in 1M *sodium hydroxide* is not more opalescent than *reference suspension II*, Appendix IV A, and is not more intensely coloured than *reference solution BY₅*, Appendix IV B, Method II.

Light absorption

Absorbance of a 0.002% w/v solution in 0.01M *methanolic hydrochloric acid* at the maximum at 279 nm, not less than 0.400 and not more than 0.445, and at the maximum at 335 nm, not less than 0.440 and not greater than 0.490, Appendix II B.

Heavy metals

1 g complies with *limit test C for heavy metals*, Appendix VII. Use 2 ml of *lead standard solution (10 ppm Pb)* to prepare the standard (20 ppm).

Related substances

Carry out the method for *liquid chromatography*, Appendix III D, using the following solutions in *absolute ethanol*. Solution (1) contains 0.0035% w/v of *ethyl meclofenamate BPCRS* (internal standard). Solution (2) contains 1.0% w/v solution of the substance being examined. Solution (3) contains 1.0% w/v of the substance being examined and 0.0035% w/v of the internal standard.

The chromatographic procedure may be carried out using (a) a stainless steel column (20 cm × 4 mm) packed with *octadecylsilyl silica gel for chromatography* (10 μm) (Spherisorb ODS 1 is suitable), (b) a mixture of 1 volume of *glacial acetic acid*, 25 volumes of *water* and 75 volumes of *methanol* as the mobile phase with a flow rate of 2 ml per minute and (c) a detection wavelength of 254 nm.

The test is not valid unless the *column efficiency* is at least 4500 theoretical plates per metre, determined using the peak due to the internal standard in the chromatogram obtained with solution (1).

In the chromatogram obtained with solution (3) the area of the peak immediately preceding the peak due to meclofenamic acid is not greater than one-seventh of the area of the peak due to the internal standard (0.05% of 2,6-dichloro-3-methylaniline). The area of any other *secondary peak* is not greater than the area of the peak due to the internal standard (0.35%).

Loss on drying

When dried at 105° to constant weight, loses not more than 0.5% of its weight. Use 1 g.

Sulphated ash

Not more than 0.1%, Appendix IX A.

ASSAY

Dissolve 0.6 g in 100 ml of warm *absolute ethanol* previously neutralised to *phenol red solution* and titrate with 0.1M *sodium hydroxide VS* using *phenol red solution* as indicator. Each ml of 0.1M *sodium hydroxide VS* is equivalent to 29.62 mg of $C_{14}H_{11}Cl_2NO_2$.

Morantel Tartrate

(Morantel Hydrogen Tartate for Veterinary Use,
Ph Eur monograph 1546)

$C_{16}H_{22}N_2O_6S$ 370.4   *26155-31-7*

Action and use
Anthelmintic.

Ph Eur

DEFINITION
1-Methyl-2-[(*E*)-2-(3-methylthiophen-2-yl)ethenyl]-1,4,5,6-tetrahydropyrimidine hydrogen tartrate.

Content
98.5 per cent to 101.5 per cent (dried substance).

CHARACTERS
Appearance
White or pale yellow, crystalline powder.

Solubility
Very soluble in water and in ethanol (96 per cent), practically insoluble in ethyl acetate.

IDENTIFICATION
First identification B.

Second identification A, C, D.

A. Melting point (*2.2.14*): 167 °C to 172 °C.

B. Infrared absorption spectrophotometry (*2.2.24*).

Comparison morantel hydrogen tartrate CRS.

C. Dissolve about 10 mg in 1 ml of a 5 g/l solution of *ammonium vanadate R*. Evaporate to dryness. Add 0.1 ml of *sulphuric acid R*. A purple colour is produced.

D. Dissolve about 10 mg in 1 ml of *0.1 M sodium hydroxide*. Transfer to a separating funnel and shake with 5 ml of *methylene chloride R*. Discard the organic layer. Neutralise the aqueous layer with a few drops of *dilute hydrochloric acid R*. The solution gives reaction (b) of tartrates (*2.3.1*).

TESTS
Solution S
Dissolve 0.25 g in *carbon dioxide-free water R* and dilute to 25.0 ml with the same solvent.

Appearance of solution
Solution S is clear (*2.2.1*) and not more intensely coloured than reference solution GY$_6$ or Y$_6$ (*2.2.2, Method II*).

pH (*2.2.3*)
3.3 to 3.9 for solution S.

Related substances
Liquid chromatography (*2.2.29*). *Carry out the test protected from light.*

Test solution Dissolve 50.0 mg of the substance to be examined in the mobile phase and dilute to 100.0 ml with the mobile phase.

Reference solution (a) Dilute 1.0 ml of the test solution to 100.0 ml with the mobile phase.

Reference solution (b) Dilute 2.0 ml of reference solution (a) to 100.0 ml with the mobile phase.

Reference solution (c) Expose 10 ml of reference solution (a) to daylight for 15 min before injection.

Reference solution (d) Dissolve 15.0 mg of *tartaric acid R* in the mobile phase and dilute to 100.0 ml with the mobile phase.

Column:
— *size: l* = 0.25 m, Ø = 4.6 mm;
— *stationary phase:* base-deactivated end-capped octadecylsilyl silica gel for chromatography R (5 μm).

Mobile phase To a mixture of 0.35 volumes of *triethylamine R* and 85 volumes of *water R* adjusted to pH 2.5 with *phosphoric acid R*, add 5 volumes of *tetrahydrofuran R* and 10 volumes of *methanol R*.

Flow rate 0.75 ml/min.

Detection Spectrophotometer at 226 nm.

Injection 20 μl.

Run time Twice the retention time of morantel.

System suitability Reference solution (c):
— *resolution:* minimum of 2 between the principal peak and the preceding peak ((*Z*)-isomer).

Limits:
— *any impurity apart from the peak due to tartaric acid:* not more than 0.5 times the area of the principal peak in the chromatogram obtained with reference solution (a) (0.5 per cent);
— *total:* not more than the area of the principal peak in the chromatogram obtained with reference solution (a) (1 per cent);
— *disregard limit:* the area of the principal peak in the chromatogram obtained with reference solution (b) (0.02 per cent).

Heavy metals (*2.4.8*)
Maximum 20 ppm.

1.0 g complies with test C. Prepare the reference solution using 2 ml of *lead standard solution (10 ppm Pb) R*.

Loss on drying (*2.2.32*)
Maximum 1.5 per cent, determined on 1.000 g by drying in an oven at 100-105 °C.

Sulphated ash (*2.4.14*)
Maximum 0.1 per cent, determined on 1.0 g.

ASSAY
Dissolve 0.280 g in 40 ml of *anhydrous acetic acid R*. Titrate with *0.1 M perchloric acid*, determining the end-point potentiometrically (*2.2.20*).

1 ml of *0.1 M perchloric acid* is equivalent to 37.04 mg of $C_{16}H_{22}N_2O_6S$.

STORAGE
Protected from light.

IMPURITIES

A. 1-methyl-2-[(*E*)-2-(4-methylthiophen-2-yl)ethenyl]-1,4,5,6-tetrahydropyrimidine,

B. 1-methyl-2-[(Z)-2-(3-methylthiophen-2-yl)ethenyl]-1,4,5,6-tetrahydropyrimidine,

C. 1,2-dimethyl-1,4,5,6-tetrahydropyrimidine,

and enantiomer

D. (1RS)-2-(1-methyl-1,4,5,6-tetrahydropyrimidin-2-yl)-1-(3-methylthiophen-2-yl)ethanol,

E. 3-methylthiophene-2-carbaldehyde.

Ph Eur

Nandrolone Laurate

$C_{30}H_{48}O_3$ 456.7   *26490-31-3*

Action and use
Anabolic steroid; androgen.

Preparation
Nandrolone Laurate Injection

DEFINITION
Nandrolone Laurate is 3-oxo-estr-4-en-17β-yl laurate. It contains not less than 97.0% and not more than 103.0% of $C_{30}H_{48}O_3$, calculated with reference to the dried substance.

CHARACTERISTICS
A white to creamy white, crystalline powder.

Practically insoluble in *water*; freely soluble in *chloroform*, in *ethanol (96%)*, in *ether*, in fixed oils and in esters of fatty acids.

IDENTIFICATION
A. The *infrared absorption spectrum*, Appendix II A, is concordant with the *reference spectrum* of nandrolone laurate *(RSV 30)*.

B. Carry out the method for *thin-layer chromatography*, Appendix III A, using a silica gel F_{254} precoated plate the surface of which has been modified by chemically-bonded octadecylsilyl groups (Whatman KC 18F plates are suitable) and a mixture of 20 volumes of *water*, 40 volumes of *acetonitrile* and 60 volumes of *propan-2-ol* as the mobile phase. Apply separately to the plate 5 μl of each of the following solutions. Solution (1) contains 0.5% w/v of the substance being examined in *chloroform*. Solution (2) contains 0.5% w/v of *nandrolone laurate BPCRS* in *chloroform*. For solution (3) mix equal volumes of solutions (1) and (2). After removal of the plate, allow it to dry in air until the odour of solvent is no longer detectable and heat at 100° for 10 minutes. Allow to cool and examine under *ultraviolet light (254 nm)*.
The principal spot in the chromatogram obtained with solution (1) corresponds to that in the chromatogram obtained with solution (2). The principal spot in the chromatogram obtained with solution (3) appears as a single, compact spot.

C. *Melting point*, about 47°, Appendix V A.

TESTS
Specific optical rotation
In a 2% w/v solution in *1,4-dioxan*, +31 to +35, calculated with reference to the dried substance, Appendix V F.

Nandrolone
Carry out the method for *thin-layer chromatography*, Appendix III A, using *silica gel G* as the coating substance and a mixture of 3 volumes of *acetone* and 7 volumes of *heptane* as the mobile phase. Apply separately to the plate 1 μl of each of two solutions in *chloroform* containing (1) 1.50% w/v of the substance being examined and (2) 0.030% w/v of *nandrolone BPCRS*. After removal of the plate, allow it to dry in air until the solvent has evaporated, spray with a 10% v/v solution of *sulphuric acid* in *ethanol (96%)*, heat at 105° for 30 minutes and examine under *ultraviolet light (365 nm)*. Any spot in the chromatogram obtained with solution (1) corresponding to nandrolone is not more intense than the spot in the chromatogram obtained with solution (2) (2%).

Loss on drying
When dried over *phosphorus pentoxide* at a pressure not exceeding 0.7 kPa for 24 hours, loses not more than 0.5% of its weight. Use 1 g.

Sulphated ash
Not more than 0.1%, Appendix IX A.

ASSAY
Dissolve 10 mg in sufficient *absolute ethanol* to produce 100 ml, dilute 5 ml to 50 ml with *absolute ethanol* and measure the *absorbance* of the resulting solution at the maximum at 240 nm, Appendix II B. Calculate the content of $C_{30}H_{48}O_3$, taking 380 as the value of A(1%, 1 cm) at the maximum at 240 nm.

STORAGE
Nandrolone Laurate should be protected from light and stored at a temperature 2° and 8°.

Nitroxinil

C$_7$H$_3$IN$_2$O$_3$ 290.0   *1689-89-0*

Action and use
Antihelminthic.

Preparation
Nitroxinil Injection

DEFINITION

Nitroxinil is 4-hydroxy-3-iodo-5-nitrobenzonitrile. It contains not less than 98.0% and not more than 101.0% of C$_7$H$_3$IN$_2$O$_3$, calculated with reference to the dried substance.

CHARACTERISTICS

A yellow to yellowish brown powder.

Practically insoluble in *water*; sparingly soluble in *ether*; slightly soluble in *ethanol (96%)*. It dissolves in solutions of alkali hydroxides.

IDENTIFICATION

A. The *infrared absorption spectrum*, Appendix II A, is concordant with the *reference spectrum* of nitroxinil *(RSV 31)*.

B. The *light absorption*, Appendix II B, in the range 220 to 350 nm of a 0.002% w/v solution in 0.01M *sodium hydroxide* exhibits maxima at 225 nm and at 271 nm. The *absorbance* at the maximum at 271 nm is about 1.3.

C. Heat with *sulphuric acid*; iodine vapour is evolved.

TESTS

Melting point
136° to 139°, Appendix V A.

Inorganic iodide
To 0.40 g add 0.35 g of N-*methylglucamine* and 10 ml of *water*, shake to dissolve and add sufficient *water* to produce 50 ml. To 10 ml of the resulting solution add 4 ml of 1M *sulphuric acid* and extract with three 10 ml quantities of *chloroform*. Add to the aqueous extract 1 ml of *hydrogen peroxide solution (100 vol)* and 1 ml of *chloroform*, shake for 2 minutes and allow to separate. Any purple colour produced in the chloroform layer is not more intense than that obtained in a solution prepared in the following manner. Add 2 ml of a 0.0026% w/v solution of *potassium iodide* to a mixture of 4 ml of 1M *sulphuric acid* and 8 ml of *water*, add 10 ml of *chloroform*, shake for 2 minutes, add to the aqueous layer 1 ml of *hydrogen peroxide solution (100 vol)* and 1 ml of *chloroform*, shake for 2 minutes and allow to separate (500 ppm of iodide).

Loss on drying
When dried to constant weight at 105°, loses not more than 1.0% of its weight. Use 1 g.

Sulphated ash
Not more than 0.1%, Appendix IX A.

ASSAY

Carry out the method for *oxygen-flask combustion for iodine*, Appendix VIII C, using 25 mg. Each ml of 0.02M *sodium thiosulphate VS* is equivalent to 0.9667 mg of C$_7$H$_3$IN$_2$O$_3$.

STORAGE

Nitroxinil should be protected from light.

Oxfendazole

(Oxfendazole for Veterinary Use, Ph Eur monograph 1458)

C$_{15}$H$_{13}$N$_3$O$_3$S   315.4   *53716-50-0*

Action and use
Antihelminthic.

Preparation
Oxfendazole Oral Suspension

Ph Eur

DEFINITION

Methyl [5-(phenylsulphinyl)-1*H*-benzimidazol-2-yl]carbamate.

Content
97.5 per cent to 100.5 per cent (dried substance).

CHARACTERS

Appearance
White or almost white powder.

Solubility
Practically insoluble in water, slightly soluble in alcohol and in methylene chloride.

It shows polymorphism.

IDENTIFICATION

Infrared absorption spectrophotometry *(2.2.24)*.

Comparison   oxfendazole CRS.

If the spectra obtained in the solid state show differences, dissolve the substance to be examined and the reference substance separately in *alcohol R*, evaporate to dryness and record new spectra using the residues.

TESTS

Related substances
Liquid chromatography *(2.2.29)*.

Test solution   Dissolve 25.0 mg of the substance to be examined in the mobile phase and dilute to 100.0 ml with the mobile phase.

Reference solution (a)   Dilute 1.0 ml of the test solution to 100.0 ml with the mobile phase.

Reference solution (b)   To 10 ml of the test solution, add 0.25 ml of *strong hydrogen peroxide solution R* and dilute to 25 ml with the mobile phase.

Reference solution (c)   Dissolve 5.0 mg of *fenbendazole CRS* and 10.0 mg of *oxfendazole impurity B CRS* in the mobile phase and dilute to 100.0 ml with the mobile phase. Dilute 1.0 ml to 20.0 ml with the mobile phase.

Reference solution (d) Dissolve 5 mg of *oxfendazole with impurity D CRS* in the mobile phase and dilute to 20 ml with the mobile phase (solution used for identification of impurity D).

Column:
— *size*: l = 0.25 m, Ø = 4.6 mm,
— *stationary phase*: spherical *end-capped octadecylsilyl silica gel for chromatography R* (5 μm) with a specific surface area of 350 m²/g, a pore size of 10 nm and a carbon loading of 14 per cent.

Mobile phase Mix 36 volumes of *acetonitrile R* and 64 volumes of a 2 g/l solution of *sodium pentanesulphonate R* adjusted to pH 2.7 with a 2.8 per cent *V/V* solution of *sulphuric acid R*.

Flow rate 1 ml/min.

Detection Spectrophotometer at 254 nm.

Injection 20 μl.

Run time 4 times the retention time of oxfendazole.

Retention time Oxfendazole = about 6.5 min.

System suitability Reference solution (b):
— *resolution*: minimum 4.0 between the 2 principal peaks corresponding to impurity C (1st peak) and oxfendazole (2nd peak).

Limits:
— *impurity A*: not more than the area of the corresponding peak in the chromatogram obtained with reference solution (c) (1.0 per cent),
— *impurity B*: not more than the area of the corresponding peak in the chromatogram obtained with reference solution (c) (2.0 per cent),
— *impurity C or D*: for each impurity, not more than the area of the principal peak in the chromatogram obtained with reference solution (a) (1.0 per cent),
— *any other impurity*: not more than 0.1 times the area of the principal peak in the chromatogram obtained with reference solution (a) (0.1 per cent),
— *total*: not more than 3 times the area of the principal peak in the chromatogram obtained with reference solution (a) (3.0 per cent),
— *disregard limit*: 0.05 times the area of the principal peak in the chromatogram obtained with reference solution (a) (0.05 per cent).

Loss on drying (2.2.32)
Maximum 0.5 per cent, determined on 1.000 g by drying in an oven at 100-105 °C at a pressure not exceeding 0.7 kPa for 2 h.

Sulphated ash (2.4.14)
Maximum 0.2 per cent, determined on 1.0 g.

ASSAY
Dissolve 0.250 g in 3 ml of *anhydrous formic acid R*. Add 40 ml of *anhydrous acetic acid R*. Titrate with *0.1 M perchloric acid*, determining the end-point potentiometrically (2.2.20).

1 ml of *0.1 M perchloric acid* is equivalent to 31.54 mg of $C_{15}H_{13}N_3O_3S$.

STORAGE
Protected from light.

IMPURITIES
A. fenbendazole,

B. X = SO₂, R = CO₂-CH₃: methyl [5-(phenylsulphonyl)-1*H*-benzimidazol-2-yl]carbamate,

C. X = SO, R = H: 5-(phenylsulphinyl)-1*H*-benzimidazol-2-amine,

D. *N,N'*-bis[5-(phenylsulphinyl)-1*H*-benzimidazol-2-yl]urea.

Ph Eur

Oxyclozanide

$C_{13}H_6Cl_5NO_3$ 401.5   *2277-92-1*

Action and use
Antihelminthic.

Preparation
Oxyclozanide Oral Suspension

DEFINITION
Oxyclozanide is 3,3',5,5',6-pentachloro-2'-hydroxysalicylanilide. It contains not less than 98.0% and not more than 101.0% of $C_{13}H_6Cl_5NO_3$, calculated with reference to the dried substance.

CHARACTERISTICS
A pale cream or cream coloured powder.

Very slightly soluble in *water*; freely soluble in *acetone*; soluble in *ethanol (96%)*; slightly soluble in *chloroform*.

IDENTIFICATION
A. The *infrared absorption spectrum*, Appendix II A, is concordant with the *reference spectrum* of oxyclozanide (*RSV 33*).

B. The *light absorption*, Appendix II B, in the range 250 to 350 nm of a 0.003% w/v solution in *acidified methanol* exhibits a maximum only at 300 nm. The *absorbance* at the maximum is about 0.76, Appendix II B.

C. *Melting point*, about 208°, Appendix V A.

TESTS

Ionisable chlorine
Dissolve 2 g in 100 ml of *methanol*, add 10 ml of 1.5M *nitric acid* and titrate with 0.1M *silver nitrate VS* determining the end point potentiometrically. Not more than 1.4 ml is required (0.25%).

Related substances
Carry out the method for *liquid chromatography*, Appendix III D, using a fixed-volume loop injector and the following solutions. Solution (1) contains 0.1% w/v of the substance being examined prepared by dissolving it in a suitable volume of *methanol* and slowly diluting with *water* containing 0.1% v/v *orthophosphoric acid* to give a solution containing about the same ratio of methanol to water as the mobile phase. For solution (2) dilute 1 volume of solution (1) to 100 volumes with the mobile phase.

The chromatographic procedure may be carried out using (a) a stainless steel column (20 cm × 5 mm) packed with *octadecylsilyl silica gel for chromatography* (5 μm) (Hypersil ODS is suitable), (b) a mixture of *methanol* and *water* containing 0.1% v/v of *orthophosphoric acid* (a mixture of 62 volumes of methanol and 38 volumes of water is usually suitable) as the mobile phase with a flow rate of 2 ml per minute and (c) a detection wavelength of 300 nm.

In the chromatogram obtained with solution (1) the area of any *secondary peak* with a retention time less than that of the principal peak is not greater than one third of the area of the principal peak in the chromatogram obtained with solution (2) (0.3%) and the area of any *secondary peak* with a retention time greater than that of the principal peak is not greater than the area of the principal peak in the chromatogram obtained with solution (2) (1%).

Loss on drying
When dried to constant weight at 60° at a pressure not exceeding 0.7 kPa, loses not more than 1.0% of its weight. Use 1 g.

Sulphated ash
Not more than 0.2%, Appendix IX A.

ASSAY
Dissolve 0.25 g in 75 ml of *anhydrous pyridine* and pass a current of *nitrogen* through the solution for 5 minutes. Carry out Method II for *non-aqueous titration*, Appendix VIII A, maintaining a current of *nitrogen* through the solution throughout the titration, using 0.1M *tetrabutylammonium hydroxide VS* as titrant and determining the end point potentiometrically. Each ml of 0.1M *tetrabutylammonium hydroxide VS* is equivalent to 20.07 mg of $C_{13}H_6Cl_5NO_3$.

Piperonyl Butoxide

$C_{19}H_{30}O_5$ 338.4   *51-03-6*

Action and use
Insecticide.

Preparation
Compound Pyrethrum Spray

DEFINITION
Piperonyl Butoxide is 5-[2-(2-butoxyethoxy)ethoxymethyl]-6-propyl-1,3-benzodioxole. It contains not less than 85.0% of $C_{19}H_{30}O_5$.

CHARACTERISTICS
A yellow or pale brown, oily liquid.

Very slightly soluble in *water*; miscible with *chloroform*, with *ethanol (96%)* with *ether* and with petroleum oils.

IDENTIFICATION
A. The *light absorption*, Appendix II B, in the range 220 to 350 nm of a 0.008% w/v solution in *absolute ethanol* exhibits well-defined maxima at 238 nm and 290 nm.
The *absorbances* at the maxima are about 1.2 and about 1.0, respectively.

B. Dissolve 0.1 mg in 0.1 ml of *acetonitrile*, add 10 mg of *gallic acid* and mix. Add 3 ml of *sulphuric acid* to form a lower layer, allow to stand for 1 minute and mix. A green colour is produced.

C. To 0.1 ml of a 0.05% w/v solution in *ethanol (96%)* add 5 ml of *tannic acid reagent*, shake vigorously for 1 minute and heat in a water bath for 5 minutes. A blue colour is produced.

TESTS
Refractive index
1.497 to 1.512, Appendix V E.

Weight per ml
1.050 to 1.065 g, Appendix V G.

Sulphated ash
Not more than 0.2%, Appendix IX A.

ASSAY
Carry out the method for *gas chromatography*, Appendix III B, using solutions in *chloroform* containing (1) 0.25% w/v of *piperonyl butoxide CRS* and 0.2% w/v of *tetraphenylethylene* (internal standard), (2) 0.25% w/v of the substance being examined and (3) 0.25% w/v of the substance being examined and 0.2% w/v of the internal standard.

The chromatographic procedure may be carried out using a glass column (1.0 m × 4 mm) packed with 3% w/w of phenyl methyl silicone fluid (50% phenyl) (OV 17 is suitable) on *acid-washed, silanised diatomaceous support* (100 to 120 mesh) and maintained at 235°.

Calculate the content of $C_{19}H_{30}O_5$ using the declared content of $C_{19}H_{30}O_5$ in *piperonyl butoxide CRS*.

Potassium Selenate

K$_2$SeO$_4$ 221.2   *7790-59-2*

Action and use
Used, with Alpha Tocopheryl Acetate, in the treatment of nutritional muscular dystrophy.

DEFINITION
Potassium Selenate contains not less than 97.0% and not more than 100.5% of K$_2$SeO$_4$, calculated with reference to the dried substance.

CHARACTERISTICS
Colourless crystals or a white, crystalline powder.

Freely soluble in *water*.

IDENTIFICATION
A. Yields the reactions characteristic of *potassium salts*, Appendix VI.

B. To a solution of 0.1 g in 3 ml of *water* add 1 ml of *hydrochloric acid* and 0.5 ml of *hydrazine hydrate* and boil. A red precipitate is produced.

C. Acidify 1 ml of a 1% w/v solution with 2M *hydrochloric acid* and add 0.15 ml of *barium chloride solution*. Wash the precipitate with *water* and boil with *hydrochloric acid*. Chlorine is evolved.

TESTS
Chloride
0.3 g complies with the *limit test for chlorides*, Appendix VII (170 ppm).

Selenite
Not more than 0.1%, calculated as SeO$_3$, when determined by the following method. Dissolve 2.0 g in 50 ml of *water*, add 50 ml of 9M *sulphuric acid*, 12 g of *disodium hydrogen orthophosphate* and 10 ml of 0.02M *potassium permanganate VS* and allow to stand for 20 minutes with occasional agitation. Titrate the excess of potassium permanganate with 0.1M *ammonium iron(II) sulphate VS*. Each ml of 0.02M *potassium permanganate VS* is equivalent to 6.348 mg of SeO$_3$.

Loss on drying
When dried to constant weight at 105°, loses not more than 0.1% of its weight. Use 1 g.

ASSAY
Dissolve 1 g in 60 ml of *water*, add 15 ml of *hydrochloric acid* and 5 ml of a 50% w/v solution of *hydrazine hydrate*, boil, heat on a water bath for 3 hours, and allow to stand overnight. Transfer the precipitated selenium to a weighed, sintered-glass crucible, wash with hot *water* until the washings are free from chloride ions, rinse with *absolute ethanol* and dry at 105° to constant weight. Correct for the amount of selenium present as selenite found in the test for selenite. Each mg of selenium is equivalent to 2.801 mg of K$_2$SeO$_4$.

Pyrethrum Flower
Dalmatian Insect Flowers
Preparations
Pyrethrum Extract
Pyrethrum Dusting Powder
Compound Pyrethrum Spray

DEFINITION
Pyrethrum Flower is the dried flower heads of *Chrysanthemum cinerariaefolium* Vis. It contains not less than 1.0% of pyrethrins of which not less than half consists of pyrethrin I.

CHARACTERISTICS
Odour, faint but characteristic.

Macroscopical
Capitula occurring loose or compressed into masses; individual capitula more or less flattened, about 6 to 12 mm in diameter, and commonly with a short piece of stalk attached; receptacle almost flat, about 5 to 10 mm in diameter, without paleae, surrounded by an involucre of 2 or 3 rows of brownish yellow lanceolate bracts; ray florets number about 15 to 23, disc florets about 200 to 300; corollas of ligulate florets pale brownish and shrivelled, oblong, about 16 mm long with three rounded apical teeth, the central tooth frequently smaller than the two lateral ones; in the middle region of the corolla about 17 veins present; corollas of the disc florets tubular, yellow, with five short lobes, and enclosing five epipetalous, syngenesious stamens; each ray and disc floret has an inferior five-ribbed oblong ovary about 5 mm long with a filiform style and bifid stigma and surmounted by a membranous tubular calyx about 1 mm long; ovaries and lower part of the corollas covered with numerous scattered shining oil glands.

Microscopical
Loosely arranged large-celled sclereids of the receptacle with moderately thickened walls and few pits; fragments of the corollas of the florets, those of the ray florets showing puckered papillae on the inner epidermis and sinuous-walled cells with a striated cuticle on the outer epidermis, those of the tubular florets composed of cells with slightly thickened walls with papillae occurring only on the lobes; ovoid to spherical glandular trichomes each composed of a short, biseriate stalk and a biseriate head with two or four cells; covering trichomes twisted, T-shaped with moderately thickened walls; numerous pollen grains, spherical, 34 to 40 µm in diameter with three pores and a warty and spiny exine; groups of small rectangular sclereids, some containing prisms of calcium oxalate, from the involucral bracts, ovaries and basal region of the calyx; parenchymatous cells of the calyx and ovaries containing tabular or diamond-shaped crystals of calcium oxalate; occasional cells containing cluster crystals from the base of the corolla of the disc florets; portions of stigmas with papillose tips.

Acid-insoluble ash
Not more than 1.0%, Appendix XI K.

ASSAY
Transfer 12.5 g in *No. 1000 powder* to an apparatus for the *continuous extraction of drugs*, Appendix XI F, and extract with *aromatic-free petroleum spirit (boiling range, 40° to 60°)* for 7 hours. Evaporate the extract to about 40 ml and allow to stand overnight at 0° to 5°. Add 20 ml of 0.5M *ethanolic potassium hydroxide* and boil under a reflux condenser for 45 minutes. Transfer the solution to a beaker and wash the flask with sufficient hot *water*, adding the washings to the

beaker, to produce a total volume of 200 ml. Boil until the volume is reduced to 150 ml, cool rapidly and transfer the solution to a stoppered flask, washing the beaker with three 20 ml quantities of *water* and transferring any gummy residue to the flask. Add 1 g of diatomaceous earth (Filtercel is suitable) and 10 ml of *barium chloride solution*, swirl gently and add sufficient *water* to produce 250 ml. Stopper the flask, shake vigorously until the separating liquid is clear and filter the suspension through a filter paper (Whatman No. 1 is suitable).

For pyrethrin I

Transfer 200 ml of the filtrate to a separating funnel, rinsing the measuring vessel with two 5 ml quantities of *water*, and add 0.05 ml of *phenolphthalein solution R1*. Neutralise the solution by the drop wise addition of *hydrochloric acid* and add 1 ml of *hydrochloric acid* in excess. Add 5 ml of a saturated solution of *sodium chloride* and 50 ml of *aromatic-free petroleum spirit (boiling range, 40° to 60°)*, shake vigorously for 1 minute, allow to separate, remove and retain the lower layer. Filter the petroleum spirit extract through absorbent cotton into a second separating funnel containing 10 ml of *water*. Return the aqueous layer to the first separating funnel and repeat the extraction with 50 ml and then with 25 ml of *aromatic-free petroleum spirit (boiling range, 40° to 60°)*, reserving the aqueous layer for the assay of pyrethrin II, and filtering the petroleum spirit extracts through the same absorbent cotton into the second separating funnel. Shake the combined petroleum spirit extracts and water for about 30 seconds and allow to separate; remove the lower layer and add it to the aqueous liquid reserved for the assay of pyrethrin II. Wash the combined petroleum spirit extracts with a further 10 ml of *water*, adding the washings to the reserved aqueous liquid.

To the petroleum spirit extracts add 5 ml of 0.1M *sodium hydroxide*, shake vigorously for 1 minute, allow to separate and remove the clear lower layer, washing the stem of the separating funnel with 1 ml of *water*. Repeat the extraction by shaking for about 30 seconds with two quantities of 2.5 ml and 1.5 ml of 0.1M *sodium hydroxide* and add the extracts to the alkaline extract. Add to the flask 10 ml of *mercury(II) sulphate solution*, stopper, swirl and allow to stand in the dark at 25° ±0.5° for exactly 60 minutes after the addition of the mercury(II) sulphate solution. Add 20 ml of *acetone* and 3 ml of a saturated solution of *sodium chloride*, heat to boiling on a water bath, allow the precipitate to settle and decant the supernatant liquid through a filter paper (Whatman No. 1 is suitable), retaining most of the precipitate in the flask. Wash the precipitate with 10 ml of *acetone*, again boil, allow to settle and decant through the same filter paper. Repeat the washing and decanting with three 10 ml quantities of hot *chloroform*. Transfer the filter paper to the flask, add 50 ml of a cooled mixture of three volumes of *hydrochloric acid* and two volumes of *water*, 1 ml of *strong iodine monochloride reagent* and 6 ml of *chloroform*. Titrate with 0.01M *potassium iodate VS*, running almost all the required volume of titrant into the flask in one portion. Continue the titration, shaking the flask vigorously for 30 seconds after each addition of the titrant, until the chloroform is colourless. Repeat the operation without the extract; the difference between the titrations represents the amount of potassium iodate required. Each ml of 0.01M *potassium iodate VS* is equivalent to 5.7 mg of pyrethrin I.

For pyrethrin II

Transfer the combined aqueous liquids reserved in the Assay for pyrethrin I to a beaker, cover with a watch glass and evaporate to 50 ml within 35 to 45 minutes. Cool, washing the underside of the watch glass with not more than 5 ml of *water* and adding the washings to the beaker. Filter through absorbent cotton into a separating funnel, washing with successive quantities of 10, 7.5, 7.5, 5 and 5 ml of *water*. Saturate the aqueous liquid with *sodium chloride*, add 10 ml of *hydrochloric acid* and 50 ml of *ether*, shake for 1 minute, allow to separate, and remove the lower layer. Repeat the extraction successively with 50, 25 and 25 ml of *ether*. Wash the combined ether extracts with three 10 ml quantities of a saturated solution of *sodium chloride* and transfer the ether layer to a flask with the aid of 10 ml of *ether*. Remove the bulk of the ether by distillation and remove the remainder with a gentle current of air and dry the residue at 100° for 10 minutes, removing any residual acid fumes with a gentle current of air. Add 2 ml of *ethanol (96%)* previously neutralised to *phenolphthalein solution R1* and 0.05 ml of *phenolphthalein solution R1*, swirl to dissolve the residue, add 20 ml of *carbon dioxide-free water* and titrate rapidly with 0.02M *sodium hydroxide VS* until the colour changes to brownish pink and persists for 30 seconds, keeping the flask stoppered between additions of alkali. Repeat the operation using the aqueous liquid reserved for the repeat operation in the Assay for pyrethrin I. The difference between the titrations represents the volume of 0.02M *sodium hydroxide VS* required. Each ml of 0.02M *sodium hydroxide VS* is equivalent to 3.74 mg of pyrethrin II.

Ronidazole

$C_6H_8N_4O_4$	200.2	7681-76-7

Action and use

Antiprotozoal.

DEFINITION

Ronidazole is (1-methyl-5-nitroimidazol-2-yl)methyl carbamate. It contains not less than 98.5% and not more than 101.0% of $C_6H_8N_4O_4$, calculated with reference to the anhydrous substance.

CHARACTERISTICS

A white to yellowish brown powder; odourless or almost odourless.

Slightly soluble in water, in chloroform and in ethanol (96%); very slightly soluble in ether.

IDENTIFICATION

A. The *infrared absorption spectrum*, Appendix II A, is concordant with the *reference spectrum* of ronidazole (*RSV 36*).

B. The *light absorption*, Appendix II B, in the range 230 to 350 nm of a 0.002% w/v solution in 0.1M *methanolic hydrochloric acid* exhibits a maximum only at 270 nm. The *absorbance* at the maximum is about 0.64.

C. *Melting point*, about 167°, Appendix V A.

TESTS

Colour of solution
A 0.5% w/v solution in *methanol* is not more intensely coloured than *reference solution Y₆, Appendix IV B*, Method II.

(1-Methyl-5-nitroimidazol-2-yl)methanol
Carry out the method for *thin-layer chromatography*, Appendix III A, using *silica gel GF₂₅₄* as the coating substance and a mixture of 5 volumes of *glacial acetic acid*, 5 volumes of *methanol* and 80 volumes of *toluene* as the mobile phase. Apply separately to the plate 20 μl of each of two solutions in *acetone* containing (1) 1.0% w/v of the substance being examined and (2) 0.0050% w/v of *(1-methyl-5-nitroimidazol-2-yl)methanol BPCRS*. After removal of the plate, allow it to dry in air and examine under *ultraviolet light (254 nm)*. Any spot in the chromatogram obtained with solution (1) corresponding to (1-methyl-5-nitroimidazol-2-yl)methanol is not more intense than the spot in the chromatogram obtained with solution (2) (0.5%).

Water
Not more than 0.5% w/w, Appendix IX C. Use 5 g.

Sulphated ash
Not more than 0.1%, Appendix IX A.

ASSAY
Carry out Method I for *non-aqueous titration*, Appendix VIII A, using 0.3 g and determining the end point potentiometrically. Each ml of 0.1M *perchloric acid VS* is equivalent to 20.02 mg C₆H₈N₄O₄.

STORAGE
Ronidazole should be protected from light.

Sodium Selenite

Na₂SeO₃   172.9   *10102-18-8*

Action and use
Used in treatment of selenium deficiency.

DEFINITION
Sodium Selenite contains not less than 44.0% and not more than 46.0% of Se, calculated with reference to the dried substance.

CHARACTERISTICS
White to slightly greyish pink, granular powder.

Freely soluble in *water*; practically insoluble in *ethanol (96%)* and in *ether*.

Dissolve 2 g in carbon dioxide-free water *prepared from distilled water and dilute to 100 ml with the same solvent (solution S)*.

IDENTIFICATION
A. Dissolve 50 mg in 5 ml of 7M *hydrochloric acid*, add 2 ml of 0.1M *sodium thiosulphate* and heat to boiling. A reddish orange precipitate is produced.

B. 1 ml of solution S yields the reactions characteristic of *sodium salts*, Appendix VI.

TESTS

Clarity of solution
Solution S is not more opalescent than *reference suspension II*, Appendix IV A.

Alkalinity
To 50 ml of solution S add 0.2 ml of *thymolphthalein solution*. Not more than 0.25 ml of 1M *hydrochloric acid VS* is required to change the colour of the solution from dark blue to very pale blue.

Chloride
Dilute 2.5 ml of solution S to 15 ml with *water*. The solution complies with the *limit test for chlorides*, Appendix VII (0.1%).

Sulphate
Dilute 3.75 ml of solution S to 15 ml with *distilled water*. The solution complies with the *limit test for sulphates*, Appendix VII (0.2%).

Loss on drying
When dried to constant weight at 100° to 105°, loses not more than 1.0% of its weight. Use 1 g.

ASSAY
Dissolve 1 g in 100 ml of *water*, add 30 ml of *hydrochloric acid* and heat just to boiling. Remove from the heat, add carefully, while shaking, 100 ml of *sulphuric acid (96% w/w)*, heat the solution to boiling, cover with a watch glass and heat in a water bath for 2 hours. Check that the precipitation of selenium is complete by adding a further 10 ml of *sulphuric acid (96% w/w)* and then allow to cool. Filter through a tared, sintered-glass filter (16) and wash the precipitate with *water* until the washings are free from chloride. Dry the filter at 100° to 105°, reweigh and determine the weight of Se obtained.

Spectinomycin Sulphate Tetrahydrate

(Spectinomycin Sulphate Tetrahydrate for Veterinary Use, Ph Eur monograph 1658)

Compound	R	R'	Molec. Formula	M_r
spectinomycin	R + R' = O		C₁₄H₂₆N₂O₁₁S,4H₂O	502.5
(4R)-dihydro-spectinomycin	OH	H	C₁₄H₂₈N₂O₁₁S,4H₂O	504.5

Ph Eur

DEFINITION
Mixture of (2R,4aR,5aR,6S,7S,8R,9S,9aR,10aS)-4a,7,9-trihydroxy-2-methyl-6,8-bis(methylamino)decahydro-4H-pyrano[2,3-b][1,4]benzodioxin-4-one sulphate tetrahydrate (spectinomycin sulphate tetrahydrate) and (2R,4R,4aS,5aR,6S,7S,8R,9S,9aR,10aS)-2-methyl-6,8-bis(methylamino)decahydro-2H-pyrano[2,3-b][1,4]benzodioxine-4,4a,7,9-tetrol sulphate tetrahydrate ((4R)-dihydrospectinomycin sulphate tetrahydrate).

It is produced by *Streptomyces spectabilis* or by any other means.

Content:
— *(4R)-dihydrospectinomycin sulphate*: maximum 2.0 per cent (anhydrous substance);

— *sum of the contents of spectinomycin sulphate and
(4R)-dihydrospectinomycin sulphate*: 93.0 per cent to
102.0 per cent (anhydrous substance).

CHARACTERS

Appearance
White or almost white powder.

Solubility
Freely soluble in water, insoluble in ethanol (96 per cent).

IDENTIFICATION

A. Infrared absorption spectrophotometry (*2.2.24*).

Comparison   spectinomycin sulphate tetrahydrate CRS.

B. Dilute 1.0 ml of solution S (see Tests) to 10 ml with
water R. The solution gives reaction (a) of sulphates (*2.3.1*).

TESTS

Solution S
Dissolve 2.50 g in *carbon dioxide-free water R* and dilute to
25.0 ml with the same solvent.

Appearance of solution
Solution S is clear (*2.2.1*) and colourless (*2.2.2, Method II*).

pH (*2.2.3*)
3.8 to 5.6 for solution S.

Specific optical rotation (*2.2.7*)
+ 10.0 to + 14.0 (anhydrous substance).

Dissolve 2.50 g in an 8 ml/l solution of *concentrated
ammonia R1* and dilute to 25.0 ml with the same solvent.
Allow the solution to stand at room temperature for not less
than 30 min and not more than 2 h prior to determination.

Related substances
Liquid chromatography (*2.2.29*). *In order to avoid the
formation of anomers, prepare the solutions immediately before use.*

Test solution   Dissolve 15.0 mg of the substance to be
examined in the mobile phase and dilute to 100.0 ml with
the mobile phase.

Reference solution (a)   Dissolve 3 mg of *spectinomycin for
system suitability CRS* in the mobile phase and dilute to 20 ml
with the mobile phase.

Reference solution (b)   Dilute 1.0 ml of the test solution to
100.0 ml with the mobile phase.

Reference solution (c)   Dilute 3.0 ml of reference solution (b)
to 10.0 ml with the mobile phase.

Column:
— *size: l = 0.25 m, Ø = 4.6 mm;*
— *stationary phase: octylsilyl silica gel for chromatography R*
(5 µm);
— *temperature:* ambient and constant.

Mobile phase   Dissolve 4.2 g of *oxalic acid R* and 2.0 ml of
heptafluorobutyric acid R in *water R* and dilute to 1000 ml
with *water R*; adjust to pH 3.2 with *sodium hydroxide
solution R*; add 105 ml of *acetonitrile R* and mix; filter through
a 0.45 µm filter and degas with *helium for chromatography R*
for 10 min.

Flow rate   1.0 ml/min.

Post-column solution   carbonate-free sodium hydroxide solution R
diluted with *carbon dioxide-free water R* to obtain a final
concentration of NaOH of 21 g/l. Degas the solution with
helium for chromatography R for 10 min before use. Add it
pulse-less to the column effluent using a 375 µl polymeric
mixing coil.

Post-column flow rate   0.5 ml/min.

Detection   Pulsed amperometric detection or equivalent with
a gold indicator electrode having preferably a diameter of

1.4 mm or greater, a suitable reference electrode and a
stainless steel counter electrode, held at + 0.12 V detection,
+ 0.70 V oxidation and − 0.60 V reduction potentials
respectively, with pulse durations according to the instrument
used. Keep the detection cell at ambient and constant
temperature. Clean the gold indicator electrode with an
eraser and damp precision wipe prior to start-up of the
system to enhance the detector sensitivity and increase the
signal-to-noise ratio.

Injection   20 µl.

Run time   1.5 times the retention time of spectinomycin.

Identification of impurities   Use the chromatogram supplied
with *spectinomycin for system suitability CRS* and the
chromatogram obtained with reference solution (a) to
identify the peaks due to impurities A, D and E.

Relative retention   With reference to spectinomycin (retention
time = 11 min to 20 min): impurity A = about 0.5;
impurity D = about 0.7; impurity E = about 0.9;
(4R)-dihydrospectinomycin = about 1.3.

System suitability   Reference solution (a):
— *resolution*: minimum 1.5 between the peaks due to
impurity E and spectinomycin.

Limits:
— *correction factor*: for the calculation of content, multiply the
peak area of impurity A by 0.4;
— *impurities A, E*: for each impurity, not more than the area
of the principal peak in the chromatogram obtained with
reference solution (b) (1.0 per cent);
— *impurity D*: not more than 4 times the area of the
principal peak in the chromatogram obtained with
reference solution (b) (4.0 per cent);
— *any other impurity*: for each impurity, not more than the
area of the principal peak in the chromatogram obtained
with reference solution (b) (1.0 per cent);
— *total*: not more than 6 times the area of the principal peak
in the chromatogram obtained with reference solution (b)
(6.0 per cent);
— *disregard limit*: the area of the principal peak in the
chromatogram obtained with reference solution (c)
(0.3 per cent); disregard the peak due to
(4R)-dihydrospectinomycin.

Water (*2.5.12*)
12.0 per cent to 16.5 per cent, determined on 0.100 g.

Sulphated ash (*2.4.14*)
Maximum 1.0 per cent, determined on 1.0 g.

Bacterial endotoxins (*2.6.14*)
Less than 0.17 IU/mg, if intended for use in the manufacture
of parenteral dosage forms without a further appropriate
procedure for the removal of bacterial endotoxins. Prepare
the solutions using a 0.42 per cent *m/m* solution of *sodium
hydrogen carbonate R*.

ASSAY
Liquid chromatography (*2.2.29*) as described in the test
for related substances with the following modifications.

Test solution   Dissolve 40.0 mg of the substance to be
examined in *water R* and dilute to 50.0 ml with the same
solvent. Allow to stand for not less than 15 h and not more
than 72 h (formation of anomers). Dilute 5.0 ml of this
solution to 50.0 ml with the mobile phase.

Reference solution   Dissolve 40.0 mg of *spectinomycin
hydrochloride CRS* (containing (4R)-dihydrospectinomycin) in
water R and dilute to 50.0 ml with the same solvent. Allow to
stand for the same period of time as the test

solution (formation of anomers). Dilute 5.0 ml of this solution to 50.0 ml with the mobile phase.

System suitability:
— *repeatability*: maximum relative standard deviation of 3.0 per cent for the principal peak after 6 injections of the reference solution.

Calculate the sum of the percentage contents of spectinomycin sulphate and (4*R*)-dihydrospectinomycin sulphate from the declared contents of $C_{14}H_{26}Cl_2N_2O_7$ and $C_{14}H_{28}Cl_2N_2O_7$ in *spectinomycin hydrochloride CRS*, applying a correction factor of 1.062.

STORAGE
In an airtight container. If the substance is sterile, store in a sterile, airtight, tamper-proof container.

IMPURITIES
Specified impurities   A, D, E.

Other detectable impurities   (The following substances would, if present at a sufficient level, be detected by one or other of the tests in the monograph. They are limited by the general acceptance criterion for other/unspecified impurities and/or by the general monograph *Substances for pharmaceutical use (2034)*. It is therefore not necessary to identify these impurities for demonstration of compliance. See also *5.10*. *Control of impurities in substances for pharmaceutical use):* B, C, F, G.

A. 1,3-dideoxy-1,3-bis(methylamino)-*myo*-inositol (actinamine),

B. (2*S*,3*RS*,5*R*)-3-hydroxy-5-methyl-2-[[(1*r*,2*R*,3*S*,4*r*,5*R*,6*S*)-2,4,6-trihydroxy-3,5-bis(methylamino)cyclohexyl]oxy] tetrahydrofuran-3-carboxylic acid (actinospectinoic acid),

C. R1 = CH₃, R2 = R4 = H, R3 = OH:
(2*R*,4*S*,4a*S*,5a*R*,6*S*,7*S*,8*R*,9*S*,9a*R*,10a*S*)-2-methyl-6,8-bis(methylamino)decahydro-2*H*-pyrano[2,3-*b*][1,4] benzodioxine-4,4a,7,9-tetrol ((4*S*)-dihydrospectinomycin),

D. R1 = CH₃, R2 = H, R3 = R4 = OH:
(2*R*,3*R*,4*S*,4a*S*,5a*R*,6*S*,7*S*,8*R*,9*S*,9a*R*,10a*S*)-2-methyl-6,8-bis(methylamino)decahydro-2*H*-pyrano[2,3-*b*][1,4] benzodioxine-3,4,4a,7,9-pentol (dihydroxyspectinomycin),

E. R1 = R4 = H, R2 + R3 = O:
(2*R*,4a*R*,5a*R*,6*S*,7*R*,8*R*,9*S*,9a*R*,10a*S*)-6-amino-4a,7,9-trihydroxy-2-methyl-8-(methylamino)decahydro-4*H*-pyrano [2,3-*b*][1,4]benzodioxin-4-one (*N*-desmethylspectinomycin),

G. R1 = CH₃, R2 + R3 = O, R4 = OH:
(2*R*,3*S*,4a*R*,5a*R*,6*S*,7*S*,8*R*,9*S*,9a*R*,10a*S*)-3,4a,7,9-tetrahydroxy-2-methyl-6,8-bis(methylamino)decahydro-4*H*-pyrano[2,3-*b*][1,4]benzodioxin-4-one (tetrahydroxyspectinomycin),

F. (2*S*,4*S*,6*R*)-4-hydroxy-6-methyl-2-[[(1*r*,2*R*,3*S*,4*r*,5*R*,6*S*)-2,4,6-trihydroxy-3,5-bis(methylamino)cyclohexyl]oxy] dihydro-2*H*-pyran-3(4*H*)-one (triol spectinomycin).

Ph Eur

Spiramycin
(Ph Eur monograph 0293)

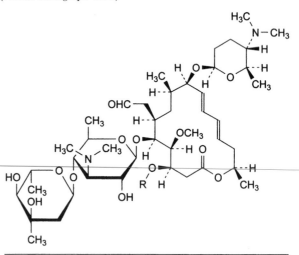

Compound	R	Molec Formula	M_r
Spiramycin I	H	$C_{43}H_{74}N_2O_{14}$	843.1
Spiramycin II	CO-CH₃	$C_{45}H_{76}N_2O_{15}$	885.1
Spiramycin III	CO-CH₂-CH₃	$C_{46}H_{78}N_2O_{15}$	899.1

8025-81-8

Action and use
Antibacterial.

Ph Eur

DEFINITION
Macrolide antibiotic produced by the growth of certain strains of *Streptomyces ambofaciens* or obtained by any other

means. The main component is (4R,5S,6S,7R,9R,10R,11E,13E,16R)-6-[[3,6-dideoxy-4-O-(2,6-dideoxy-3-C-methyl-α-L-*ribo*-hexopyranosyl)-3-(dimethylamino)-β-D-glucopyranosyl]oxy]-4-hydroxy-5-methoxy-9,16-dimethyl-7-(2-oxoethyl)-10-[[2,3,4,6-tetradeoxy-4-(dimethylamino)-D-*erythro*-hexopyranosyl]oxy]oxacyclohexadeca-11,13-dien-2-one (spiramycin I; M_r 843). Spiramycin II (4-O-acetylspiramycin I) and spiramycin III (4-O-propanoylspiramycin I) are also present.

Potency
Minimum 4100 IU/mg (dried substance).

CHARACTERS

Appearance
White or slightly yellowish powder, slightly hygroscopic.

Solubility
Slightly soluble in water, freely soluble in acetone, in ethanol (96 per cent) and in methanol.

IDENTIFICATION

A. Dissolve 0.10 g in *methanol R* and dilute to 100.0 ml with the same solvent. Dilute 1.0 ml of the solution to 100.0 ml with *methanol R*. Examined between 220 nm and 350 nm (*2.2.25*), the solution shows an absorption maximum at 232 nm. The specific absorbance at the absorption maximum is about 340.

B. Thin-layer chromatography (*2.2.27*).

Test solution Dissolve 40 mg of the substance to be examined in *methanol R* and dilute to 10 ml with the same solvent.

Reference solution (a) Dissolve 40 mg of *spiramycin CRS* in *methanol R* and dilute to 10 ml with the same solvent.

Reference solution (b) Dissolve 40 mg of *erythromycin A CRS* in *methanol R* and dilute to 10 ml with the same solvent.

Plate TLC silica gel G plate R.

Mobile phase The upper layer of a mixture of 4 volumes of *2-propanol R*, 8 volumes of a 150 g/l solution of *ammonium acetate R* previously adjusted to pH 9.6 with *strong sodium hydroxide solution R*, and 9 volumes of *ethyl acetate R*.

Application 5 µl.

Development Over 3/4 of the plate.

Drying In air.

Detection Spray with *anisaldehyde solution R1* and heat at 110 °C for 5 min.

Results The principal spot in the chromatogram obtained with the test solution is similar in position, colour and size to the principal spot in the chromatogram obtained with reference solution (a). If in the chromatogram obtained with the test solution 1 or 2 spots occur with R_f values slightly higher than that of the principal spot, these spots are similar in position and colour to the secondary spots in the chromatogram obtained with reference solution (a) and differ from the spots in the chromatogram obtained with reference solution (b).

C. Dissolve 0.5 g in 10 ml of *0.05 M sulphuric acid* and add 25 ml of *water R*. Adjust to about pH 8 with *0.1 M sodium hydroxide* and dilute to 50 ml with *water R*. To 5 ml of this solution add 2 ml of a mixture of 1 volume of *water R* and 2 volumes of *sulphuric acid R*. A brown colour develops.

TESTS

pH (*2.2.3*)
8.5 to 10.5.
Dissolve 0.5 g in 5 ml of *methanol R* and dilute to 100 ml with *carbon dioxide-free water R*.

Specific optical rotation (*2.2.7*)
− 80 to − 85 (dried substance).
Dissolve 1.00 g in a 10 per cent *V/V* solution of *dilute acetic acid R* and dilute to 50.0 ml with the same acid solution.

Composition
Liquid chromatography (*2.2.29*) as described in the test for related substances.

Injection Test solution and reference solution (a).

Calculate the percentage content using the declared content of spiramycins I, II and III in *spiramycin CRS*.

Composition of spiramycins (dried substance):
— *spiramycin I*: minimum 80.0 per cent,
— *spiramycin II*: maximum 5.0 per cent,
— *spiramycin III*: maximum 10.0 per cent,
— *sum of spiramycins I, II and III*: minimum 90.0 per cent.

Related substances
Liquid chromatography (*2.2.29*).

Prepare the solutions immediately before use.

Test solution Dissolve 25.0 mg of the substance to be examined in a mixture of 3 volumes of *methanol R* and 7 volumes of *water R* and dilute to 25.0 ml with the same mixture of solvents.

Reference solution (a) Dissolve 25.0 mg of *spiramycin CRS* in a mixture of 3 volumes of *methanol R* and 7 volumes of *water R* and dilute to 25.0 ml with the same mixture of solvents.

Reference solution (b) Dilute 2.0 ml of reference solution (a) to 100.0 ml with a mixture of 3 volumes of *methanol R* and 7 volumes of *water R*.

Reference solution (c) Dissolve 5 mg of *spiramycin CRS* in 15.0 ml of *buffer solution pH 2.2 R* and dilute to 25.0 ml with *water R*, then heat in a water-bath at 60 °C for 30 min.

Blank solution methanol R, water R (3:7 *V/V*).

Column:
— *size*: l = 0.25 m, Ø = 4.6 mm,
— *stationary phase*: octadecylsilyl silica gel for chromatography R (5 µm) (polar embedded octadecylsilyl methylsilica gel), with a pore size of 12.5 nm and a carbon loading of 15 per cent,
— *temperature*: 70 °C.

Mobile phase Mix 5 volumes of a 34.8 g/l solution of *dipotassium hydrogen phosphate R* previously adjusted to pH 6.5 with a 27.2 g/l solution of *potassium dihydrogen phosphate R*, 40 volumes of *acetonitrile R* and 55 volumes of *water R*.

Flow rate 1.0 ml/min.

Detection Spectrophotometer at 232 nm.

Injection 20 µl of the blank solution, the test solution and reference solutions (b) and (c).

Run time 3 times the retention time of spiramycin I.

Identification of spiramycins Use the chromatogram supplied with *spiramycin CRS* and the chromatogram obtained with reference solution (a) to identify the peaks due to spiramycins I, II and III.

Relative retention With reference to spiramycin I (retention time = 20 min to 30 min):
spiramycin II = about 1.4; spiramycin III = about 2.0;

impurity F = about 0.41; impurity A = about 0.45; impurity D = about 0.50; impurity G = 0.66; impurity B = about 0.73; impurity H = about 0.87; impurity E = about 2.5.

If necessary adjust the composition of the mobile phase by changing the amount of acetonitrile.

System suitability   Reference solution (c):
— *resolution*: minimum 10.0 between the peaks due to impurity A and spiramycin I.

Limits:
— *impurities A, B, C, D, E, F, G, H*: for each impurity, not more than the area of the principal peak in the chromatogram obtained with reference solution (b) (2.0 per cent),
— *any other impurity*: for each impurity, not more than the area of the principal peak in the chromatogram obtained with reference solution (b) (2.0 per cent),
— *total*: not more than 5 times the area of the principal peak in the chromatogram obtained with reference solution (b) (10.0 per cent),
— *disregard limit*: 0.05 times the area of the principal peak in the chromatogram obtained with reference solution (b) (0.1 per cent); disregard any peak due to the blank and the peaks due to spiramycins I, II and III.

Heavy metals (*2.4.8*)
Maximum 20 ppm.

1.0 g complies with limit test F. Prepare the reference solution using 2 ml of *lead standard solution (10 ppm Pb) R*.

Loss on drying (*2.2.32*)
Maximum 3.5 per cent, determined on 0.500 g by drying at 80 °C over *diphosphorus pentoxide R* at a pressure not exceeding 670 Pa for 6 h.

Sulphated ash (*2.4.14*)
Maximum 0.1 per cent, determined on 1.0 g.

ASSAY
Carry out the microbiological assay of antibiotics (*2.7.2*).

STORAGE
In an airtight container.

IMPURITIES
Specified impurities   A, B, C, D, E, F, G, H.

B. R1 = H, R2 = osyl, R3 = CH$_2$-CH$_2$OH:
(4R,5S,6S,7R,9R,10R,11E,13E,16R)-6-[[3,6-dideoxy-4-O-(2,6-dideoxy-3-C-methyl-α-L-*ribo*-hexopyranosyl)-3-(dimethylamino)-β-D-glucopyranosyl]oxy]-4-hydroxy-7-(2-hydroxyethyl)-5-methoxy-9,16-dimethyl-10-[[2,3,4,6-tetradeoxy-4-(dimethylamino)-β-D-*erythro*-hexopyranosyl]oxy]oxacyclohexadeca-11,13-dien-2-one (spiramycin IV),

C. R1 = H, R2 = osyl, R3 = C(=CH$_2$)-CHO:
(4R,5S,6S,7S,9R,10R,11E,13E,16R)-6-[[3,6-dideoxy-4-O-(2,6-dideoxy-3-C-methyl-α-L-*ribo*-hexopyranosyl)-3-(dimethylamino)-β-D-glucopyranosyl]oxy]-7-(1-formylethenyl)-4-hydroxy-5-methoxy-9,16-dimethyl-10-[[2,3,4,6-tetradeoxy-4-(dimethylamino)-β-D-*erythro*-hexopyranosyl]oxy]oxacyclohexadeca-11,13-dien-2-one (17-methylenespiramycin I),

E. R1 = H, R2 = osyl, R3 = CH$_2$-CH$_3$:
(4R,5S,6S,7S,9R,10R,11E,13E,16R)-6-[[3,6-dideoxy-4-O-(2,6-dideoxy-3-C-methyl-α-L-*ribo*-hexopyranosyl)-3-(dimethylamino)-β-D-glucopyranosyl]oxy]-7-ethyl-4-hydroxy-5-methoxy-9,16-dimethyl-10-[[2,3,4,6-tetradeoxy-4-(dimethylamino)-β-D-erythro-hexopyranosyl]oxy]oxacyclohexadeca-11,13-dien-2-one (18-deoxy-18-dihydrospiramycin I or DSPM),

G. R1 = CO-CH$_3$, R2 = OH, R3 = CH$_2$-CHO:
(4R,5S,6S,7R,9R,10R,11E,13E,16R)-6-[[3,6-dideoxy-3-(dimethylamino)-β-D-glucopyranosyl]oxy]-5-methoxy-9,16-dimethyl-2-oxo-7-(2-oxoethyl)-10-[[2,3,4,6-tetradeoxy-4-(dimethylamino)-β-D-*erythro*-hexopyranosyl]oxy]oxacyclohexadeca-11,13-dien-4-yl acetate (neospiramycin II),

H. R1 = CO-C$_2$H$_5$, R2 = OH, R3 = CH$_2$-CHO:
(4R,5S,6S,7R,9R,10R,11E,13E,16R)-6-[[3,6-dideoxy-3-(dimethylamino)-β-D-glucopyranosyl]oxy]-5-methoxy-9,16-dimethyl-2-oxo-7-(2-oxoethyl)-10-[[2,3,4,6-tetradeoxy-4-(dimethylamino)-β-D-*erythro*-hexopyranosyl]oxy]oxacyclohexadeca-11,13-dien-4-yl propanoatate (neospiramycin III),

D. (4R,5S,6S,7R,9R,10R,11E,13E,16R)-6-[[3,6-dideoxy-4-O-(2,6-dideoxy-3-C-methyl-α-L-*ribo*-hexopyranosyl)-3-(dimethylamino)-β-D-glucopyranosyl]oxy]-10-[(2,6-dideoxy-3-C-methyl-α-L-*ribo*-hexopyranosyl)oxy]-4-hydroxy-5-methoxy-9,16-dimethyl-7-(2-oxoethyl)oxacyclohexadeca-11,13-dien-2-one (spiramycin V),

A. R1 = H, R2 = OH, R3 = CH$_2$-CHO:
(4R,5S,6S,7R,9R,10R,11E,13E,16R)-6-[[3,6-dideoxy-3-(dimethylamino)-β-D-glucopyranosyl]oxy]-4-hydroxy-5-methoxy-9,16-dimethyl-7-(2-oxoethyl)-10-[[2,3,4,6-tetradeoxy-4-(dimethylamino)-β-D-*erythro*-hexopyranosyl]oxy]oxacyclohexadeca-11,13-dien-2-one (neospiramycin I),

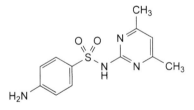

F. spiramycin dimer.

Ph Eur

Sulfadimidine

(Ph Eur monograph 0295)

$C_{12}H_{14}N_4O_2S$ 278.3   57-68-1

Action and use
Sulfonamide antibacterial.

Preparation
Sulfadimidine Injection
Sulfadimidine Tablets

Ph Eur

DEFINITION
Sulfadimidine contains not less than 99.0 per cent and not more than the equivalent of 101.0 per cent of 4-amino-*N*-(4,6-dimethylpyrimidin-2-yl)benzenesulphonamide, calculated with reference to the dried substance.

CHARACTERS
White or almost white powder or crystals, very slightly soluble in water, soluble in acetone, slightly soluble in alcohol. It dissolves in solutions of alkali hydroxides and in dilute mineral acids.

It melts at about 197 °C, with decomposition.

IDENTIFICATION
First identification   A, B.
Second identification   B, C, D.

A. Examine by infrared absorption spectrophotometry *(2.2.24)*, comparing with the spectrum obtained with *sulfadimidine CRS*. Examine the substances prepared as discs.

B. Examine the chromatograms obtained in the test for related substances. The principal spot in the chromatogram obtained with test solution (a) corresponds in position and size to the principal spot in the chromatogram obtained with reference solution (a).

C. Place 3 g in a dry tube. Immerse the lower part of the tube, inclined at 45°, in a silicone oil bath and heat to about 270 °C. The substance to be examined decomposes and a white or yellowish-white sublimate is formed which, after recrystallisation from *toluene R* and drying at 100 °C, melts *(2.2.14)* at 150 °C to 154 °C.

D. Dissolve about 5 mg in 10 ml of *1 M hydrochloric acid*. Dilute 1 ml of the solution to 10 ml with *water R*. The solution, without further acidification, gives the reaction of primary aromatic amines *(2.3.1)*.

TESTS
Appearance of solution
Dissolve 0.5 g in a mixture of 5 ml of *dilute sodium hydroxide solution R* and 5 ml of *water R*. The solution is not more intensely coloured than reference solution Y_5, BY_5 or GY_5 *(2.2.2, Method II)*.

Acidity
To 1.25 g, finely powdered, add 25 ml of *carbon dioxide-free water R*. Heat at about 70 °C for 5 min. Cool in iced water for about 15 min and filter. To 20 ml of the filtrate add 0.1 ml of *bromothymol blue solution R1*. Not more than 0.2 ml of *0.1 M sodium hydroxide* is required to change the colour of the indicator.

Related substances
Examine by thin-layer chromatography *(2.2.27)*, using *silica gel GF_{254} R* as the coating substance.

Test solution (a)   Dissolve 20 mg of the substance to be examined in 3 ml of a mixture of 2 volumes of *concentrated ammonia R* and 48 volumes of *methanol R* and dilute to 5.0 ml with the same mixture of solvents.

Test solution (b)   Dissolve 0.10 g of the substance to be examined in 0.5 ml of *concentrated ammonia R* and dilute to 5.0 ml with *methanol R*. If the solution is not clear, heat gently until dissolution is complete.

Reference solution (a)   Dissolve 20 mg of *sulfadimidine CRS* in 3 ml of a mixture of 2 volumes of *concentrated ammonia R* and 48 volumes of *methanol R* and dilute to 5.0 ml with the same mixture of solvents.

Reference solution (b)   Dilute 1.25 ml of test solution (a) to 50 ml with a mixture of 2 volumes of *concentrated ammonia R* and 48 volumes of *methanol R*.

Apply to the plate 5 µl of each solution. Develop over a path of 15 cm using a mixture of 3 volumes of *dilute ammonia R1*, 5 volumes of *water R*, 40 volumes of *nitromethane R* and 50 volumes of *dioxan R*. Dry the plate at 100 °C to 105 °C and examine in ultraviolet light at 254 nm. Any spot in the chromatogram obtained with test solution (b), apart from the principal spot, is not more intense than the spot in the chromatogram obtained with reference solution (b) (0.5 per cent).

Heavy metals (2.4.8)
1.0 g complies with limit test D for heavy metals (20 ppm).
Prepare the standard using 2 ml of *lead standard solution (10 ppm Pb) R*.

Loss on drying (2.2.32)
Not more than 0.5 per cent, determined on 1.00 g by drying in an oven at 100 °C to 105 °C.

Sulphated ash (2.4.14)
Not more than 0.1 per cent, determined on 1.0 g.

ASSAY
Dissolve 0.250 g in a mixture of 20 ml of *dilute hydrochloric acid R* and 50 ml of *water R*. Cool the solution in iced water. Carry out the determination of primary aromatic amino-nitrogen (2.5.8), determining the end-point electrometrically.

1 ml of *0.1 M sodium nitrite* is equivalent to 27.83 mg of $C_{12}H_{14}N_4O_2S$.

STORAGE
Store protected from light.

Ph Eur

Sulfamerazine

(Ph Eur monograph 0358)

$C_{11}H_{12}N_4O_2S$ 264.3   *127-79-7*

Action and use
Antibacterial.

Ph Eur

DEFINITION
Sulfamerazine contains not less than 99.0 per cent and not more than the equivalent of 101.0 per cent of 4-amino-N-(4-methyl-2-pyrimidinyl)benzenesulphonamide, calculated with reference to the dried substance.

CHARACTERS
White, yellowish-white or pinkish-white, crystalline powder or crystals, very slightly soluble in water, sparingly soluble in acetone, slightly soluble in alcohol, very slightly soluble in methylene chloride. It dissolves in solutions of alkali hydroxides and in dilute mineral acids.

It melts at about 235 °C, with decomposition.

IDENTIFICATION
First identification   A, B.
Second identification   B, C, D.

A. Examine by infrared absorption spectrophotometry (2.2.24), comparing with the spectrum obtained with *sulfamerazine CRS*. Examine the substances as discs.

B. Examine the chromatograms obtained in the test for related substances. The principal spot in the chromatogram obtained with test solution (b) is similar in position, colour and size to the principal spot in the chromatogram obtained with reference solution (a).

C. Place 3 g in a dry tube. Incline the tube by about 45°, immerse the bottom of the tube in a silicone-oil bath and heat to about 270 °C. The substance decomposes, producing a white or yellowish-white sublimate which, after recrystallisation from *toluene R* and drying at 100 °C, melts (2.2.14) at 157 °C to 161 °C.

D. Dissolve about 20 mg in 0.5 ml of *dilute hydrochloric acid R* and add 1 ml of *water R*. The solution gives, without further addition of acid, the identification reaction of primary aromatic amines (2.3.1).

TESTS
Appearance of solution
Dissolve 0.8 g in a mixture of 5 ml of *dilute sodium hydroxide solution R* and 5 ml of *water R*. The solution is not more intensely coloured than reference solution Y_4, BY_4 or GY_4 (2.2.2, Method II).

Acidity
To 1.25 g, finely powdered, add 40 ml of *carbon dioxide-free water R* and heat at about 70 °C for 5 min. Cool for about 15 min in iced water and filter. To 20 ml of the filtrate add 0.1 ml of *bromothymol blue solution R1*. Not more than 0.2 ml of *0.1 M sodium hydroxide* is required to change the colour of the indicator.

Related substances
Examine by thin-layer chromatography (2.2.27) using *silica gel GF$_{254}$ R* as the coating substance.

Test solution (a)   Dissolve 0.10 g of the substance to be examined in 3 ml of a mixture of 2 volumes of *concentrated ammonia R* and 48 volumes of *methanol R* and dilute to 5 ml with the same mixture of solvents.

Test solution (b)   Dilute 1 ml of test solution (a) to 10 ml with a mixture of 2 volumes of *concentrated ammonia R* and 48 volumes of *methanol R*.

Reference solution (a)   Dissolve 10 mg of *sulfamerazine CRS* in 3 ml of a mixture of 2 volumes of *concentrated ammonia R* and 48 volumes of *methanol R* and dilute to 5 ml with the same mixture of solvents.

Reference solution (b)   Dilute 2.5 ml of test solution (b) to 50 ml with a mixture of 2 volumes of *concentrated ammonia R* and 48 volumes of *methanol R*.

Apply to the plate 5 µl of each solution. Develop over a path of 15 cm with a mixture of 3 volumes of *dilute ammonia R1*, 5 volumes of *water R*, 40 volumes of *nitromethane R* and 50 volumes of *dioxan R*. Dry the plate at 100 °C to 105 °C and examine in ultraviolet light at 254 nm. Any spot in the chromatogram obtained with test solution (a), apart from the principal spot, is not more intense that the spot in the chromatogram obtained with reference solution (b) (0.5 per cent).

Heavy metals (2.4.8)
1.0 g complies with limit test C for heavy metals (20 ppm). Prepare the standard using 2 ml of *lead standard solution (10 ppm Pb) R*.

Loss on drying (2.2.32)
Not more than 0.5 per cent, determined on 1.000 g by drying in an oven at 100 °C to 105 °C.

Sulphated ash (2.4.14)
Not more than 0.1 per cent, determined on 1.0 g.

ASSAY
Dissolve 0.2500 g in a mixture of 20 ml of *dilute hydrochloric acid R* and 50 ml of *water R*. Cool the solution in iced water.

Carry out the determination of primary aromatic amino-nitrogen (2.5.8), determining the end-point electrometrically.

1 ml of *0.1 M sodium nitrite* is equivalent to 26.43 mg of $C_{11}H_{12}N_4O_2S$.

STORAGE
Store protected from light.

—— Ph Eur

Sulfametoxypyridazine

(*Sulfamethoxypyridazine for Veterinary Use,
Ph Eur monograph 0638*)

$C_{11}H_{12}N_4O_3S$ 280.3   *80-35-3*

Action and use
Sulfonamide antibacterial.

Preparation
Sulfametoxypyridazine Injection

Ph Eur

DEFINITION
Sulfamethoxypyridazine for veterinary use contains not less than 99.0 per cent and not more than the equivalent of 101.0 per cent of 4-amino-*N*-(6-methoxypyridazin-3-yl)benzenesulphonamide, calculated with reference to the dried substance.

CHARACTERS
A white or slightly yellowish, crystalline powder, colouring slowly on exposure to light, practically insoluble in water, sparingly soluble in acetone, slightly soluble in alcohol, very slightly soluble in methylene chloride. It dissolves in solutions of alkali hydroxides and in dilute mineral acids.

It melts at about 180 °C, with decomposition.

IDENTIFICATION
First identification   A, B.
Second identification   B, C, D.

A. Examine by infrared absorption spectrophotometry (2.2.24), comparing with the spectrum obtained with *sulfamethoxypyridazine CRS*. Examine the substances prepared as discs.

B. Examine the chromatograms obtained in the test for related substances. The principal spot in the chromatogram obtained with test solution (b) is similar in position and size to the principal spot in the chromatogram obtained with reference solution (a).

C. Dissolve 0.5 g in 1 ml of a 40 per cent *V/V* solution of *sulphuric acid R*, heating gently. Continue heating until a crystalline precipitate appears (about 2 min). Cool and add 10 ml of *dilute sodium hydroxide solution R*. Cool again, add 25 ml of *ether R* and shake the solution for 5 min. Separate the ether layer, dry over *anhydrous sodium sulphate R* and filter. Evaporate the ether by heating in a water-bath. An oily residue is obtained which becomes crystalline on cooling;

if necessary, scratch the wall of the container with a glass rod. The residue melts (2.2.14) at 102 °C to 106 °C.

D. Dissolve about 5 mg in 10 ml of *1 M hydrochloric acid*. Dilute 1 ml of the solution to 10 ml with *water R*. The solution, without further acidification, gives the reaction of primary aromatic amines (2.3.1).

TESTS
Appearance of solution
Dissolve 1.0 g in a mixture of 10 ml of *1 M sodium hydroxide* and 15 ml of *water R*. The solution is clear (2.2.1) and not more intensely coloured than reference solution Y_4 or BY_4 (2.2.2, Method II).

Acidity
To 1.25 g, finely powdered, add 25 ml of *carbon dioxide-free water R*. Heat at 70 °C for 5 min. Cool in iced water for about 15 min and filter. To 20 ml of the filtrate add 0.1 ml of *bromothymol blue solution R1*. Not more than 0.5 ml of *0.1 M sodium hydroxide* is required to change the colour of the indicator.

Related substances
Examine by thin layer chromatography (2.2.27), using *TLC silica gel GF₂₅₄ plate R*.

Test solution (a)   Dissolve 0.10 g of the substance to be examined in *acetone R* and dilute to 5 ml with the same solvent.

Test solution (b)   Dilute 1 ml of test solution (a) to 10 ml with *acetone R*.

Reference solution (a)   Dissolve 20 mg of *sulfamethoxypyridazine CRS* in *acetone R* and dilute to 10 ml with the same solvent.

Reference solution (b)   Dilute 2.5 ml of test solution (b) to 50 ml with *acetone R*.

Apply separately to the plate 5 μl of each solution. Develop over a path of 15 cm using a mixture of 1 volume of *dilute ammonia R1*, 9 volumes of *water R*, 30 volumes of *2-propanol R* and 50 volumes of *ethyl acetate R*. Dry the plate at 100-105 °C and examine in ultraviolet light at 254 nm. Any spot in the chromatogram obtained with test solution (a), apart from the principal spot, is not more intense than the spot in the chromatogram obtained with reference solution (b) (0.5 per cent).

Heavy metals (2.4.8)
1.0 g complies with limit test D for heavy metals (20 ppm). Prepare the standard using 2 ml of *lead standard solution (10 ppm Pb) R*.

Loss on drying (2.2.32)
Not more than 0.5 per cent, determined on 1.000 g by drying in an oven at 100-105 °C.

Sulphated ash (2.4.14)
Not more than 0.1 per cent, determined on 1.0 g.

ASSAY
Carry out the assay of primary aromatic amino-nitrogen (2.5.8), using 0.2500 g, determining the end-point electrometrically.

1 ml of *0.1 M sodium nitrite* is equivalent to 28.03 mg of $C_{11}H_{12}N_4O_3S$.

STORAGE
Protected from light.

—— Ph Eur

Sulfanilamide

(Ph Eur monograph 1571)

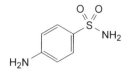

$C_6H_8N_2O_2S$ 172.2   *63-74-1*

Action and use
Antibacterial.

Ph Eur

DEFINITION
Sulfanilamide contains not less than 99.0 per cent and not more than the equivalent of 101.0 per cent of 4-aminobenzenesulphonamide, calculated with reference to the dried substance.

CHARACTERS
White or yellowish-white crystals or fine powder, slightly soluble in water, freely soluble in acetone, sparingly soluble in alcohol, practically insoluble in methylene chloride.
It dissolves in solutions of alkali hydroxides and in dilute mineral acids.

IDENTIFICATION
First identification   B.
Second identification   A, C, D.

A. Melting point (*2.2.14*): 164.5 °C to 166.0 °C.

B. Examine by infrared absorption spectrophotometry (*2.2.24*), comparing with the spectrum obtained with *sulfanilamide CRS*. Examine the substances prepared as discs.

C. Examine the chromatograms obtained in the test for related substances. The principal spot in the chromatogram obtained with test solution (a) is similar in position and size to the principal spot in the chromatogram obtained with reference solution (a).

D. Dissolve about 5 mg in 10 ml of *1 M hydrochloric acid*. Dilute 1 ml of the solution to 10 ml with *water R*. The solution, without further acidification, gives the reaction of primary aromatic amines (*2.3.1*).

TESTS
Solution S
To 2.5 g add 50 ml of *carbon dioxide-free water R*. Heat at about 70 °C for about 5 min. Cool in iced water for about 15 min and filter.

Acidity
To 20 ml of solution S add 0.1 ml of *bromothymol blue solution R1*. Not more than 0.2 ml of *0.1 M sodium hydroxide* is required to change the colour of the indicator.

Related substances
Examine by thin-layer chromatography (*2.2.27*), using a *TLC silica gel F₂₅₄ plate R*.

Test solution (a)   Dissolve 20 mg of the substance to be examined in 3 ml of a mixture of 2 volumes of *concentrated ammonia R* and 48 volumes of *methanol R* and dilute to 5 ml with the same mixture of solvents.

Test solution (b)   Dissolve 0.10 g of the substance to be examined in 0.5 ml of *concentrated ammonia R* and dilute to 5 ml with *methanol R*. If the solution is not clear, heat gently until dissolution is complete.

Reference solution (a)   Dissolve 20 mg of *sulfanilamide CRS* in 3 ml of a mixture of 2 volumes of *concentrated ammonia R* and 48 volumes of *methanol R* and dilute to 5 ml with the same mixture of solvents.

Reference solution (b)   Dilute 1.25 ml of test solution (a) to 50 ml with a mixture of 2 volumes of *concentrated ammonia R* and 48 volumes of *methanol R*.

Reference solution (c)   Dissolve 20 mg of the substance to be examined and 20 mg of *sulfamerazine CRS* in 3 ml of a mixture of 2 volumes of *concentrated ammonia R* and 48 volumes of *methanol R* and dilute to 5 ml with the same mixture of solvents.

Apply to the plate 5 μl of each solution. Develop over a path corresponding to two-thirds of the plate height using a mixture of 3 volumes of *dilute ammonia R1*, 5 volumes of *water R*, 40 volumes of *nitromethane R* and 50 volumes of *dioxan R*. Dry the plate at 100 °C to 105 °C and examine in ultraviolet light at 254 nm. Any spot in the chromatogram obtained with test solution (b), apart from the principal spot, is not more intense than the spot in the chromatogram obtained with reference solution (b) (0.5 per cent). The test is not valid unless the chromatogram obtained with reference solution (c) shows two clearly separated principal spots.

Heavy metals (*2.4.8*)
12 ml of solution S complies with limit test A for heavy metals (20 ppm). Prepare the standard using *lead standard solution (1 ppm Pb) R*.

Loss on drying (*2.2.32*)
Not more than 0.5 per cent, determined on 1.000 g by drying in an oven at 100 °C to 105 °C.

Sulphated ash (*2.4.14*)
Not more than 0.1 per cent, determined on 1.0 g.

ASSAY
Carry out the determination of primary aromatic amino-nitrogen (*2.5.8*), using 0.140 g and determining the end-point electrometrically.

1 ml of *0.1 M sodium nitrite* is equivalent to 17.22 mg of $C_6H_8N_2O_2S$.

STORAGE
Store protected from light.

Ph Eur

Sulfaquinoxaline

$C_{14}H_{12}N_4O_2S$ 300.3   *59-40-5*

Action and use
Sulfonamide antibacterial.

DEFINITION
Sulfaquinoxaline is N^1-quinoxalin-2-ylsulphanilamide.
It contains not less than 98.0% and not more than 101.0%

of $C_{14}H_{12}N_4O_2S$, calculated with reference to the dried substance.

CHARACTERISTICS

A yellow powder.

Practically insoluble in water; very slightly soluble in ethanol (96%); practically insoluble in ether. It dissolves in aqueous solutions of alkalis.

IDENTIFICATION

A. The *infrared absorption spectrum*, Appendix II A, is concordant with the *reference spectrum* of sulfaquinoxaline *(RSV 41)*.

B. The *light absorption*, Appendix II B, in the range 230 to 350 nm of a 0.001% w/v solution in 0.01M *sodium hydroxide* exhibits a maximum only at 252 nm. The *absorbance* at 252 nm is about 1.1.

C. Yields the reaction characteristic of *primary aromatic amines*, Appendix VI, dissolving 4 mg in 2 ml of warm 2M *hydrochloric acid*. An orange-red precipitate is produced.

TESTS

Acidity

To 2 g add 100 ml of *water*, heat at 70° for 5 minutes, cool to 20° and filter. 50 ml of the filtrate requires for titration to pH 7.0 not more than 0.2 ml of 0.1M *sodium hydroxide VS*, Appendix V L.

Heavy metals

Dissolve the residue obtained in the test for Sulphated ash in 1 ml of 2M *hydrochloric acid* and dilute to 14 ml with *water*. 12 ml of the solution complies with *limit test A for heavy metals*, Appendix VII. Use *lead standard solution (2 ppm Pb)* to prepare the standard (20 ppm).

Related substances

Carry out the method for *thin-layer chromatography*, Appendix III A, using a silica gel F_{254} precoated plate (Merck silica gel 60 F_{254} plates are suitable) and a mixture of 20 volumes of 18M *ammonia*, 40 volumes of *methanol* and 60 volumes of *chloroform* as the mobile phase. Apply separately to the plate 5 μl of each of the following solutions. For solution (1) dissolve 0.40 g of the substance being examined in 4 ml of 1M *sodium hydroxide* and add sufficient *methanol* to produce 100 ml. Solution (2) contains 0.012% w/v of N^1,N^2-*diquinoxalin-2-ylsulphanilamide BPCRS* in *methanol*. Solution (3) contains 0.0040% w/v of *sulphanilamide* in *methanol*. After removal of the plate, allow it to dry in air until the solvent has evaporated and examine under *ultraviolet light (254 nm)*. Any spot corresponding to N^1,N^2-*diquinoxalin-2-ylsulphanilamide* in the chromatogram obtained with solution (1) is not more intense than the spot in the chromatogram obtained with solution (2) (3%). Any other *secondary spot* in the chromatogram obtained with solution (1) is not more intense than the spot in the chromatogram obtained with solution (3) (1%).

Loss on drying

When dried to constant weight at 105°, loses not more than 1.0% of its weight. Use 1 g.

Sulphated ash

Not more than 0.1%, Appendix IX A. Ignite at 600° and use 1.5 g.

ASSAY

Dissolve 0.65 g in 10 ml of a mixture of equal volumes of 1M *sodium hydroxide* and *water*. Add 20 ml of *glycerol*, 20 ml of 9M *sulphuric acid* and 5 g of *potassium bromide*, cool in ice and titrate slowly with 0.1M *sodium nitrate VS*, stirring constantly and determining the end point electrometrically.

Each ml of 0.1M *sodium nitrite VS* is equivalent to 30.03 mg of $C_{14}H_{12}N_4O_2S$.

STORAGE

Sulfaquinoxaline should be protected from light.

Sulfathiazole Sodium

$C_9H_8N_3NaO_2S_2,1\frac{1}{2}H_2O$	304.3	*144-74-1(anhydrous)*
$C_9H_8N_3NaO_2S_2,5H_2O$	367.4	*6791-71-5*

Action and use
Sulfonamide antibacterial.

Preparation
Tylosin Tartrate and Sulfathiazole Sodium Veterinary Oral Powder

DEFINITION

Sulfathiazole Sodium is the hydrated sodium salt of N^1-thiazol-2-yl sulphanilamide, either the sesquihydrate or the pentahydrate. It contains not less than 99.0% and not more than 101.0% of $C_9H_8N_3NaO_2S_2$, calculated with reference to the dried substance.

CHARACTERISTICS

A white or yellowish white, crystalline powder or granules.

Freely soluble in *water*; soluble in *ethanol (96%)*.

IDENTIFICATION

A. The *infrared absorption spectrum* of the dried substance, Appendix II A, is concordant with the *reference spectrum* of sulfathiazole sodium *(RSV 42)*.

B. Dissolve 1 g in 25 ml of *water* and add 2 ml of 6M *acetic acid*. The *melting point* of the precipitate, after washing with *water* and drying for 4 hours at 105°, is about 201°, Appendix V A.

C. The precipitate obtained in test B yields the reaction characteristic of primary aromatic amines, Appendix VI, giving an orange-red precipitate.

TESTS

Alkalinity

pH of a solution containing the equivalent of 1.0% w/v of the anhydrous substance, 9.0 to 10.0, Appendix V L.

Heavy metals

Dissolve a quantity containing the equivalent of 2.5 g of the anhydrous substance in 10 ml of *water*, add 15 ml of 2M *acetic acid*, shake for 30 minutes and filter. 12 ml of the resulting solution complies with *limit test A for heavy metals*, Appendix VII. Use *lead standard solution (2 ppm Pb)* to prepare the standard (20 ppm).

Related substances

Carry out the method for *thin-layer chromatography*, Appendix III A, using *silica gel H* as the coating substance and a mixture of 18 volumes of 10M *ammonia* and 90 volumes of *butan-1-ol* as the mobile phase. Apply separately to the plate 10 μl of each of two solutions in a mixture of 1 volume of 13.5M *ammonia* and 9 volumes of *ethanol (96%)* containing (1) 1.0% w/v of the substance being examined and (2) 0.0050% w/v of *sulfanilamide*. After removal of the plate, heat it at 105° for 10 minutes and spray with a 0.1% w/v solution of *4-dimethylaminobenzaldehyde* in *ethanol (96%)* containing 1% v/v of *hydrochloric acid*. Any *secondary spot* in the chromatogram obtained with solution (1) is not more intense than the spot in the chromatogram obtained with solution (2) (0.5%).

Loss on drying
When dried to constant weight at 105°, loses not less than 6.0% and not more than 10.0% of its weight (sesquihydrate) or not less than 22.0% and not more than 27.0% of its weight (pentahydrate).

ASSAY
Dissolve 0.5 g in a mixture of 75 ml of *water* and 10 ml of *hydrochloric acid*, add 3 g of *potassium bromide*, cool in ice and titrate slowly with 0.1M *sodium nitrite VS*, stirring constantly and determining the end point electrometrically. Each ml of 0.1M *sodium nitrite VS* is equivalent to 27.73 mg of $C_9H_8N_3NaO_2S_2$.

STORAGE
Sulfathiazole Sodium should be protected from light.

LABELLING
The label states whether the substance is the sesquihydrate or the pentahydrate.

Testosterone Phenylpropionate

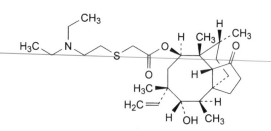

$C_{28}H_{36}O_3$ 420.6   *1255-49-8*

Action and use
Androgen.

Preparation
Testosterone Phenylpropionate Injection

DEFINITION
Testosterone Phenylpropionate is 3-oxo-androst-4-en-17β-yl 3-phenylpropionate. It contains not less than 97.0% and not more than 103.0% of $C_{28}H_{36}O_3$, calculated with reference to the dried substance.

CHARACTERISTICS
A white to almost white, crystalline powder.

Practically insoluble in *water*; sparingly soluble in *ethanol (96%)*.

IDENTIFICATION
A. The *infrared absorption spectrum*, Appendix II A, is concordant with the *reference spectrum* of testosterone phenylpropionate *(RSV 43)*. If the spectra are not concordant, dissolve the substances in the minimum volume

of *dichloromethane*, evaporate to dryness and prepare a new spectrum of the residue.

B. Complies with the test for *identification of steroids*, Appendix III A, using *impregnating solvent III* and *mobile phase F*.

C. Dissolve 25 mg in 1 ml of *methanol*, add 2 ml of *semicarbazide acetate solution*, heat under a reflux condenser for 30 minutes and cool. The *melting point* of the resulting precipitate is about 218°, Appendix V A.

TESTS
Melting point
114° to 117°, Appendix V A.

Specific optical rotation
In a 1% w/v solution in *1,4-dioxan*, +86 to +91, calculated with reference to the dried substance, Appendix V F.

Loss on drying
When dried to constant weight at 105°, loses not more than 0.5% of its weight. Use 1 g.

Sulphated ash
Not more than 0.1%, Appendix IX A.

ASSAY
Dissolve 10 mg in sufficient *absolute ethanol* to produce 100 ml, dilute 5 ml to 50 ml with *absolute ethanol* and measure the *absorbance* of the resulting solution at the maximum at 240 nm, Appendix II B. Calculate the content of $C_{28}H_{36}O_3$ taking 395 as the value of A(1%, 1 cm) at the maximum at 240 nm.

STORAGE
Testosterone Phenylpropionate should be protected from light.

Tiamulin

(Tiamulin for Veterinary Use, Ph Eur monograph 1660)

$C_{28}H_{47}NO_4S$ 493.8   *56142-71-3*

Action and use
Antibacterial.

Ph Eur

DEFINITION
(3a*S*,4*R*,5*S*,6*S*,8*R*,9*R*,9a*R*,10*R*)-6-Ethenyl-5-hydroxy-4,6,9,10-tetramethyl-1-oxodecahydro-3a,9-propano-3a*H*-cyclopentacycloocten-8-yl [[2-(diethylamino)ethyl] sulphanyl]acetate.

Content
96.5 per cent to 102.0 per cent (dried substance).

CHARACTERS

Appearance

Sticky, translucent yellowish mass, slightly hygroscopic.

Solubility

Practically insoluble in water, very soluble in methylene chloride, freely soluble in anhydrous ethanol.

IDENTIFICATION

Infrared absorption spectrophotometry (2.2.24).

Comparison Ph. Eur. reference spectrum of tiamulin.

TESTS

Appearance of solution

The solution is clear (2.2.1) and its absorbance (2.2.25) at 420 nm is maximum 0.050.

Dissolve 2.5 g in 50 ml of *methanol R*.

Related substances

Liquid chromatography (2.2.29).

Ammonium carbonate buffer solution pH 10.0 Dissolve 10.0 g of *ammonium carbonate R* in *water R*, add 22 ml of *perchloric acid solution R* and dilute to 1000.0 ml with *water R*. Adjust to pH 10.0 with *concentrated ammonia R1*.

Solvent mixture ammonium carbonate buffer solution pH 10.0, *acetonitrile R1* (50:50 *V/V*).

Test solution Dissolve 0.200 g of the substance to be examined in the solvent mixture and dilute to 50.0 ml with the solvent mixture.

Reference solution (a) Dissolve 0.250 g of *tiamulin hydrogen fumarate CRS* in the solvent mixture and dilute to 50.0 ml with the solvent mixture.

Reference solution (b) Dilute 1.0 ml of the test solution to 100.0 ml with the solvent mixture.

Reference solution (c) Dilute 0.1 ml of *toluene R* to 100 ml with *acetonitrile R*. Dilute 0.1 ml of this solution to 100.0 ml with the solvent mixture.

Column:
— *size*: l = 0.15 m, Ø = 4.6 mm,
— *stationary phase: end-capped octadecylsilyl silica gel for chromatography R* (5 μm),
— *temperature*: 30 °C.

Mobile phase acetonitrile R1, ammonium carbonate buffer solution pH 10.0, *methanol R1* (21:30:49 *V/V/V*).

Flow rate 1.0 ml/min.

Detection Spectrophotometer at 212 nm.

Injection 20 μl.

Run time 3 times the retention time of tiamulin.

Relative retention with reference to tiamulin (retention time = about 18 min): impurity A = about 0.22; impurity B = about 0.5; impurity C = about 0.66; impurity D = about 1.1; impurity F = about 1.6; impurity E = about 2.4.

System suitability Reference solution (a):
— baseline separation between the peaks due to tiamulin and impurity D.

Limits:
— *impurities A, B, C, D, E, F*: for each impurity, not more than the area of the principal peak in the chromatogram obtained with reference solution (b) (1.0 per cent),
— *any other impurity*: for each impurity, not more than 0.2 times the area of the principal peak in the chromatogram obtained with reference solution (b) (0.2 per cent),

— *total*: not more than 3 times the area of the principal peak in the chromatogram obtained with reference solution (b) (3.0 per cent),
— *disregard limit*: 0.1 times the area of the principal peak in the chromatogram obtained with reference solution (b) (0.1 per cent); disregard any peak present in the chromatogram obtained with reference solution (c).

Loss on drying (2.2.32)

Maximum 1.0 per cent, determined on 1.000 g by drying in an oven at 80 °C.

Bacterial endotoxins (2.6.14, Method D)

Less than 0.4 IU/mg, determined in a 1 mg/ml solution in *anhydrous ethanol R* (endotoxin free) diluted 1:40 with water for bacterial endotoxins test.

ASSAY

Liquid chromatography (2.2.29) as described in the test for related substances with the following modification.

Injection Test solution and reference solution (a).

Calculate the percentage content of $C_{28}H_{47}NO_4S$, from the declared content of *tiamulin hydrogen fumarate CRS*.

STORAGE

Protected from light.

LABELLING

The label states where appropriate that the substance is free from bacterial endotoxins.

IMPURITIES

Specified impurities A, B, C, D, E, F.

Other detectable impurities G, H, I, J, K, L, M, N, O, P, Q, R.

A. R1 = R2 = H: (3aS,4R,5S,6S,8R,9R,9aR,10R)-6-ethenyl-5,8-dihydroxy-4,6,9,10-tetramethyloctahydro-3a,9-propano-3aH-cyclopentacycloocten-1(4H)-one (mutilin),

G. R1 = CO-CH$_2$OH, R2 = H: (3aS,4R,5S,6S,8R,9R,9aR,10R)-6-ethenyl-5-hydroxy-4,6,9,10-tetramethyl-1-oxodecahydro-3a,9-propano-3aH-cyclopentacycloocten-8-yl hydroxyacetate (pleuromutilin),

J. R1 = CO-CH$_3$, R2 = H: (3aS,4R,5S,6S,8R,9R,9aR,10R)-6-ethenyl-5-hydroxy-4,6,9,10-tetramethyl-1-oxodecahydro-3a,9-propano-3aH-cyclopentacycloocten-8-yl acetate (mutilin 14-acetate),

K. R1 = H, R2 = CO-CH$_3$: (3aS,4R,5S,6S,8R,9R,9aR,10R)-6-ethenyl-8-hydroxy-4,6,9,10-tetramethyl-1-oxodecahydro-3a,9-propano-3aH-cyclopentacycloocten-5-yl acetate (mutilin 11-acetate),

L. R1 = CO-CH$_2$-O-SO$_2$-C$_6$H$_4$-pCH$_3$, R2 = H: (3aS,4R,5S,6S,8R,9R,9aR,10R)-6-ethenyl-5-hydroxy-4,6,9,10-tetramethyl-1-oxodecahydro-3a,9-propano-3aH-cyclopentacycloocten-8-yl [[(4-methylphenyl)sulphonyl]oxy]acetate (pleuromutilin 22-tosylate),

M. R1 = R2 = CO-CH$_3$: (3aS,4R,5S,6S,8R,9R,9aR,10R)-6-
ethenyl-4,6,9,10-tetramethyl-1-oxodecahydro-3a,9-propano-
3aH-cyclopentacyclooocten-5,8-diyl diacetate (mutilin 11,14-
diacetate),

P. R1 = CO-CH$_2$-O-SO$_2$-C$_6$H$_5$, R2 = H:
(3aS,4R,5S,6S,8R,9R,9aR,10R)-6-ethenyl-5-hydroxy-
4,6,9,10-tetramethyl-1-oxodecahydro-3a,9-propano-3aH-
cyclopentacyclooocten-8-yl [(phenylsulphonyl)oxy]acetate,

B. R = CH$_2$-C$_6$H$_5$:
2-(benzylsulphanyl)-N,N-diethylethanamine,

C. R = S-CH$_2$-CH$_2$-N(C$_2$H$_5$)$_2$:
2,2′-(disulphane-1,2-diyl)bis(N,N-diethylethanamine),

O. R = H: 2-(diethylamino)ethanethiol,

D. (3aR,4R,6S,8R,9R,9aR,10R)-6-ethenylhydroxy-4,6,9,10-
tetramethyl-5-oxodecahydro-3a,9-propano-3aH-
cyclopentacyclooocten-8-yl [[2-(diethylamino)ethyl]
sulphanyl]acetate,

E. (3aS,4R,6S,8R,9R,9aR,10R)-6-ethenyl-4,6,9,10-
tetramethyl-1,5-dioxodecahydro-3a,9-propano-3aH-
cyclopentacyclooocten-8-yl [[2-(diethylamino)ethyl]
sulphanyl]acetate (11-oxotiamulin),

F. (1RS,3aR,4R,6S,8R,9R,9aR,10R)-6-ethenyl-1-hydroxy-
4,6,9,10-tetramethyl-5-oxodecahydro-3a,9-propano-3aH-
cyclopentacyclooocten-8-yl [[2-(diethylamino)ethyl]
sulphanyl]acetate (1-hydroxy-11-oxotiamulin),

H. (2E)-4-[(2RS)-2-[(3aS,4R,5S,6R,8R,9R,9aR,10R)-8-[[[2-
(diethylamino)ethyl]sulphanyl]acetyl]oxy]-5-hydroxy-
4,6,9,10-tetramethyl-1-oxodecahydro-3a,9-propano-3aH-
cyclopentacyclooocten-6-yl]-2-hydroxyethoxy]-4-oxobut-2-
enoic acid (19,20-dihydroxytiamulin 20-fumarate),

I. (2E)-4-[[(3aS,4R,5S,6S,8R,9R,9aR,10R)-8-[[[2-
(diethylamino)ethyl]sulphanyl]acetyl]oxy]-6-ethenyl-1,5-
dihydroxy-4,6,9,10-tetramethyldecahydro-3a,9-propano-3aH-
cyclopentacyclooocten-2-yl]oxy]-4-oxobut-2-enoic acid (2,3-
dihydroxytiamulin 2-fumarate),

N. (2E)-4-[2-[[(3aS,4R,5S,6S,8R,9R,9aR,10R)-6-ethenyl-5-
hydroxy-4,6,9,10-tetramethyl-1-oxodecahydro-3a,9-propano-
3aH-cyclopentacyclooocten-8-yl]oxy]-2-oxoethoxy]-4-oxobut-
2-enoic acid (pleuromutilin 22-fumarate),

Q. (3aS,4R,5S,6S,8R,9R,10R)-6-ethenyl-2,5-dihydroxy-
4,6,9,10-tetramethyl-2,3,4,5,6,7,8,9-octahydro-3a,9-propano-
3aH-cyclopentacyclooocten-8-yl [[2-(diethylamino)ethyl]
sulphanyl]acetate (3,4-didehydro-2-hydroxytiamulin),

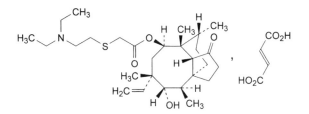

R. *N*-benzyl-*N*,*N*-dibutylbutan-1-aminium.

_____ *Ph Eur*

Tiamulin Hydrogen Fumarate

(*Tiamulin Hydrogen Fumarate for Veterinary Use,*
Ph Eur monograph 1659)

$C_{32}H_{51}NO_8S$ 610   55297-96-6

Action and use
Antibacterial.

Ph Eur _____

DEFINITION
(3a*S*,4*R*,5*S*,6*S*,8*R*,9*R*,9a*R*,10*R*)-6-Ethenyl-5-hydroxy-
4,6,9,10-tetramethyl-1-oxodecahydro-3a,9-propano-3a*H*-
cyclopentacyclooocten-8-yl [[2-(diethylamino)ethyl]
sulphanyl]acetate hydrogen (*E*)-but-2-enedioate.

Content
96.5 per cent to 102.0 per cent (dried substance).

CHARACTERS
Appearance
White or light yellow, crystalline powder.

Solubility
Soluble in water, freely soluble in anhydrous ethanol
and soluble in methanol.

IDENTIFICATION
Infrared absorption spectrophotometry (*2.2.24*).

Comparison   *tiamulin hydrogen fumarate CRS.*

TESTS
pH (*2.2.3*)
3.1 to 4.1.

Dissolve 0.5 g in *carbon dioxide-free water R* and dilute to
50 ml with the same solvent.

Related substances
Liquid chromatography (*2.2.29*).

Ammonium carbonate buffer solution pH 10.0   Dissolve 10.0 g
of *ammonium carbonate R* in *water R*, add 22 ml of *perchloric
acid solution R* and dilute to 1000.0 ml with *water R*. Adjust
to pH 10.0 with *concentrated ammonia R1*.

Solvent mixture   amonium carbonate buffer
solution pH 10.0, *acetonitrile R1* (50:50 *V/V*).

Test solution   Dissolve 0.200 g of the substance to be
examined in the solvent mixture and dilute to 50.0 ml with
the solvent mixture.

Reference solution (a)   Dissolve 0.200 g of *tiamulin hydrogen
fumarate CRS* in the solvent mixture and dilute to 50.0 ml
with the solvent mixture.

Reference solution (b)   Dilute 1.0 ml of the test solution to
100.0 ml with the solvent mixture.

Reference solution (c)   Dissolve 40.0 mg of *fumaric acid R* in
the solvent mixture and dilute to 50.0 ml with the solvent
mixture.

Reference solution (d)   Dissolve 4 mg of *tiamulin for peak
identification CRS* (tiamulin hydrogen fumarate containing
impurities B, C, D, F, H and I) in the solvent mixture and
dilute to 1 ml with the solvent mixture.

Column:
— *size: l* = 0.15 m, Ø = 4.6 mm,
— *stationary phase:* end-capped octadecylsilyl silica gel for
   chromatography R (5 µm),
— *temperature:* 30 °C.

Mobile phase   acetonitrile R1, ammonium carbonate buffer
solution pH 10.0, methanol R1 (21:30:49 *V/V/V*).

Flow rate   1.0 ml/min.

Detection   Spectrophotometer at 212 nm.

Injection   20 µl.

Run time   3 times the retention time of tiamulin.

Identification of impurities   Use the chromatogram supplied
with *tiamulin for peak identification CRS* and the
chromatogram obtained with reference solution (d) to
identify the peaks due to impurities B and H.

Relative retention with reference to tiamulin (retention
time = about 18 min): impurity G = about 0.2;
impurity A = about 0.22; impurity H = about 0.23;
impurity I = about 0.3; impurity J = about 0.4;
impurity K = about 0.45; impurity B = about 0.5;
impurity L = about 0.65; impurity C = about 0.66;
impurity F = about 0.8; impurity M = about 0.85;
impurity D = about 1.1; impurity S = about 1.4;
impurity T = about 1.6; impurity E = 2.4.

System suitability   Reference solution (a):
— baseline separation between the peaks due to tiamulin
   and impurity D.

Limits:
— *impurities B, H:* for each impurity, not more than
   1.5 times the area of the principal peak in the
   chromatogram obtained with reference solution (b)
   (1.5 per cent),
— *impurities A, C, D, E, F, G, I, J, K, L, M, S, T:* for each
   impurity, not more than the area of the principal peak in
   the chromatogram obtained with reference solution (b)
   (1.0 per cent),
— *any other impurity:* for each impurity, not more than
   0.2 times the area of the principal peak in the
   chromatogram obtained with reference solution (b)
   (0.2 per cent),
— *total:* not more than 3 times the area of the principal peak
   in the chromatogram obtained with reference solution (b)
   (3.0 per cent),
— *disregard limit:* 0.1 times the area of the principal peak in
   the chromatogram obtained with reference solution (b)
   (0.1 per cent); disregard any peak present in reference
   solution (c).

Loss on drying (*2.2.32*)
Maximum 0.5 per cent, determined on 1.000 g by drying in an oven at 100-105 °C.

ASSAY
Liquid chromatography (*2.2.29*) as described in the test for related substances with the following modification.

Injection Test solution and reference solution (a).

Calculate the percentage content of $C_{32}H_{51}NO_8S$ from the declared content of *tiamulin hydrogen fumarate CRS*.

STORAGE
Protected from light.

IMPURITIES
Specified impurities A, B, C, D, E, F, G, H, I, J, K, L, M, S, T.

Other detectable impurities N, O, P, Q, R.

A. R1 = R2 = H: (3a*S*,4*R*,5*S*,6*S*,8*R*,9*R*,9a*R*,10*R*)-6-ethenyl-5,8-dihydroxy-4,6,9,10-tetramethyloctahydro-3a,9-propano-3a*H*-cyclopentacycloocten-1(4*H*)-one (mutilin),

G. R1 = CO-CH₂OH, R2 = H: (3a*S*,4*R*,5*S*,6*S*,8*R*,9*R*,9a*R*,10*R*)-6-ethenyl-5-hydroxy-4,6,9,10-tetramethyl-1-oxodecahydro-3a,9-propano-3a*H*-cyclopentacycloocten-8-yl hydroxyacetate (pleuromutilin),

J. R1 = CO-CH₃, R2 = H: (3a*S*,4*R*,5*S*,6*S*,8*R*,9*R*,9a*R*,10*R*)-6-ethenyl-5-hydroxy-4,6,9,10-tetramethyl-1-oxodecahydro-3a,9-propano-3a*H*-cyclopentacycloocten-8-yl acetate (mutilin 14-acetate),

K. R1 = H, R2 = CO-CH₃: (3a*S*,4*R*,5*S*,6*S*,8*R*,9*R*,9a*R*,10*R*)-6-ethenyl-8-hydroxy-4,6,9,10-tetramethyl-1-oxodecahydro-3a,9-propano-3a*H*-cyclopentacycloocten-5-yl acetate (mutilin 11-acetate),

L. R1 = CO-CH₂-O-SO₂-C₆H₄-*p*CH₃, R2 = H: (3a*S*,4*R*,5*S*,6*S*,8*R*,9*R*,9a*R*,10*R*)-6-ethenyl-5-hydroxy-4,6,9,10-tetramethyl-1-oxodecahydro-3a,9-propano-3a*H*-cyclopentacycloocten-8-yl [[(4-methylphenyl)sulphonyl]oxy]acetate (pleuromutilin 22-tosylate),

M. R1 = R2 = CO-CH₃: (3a*S*,4*R*,5*S*,6*S*,8*R*,9*R*,9a*R*,10*R*)-6-ethenyl-4,6,9,10-tetramethyl-1-oxodecahydro-3a,9-propano-3a*H*-cyclopentacycloocten-5,8-diyl diacetate (mutilin 11,14-diacetate),

P. R1 = CO-CH₂-O-SO₂-C₆H₅, R2 = H: (3a*S*,4*R*,5*S*,6*S*,8*R*,9*R*,9a*R*,10*R*)-6-ethenyl-5-hydroxy-4,6,9,10-tetramethyl-1-oxodecahydro-3a,9-propano-3a*H*-cyclopentacycloocten-8-yl [(phenylsulphonyl)oxy]acetate,

T. R1 = CO-CH₂-[S-CH₂-CH₂-]₂N(C₂H₅)₂, R2 = H: (3a*S*,4*R*,5*S*,6*S*,8*R*,9*R*,9a*R*,10*R*)-6-ethenyl-5-hydroxy-4,6,9,10-tetramethyl-1-oxodecahydro-3a,9-propano-3a*H*-cyclopentacycloocten-8-yl [[2-[[2-(diethylamino)ethyl]sulphanyl]ethyl]sulphanyl]acetate,

B. R = CH₂-C₆H₅: 2-(benzylsulphanyl)-*N*,*N*-diethylethanamine,

C. R = S-CH₂-CH₂-N(C₂H₅)₂: 2,2'-(disulphane-1,2-diyl)bis(*N*,*N*-diethylethanamine),

O. R = H: 2-(diethylamino)ethanethiol,

D. (3a*R*,4*R*,6*S*,8*R*,9*R*,9a*R*,10*R*)-6-ethenylhydroxy-4,6,9,10-tetramethyl-5-oxodecahydro-3a,9-propano-3a*H*-cyclopentacycloocten-8-yl [[2-(diethylamino)ethyl]sulphanyl]acetate,

E. (3a*S*,4*R*,6*S*,8*R*,9*R*,9a*R*,10*R*)-6-ethenyl-4,6,9,10-tetramethyl-1,5-dioxodecahydro-3a,9-propano-3a*H*-cyclopentacycloocten-8-yl [[2-(diethylamino)ethyl]sulphanyl]acetate (11-oxotiamulin),

F. impurity of unknown structure with a relative retention of about 0.8,

H. (2*E*)-4-[(2*RS*)-2-[(3a*S*,4*R*,5*S*,6*R*,8*R*,9*R*,9a*R*,10*R*)-8-[[[[2-(diethylamino)ethyl]sulphanyl]acetyl]oxy]-5-hydroxy-4,6,9,10-tetramethyl-1-oxodecahydro-3a,9-propano-3a*H*-cyclopentacycloocten-6-yl]-2-hydroxyethoxy]-4-oxobut-2-enoic acid (19,20-dihydroxytiamulin 20-fumarate),

I. (2E)-4-[[(3aS,4R,5S,6S,8R,9R,9aR,10R)-8-[[[[2-
(diethylamino)ethyl]sulphanyl]acetyl]oxy]-6-ethenyl-1,5-
dihydroxy-4,6,9,10-tetramethyldecahydro-3a,9-propano-3aH-
cyclopentacycloocten-2-yl]oxy]-4-oxobut-2-enoic acid (2,3-
dihydroxytiamulin 2-fumarate),

N. (2E)-4-[2-[[(3aS,4R,5S,6S,8R,9R,9aR,10R)-6-ethenyl-5-
hydroxy-4,6,9,10-tetramethyl-1-oxodecahydro-3a,9-propano-
3aH-cyclopentacycloocten-8-yl]oxy]-2-oxoethoxy]-4-oxobut-
2-enoic acid (pleuromutilin 22-fumarate),

Q. (3aS,4R,5S,6S,8R,9R,10R)-6-ethenyl-2,5-dihydroxy-
4,6,9,10-tetramethyl-2,3,4,5,6,7,8,9-octahydro-3a,9-propano-
3aH-cyclopentacycloocten-8-yl [[2-(diethylamino)ethyl]
sulphanyl]acetate (3,4-didehydro-2-hydroxytiamulin),

R. N-benzyl-N,N-dibutylbutan-1-aminium,

S. (1RS,3aR,4R,5S,6S,8R,9R,9aR,10R)-6-ethenyl-1-ethyl-
1,5-dihydroxy-4,6,9,10,12,12-hexamethyldecahydro-3a,9-
propano-3aH-cyclopentacycloocten-8-yl [[2-
(diethylamino)ethyl]sulphanyl]acetate.

Ph Eur

Tylosin

(Tylosin for Veterinary Use, Ph Eur monograph 1273)

Name	Mol. Formula	R1	R2	R3
tylosin A	$C_{46}H_{77}NO_{17}$	osyl	OCH_3	CHO
tylosin B	$C_{39}H_{65}NO_{14}$	H	OCH_3	CHO
tylosin C	$C_{45}H_{75}NO_{17}$	osyl	OH	CHO
tylosin D	$C_{46}H_{79}NO_{17}$	osyl	OCH_3	CH_2OH

Action and use
Macrolide antibacterial.

Preparations
Tylosin Injection
Tylosin Tablets

Ph Eur

DEFINITION
Tylosin for veterinary use is a mixture of macrolide
antibiotics produced by a strain of *Streptomyces fradiae* or by
any other means. The main component of the mixture is
(4R,5S,6S,7R,9R,11E,13E,15R,16R)-15-[[(6-deoxy-2,3-di-O-
methyl-β-D-allopyranosyl)oxy]methyl]-6-[[3,6-dideoxy-4-O-
(2,6-dideoxy-3-C-methyl-α-L-ribo-hexopyranosyl)-3-
(dimethylamino)-β-D-glucopyranosyl]oxy]-16-ethyl-4-
hydroxy-5,9,13-trimethyl-7-(2-oxoethyl)oxacyclohexadeca-
11,13-diene-2,10-dione (tylosin A, M_r 916). Tylosin B
(desmycosin, M_r 772), tylosin C (macrocin, M_r 902) and
tylosin D (relomycin, M_r 918) may also be present. They
contribute to the potency of the substance to be examined,
which is not less than 900 IU/mg, calculated with reference
to the dried substance.

CHARACTERS

An almost white or slightly yellow powder, slightly soluble in water, freely soluble in anhydrous ethanol and in methylene chloride. It dissolves in dilute solutions of mineral acids.

IDENTIFICATION

A. Examine by infrared absorption spectrophotometry (2.2.24), comparing with the spectrum obtained with *tylosin CRS*.

B. Examine the chromatograms obtained in the test for composition. The retention time and size of the principal peak in the chromatogram obtained with the test solution are the same as those of the principal peak in the chromatogram obtained with reference solution (a).

C. Dissolve about 30 mg in a mixture of 0.15 ml of *water R*, 2.5 ml of *acetic anhydride R* and 7.5 ml of *pyridine R*. Allow to stand for about 10 min. No green colour develops.

TESTS

pH (2.2.3)

Suspend 0.25 g in 10 ml of *carbon dioxide-free water R*. The pH of the suspension is 8.5 to 10.5.

Composition

Examine by liquid chromatography (2.2.29). *Prepare the solutions immediately before use.*

The content of tylosin A is not less than 80.0 per cent and the sum of the contents of tylosin A, tylosin B, tylosin C and tylosin D is not less than 95.0 per cent.

Test solution   Dissolve 20.0 mg of the substance to be examined in a mixture of equal volumes of *acetonitrile R* and *water R* and dilute to 100.0 ml with the same mixture of solvents.

Reference solution (a)   Dissolve 2 mg of *tylosin phosphate for peak identification CRS* (containing tylosins A, B, C and D) in a mixture of equal volumes of *acetonitrile R* and *water R* and dilute to 10 ml with the same mixture of solvents.

Reference solution (b)   Dissolve 2 mg of *tylosin CRS* and 2 mg of *tylosin D CRS* in a mixture of equal volumes of *acetonitrile R* and *water R* and dilute to 10 ml with the same mixture of solvents.

The chromatographic procedure may be carried out using:
— a stainless steel column 0.20 m long and 4.6 mm in internal diameter packed with *octadecylsilyl silica gel for chromatography R* (5 μm),
— as mobile phase at a flow rate of 1.0 ml/min a mixture of 40 volumes of *acetonitrile R* and 60 volumes of a 200 g/l solution of *sodium perchlorate R* previously adjusted to pH 2.5 using *1 M hydrochloric acid*,
— as detector a spectrophotometer set at 290 nm,

maintaining the temperature of the column at 35 °C.

Inject 20 μl of reference solution (b). When the chromatograms are recorded in the prescribed conditions, the retention time of tylosin A is about 12 min. The test is not valid unless, in the chromatogram obtained, the resolution between the peaks due to tylosin A and tylosin D is at least 2.0. Inject 20 μl of the test solution and 20 μl of reference solution (a). Use the chromatogram supplied with *tylosin phosphate for peak identification CRS* and the chromatogram obtained with reference solution (a) to identify the peaks due to tylosins A, B, C and D. Calculate the percentage content of the constituents from the areas of the peaks in the chromatogram obtained with the test solution by the normalisation procedure.

Tyramine

In a 25.0 ml volumetric flask, dissolve 50.0 mg of the substance to be examined in 5.0 ml of a 3.4 g/l solution of *phosphoric acid R*. Add 1.0 ml of *pyridine R* and 2.0 ml of a saturated solution of *ninhydrin R* (about 40 g/l). Close the flask with a piece of aluminium foil and heat in a water-bath at 85 °C for 30 min. Cool the solution rapidly and dilute to 25.0 ml with *water R*. Mix and measure immediately the absorbance (2.2.25) of the solution at 570 nm using a blank solution as the compensation liquid. The absorbance is not greater than that of a standard prepared at the same time and in the same manner using 5.0 ml of a 35 mg/l solution of *tyramine R* in a 3.4 g/l solution of *phosphoric acid R* (0.35 per cent). If intended for use in the manufacture of parenteral dosage forms, the absorbance is not greater than that of a standard prepared at the same time and in the same manner using 5.0 ml of a 15 mg/l solution of *tyramine R* in a 3.4 g/l solution of *phosphoric acid R* (0.15 per cent).

Loss on drying (2.2.32)

Not more than 5.0 per cent, determined on 1.000 g by drying in an oven at 60 °C at a pressure not exceeding 0.7 kPa for 3 h.

Sulphated ash (2.4.14)

Not more than 3.0 per cent, determined on 1.0 g.

ASSAY

Carry out the microbiological assay of antibiotics (2.7.2). Use *tylosin CRS* as the reference substance.

STORAGE

Store protected from light.

IMPURITIES

A. desmycinosyltylosin,

B. tylosin A aldol.

Tylosin Phosphate

(Tylosin Phosphate Bulk Solution for Veterinary Use, Ph Eur monograph 1661)

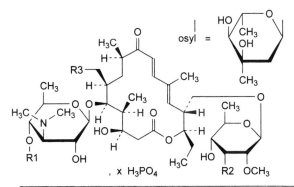

Tylosin	R1	R2	R3	Mol. Formula	M_r
A	osyl	OCH_3	CHO	$C_{46}H_{77}NO_{17}$	916
B	H	OCH_3	CHO	$C_{39}H_{65}NO_{14}$	772
C	osyl	OH	CHO	$C_{45}H_{75}NO_{17}$	902
D	osyl	OCH_3	CH_2OH	$C_{46}H_{79}NO_{17}$	918

Action and use
Macrolide antibacterial.

Ph Eur _____

DEFINITION
Solution of the dihydrogen phosphate of a mixture of macrolide antibiotics produced by a strain of *Streptomyces fradiae* or by any other means.

The main component is the phosphate of (4R,5S,6S,7R,9R,11E,13E,15R,16R)-15-[[(6-deoxy-2,3-di-O-methyl-β-D-allopyranosyl)oxy]methyl]-6-[[3,6-dideoxy-4-O-(2,6-dideoxy-3-C-methyl-α-L-*ribo*-hexopyranosyl)-3-(dimethylamino)-β-D-glucopyranosyl]oxy]-16-ethyl-4-hydroxy-5,9,13-trimethyl-7-(2-oxoethyl)oxacyclohexadeca-11,13-diene-2,10-dione (tylosin A phosphate).

The phosphates of tylosin B (desmycosin phosphate), tylosin C (macrocin phosphate) and tylosin D (relomycin phosphate) may also be present. The solution also contains sodium dihydrogen phosphate.

Potency
Minimum 800 IU per milligram of dry residue. Tylosins A, B, C and D contribute to the potency.

CHARACTERS
Appearance
Yellow or brownish-yellow, viscous liquid.

Solubility
Miscible with water.

IDENTIFICATION
A. Ultraviolet and visible absorption spectrophotometry *(2.2.25)*.

Test solution Dilute an amount of the preparation to be examined equivalent to 400 000 IU of tylosin phosphate to 100.0 ml with *water R*. Dilute 1.0 ml of this solution to 100.0 ml with *water R*.

Spectral range 230-350 nm.

Absorption maximum At 290 nm.

Absorbance at the absorption maximum Minimum 0.70.

B. Examine the chromatograms obtained in the test for composition.

Results The principal peak in the chromatogram obtained with the test solution is similar in retention time and size to the principal peak in the chromatogram obtained with reference solution (a).

C. Dilute an amount of the preparation to be examined equivalent to 400 000 IU of tylosin phosphate in 10 ml of water R. The solution gives reaction (a) of *phosphates (2.3.1)*.

TESTS
pH *(2.2.3)*
5.5 to 6.5.

Dilute 1.0 g in 10 ml of *carbon dioxide-free water R*.

Composition
Liquid chromatography *(2.2.29)*: use the normalisation procedure. *Prepare the solutions immediately before use.*

Test solution Dilute an amount of the preparation to be examined equivalent to 50 000 IU of tylosin phosphate to 200 ml with a mixture of equal volumes of *acetonitrile R* and *water R*.

Reference solution (a) Dissolve 2 mg of *tylosin phosphate for peak identification CRS* (containing tylosins A, B, C and D) in a mixture of equal volumes of *acetonitrile R* and *water R* and dilute to 10 ml with the same mixture of solvents.

Reference solution (b) Dissolve 2 mg of *tylosin CRS* and 2 mg of *tylosin D CRS* in a mixture of equal volumes of *acetonitrile R* and *water R* and dilute to 10 ml with the same mixture of solvents.

Reference solution (c) Dilute 1.0 ml of reference solution (a) to 100.0 ml with a mixture of equal volumes of *acetonitrile R* and *water R*. Dilute 1.0 ml of this solution to 10.0 ml with a mixture of equal volumes of *acetonitrile R* and *water R*.

Column:
— *size*: l = 0.20 m, Ø = 4.6 mm;
— *stationary phase*: octadecylsilyl silica gel for chromatography R (5 μm);
— *temperature*: 35 °C.

Mobile phase Mix 40 volumes of *acetonitrile R* and 60 volumes of a 200 g/l solution of *sodium perchlorate R* previously adjusted to pH 2.5 using a 36.5 g/l solution of *hydrochloric acid R*.

Flow rate 1.0 ml/min.

Detection Spectrophotometer at 290 nm.

Injection 20 μl.

Run time 1.8 times the retention time of tylosin A.

Identification of tylosins Use the chromatogram supplied with *tylosin phosphate for peak identification CRS* and the chromatogram obtained with reference solution (a) to identify the peaks due to tylosins A, B, C and D.

Relative retention With reference to tylosin A (retention time = about 12 min): impurity A = about 0.35; tylosin C = about 0.5; tylosin B = about 0.6; tylosin D = about 0.85; impurity B = about 0.9.

System suitability Reference solution (b):
— resolution: minimum 2.0 between the peaks due to tylosin D and tylosin A.

Limits:
— *tylosin A*: minimum 80.0 per cent;
— *sum of the contents of tylosin A, tylosin B, tylosin C and tylosin D*: minimum 95.0 per cent;
— *disregard limit*: area of the principal peak in the chromatogram obtained with reference solution (c).

Tyramine

In a 25.0 ml volumetric flask, dissolve an amount of the preparation to be examined equivalent to 50 000 IU of tylosin phosphate in 5.0 ml of a 3.4 g/l solution of *phosphoric acid R*. Add 1.0 ml of *pyridine R* and 2.0 ml of a saturated solution of *ninhydrin R* (about 40 g/l). Close the flask with aluminium foil and heat in a water-bath at 85 °C for 20-30 min. Cool the solution rapidly and dilute to 25.0 ml with *water R*. Mix and measure immediately the *absorbance* (*2.2.25*) of the solution at 570 nm using a blank solution as the compensation liquid.

The absorbance is not greater than that of a standard prepared at the same time and in the same manner using 5.0 ml of a 35 mg/l solution of *tyramine R* in a 3.4 g/l solution of *phosphoric acid R*.

Phosphate

8.5 per cent to 10.0 per cent of PO_4, calculated with reference to the dry residue (see Assay).

Test solution Dissolve an amount of the preparation to be examined equivalent to 200 000 IU of tylosin phosphate in 50 ml of *water R*. Add 5.0 ml of *dilute sulphuric acid R* and dilute to 100.0 ml with *water R*. To 2.0 ml of this solution add successively, mixing after each addition, 10.0 ml of water R, 5.0 ml of *ammonium molybdate reagent R2*, 1.0 ml of *hydroquinone solution R* and 1.0 ml of a 200 g/l solution of *sodium metabisulphite R*. Allow to stand for at least 20 min and dilute to 50.0 ml with *water R*. Mix thoroughly.

Reference solution (a) To 1.0 ml of a standard solution containing 0.430 g/l of *potassium dihydrogen phosphate R* (corresponds to 300 ppm of PO_4) add successively, mixing after each addition, 10.0 ml of *water R*, 5.0 ml of *ammonium molybdate reagent R2*, 1.0 ml of *hydroquinone solution R* and 1.0 ml of a 200 g/l solution of *sodium metabisulphite R*. Allow to stand for at least 20 min and dilute to 50.0 ml with *water R*. Mix thoroughly.

Reference solution (b) Prepare as reference solution (a) but using 2.0 ml of the standard solution.

Reference solution (c) Prepare as reference solution (a) but using 5.0 ml of the standard solution.

Compensation liquid Prepare as reference solution (a) but omitting the standard solution.

Measure the absorbance (*2.2.25*) of the test solution and of the reference solutions at 650 nm. Draw a calibration curve with the absorbances of the 3 reference solutions as a function of the quantity of phosphate in the solutions and read from the curve the quantity of phosphate in the test solution. Determine the percentage content of PO_4, calculated with reference to the dry residue (see Assay).

ASSAY

Carry out the microbiological assay of antibiotics (*2.7.2*).

Use *tylosin CRS* as the reference substance. Calculate the potency from the mass of the dry residue and the activity of the solution.

Dry residue Dry 3.0 g of the preparation to be examined *in vacuo* at 60 °C for 3 h and weigh.

STORAGE

Protected from light, at a temperature of 2 °C to 8 °C.

LABELLING

The label states the concentration of the solution in International Units per milligram of preparation.

IMPURITIES

A. desmycinosyltylosin A,

and epimer at C*

B. (1R,2S,3S,4R,8R,9R,10E,12E,15R,16RS)-9-[[(6-deoxy-2,3-di-O-methy-β-D-allopyranosyl)oxy]methyl]-2-[[3,6-dideoxy-4-O-(2,6-dideoxy-3-C-methyl-α-L-*ribo*-hexopyranosyl)-3-(dimethylamino)-β-D-glucopyranosyl]oxy]-8-ethyl-4,16-dihydroxy-3,11,15-trimethyl-7-oxabicyclo[13.2.1]octadeca-10,12-diene-6,14-dione (tylosin A aldol).

Ph Eur

Tylosin Tartrate

(Tylosin Tartrate for Veterinary Use,
Ph Eur monograph 1274)

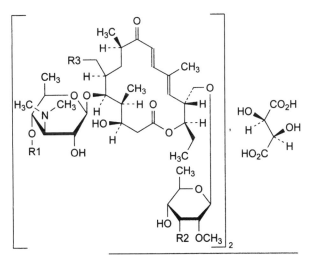

Tylosin	Mol. Form.	R1	R2	R3
A	$C_{46}H_{77}NO_{17}$	osyl	OCH_3	CHO
B	$C_{39}H_{65}NO_{14}$	H	OCH_3	CHO
C	$C_{45}H_{75}NO_{17}$	osyl	OH	CHO
D	$C_{46}H_{79}NO_{17}$	osyl	OCH_3	CH_2OH

Action and use

Macrolide antibacterial.

Preparation

Tylosin Tartrate and Sulfathiazole Sodium Veterinary Oral Powder

Ph Eur _____

DEFINITION

Tylosin tartrate for veterinary use is a tartrate of a mixture of macrolide antibiotics produced by a strain of *Streptomyces fradiae* or by any other means. The main component of the mixture is (4R,5S,6S,7R,9R,11E,13E,15R,16R)-15-[[(6-deoxy-2,3-di-*O*-methyl-β-D-allopyranosyl)oxy]methyl]-6-[[3,6-dideoxy-4-*O*-(2,6-dideoxy-3-*C*-methyl-α-L-*ribo*-hexopyranosyl)-3-(dimethylamino)-β-D-glucopyranosyl]oxy]-16-ethyl-4-hydroxy-5,9,13-trimethyl-7-(2-oxoethyl)oxacyclohexadeca-11,13-diene-2,10-dione (tylosin A, tartrate M_r 1982). Tylosin B (desmycosin, tartrate M_r 1694), tylosin C (macrocin, tartrate M_r 1954) and tylosin D (relomycin, tartrate M_r 1986) may also be present. They contribute to the potency of the substance to be examined, which is not less than 800 IU/mg, calculated with reference to the dried substance.

CHARACTERS

An almost white or slightly yellow, hygroscopic powder, freely soluble in water and in methylene chloride, slightly soluble in anhydrous ethanol. It dissolves in dilute solutions of mineral acids.

IDENTIFICATION

A. Examine by infrared absorption spectrophotometry (2.2.24), comparing with the *Ph. Eur. reference spectrum* of *tylosin tartrate*.

B. Examine the chromatograms obtained in the test for composition. The retention time and size of the principal peak in the chromatogram obtained with the test solution are the same as those of the principal peak in the chromatogram obtained with reference solution (a).

C. Dissolve about 30 mg in a mixture of 0.15 ml of *water R*, 2.5 ml of *acetic anhydride R* and 7.5 ml of *pyridine R*. Allow to stand for about 10 min. A green colour is produced.

TESTS

pH (2.2.3)

Dissolve 0.25 g in 10 ml of *carbon dioxide-free water R*. The pH of the solution is 5.0 to 7.2.

Composition

Examine by liquid chromatography (2.2.29). *Prepare the solutions immediately before use.*

The content of tylosin A is not less than 80.0 per cent and the sum of the contents of tylosin A, tylosin B, tylosin C and tylosin D is not less than 95.0 per cent.

Test solution Dissolve 20.0 mg of the substance to be examined in a mixture of equal volumes of *acetonitrile R* and *water R* and dilute to 100.0 ml with the same mixture of solvents.

Reference solution (a) Dissolve 2 mg of *tylosin phosphate for peak identification CRS* (containing tylosins A, B, C and D) in a mixture of equal volumes of *acetonitrile R* and *water R* and dilute to 10 ml with the same mixture of solvents.

Reference solution (b) Dissolve 2 mg of *tylosin CRS* and 2 mg of *tylosin D CRS* in a mixture of equal volumes of *acetonitrile R* and *water R* and dilute to 10 ml with the same mixture of solvents.

The chromatographic procedure may be carried out using:
— a stainless steel column 0.20 m long and 4.6 mm in internal diameter packed with *octadecylsilyl silica gel for chromatography R* (5 μm),
— as mobile phase at a flow rate of 1.0 ml/min a mixture of 40 volumes of *acetonitrile R* and 60 volumes of a 200 g/l solution of *sodium perchlorate R* previously adjusted to pH 2.5 using *1 M hydrochloric acid*,
— as detector a spectrophotometer set at 290 nm,

maintaining the temperature of the column at 35 °C.

Inject 20 μl of reference solution (b). When the chromatograms are recorded in the prescribed conditions, the retention time of tylosin A is about 12 min. The test is not valid unless, in the chromatogram obtained, the *resolution* between the peaks corresponding to tylosin A and tylosin D is at least 2.0. Inject 20 μl of the test solution and 20 μl of reference solution (a). Use the chromatogram supplied with *tylosin phosphate for peak identification CRS* and the chromatogram obtained with reference solution (a) to identify the peaks due to tylosins A, B, C and D. Calculate the percentage content of the constituents from the areas of the peaks in the chromatogram obtained with the test solution by the normalisation procedure.

Tyramine

In a 25.0 ml volumetric flask, dissolve 50.0 mg of the substance to be examined in 5.0 ml of a 3.4 g/l solution of *phosphoric acid R*. Add 1.0 ml of *pyridine R* and 2.0 ml of a saturated solution of *ninhydrin R* (about 40 g/l). Close the flask with a piece of aluminium foil and heat in a water-bath at 85 °C for 30 min. Cool the solution rapidly and dilute to 25.0 ml with *water R*. Mix and measure immediately the absorbance (2.2.25) of the solution at 570 nm using a blank solution as the compensation liquid. The absorbance is not greater than that of a standard prepared at the same time and in the same manner using 5.0 ml of a 35 mg/l solution of *tyramine R* in a 3.4 g/l solution of *phosphoric acid R*

(0.35 per cent). If intended for use in the manufacture of parenteral dosage forms, the absorbance is not greater than that of a standard prepared at the same time and in the same manner using 5.0 ml of a 15 mg/l solution of *tyramine R* in a 3.4 g/l solution of *phosphoric acid R* (0.15 per cent).

Loss on drying (*2.2.32*)
Not more than 4.5 per cent, determined on 1.000 g by drying at 60 °C at a pressure not exceeding 0.7 kPa for 3 h.

Sulphated ash (*2.4.14*)
Not more than 2.5 per cent, determined on 1.0 g.

ASSAY
Carry out the microbiological assay of antibiotics (*2.7.2*). Use *tylosin CRS* as the reference substance.

STORAGE
Store in an airtight container, protected from light.

IMPURITIES

A. desmycinosyltylosin,

B. tylosin A aldol.

Ph Eur

Valnemulin Hydrochloride

(*Valnemulin Hydrochloride for Veterinary Use, Ph Eur monograph 2137*)

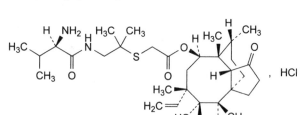

$C_{31}H_{52}N_2O_5S,HCl$ 601   *101312-92-9*

Action and use
Antibacterial.

Ph Eur

DEFINITION
(3aS,4R,5S,6S,8R,9R,9aR,10R)-6-Ethenyl-5-hydroxy-4,6,9,10-tetramethyl-1-oxodecahydro-3a,9-propano-3aH-cyclopenta[8]annulen-8-yl [[2-[[(2R)-2-amino-3-methylbutanoyl]amino]-1,1-dimethylethyl]sulphanyl]acetate hydrochloride.

Semi-synthetic product derived from a fermentation product.

Content
96.0 per cent to 102.0 per cent (anhydrous substance).

CHARACTERS
Appearance
White or yellowish, amorphous powder, hygroscopic.

Solubility
Freely soluble in water and in anhydrous ethanol, practically insoluble in *tert*-butyl methyl ether.

IDENTIFICATION
A. Infrared absorption spectrophotometry (*2.2.24*).
Comparison   valnemulin hydrochloride CRS.
B. It gives reaction (a) of chlorides (*2.3.1*).

TESTS
pH (*2.2.3*)
3.0 to 6.0.
Dissolve 2.0 g in *carbon dioxide-free water R* and dilute to 20 ml with the same solvent.

Specific optical rotation (*2.2.7*)
+ 15.5 to + 18.0 (anhydrous substance).
Dissolve 0.250 g in *water R* and dilute to 25.0 ml with the same solvent.

Related substances
Liquid chromatography (*2.2.29*).

Phosphate buffer solution pH 2.5   Dissolve 8.0 g of *disodium hydrogen phosphate R* and 3.0 g of *potassium dihydrogen phosphate R* in *water for chromatography R* and dilute to 1000.0 ml with the same solvent. Adjust to pH 2.5 with *phosphoric acid R*.

Solvent mixture   Mix equal volumes of *acetonitrile R1* and *water for chromatography R*.

Test solution   Dissolve 0.100 g of the substance to be examined in the solvent mixture and dilute to 10.0 ml with the solvent mixture.

Reference solution (a)   Dilute 1.0 ml of the test solution to 100.0 ml with the solvent mixture.

Reference solution (b) Dissolve 5 mg of *valnemulin impurity E CRS* and 5 mg of the substance to be examined in the solvent mixture and dilute to 25 ml with the solvent mixture.

Reference solution (c) Dissolve the contents of a vial of *valnemulin for peak identification CRS* (containing impurities A, B and C) in 1 ml of the solvent mixture.

Column:
— *size:* l = 0.15 m, Ø = 4.6 mm;
— *stationary phase: octadecylsilyl silica gel for chromatography R* (3 μm);
— *temperature:* 50 °C.

Mobile phase:
— *mobile phase A*: phosphate buffer solution pH 2.5, *water R* (25:75 V/V);
— *mobile phase B*: phosphate buffer solution pH 2.5, *acetonitrile R1* (25:75 V/V);

Time (min)	Mobile phase A (per cent V/V)	Mobile phase B (per cent V/V)
0 - 2	95 → 55	5 → 45
2 - 4.5	55 → 50	45 → 50
4.5 - 5.5	50 → 35	50 → 65
5.5 - 6.85	35	65
6.85 - 10	35 → 0	65 → 100
10 - 13	0	100
13 - 14	0 → 95	100 → 5
14 - 20	95	5

Flow rate 1.5 ml/min.

Detection Spectrophotometer at 200 nm.

Injection 5 μl.

Identification of impurities Use the chromatogram supplied with *valnemulin for peak identification CRS* and the chromatogram obtained with reference solution (c) to identify the peaks due to impurities A, B and C.

Relative retention With reference to valnemulin (retention time = about 7 min): impurity D = about 0.2; impurity A = about 0.7; impurity B = about 0.85; impurity E = about 0.9; impurity C = about 1.1.

System suitability Reference solution (b):
— *resolution*: minimum 1.5 between the peaks due to impurity E and valnemulin.

Limits:
— *correction factors*: for the calculation of content multiply the peak areas of the following impurities by the corresponding correction factor: impurity B = 3.2; impurity E = 4.2;
— *impurity A*: not more than 0.5 times the area of the principal peak in the chromatogram obtained with reference solution (a) (0.5 per cent);
— *impurity B*: not more than twice the area of the principal peak in the chromatogram obtained with reference solution (a) (2.0 per cent);
— *impurity C*: not more than the area of the principal peak in the chromatogram obtained with reference solution (a) (1.0 per cent);
— *any other impurity*: for each impurity, not more than 0.2 times the area of the principal peak in the chromatogram obtained with reference solution (a) (0.2 per cent);

— *total*: not more than 3 times the area of the principal peak in the chromatogram obtained with reference solution (a) (3.0 per cent);
— *disregard limit*: 0.1 times the area of the principal peak in the chromatogram obtained with reference solution (a) (0.1 per cent); disregard the peak due to the chloride ion.

Water (*2.5.12*)
Maximum 4.0 per cent, determined on 0.500 g.

ASSAY
Liquid chromatography (*2.2.29*).

Test solution Dissolve 40.0 mg of the substance to be examined in a mixture of equal volumes of *acetonitrile R1* and *water R* and dilute to 50.0 ml with the same mixture of solvents.

Reference solution Dissolve 50.0 mg of *valnemulin hydrogen tartrate CRS* in a mixture of equal volumes of *acetonitrile R1* and *water R* and dilute to 50.0 ml with the same mixture of solvents.

Column:
— *size:* l = 0.125 m, Ø = 4.6 mm;
— *stationary phase: octadecylsilyl silica gel for chromatography R* (3 μm);
— *temperature*: 45 °C.

Mobile phase Mix 43 volumes of *acetonitrile R1* and 57 volumes of a solution containing 0.94 g/l of *disodium hydrogen phosphate R* and 8.7 g/l of *potassium dihydrogen phosphate R* previously adjusted to pH 2.5 with *phosphoric acid R*.

Flow rate 1.2 ml/min.

Detection Spectrophotometer at 210 nm.

Injection 5 μl.

Run time 3 times the retention time of valnemulin (retention time = about 2.4 min).

Calculate the percentage content of $C_{31}H_{53}ClN_2O_5S$, using the declared content of *valnemulin hydrogen tartrate CRS* and by multiplying by 0.841.

STORAGE
In an airtight container, protected from light.

IMPURITIES
Specified impurities A, B, C.

Other detectable impurities (the following substances would, if present at a sufficient level, be detected by one or other of the tests in the monograph. They are limited by the general acceptance criterion for other/unspecified impurities and/or by the general monograph *Substances for pharmaceutical use* (*2034*). It is therefore not necessary to identify these impurities for demonstration of compliance. See also *5.10. Control of impurities in substances for pharmaceutical use*): D, E.

A. R = D-Val, X = SO: (3aS,4R,5S,6S,8R,9R,9aR,10R)-6-ethenyl-5-hydroxy-4,6,9,10-tetramethyl-1-oxodecahydro-3a,9-propano-3aH-cyclopenta[8]annulen-8-yl [[2-[[(2R)-2-amino-3-methylbutanoyl]amino]-1,1-dimethylethyl]sulphinyl]acetate (valnemulin sulphoxide),

B. R = H, X = S: (3aS,4R,5S,6S,8R,9R,9aR,10R)-6-ethenyl-5-hydroxy-4,6,9,10-tetramethyl-1-oxodecahydro-3a,9-propano-3aH-cyclopenta[8]annulen-8-yl [(2-amino-1,1-dimethylethyl)sulphanyl]acetate (dimethyl cysteaminyl pleuromulin),

C. R = D-Val-D-Val, X = S: (3aS,4R,5S,6S,8R,9R,9aR,10R)-6-ethenyl-5-hydroxy-4,6,9,10-tetramethyl-1-oxodecahydro-3a,9-propano-3aH-cyclopenta[8]annulen-8-yl [[2-[[(2R)-2-[[(2R)-2-amino-3-methylbutanoyl]amino]-3-methylbutanoyl]amino]-1,1-dimethylethyl]sulphanyl]acetate (valyl-valneumulin),

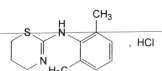

D. (2R)-2-amino-3-methylbutanoic acid (D-valine),

E. (3aS,4R,5S,6S,8R,9R,9aR,10R)-6-ethenyl-5-hydroxy-4,6,9,10-tetramethyl-1-oxodecahydro-3a,9-propano-3aH-cyclopenta[8]annulen-8-yl 2-hydroxyacetate (pleuromulin).

_____ Ph Eur

Xylazine Hydrochloride

(*Xylazine Hydrochloride for Veterinary Use, Ph Eur monograph 1481*)

$C_{12}H_{17}ClN_2S$ 256.8   7361-61-7

Action and use

Analgesic.

Ph Eur _____

DEFINITION

N-(2,6-Dimethylphenyl)-5,6-dihydro-4H-1,3-thiazin-2-amine hydrochloride.

Content

98.0 per cent to 102.0 per cent (dried substance).

CHARACTERS

Appearance

White or almost white, crystalline powder, hygroscopic.

Solubility

Freely soluble in water, very soluble in methanol, freely soluble in methylene chloride.

IDENTIFICATION

A. Infrared absorption spectrophotometry (*2.2.24*).

Preparation Discs.

Comparison xylazine hydrochloride CRS.

B. It gives reaction (b) of chlorides (*2.3.1*).

TESTS

Solution S

Dissolve 5.0 g in *carbon dioxide-free water R* prepared from *distilled water R*, heating at 60 °C if necessary; allow to cool and dilute to 50.0 ml with the same solvent.

Appearance of solution

Solution S is not more opalescent than reference suspension II (*2.2.1*) and is colourless (*2.2.2, Method II*).

pH (*2.2.3*)

4.0 to 5.5 for solution S.

Impurity A

Maximum 100 ppm.

Solution A Dissolve 0.25 g of the substance to be examined in *methanol R* and dilute to 10 ml with the same solvent. This solution is used to prepare the test solution.

Solution B Dissolve 50 mg of *2,6-dimethylaniline R* in *methanol R* and dilute to 100 ml with the same solvent. Dilute 1 ml of the solution to 100 ml with *methanol R*. This solution is used to prepare the reference solution.

Using 2 flat-bottomed tubes with an inner diameter of about 10 mm, place in the first tube 2 ml of solution A, and in the second tube 1 ml of solution B and 1 ml of *methanol R*. To each tube add 1 ml of a freshly prepared 10 g/l solution of *dimethylaminobenzaldehyde R* in *methanol R* and 2 ml of *glacial acetic acid R* and allow to stand at room temperature for 10 min. Compare the colours in diffused daylight, viewing vertically against a white background. Any yellow colour in the test solution is not more intense than that in the reference solution.

Related substances

Liquid chromatography (*2.2.29*). *Prepare the solutions immediately before use.*

Solvent mixture Mix 8 volumes of *acetonitrile R*, 30 volumes of *methanol R* and 62 volumes of a 2.72 g/l solution of *potassium dihydrogen phosphate R* adjusted to pH 7.2 with *dilute sodium hydroxide solution R.*

Test solution Dissolve 0.100 g of the substance to be examined in the solvent mixture and dilute to 20.0 ml with the solvent mixture.

Reference solution Dissolve 5.0 mg of the substance to be examined, 5.0 mg of *2,6-dimethylaniline R*, 5.0 mg of *xylazine impurity C CRS* and 5.0 mg of *xylazine impurity E CRS* in *acetonitrile R* and dilute to 100.0 ml with the same solvent. Dilute 1.0 ml of this solution to 10.0 ml with the solvent mixture.

Column:

— *size*: l = 0.15 m, Ø = 3.9 mm,

— *stationary phase*: end-capped octylsilyl silica gel for chromatography with polar incorporated groups R (5 μm),

— *temperature*: 40 °C.

Mobile phase:

— *mobile phase A*: mix 30 volumes of *methanol R* and 70 volumes of a 2.72 g/l solution of *potassium dihydrogen phosphate R* adjusted to pH 7.2 with *dilute sodium hydroxide solution R*,

— *mobile phase B*: *methanol R*, *acetonitrile R* (30:70 *V/V*),

Time (min)	Mobile phase A (per cent *V/V*)	Mobile phase B (per cent *V/V*)
0 - 15	89 → 28	11 → 72
15 - 21	28	72
21 - 22	28 → 89	72 → 11
22 - 33	89	11

Flow rate 1.0 ml/min.

Detection Spectrophotometer at 230 nm.

Equilibration For at least 30 min with a mixture of 28 volumes of mobile phase A and 72 volumes of mobile phase B.

Injection 20 µl.

Relative retention with reference to xylazine (retention time = about 7.5 min): impurity A = about 0.8; impurity E = about 1.6; impurity C = about 2.2.

System suitability Reference solution:
— *resolution*: minimum 4.0 between the peaks due to impurity A and xylazine.

Limits:
— *impurities C, E*: for each impurity, not more than twice the area of the corresponding peak in the chromatogram obtained with the reference solution (0.2 per cent),
— *impurities B, D*: for each impurity, not more than twice the area of the peak due to xylazine in the chromatogram obtained with the reference solution (0.2 per cent),
— *any other impurity*: for each impurity, not more than twice the area of the peak due to xylazine in the chromatogram obtained with the reference solution (0.2 per cent),
— *total of impurities other than B, C, D and E*: not more than twice the area of the peak due to xylazine in the chromatogram obtained with the reference solution (0.2 per cent),
— *disregard limit*: 0.5 times the area of the peak due to xylazine in the chromatogram obtained with the reference solution (0.05 per cent); disregard any peak due to the blank.

Heavy metals (*2.4.8*)
Maximum 10 ppm.

12 ml of solution S complies with limit test A. Prepare the standard using 10 ml of *lead standard solution (1 ppm Pb) R*.

Loss on drying (*2.2.32*)
Maximum 0.5 per cent, determined on 1.000 g by drying in an oven at 100-105 °C for 2 h.

Sulphated ash (*2.4.14*)
Maximum 0.1 per cent, determined on 1.0 g.

ASSAY
Dissolve 0.200 g in 25 ml of *alcohol R*. Add 25 ml of *water R*. Titrate with *0.1 M sodium hydroxide*, determining the end-point potentiometrically (*2.2.20*).

1 ml of *0.1 M sodium hydroxide* is equivalent to 25.68 mg of $C_{12}H_{17}ClN_2S$.

STORAGE
In an airtight container, protected from light.

IMPURITIES
Specified impurities A, B, C, D, E.

A. R = NH$_2$: 2,6-dimethylaniline (2,6-xylidine),
C. R = N=C=S: 2,6-dimethylphenyl isothiocyanate,
D. R = NH-CS-NH-[CH$_2$]$_3$-OH:
N-(2,6-dimethylphenyl)-N'-(3-hydroxypropyl)thiourea,
E. R = NH-CS-S-CH$_3$:
methyl (2,6-dimethylphenyl)carbamodithioate,

B. N,N'-bis(2,6-dimethylphenyl)thiourea.

Ph Eur

Monographs

Formulated Preparations

Attention is drawn to the General Notices of the British Pharmacopoeia
(Veterinary) governing this section

FORMULATED PREPARATIONS: GENERAL MONOGRAPHS

The general provisions of the European Pharmacopoeia relating to a specific type of dosage form apply to all veterinary dosage forms of the type defined, whether or not an individual monograph is included in the British Pharmacopoeia (Veterinary). These provisions are reproduced in the general monographs of the British Pharmacopoeia listed below:

Capsules

Liquids for Cutaneous Application†

Ear Preparations

Extracts

Eye Preparations

Medicated Foams

Granules*

Preparations for Inhalation

Preparations for Irrigation

Nasal Preparations

Oral Liquids*

Parenteral Preparations*

Pressurised Pharmaceutical Preparations

Rectal Preparations

Sticks

Tablets*

Medicated Tampons

Topical Powders*

Topical Semi-solid Preparations

Tinctures

Transdermal Patches

Vaginal Preparations

Where a general monograph of the British Pharmacopoeia listed above includes additional statements and requirements applicable to the individual monographs of the British Pharmacopoeia, such statements, modified where appropriate as described below, apply unless otherwise indicated to any individual monograph for that dosage form in the British Pharmacopoeia (Veterinary).

Individual monographs of the British Pharmacopoeia (Veterinary) for each type of dosage form are listed for information at the end of each general monograph in the British Pharmacopoeia (Veterinary).

---

*Where justified and authorised, the requirements of the European Pharmacopoeia reproduced in the general monograph do not necessarily apply to formulated preparations for veterinary use.
† Where justified and authorised, the requirements of the European Pharmacopoeia reproduced in the general monograph do not necessarily apply to formulated preparations for systemic and veterinary use.

Glossary

A glossary of terms relating to formulated preparations is included in the British Pharmacopoeia.

VETERINARY LIQUID PREPARATIONS FOR CUTANEOUS APPLICATION

(Ph Eur monograph 1808)

Veterinary Liquid Preparations for Cutaneous Application comply with the requirements of the European Pharmacopoeia. These requirements are reproduced below.

Ph Eur _____

Unless otherwise justified and authorised, veterinary liquid preparations for cutaneous application comply with the requirements of the monograph on Liquid preparations for cutaneous application (0927). In addition to these requirements, the following statements apply to veterinary liquid preparations for cutaneous application.

DEFINITION

Veterinary liquid preparations for cutaneous application are liquid preparations intended to be applied to the skin to obtain a local and/or systemic effect. They are solutions, suspensions or emulsions which may contain one or more active substances in a suitable vehicle. They may be presented as concentrates in the form of wettable powders, pastes, solutions or suspensions, which are used to prepare diluted suspensions or emulsions of active substances. They may contain suitable antimicrobial preservatives, antioxidants and other excipients such as stabilisers, emulsifiers and thickeners.

Several categories of veterinary liquid preparations for cutaneous application may be distinguished:
— cutaneous foams (see *Liquid preparations for cutaneous application (0927)*),
— dip concentrates,
— pour-on preparations,
— shampoos (see *Liquid preparations for cutaneous application (0927)*),
— spot-on preparations,
— sprays,
— teat dips,
— teat sprays,
— udder-washes.

DIP CONCENTRATES

DEFINITION

Dip concentrates are preparations containing one or more active substances, usually in the form of wettable powders, pastes, solutions or suspensions, which are used to prepare diluted solutions, suspensions or emulsions of active substances. The diluted preparations are applied by complete immersion of the animal.

POUR-ON PREPARATIONS

DEFINITION

Pour-on preparations contain one or more active substances for the prevention and treatment of ectoparasitic and/or endoparasitic infestations of animals. They are applied in volumes which are usually greater than 5 ml by pouring along the animal's dorsal midline.

SPOT-ON PREPARATIONS

DEFINITION
Spot-on preparations contain one or more active substances for the prevention and treatment of ectoparasitic and/or endoparasitic infestations of animals. They are applied in volumes which are usually less than 10 ml, to a small area on the head or back, as appropriate, of the animal.

SPRAYS

DEFINITION
Sprays contain one or more active substances that are intended to be applied externally for therapeutic or prophylactic purposes. They are delivered in the form of an aerosol by the actuation of an appropriate valve or by means of a suitable atomising device that is either an integral part of the container or is supplied separately.

Sprays may be presented in pressurised containers (see *Pressurised pharmaceutical preparations (0523)*). When so presented, sprays usually consist of one or more active substances in a suitable vehicle held under pressure with suitable propellants or suitable mixtures of propellants. When otherwise presented, sprays are supplied in well-closed containers.

PRODUCTION
During the development and manufacture of a spray, measures are taken to ensure that the assembled product conforms to a defined spray rate and spray pattern.

TEAT DIPS

DEFINITION
Teat dips contain one or more disinfectant active substances, usually in the form of solutions into which the teats of an animal are dipped pre- and, where necessary, post-milking to reduce the population of pathogenic micro-organisms on the surfaces. Teat dips may be supplied/presented as ready-to-use preparations or they may be prepared by dilution of teat dip concentrates. Pre- and post-milking teat dips often differ in formulation. Teat dips usually contain emollients to promote skin hydration, to soften the skin and allow healing of lesions that would otherwise harbour bacteria.

TEAT SPRAYS

DEFINITION
Teat sprays contain one or more disinfectant active substances, usually in the form of solutions which are sprayed onto the teats of an animal pre- and, where necessary, post-milking to reduce the population of pathogenic micro-organisms on the surfaces. Teat sprays may be supplied/presented as ready-to-use preparations or they may be prepared by dilution of teat spray concentrates. Pre- and post-milking sprays often differ in formulation. Teat sprays usually contain emollients to promote skin hydration, to soften the skin and allow healing of lesions that would otherwise harbour bacteria.

UDDERWASHES

DEFINITION
Udder-washes contain one or more disinfectant active substances, usually in the form of solutions which are sprayed onto the udder and teats of an animal to remove mud and faecal contamination before the application of teat dips or sprays. Udder-washes are usually prepared by the dilution either of concentrated preparations or of ready-to-use teat dips or teat sprays.

Ph Eur

Liquid Preparations for Cutaneous Application of the British Pharmacopoeia (Veterinary)

In addition to the above requirements of the European Pharmacopoeia, the following statements apply to any dip concentrate, pour-on or spray that is the subject of an individual monograph in the British Pharmacopoeia (Veterinary).

DIP CONCENTRATES

DEFINITION
When diluted, Dip Concentrates are used for the prevention and treatment of ectoparasitic infestations of animals. The diluted preparations are applied by complete immersion of the animal or, where appropriate, by spraying.

LABELLING
The label states (1) the name and concentration of the active ingredient or ingredients; (2) the name and proportion of any antimicrobial preservative; (3) the species of animal for which the preparation is intended; (4) the name and quantity of diluent and the directions for preparation of the diluted dip for use; (5) the date after which the Dip Concentrate should not be used; (6) the conditions under which it should be stored; (7) any special precautions associated with use of the Dip Concentrate; (8) where appropriate, the time(s) that must elapse between treatment and harvesting of material for human consumption.

POUR-ONS

LABELLING
The label states (1) the name and concentration of the active ingredient or ingredients; (2) the species of animal for which the preparation is intended; (3) that the Pour-on is intended for external use only; (4) the date after which the Pour-on should not be used; (5) the conditions under which it should be stored; (6) the directions for using the Pour-on; (7) any special precautions associated with its use; (8) where appropriate, the time(s) that must elapse between treatment and harvesting of material for human consumption.

SPRAYS

LABELLING
The label states (1) the name and concentration of the active ingredient or ingredients; (2) that the Spray is intended for external use only; (3) the date after which the Spray should not be used; (4) the conditions under which it should be stored; (5) the directions for using the Spray; (6) any special precautions associated with its use.

EXTRACTS

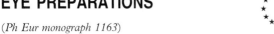

(Ph Eur monograph 0765)

Extracts comply with the requirements of the European Pharmacopoeia. These requirements are reproduced in the British Pharmacopoeia.

EYE PREPARATIONS

(Ph Eur monograph 1163)

Eye Preparations comply with the requirements of the European Pharmacopoeia. These requirements are reproduced in the British Pharmacopoeia.

Eye Preparations of the British Pharmacopoeia (Veterinary)

In addition to the requirements of the European Pharmacopoeia, the statements applicable to Eye Preparations of the British Pharmacopoeia apply to those eye ointments that are the subject of an individual monograph in the British Pharmacopoeia (Veterinary).

GRANULES

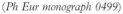

(Ph Eur monograph 0499)

Unless otherwise justified and authorised, Granules comply with the appropriate requirements of the European Pharmacopoeia. These requirements are reproduced in the British Pharmacopoeia.

Granules of the British Pharmacopoeia (Veterinary)

In addition to the requirements of the European Pharmacopoeia, the statements applicable to Granules of the British Pharmacopoeia apply to those granules that are the subject of an individual monograph in the British Pharmacopoeia (Veterinary).

INTRAMAMMARY INFUSIONS

INTRAMAMMARY INJECTIONS

(Intramammary Preparations for Veterinary Use, Ph Eur monograph 0945)

Intramammary Infusions comply with the requirements of the European Pharmacopoeia monograph for Intramammary Preparations for Veterinary Use. These requirements are reproduced below.

Ph Eur _____

DEFINITION

Intramammary preparations for veterinary use are sterile preparations intended for introduction into the mammary gland via the teat canal. There are two main categories: those intended for administration to lactating animals, and those intended for administration to animals at the end of lactation or to non-lactating animals for the treatment or prevention of infection.

Intramammary preparations for veterinary use are solutions, emulsions or suspensions or semi-solid preparations containing one or more active substances in a suitable vehicle. They may contain excipients such as stabilising, emulsifying, suspending and thickening agents. Suspensions may show a sediment which is readily dispersed on shaking. Emulsions may show evidence of phase separation but are readily redispersed on shaking.

Unless otherwise justified and authorised, intramammary preparations for veterinary use are supplied in containers for use on one occasion only for introduction in a single teat canal of an animal.

If supplied in multidose containers, aqueous preparations contain a suitable antimicrobial preservative at a suitable concentration, except where the preparation itself has adequate antimicrobial properties. Precautions for administration and for storage between administrations must be taken.

Where applicable, containers for intramammary preparations for veterinary use comply with the requirements of *Materials used for the manufacture of containers (3.1 and subsections)* and *Containers (3.2 and subsections)*.

PRODUCTION

During the development of a intramammary preparation for veterinary use, the formulation for which contains an antimicrobial preservative, the effectiveness of the chosen preservative shall be demonstrated to the satisfaction of the competent authority. A suitable test method together with criteria for judging the preservative properties of the formulation are provided in the text on *Efficacy of antimicrobial preservation (5.1.3)*.

Intramammary preparations for veterinary use are prepared using materials and methods designed to ensure sterility and to avoid the introduction of contaminants and the growth of micro-organisms; recommendations on this aspect are provided in the text on *Methods of preparation of sterile products (5.1.1)*.

In the manufacture of intramammary preparations for veterinary use containing dispersed particles, measures are taken to ensure a suitable and controlled particle size with regard to the intended use.

TESTS

Deliverable mass or volume

Squeeze out as much as possible of the contents of ten containers according to the instructions on the label. The mean mass or volume does not differ by more than 10 per cent from the nominal mass or volume.

Sterility *(2.6.1)*

Intramammary preparations for veterinary use comply with the test for sterility; use the technique of membrane filtration or, in justified cases, direct inoculation of the culture media. Squeeze out the contents of ten containers and mix thoroughly. For each medium, use 0.5 g to 1 g (or 0.5 ml to 1 ml as appropriate) taken from the mixed sample.

STORAGE

Store in a sterile, airtight, tamper-proof container.

LABELLING

The label states:
— the name of the active substance(s) and the mass or number of International Units of the active substance(s)

that may be delivered from the container using normal technique,
— whether the preparation is intended for use in a lactating animal or a non-lactating animal,
— in the case of multidose containers, the name of any added antimicrobial preservative.

Intramammary Infusions of the British Pharmacopoeia (Veterinary)

In addition to the above requirements of the European Pharmacopoeia, the following statements apply to those intramammary infusions that are the subject of an individual monograph in the British Pharmacopoeia (Veterinary).

DEFINITION

Intramammary Infusions intended for administration to lactating animals are described as Intramammary Infusions (Lactating Cow) and those intended for administration to animals at the end of lactation or during the non-lactating period for the prevention or treatment of infections during the dry period are described as Intramammary Infusions (Dry Cow).

PRODUCTION

Intramammary Infusions are prepared by dissolving or suspending the sterile medicaments in the sterilised vehicle using aseptic technique, unless a process of terminal sterilisation is employed.

When Intramammary Infusions are supplied in single-dose containers, these are sealed so as to exclude micro-organisms and are fitted with a smooth, tapered nozzle to facilitate the introduction of the infusion into the teat canal.

The containers are sterilised before being filled aseptically unless the intramammary infusion is to be subjected to a process of terminal sterilisation.

Sterility

Guidance to manufacturers on the number of containers to be tested is provided in the Annex to this monograph.

LABELLING

The label states (1) whether the preparation is an Intramammary Infusion (Lactating Cow) or an Intra-mammary Infusion (Dry Cow); (2) for Intramammary Infusions (Dry Cow), that the preparation is not intended for use in lactating animals; (3) the conditions under which the preparation should be stored; (4) the date after which the preparation is not intended to be used.

ANNEX

Guidance to manufacturers in performing the test for sterility

In determining the number of containers to be tested, the manufacturer should have regard to the environmental conditions of manufacture, the quantity (volume) of preparation per container and any other special considerations applying to the preparation concerned. With respect to intramammary infusions, 1% of the containers in a batch, with a minimum of three and a maximum of ten is considered a suitable number assuming that the preparation has been manufactured under appropriately validated conditions designed to exclude contamination.

INTRARUMINAL DEVICES

(*Ph Eur monograph 1228*)

Intraruminal Devices comply with the requirements of the European Pharmacopoeia. These requirements are reproduced below.

Ph Eur

The requirements of this monograph do not apply to preparations (sometimes known as boluses), such as large conventional tablets, capsules or moulded dosage forms which give immediate or prolonged release of the active substance(s). Such preparations comply with the relevant parts of the monographs on Capsules (0016) or Tablets (0478).

DEFINITION

Intraruminal devices are solid preparations each containing one or more active substances. They are intended for oral administration to ruminant animals and are designed to be retained in the rumen to deliver the active substance(s) in a continuous or pulsatile manner. The period of release of the active substance(s) may vary from days to weeks according to the nature of the formulation and/or the delivery device.

Intraruminal devices may be administered using a balling gun. Some intraruminal devices are intended to float on the surface of the ruminal fluid while others are intended to remain on the floor of the rumen or reticulum. Each device has a density appropriate for its intended purpose.

PRODUCTION

For continuous release, the intraruminal device is designed to release the active substance(s) at a defined rate over a defined period of time. This may be achieved by erosion, corrosion, diffusion, osmotic pressure or any other suitable chemical, physical or physico-chemical means.

For pulsatile-release, the intraruminal device is designed to release a specific quantity of active substance(s) at one or several defined intermediate times. This may be achieved by corrosion by ruminal fluids of the metallic elements of the intraruminal device which leads to sequential release of the constituent units which are usually in the form of tablets.

In the manufacture of intraruminal devices, means are taken to ensure an appropriate release of the active substance(s).

In the manufacture, packaging, storage and distribution of intraruminal devices, suitable means are taken to ensure their microbial quality; recommendations on this aspect are provided in the text on *Microbiological quality of pharmaceutical preparations (5.1.4)*.

TESTS

Uniformity of dosage units

Constituent tablet units of intraruminal devices comply with the test for uniformity of dosage units (*2.9.40*) or, where justified and authorised, with the tests for uniformity of content and/or uniformity of mass shown below. Herbal drugs and herbal drug preparations present in the dosage form are not subject to the provisions of this paragraph.

Uniformity of content (*2.9.6*)

Unless otherwise justified and authorised, constituent tablet units of intraruminal devices in which the active substances are present at levels less than 2 mg or less than 2 per cent of the total mass comply with test A for uniformity of content of single-dose preparations. If the preparation contains more than one active substance, the requirement applies only to those substances which correspond to the above conditions.

Uniformity of mass (*2.9.5*)
Unless otherwise justified and authorised, the constituent tablet units of intraruminal devices comply with the test for uniformity of mass. If the test for uniformity of content is prescribed for all active substances, the test for uniformity of mass is not required.

LABELLING
The label states:
— for continuous-release devices, the dose released per unit time,
— for pulsatile-release devices, the dose released at specified times.

Ph Eur

INTRAUTERINE PREPARATIONS

(*Intrauterine Preparations for Veterinary Use,
Ph Eur monograph 1806*)

Intrauterine Preparations comply with the requirements of the European Pharmacopoeia. These requirements are reproduced below.

Ph Eur

DEFINITION
Intrauterine preparations for veterinary use are liquid, semi-solid or solid preparations intended for the direct administration to the uterus (cervix, cavity or fundus), usually in order to obtain a local effect. They contain 1 or more active substances in a suitable basis.

Where appropriate, containers for intrauterine preparations for veterinary use comply with the requirements for *Materials used for the manufacture of containers* (*3.1 and subsections*) and *Containers* (*3.2 and subsections*).

Several categories of intrauterine preparations for veterinary use may be distinguished:
— intrauterine tablets,
— intrauterine capsules,
— intrauterine solutions, emulsions and suspensions, concentrates for intrauterine solutions,
— tablets for intrauterine solutions and suspensions,
— semi-solid intrauterine preparations,
— intrauterine foams,
— intrauterine sticks.

PRODUCTION
During the development of an intrauterine preparation for veterinary use, the effectiveness of any added antimicrobial preservative shall be demonstrated to the satisfaction of the competent authority. A suitable test method together with criteria for judging the preservative properties of the formulation are provided under *Efficacy of antimicrobial preservation* (*5.1.3*).

In the manufacture, packaging, storage and distribution of intrauterine preparations for veterinary use, suitable means are taken to ensure their microbial quality; recommendations on this aspect are provided in the text on *Microbiological quality of pharmaceutical preparations* (*5.1.4, Category 2*).

Sterile intrauterine preparations for veterinary use are prepared using materials and methods designed to ensure sterility and to avoid the introduction of contaminants and the growth of microorganisms; recommendations on this aspect are provided in the text on *Methods of preparation of sterile products* (*5.1.1*).

During development, it must be demonstrated that the nominal content can be withdrawn from the container of liquid and semi-solid intrauterine preparations for veterinary use presented in single-dose containers.

TESTS
Uniformity of dosage units
Single-dose intrauterine preparations for veterinary use comply with the test for uniformity of dosage units (*2.9.40*) or, where justified and authorised, with the tests for uniformity of content and/or uniformity of mass shown below. Herbal drugs and herbal drug preparations present in the dosage form are not subject to the provisions of this paragraph.

Uniformity of content (*2.9.6*)
Unless otherwise prescribed or justified and authorised, solid single-dose preparations with a content of active substance less than 2 mg or less than 2 per cent of the total mass comply with test A (intrauterine tablets) or test B (intrauterine capsules) for uniformity of content of single-dose preparations. If the preparation has more than 1 active substance, the requirement applies only to those substances which correspond to the above conditions.

Uniformity of mass (*2.9.5*)
Solid single-dose intrauterine preparations for veterinary use comply with the test for uniformity of mass of single-dose preparations. If the test for uniformity of content is prescribed or justified and authorised for all the active substances, the test for uniformity of mass is not required.

Dissolution
A suitable test may be carried out to demonstrate the appropriate release of the active substance(s) from solid single-dose intrauterine preparations for veterinary use, for example one of the tests described in *Dissolution test for solid dosage forms* (*2.9.3*).

When a dissolution test is prescribed, a disintegration test may not be required.

Sterility (*2.6.1*)
Sterile intrauterine preparations for veterinary use comply with the test for sterility. Applicators supplied with the preparation also comply with the test for sterility. Remove the applicator with aseptic precautions from its package and transfer it to a tube of culture medium so that it is completely immersed. Incubate and interpret the results as described in the test for sterility.

LABELLING
The label states:
— the name of any added antimicrobial preservative,
— where applicable, that the preparation is sterile.

INTRAUTERINE TABLETS

DEFINITION
Intrauterine tablets are solid preparations each containing a single dose of 1 or more active substances. They generally conform to the definition given in the monograph on *Tablets (0478)*.

A suitable applicator may be used for application into the uterus.

TESTS
Disintegration
Unless intended for prolonged local action, they comply with the test for disintegration of suppositories and pessaries (*2.9.2*). Examine the state of the tablets after 30 min, unless otherwise justified and authorised.

INTRAUTERINE CAPSULES

DEFINITION
Intrauterine capsules are solid, single-dose preparations. They are generally similar to soft capsules, differing only in their shape and size. Intrauterine capsules have various shapes, usually ovoid. They are smooth and have a uniform external appearance.

A suitable applicator may be used for application into the uterus.

TESTS
Disintegration
Unless intended for prolonged local action, they comply with the test for disintegration of suppositories and pessaries (2.9.2). Examine the state of the capsules after 30 min, unless otherwise justified and authorised.

INTRAUTERINE SOLUTIONS, SUSPENSIONS AND EMULSIONS CONCENTRATES FOR INTRAUTERINE SOLUTIONS

DEFINITION
Intrauterine solutions, suspensions and emulsions are liquid preparations. Concentrates for intrauterine solutions are intended for administration after dilution.

They may contain excipients, for example to adjust the viscosity of the preparation, to adjust or stabilise the pH, to increase the solubility of the active substance(s) or to stabilise the preparation. The excipients do not adversely affect the intended medical action, or, at the concentrations used, cause undue local irritation.

Intrauterine emulsions may show evidence of phase separation, but are readily redispersed on shaking. Intrauterine suspensions may show a sediment that is readily dispersed on shaking to give a suspension which remains sufficiently stable to enable a homogeneous preparation to be delivered.

They may be supplied in single-dose containers.
The container is adapted to deliver the preparation to the uterus or it may be accompanied by a suitable applicator.

PRODUCTION
In the manufacture of intrauterine suspensions, measures are taken to ensure a suitable and controlled particle size with regard to the intended use.

TABLETS FOR INTRAUTERINE SOLUTIONS AND SUSPENSIONS

DEFINITION
Tablets intended for the preparation of intrauterine solutions and suspensions are single-dose preparations which are dissolved or dispersed in water at the time of administration. They may contain excipients to facilitate dissolution or dispersion or to prevent caking.

Tablets for intrauterine solutions or suspensions conform with the definition given in the monograph on *Tablets (0478)*.

After dissolution or dispersion, they comply with the requirements for intrauterine solutions or intrauterine suspensions, as appropriate.

TESTS
Disintegration
Tablets for intrauterine solutions or suspensions disintegrate within 3 min when tested according to the test for

disintegration of tablets and capsules (2.9.1), but using *water R* at 15-25 °C.

LABELLING
The label states:
— the method of preparation of the intrauterine solution or suspension,
— the conditions and duration of storage of the solution or suspension after reconstitution.

SEMI-SOLID INTRAUTERINE PREPARATIONS

DEFINITION
Semi-solid preparations for intrauterine use are ointments, creams or gels.

Semi-solid preparations for intrauterine use comply with the requirements of the monograph on *Semi-solid preparations for cutaneous application (0132)*.

They are often supplied in single-dose containers.
The container is adapted to deliver the preparation to the uterus or it may be accompanied by a suitable applicator.

INTRAUTERINE FOAMS

DEFINITION
Intrauterine foams comply with the requirements of the monograph on *Medicated foams (1105)*.

They are supplied in multi-dose containers. The container is adapted to deliver the preparation to the uterus or it may be accompanied by a suitable applicator.

INTRAUTERINE STICKS

DEFINITION
Intrauterine sticks comply with the requirements of the monograph on *Sticks (1154)*. They often produce a foam when coming into contact with physiological fluids.

Ph Eur

ORAL LIQUIDS

LIQUID PREPARATIONS FOR ORAL USE
(*Ph Eur monograph 0672*)

Unless otherwise justified and authorised, Oral Liquids comply with the appropriate requirements of the European Pharmacopoeia monograph for Liquid Preparations for Oral Use. These requirements are reproduced in the British Pharmacopoeia.

Oral Liquids of the British Pharmacopoeia (Veterinary)

In addition to the requirements of the European Pharmacopoeia, the statements applicable to Oral Liquids of the British Pharmacopoeia apply to any oral solution or oral suspension that is the subject of an individual monograph in the British Pharmacopoeia (Veterinary).

PARENTERAL PREPARATIONS

(Ph Eur monograph 0520)

Unless otherwise justified and authorised, Parenteral Preparations comply with the appropriate requirements of the European Pharmacopoeia. These requirements are reproduced in the British Pharmacopoeia or, where they apply to veterinary preparations only, below.

Ph Eur ___

Special requirements may apply to preparations for veterinary use depending on the species of animal for which the preparation is intended.

TESTS

Particulate contamination: sub-visible particles *(2.9.19)*
In the case of preparations for subcutaneous or intramuscular injection, higher limits may be appropriate.
Radiopharmaceutical preparations are exempt from these requirements. Preparations for which the label states that the product is to be used with a final filter are exempt from these requirements, providing it has been demonstrated that the filter delivers a solution that complies with the test.

For preparations for veterinary use, when supplied in containers with a nominal content of more than 100 ml and when the content is equivalent to a dose of more than 1.4 ml per kilogram of body mass, solutions for infusion or solutions for injection comply with the test for particulate contamination: sub-visible particles.

INJECTIONS

TESTS

Bacterial endotoxins - pyrogens
A test for bacterial endotoxins *(2.6.14)* is carried out or, where justified and authorised, the test for pyrogens *(2.6.8)*. Recommendations on the limits for bacterial endotoxins are given in chapter *2.6.14*.

When the volume to be injected in a single dose is 15 ml or more and is equivalent to a dose of 0.2 ml or more per kilogram of body mass, the preparation complies with a test for bacterial endotoxins *(2.6.14)* or with the test for pyrogens *(2.6.8)*.

Where the label states that the preparation is free from bacterial endotoxins or apyrogenic, respectively, the preparation complies with a test for bacterial endotoxins *(2.6.14)* or with the test for pyrogens *(2.6.8)*, respectively.

_____ *Ph Eur*

Parenteral Preparations of the British Pharmacopoeia (Veterinary)

In addition to the requirements of the European Pharmacopoeia, the statements applicable to Parenteral Preparations of the British Pharmacopoeia, modified as stated below, apply to those injections and intravenous infusions that are the subject of an individual monograph in the British Pharmacopoeia (Veterinary).

DEFINITION

Parenteral Preparations prepared with an oily vehicle are suitable for intramuscular or subcutaneous administration only and are not given intravenously.

Veterinary Oral Pastes

Unless otherwise authorised and justified, Veterinary Oral Pastes comply with the requirements of the monograph on Oromucosal Preparations. In addition, the following statements apply to Veterinary Oral Pastes that are the subject of an individual monograph in the British Pharmacopoeia (Veterinary).

DEFINITION

Veterinary Oral Pastes are semi-solid preparations containing one or more active substances in a suitable vehicle. They are administered to the oral cavity and are intended to be swallowed for delivery of active substances to the gastrointestinal tract.

Veterinary Oral Pastes may contain suitable antimicrobial preservatives and other excipients such as dispersing, suspending, thickening, emulsifying, buffering, wetting, solubilising, stabilising, flavouring and sweetening agents.

Where applicable, containers for Veterinary Oral Pastes comply with the requirements for *Materials used for the manufacture of containers* (Appendix XX) and *Containers* (Appendix XIX A to C).

Veterinary Oral Pastes are presented in multi-dose containers which are designed to allow the accurate dosing of animals according to their bodyweight.

TESTS

Dissolution
A suitable test may be carried out to demonstrate the appropriate release of the active substance(s), for example, the test using Apparatus 2 described under *dissolution test for tablets and capsules*, Appendix XII B1.

Uniformity of mass of delivered doses from multi-dose containers
Veterinary Oral Pastes supplied in multi-dose containers comply with Appendix XII C2.

STORAGE

If the preparation contains water or other volatile ingredients, store in an airtight container.

LABELLING

The label states the name and quantity of active substance in a suitable amount by weight or volume.

The label also states the directions for use of the Veterinary Oral Paste.

TOPICAL POWDERS

POWDERS FOR CUTANEOUS APPLICATION

(Ph Eur monograph 1166)

Unless otherwise justified and authorised, Topical Powders comply with the requirements of the European Pharmacopoeia monograph for Powders for Cutaneous Application. These requirements are reproduced in the British Pharmacopoeia.

Topical Powders of the British Pharmacopoeia (Veterinary)

In addition to the requirements of the European Pharmacopoeia, the statements applicable to Topical Powders of the British Pharmacopoeia apply to any dusting powder that is the subject of an individual monograph in the British Pharmacopoeia (Veterinary).

VETERINARY ORAL POWDERS

Unless otherwise justified and authorised, Veterinary Oral Powders comply with the requirements of the European Pharmacopoeia monograph for Oral Powders (1165). In addition to these requirements, reproduced in the British Pharmacopoeia, the following statements apply to those veterinary oral powders that are the subject of an individual monograph in the British Pharmacopoeia (Veterinary).

DEFINITION

Veterinary Oral Powders are finely divided powders that contain one or more active ingredients with or without excipients such as antimicrobial preservatives, dispersing, suspending or wetting agents and, where necessary, authorised flavouring agents and colouring matter. They are intended for oral administration, usually after dilution in the feed or drinking water. Veterinary Oral Powders may be in the form of soluble or wettable powders.

STORAGE

Veterinary Oral Powders should be stored in airtight containers.

LABELLING

For single-dose containers the label states the name and quantity of active ingredient per container. For multi-dose containers the label states the name and quantity of active ingredient in a suitable amount by weight.

The label also states (1) the name and proportion of any antimicrobial preservative; (2) the directions for use of the Veterinary Oral Powder; (3) the date after which the Veterinary Oral Powder is not intended to be used; (4) the conditions under which the Veterinary Oral Powder should be stored.

PREMIXES

(Premixes for Medicated Feeding Stuffs for Veterinary Use, Ph Eur monograph 1037)

Premixes comply with the requirements of the European Pharmacopoeia monograph for Premixes for Medicated Feeding Stuffs for Veterinary Use. These requirements are reproduced below.

Ph Eur

DEFINITION

Mixtures of one or more active substances, usually in suitable bases, that are prepared to facilitate feeding the active substances to animals. They are used exclusively in the preparation of medicated feeding stuffs.

Premixes occur in granulated, powdered, semi-solid or liquid form. Used as powders or granules, they are free-flowing and homogeneous; any aggregates break apart during normal handling. Used in liquid form, they are homogeneous suspensions or solutions which may be obtained from thixotropic gels or structured liquids. The particle size and other properties are such as to ensure uniform distribution of the active substance(s) in the final feed. Unless otherwise justified and authorised, the instructions for use state that the concentration of a premix in granulated or powdered form is at least 0.5 per cent in the medicated feeding stuff.

PRODUCTION

Active substance

An active substance intended for incorporation into a medicated premix complies with the requirements of the relevant monograph of the European Pharmacopoeia, unless already otherwise justified and authorised for existing premixes.

TESTS

Loss on drying *(2.2.32)*

Unless otherwise justified and authorised, for premixes occurring in granulated or powdered form, maximum 15.0 per cent, determined on 3.000 g by drying in an oven at 100-105 °C for 2 h.

LABELLING

The label states:

— the category of animal for which the premix is intended,
— the instructions for the preparation of the medicated feeding stuffs from the premix and the basic feed,
— where applicable, the time that must elapse between the cessation of feeding of the medicated feeding stuff and collection of the material intended for human consumption.

Ph Eur

Premixes of the British Pharmacopoeia (Veterinary)

DEFINITION

Premixes may occur in pelleted form.

LABELLING

The label states (1) any special precautions associated with the use of the Premix; (2) the date after which the Premix is not intended to be used; (3) the conditions under which it should be stored; (4) the time that the preparation will remain stable following incorporation into finished feed and into pelleted feed.

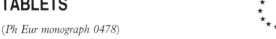

TABLETS

(*Ph Eur monograph 0478*)

Unless otherwise justified and authorised, Tablets comply with the appropriate requirements of the European Pharmacopoeia. These requirements are reproduced in the British Pharmacopoeia.

Tablets of the British Pharmacopoeia (Veterinary)

In addition to the requirements of the European Pharmacopoeia, the statements applicable to Tablets of the British Pharmacopoeia, modified as stated below, apply to those tablets that are the subject of an individual monograph in the British Pharmacopoeia (Veterinary).

DEFINITION

Tablets of the British Pharmacopoeia (Veterinary) are usually solid, right circular cylinders the end surfaces of which are flat or convex and the edges of which may be bevelled except that those that weigh 5 g or more are frequently elongated or biconical.

Disintegration

Apply test A or test B, Appendix XII A1, as appropriate. When using test B, test 6 tablets either by using two basket-rack assemblies in parallel or by repeating the procedure. To pass the test, all six of the tablets must have disintegrated.

FORMULATED PREPARATIONS: SPECIFIC MONOGRAPHS

Acepromazine Injection

Action and use
Dopamine receptor antagonist; neuroleptic.

DEFINITION

Acepromazine Injection is a sterile solution of Acepromazine Maleate in Water for Injections. The pH of the solution is adjusted to about 5 by the addition of Sodium Hydroxide.

The injection complies with the requirements stated under Parenteral Preparations and with the following requirements.

Content of acepromazine, $C_{19}H_{22}N_2OS$
92.5 to 107.5% of the stated amount.

IDENTIFICATION

A. To a volume containing the equivalent of 20 mg of acepromazine add 2 ml of *water* and 3 ml of 2M *sodium hydroxide*, extract with two 5 ml quantities of *cyclohexane* and evaporate to dryness under reduced pressure. The *infrared absorption spectrum* of the residue, Appendix II A, is concordant with the *reference spectrum* of acepromazine (*RSV 01*).

B. Complies with the test for *identification of phenothiazines*, Appendix III A, applying to the plate 1 µl of each of the following solutions. For solution (1) extract a volume containing the equivalent of 20 mg of acepromazine with two 5 ml quantities of *chloroform* and use the combined extracts. Solution (2) is a solution of *acepromazine maleate BPCRS* in *chloroform* containing the equivalent of 0.2% w/v of acepromazine.

C. To 5 mg of the residue obtained in test A add 2 ml of *sulphuric acid*. A yellow colour is produced which becomes deep orange on warming for 2 minutes.

D. To a volume of the injection containing the equivalent of 25 mg of acepromazine add 2 ml of 5M sodium hydroxide and shake with three 3 ml quantities of ether. Add 2 ml of bromine solution to the aqueous solution, warm in a water bath for 10 minutes, heat to boiling and cool. Add 0.25 ml to a solution of 10 mg of resorcinol in 3 ml of sulphuric acid and heat for 15 minutes in a water bath. A bluish black colour develops.

TESTS
Acidity
pH, 4.5 to 5.5, Appendix V L.

ASSAY

To a volume containing the equivalent of 40 mg of acepromazine add 5 ml of 1M *sodium hydroxide* and extract with 50 ml quantities of *chloroform* until the chloroform extract is colourless. Wash the extracts with the same 10 ml of *water* and filter through a plug of absorbent cotton previously moistened with *chloroform*. Evaporate the combined extracts to dryness and dissolve the residue in 15 ml of *acetic anhydride*. Carry out Method I for *non-aqueous titration*, Appendix VIII A, using 0.02M *perchloric acid VS* as titrant and *crystal violet solution* as indicator. Each ml of 0.02M *perchloric acid VS* is equivalent to 6.529 mg of $C_{19}H_{22}N_2OS$.

STORAGE
Acepromazine Injection should be protected from light.

LABELLING
The strength is stated as the equivalent amount of acepromazine in a suitable dose-volume.

Acepromazine Tablets

Action and use
Dopamine receptor antagonist; neuroleptic.

DEFINITION
Acepromazine Tablets contain Acepromazine Maleate.

The tablets comply with the requirements stated under Tablets and with the following requirements.

Content of acepromazine, $C_{19}H_{22}N_2OS$
92.5 to 107.5% of the stated amount.

IDENTIFICATION
A. To a quantity of the powdered tablets containing the equivalent of 20 mg of acepromazine add 2 ml of *water* and 3 ml of 2M *sodium hydroxide*. Extract with two 5 ml quantities of *cyclohexane* and evaporate to dryness under reduced pressure. The *infrared absorption spectrum* of the residue, Appendix II A, is concordant with the *reference spectrum* of acepromazine *(RSV 01)*.

B. Complies with the test for *identification of phenothiazines*, Appendix III A, applying to the plate 1 μl of each of the following solutions. For solution (1) extract a quantity of the powdered tablets containing the equivalent of 20 mg of acepromazine with two 5 ml quantities of *chloroform*. Solution (2) is a solution of *acepromazine maleate BPCRS* in *chloroform* containing the equivalent of 0.2% w/v of acepromazine.

C. To a quantity of the powdered tablets containing the equivalent of 5 mg of acepromazine add 2 ml of *sulphuric acid*. A yellow colour is produced which becomes deep orange on warming for 2 minutes.

D. Dissolve as completely as possible a quantity of the powdered tablets containing the equivalent of 25 mg of acepromazine in a mixture of 3 ml of *water* and 2 ml of 5M *sodium hydroxide* and shake with three 3 ml quantities of *ether*. Add 2 ml of *bromine solution* to the aqueous solution, warm in a water bath for 10 minutes, heat to boiling and cool. Add 0.25 ml to a solution of 10 mg of *resorcinol* in 3 ml of *sulphuric acid* and heat for 15 minutes on a water bath. A bluish black colour develops.

TESTS
Related substances
Comply with the test for *related substances in phenothiazines*, Appendix III A, but using a mixture of 8 volumes of *diethylamine*, 17 volumes of *butan-2-one* and 75 volumes of n-hexane as the mobile phase and using the following solutions. For solution (1) shake a quantity of the powdered tablets containing the equivalent of 50 mg of acepromazine with 10 ml of *chloroform*, filter, evaporate to dryness and dissolve the residue in 5 ml of *methanol* containing 0.5% v/v of 13.5M *ammonia*. For solution (2) dilute 1 volume of solution (1) to 100 volumes with *methanol* containing 0.5% v/v of 13.5M *ammonia*.

ASSAY
Weigh and powder 20 tablets. To a quantity of the powder containing the equivalent of 60 mg of acepromazine add 5 ml of *water* and extract with three or more 50 ml quantities of *chloroform* or until the chloroform extract is colourless. Evaporate to dryness and dissolve the residue in 15 ml of *acetic anhydride*. Carry out Method I for *non-aqueous titration*, Appendix VIII A, using 0.02M *perchloric acid VS* as titrant and *crystal violet solution* as indicator. Each ml of 0.02M *perchloric acid VS* is equivalent to 6.529 mg of $C_{19}H_{22}N_2OS$.

LABELLING
The quantity of the active ingredient is stated in terms of the equivalent amount of acepromazine.

Amitraz Dip Concentrate (Liquid)

Action and use
Topical parasiticide; acaricide.

DEFINITION
Amitraz Dip Concentrate (Liquid) contains Amitraz in a suitable emulsifiable vehicle. It may contain a suitable stabilising agent.

The dip concentrate complies with the requirements stated under Veterinary Liquid Preparations for Cutaneous Application and with the following requirements.

Content of amitraz, $C_{19}H_{23}N_3$
94.0 to 106.0% of the stated amount.

IDENTIFICATION
A. In the test for Related substances, the principal spot in the chromatogram obtained with solution (2) corresponds to that in the chromatogram obtained with solution (3).

B. In the Assay, the chromatogram obtained with solution (1) shows a peak with the same retention time as the peak due to amitraz in the chromatogram obtained with solution (3).

Related substances
Carry out the method for *thin-layer chromatography*, Appendix III A, using *silica gel HF$_{254}$* as the coating substance and a mixture of 2 volumes of *triethylamine*, 3 volumes of *ethyl acetate* and 5 volumes of *cyclohexane* as the mobile phase. Stand the plate to a depth of 3.5 cm in a solution prepared by dissolving 35 g of *acetamide* in 100 ml of *methanol*, adding 100 ml of *triethylamine* and diluting to 250 ml with *methanol* before standing the plate in a stream of cold air for about 30 seconds. Immediately apply separately to the plate, at a level 1 cm below the top of the impregnated zone, 2 μl of each of the following solutions. For solution (1) dilute the dip concentrate with *toluene* to produce a solution containing 5.0% w/v of Amitraz. For solution (2) dilute 1 volume of solution (1) to 10 volumes with *toluene*. Solution (3) contains 0.5% w/v of *amitraz BPCRS* in *toluene*. Solution (4) contains 0.10% w/v of *amitraz BPCRS* in *toluene*. Solution (5) contains 0.005% w/v of *2,4-dimethylaniline* in *toluene*. Develop the chromatograms without delay. After removal of the plate, allow it to dry in air and examine under *ultraviolet light (254 nm)*. Any *secondary spot* in the chromatogram obtained with solution (1) is not more intense than the spot in the chromatogram obtained with solution (4) (2%). Expose the plate to the vapour of hydrochloric acid until the coating is impregnated. Expose to the vapour of nitrogen dioxide (prepared by the

action of nitric acid on zinc) for 10 minutes, remove any excess nitrogen dioxide with air and spray with a 0.5% w/v solution of N-*(1-naphthyl) ethylenediamine dihydrochloride* in *methanol (50%)*. In the chromatogram obtained with solution (1) any spot corresponding to 2,4-dimethylaniline is not more intense than the spot in the chromatogram obtained with solution (5) (0.1%).

Water

Not more than 0.15% w/v, Appendix IX C, Method IA. Use 5 ml of the dip concentrate and a mixture of equal volumes of *chloroform* and *2-chloroethanol* in place of anhydrous methanol.

ASSAY

Prepare a 2% v/v solution of *squalane* (internal standard) in *methyl acetate* (solution A) and carry out the method for *gas chromatography*, Appendix III B, using the following solutions. For solution (1) dissolve a quantity of the dip concentrate containing 0.15 g of Amitraz in sufficient *methyl acetate* to produce 30 ml. For solution (2) dissolve a quantity of the dip concentrate containing 0.15 g of Amitraz in 10 ml of solution A and add sufficient *methyl acetate* to produce 30 ml. For solution (3) dissolve 0.15 g of *amitraz BPCRS* in 10 ml of solution A and add sufficient *methyl acetate* to produce 30 ml.

The chromatographic procedure may be carried out using a fused silica capillary column (15 m × 0.53 mm) coated with a 1.5 μm film of methyl silicone gum (Chrompack CP-Sil 5 CB is suitable) and maintained at 220° with the inlet port at 230° and the detector at 300° and a flow rate of 12 ml per minute for the carrier gas. Inject 1 μl of each solution.

The assay is not valid unless, in the chromatogram obtained with solution (3), the *resolution factor* between the peaks corresponding to squalane and amitraz is at least 3.0.

Calculate the content of $C_{19}H_{23}N_3$ from the chromatograms obtained and using the declared content of $C_{19}H_{23}N_3$ in *amitraz BPCRS*.

Amitraz Dip Concentrate (Powder)

Action and use
Topical parasiticide; acaricide.

DEFINITION

Amitraz Dip Concentrate (Powder) consists of Amitraz mixed with suitable wetting, dispersing and suspending agents. It may contain a suitable stabilising agent.

The dip concentrate complies with the requirements stated under Veterinary Liquid Preparations for Cutaneous Application and with the following requirements.

Content of amitraz, $C_{19}H_{23}N_3$
95.0 to 105.0% of the stated amount.

IDENTIFICATION

Shake a quantity of the powder containing 0.1 g of Amitraz with 10 ml of *acetone* for 5 minutes, filter and evaporate the filtrate to dryness. The *infrared absorption spectrum* of the residue, Appendix II A, is concordant with the *reference spectrum* of amitraz *(RSV 04)*.

TESTS
Related substances

Carry out the method for *thin-layer chromatography*, Appendix III A, using *silica gel HF254* as the coating substance and a mixture of 2 volumes of *triethylamine*, 3 volumes of *ethyl*

acetate and 5 volumes of *cyclohexane* as the mobile phase. Stand the plate to a depth of 3.5 cm in a solution prepared by dissolving 35 g of *acetamide* in 100 ml of *methanol*, adding 100 ml of *triethylamine* and diluting to 250 ml with *methanol* before standing the plate in a stream of cold air for about 30 seconds. Immediately apply separately to the plate, at a level 1 cm below the top of the impregnated zone, 2 μl of each of the following solutions. For solution (1) use the supernatant liquid obtained after centrifuging a suspension of the powder in *toluene* containing 5.0% w/v of Amitraz. Solution (2) contains 0.10% w/v of *amitraz BPCRS* in *toluene*. Solution (3) contains 0.005% w/v of *2,4-dimethylaniline* in *toluene*. Develop the chromatograms without delay. After removal of the plate, allow it to dry in air and examine under *ultraviolet light (254 nm)*. Any *secondary spot* in the chromatogram obtained with solution (1) is not more intense than the spot in the chromatogram obtained with solution (2) (2%). Expose the plate to the vapour of hydrochloric acid until the coating is impregnated. Expose to the vapour of nitrogen dioxide (prepared by the action of nitric acid on zinc) for 10 minutes, remove any excess nitrogen dioxide with air and spray with a 0.5% w/v solution of N-*(1-naphthyl)- ethylenediamine dihydrochloride* in *methanol (50%)*. In the chromatogram obtained with solution (1) any spot corresponding to 2,4-dimethylaniline is not more intense than the spot in the chromatogram obtained with solution (3) (0.1%).

ASSAY

Carry out the Assay described under Amitraz Dip Concentrate (Liquid) preparing solutions (1) and (2) in the following manner. For solution (1) shake a quantity of the powder containing 0.15 g of Amitraz with 30 ml of *methyl acetate*, centrifuge and use the supernatant liquid.
For solution (2) shake a quantity of the powder containing 0.15 g of Amitraz in a mixture of 10 ml of solution A and 20 ml of *methyl acetate*, centrifuge and use the supernatant liquid.

Amitraz Pour-on

Action and use
Topical parasiticide; acaricide.

DEFINITION

Amitraz Pour-on is a *pour-on solution*. It contains Amitraz in a suitable vehicle. It may contain a suitable stabilising agent.

The pour-on complies with the requirements stated under Veterinary Liquid Preparations for Cutaneous Application and with the following requirements.

Content of amitraz, $C_{19}H_{23}N_3$
90.0 to 105.0% of the stated amount.

IDENTIFICATION

In the Assay, the chromatogram obtained with solution (1) shows a peak with the same retention time as the peak due to Amitraz in the chromatogram obtained with solution (3).

Water

Not more than 0.05% w/v, Appendix IX C, Method IA. Use 5 ml of the preparation being examined and a mixture of equal volumes of *chloroform* and *2-chloroethanol* in place of anhydrous methanol.

ASSAY

Prepare a 0.1% w/v solution of *benzyl butyl phthalate* (internal standard) in *methyl acetate* (solution A) and carry out the method for *gas chromatography*, Appendix III B, using the following solutions. For solution (1) dilute a quantity of the preparation being examined containing 12.5 mg of Amitraz in sufficient *methyl acetate* to produce 20 ml. For solution (2) dilute a quantity of the preparation being examined containing 12.5 mg of Amitraz in 10 ml of solution A and add sufficient *methyl acetate* to produce 20 ml.

For solution (3) dissolve 12.5 mg of *amitraz BPCRS* in 10 ml of solution A and add sufficient *methyl acetate* to produce 20 ml.

The chromatographic procedure may be carried out using a fused silica capillary column (15 m × 0.53 mm) coated with a 1.2 μm film of *poly [(cyanopropyl) methylphenyl-methylsiloxane]* (Chrompack CP-Sil 43 CB is suitable) at an initial temperature of 145°, maintained at 145° for 15 minutes, increasing linearly to 195° at a rate of 16° per minute and maintained at 195° for 30 minutes with the inlet port at 220° and the detector at 250° and a flow rate of 13 ml per minute for the carrier gas. Inject 1.5 μl of each solution.

The assay is not valid unless, in the chromatogram obtained with solution (3), the *resolution factor* between the peaks corresponding to benzyl butyl phthalate and amitraz is at least 3.0.

Calculate the content of $C_{19}H_{23}N_3$ from the chromatograms obtained and using the declared content of $C_{19}H_{23}N_3$ in *amitraz BPCRS*.

Amoxicillin Oily Injections

Action and use
Penicillin antibacterial.

DEFINITION
Amoxicillin Oily Injections are sterile suspensions of Amoxicillin Trihydrate in oily vehicles appropriate to their intended use. Injections intended for use as long acting preparations are described as Amoxicillin Oily Injection (Long Acting).

The injections comply with the requirements stated under Parenteral Preparations and with the following requirements.

Content of amoxicillin, $C_{16}H_{19}N_3O_5S$
90.0 to 105.0% of the stated amount.

CHARACTERISTICS
A white or almost white, oily suspension.

IDENTIFICATION
Extract a quantity containing the equivalent of 0.25 g of amoxicillin with three 20 ml quantities of *petroleum spirit (boiling range, 120° to 160°)* and discard the extracts. Wash the residue with *ether* and dry in a current of air. The residue complies with the following tests.

A. The *infrared absorption spectrum*, Appendix II A, is concordant with the *reference spectrum* of amoxicillin trihydrate *(RSV 05)*.

B. Carry out the method for *thin-layer chromatography*, Appendix III A, using a *TLC silica gel silanised plate* (Merck silanised silica gel 60 F_{254s} (RP-18) plates are suitable) and a mixture of 10 volumes of *acetone* and 90 volumes of a 15.4% w/v solution of *ammonium acetate* adjusted to pH 5.0 with *glacial acetic acid* as the mobile phase. Apply separately to the plate 1 μl of each of the following solutions. For solution (1) dissolve a quantity of the residue in

sufficient *sodium hydrogen carbonate solution* to produce a solution containing the equivalent of 0.25% w/v of amoxicillin. Solution (2) contains 0.25% w/v of *amoxicillin trihydrate EPCRS* in *sodium hydrogen carbonate solution*. Solution (3) contains 0.25% w/v of each of *amoxicillin trihydrate EPCRS* and *ampicillin trihydrate EPCRS* in *sodium hydrogen carbonate solution*. After removal of the plate, allow it to dry in air, expose it to iodine vapour until spots appear and examine in daylight. The principal spot in the chromatogram obtained with solution (1) is similar in position, colour and size to that in the chromatogram obtained with solution (2). The test is not valid unless the chromatogram obtained with solution (3) shows two clearly separated spots.

TESTS
Pyrogens
The requirement for Pyrogens does not apply to Amoxicillin Oily Injections.

ASSAY
Carry out the method for *liquid chromatography*, Appendix III D, injecting 50 μl of each of the following solutions. For solution (1) shake a quantity containing the equivalent of 60 mg of amoxicillin with 15 ml of *petroleum spirit (boiling range, 120° to 160°)*, centrifuge and discard the supernatant liquid. Repeat the extraction twice using a further 15 ml of *petroleum spirit (boiling range, 120° to 160°)* each time. Dissolve the residue in 20 ml of *ether*, centrifuge, discard the supernatant liquid and allow the residue remaining to dry in air until the solvents have evaporated. Dissolve the dried residue in mobile phase A, add sufficient mobile phase A to produce 100 ml, mix and filter (Whatman GF/C filter paper is suitable). Solution (2) contains 0.070% w/v of *amoxicillin trihydrate EPCRS* in mobile phase A. Solution (3) contains 0.0004% w/v of *cefadroxil EPCRS* and 0.003% w/v of *amoxicillin trihydrate EPCRS* in mobile phase A.

The chromatographic procedure may be carried out using (a) a stainless steel column (25 cm × 4.6 mm) packed with *octadecylsilyl silica gel for chromatography* (5 μm) (Hypersil 5 ODS is suitable), (b) as the mobile phase with a flow rate of 1 ml per minute a mixture of 8 volumes of mobile phase B and 92 volumes of mobile phase A as described below and (c) a detection wavelength of 254 nm.

Mobile phase A: Mix 1 volume of *acetonitrile* and 99 volumes of a 25% v/v solution of 0.2M *potassium dihydrogen orthophosphate* adjusted to pH 5.0 with 2M *sodium hydroxide*.

Mobile phase B: Mix 20 volumes of *acetonitrile* and 80 volumes of a 25% v/v solution of 0.2M *potassium dihydrogen orthophosphate* adjusted to pH 5.0 with 2M *sodium hydroxide*.

The test is not valid unless, in the chromatogram obtained with solution (3), the *resolution factor* between the peaks due to amoxicillin and cefadroxil is at least 2.0. If necessary, adjust the composition of the mobile phase to achieve the required resolution.

Calculate the content of $C_{16}H_{19}N_3O_5S$ in the injection from the chromatograms obtained and from the declared content of $C_{16}H_{19}N_3O_5S$ in *amoxicillin trihydrate EPCRS*.

LABELLING
The label states (1) the strength in terms of the equivalent amount of amoxicillin in a suitable dose-volume; (2) where appropriate, that the preparation is Amoxicillin Oily Injection (Long Acting).

Amoxicillin Veterinary Oral Powder

Action and use
Penicillin antibacterial.

DEFINITION

Amoxicillin Veterinary Oral Powder is a mixture of Amoxicillin Trihydrate, Lactose or other suitable diluent and a stabilising agent.

The veterinary oral powder complies with the requirements stated under Veterinary Oral Powders and with the following requirements.

Content of amoxicillin, $C_{16}H_{19}N_3O_5S$
90.0 to 110.0% of the stated amount.

IDENTIFICATION

A. Carry out the method for *thin-layer chromatography*, Appendix III A, using a *TLC silica gel silanised plate* (Merck silanised silica gel 60 F_{254s} (RP-18) plates are suitable) and a mixture of 10 volumes of *acetone* and 90 volumes of a 15.4% w/v solution of *ammonium acetate* adjusted to pH 5.0 with *glacial acetic acid* as the mobile phase. Apply separately to the plate 1 µl of each of the following solutions. For solution (1) dissolve a quantity of the veterinary oral powder containing the equivalent of 0.25 g of amoxicillin in sufficient *sodium hydrogen carbonate solution* to produce 100 ml. Solution (2) contains 0.25% w/v of *amoxicillin trihydrate EPCRS* in *sodium hydrogen carbonate solution*. Solution (3) contains 0.25% w/v of each of *amoxicillin trihydrate EPCRS* and *ampicillin trihydrate EPCRS* in *sodium hydrogen carbonate solution*. After removal of the plate, allow it to dry in air, expose it to iodine vapour until spots appear and examine in daylight. The principal spot in the chromatogram obtained with solution (1) is similar in position, colour and size to that in the chromatogram obtained with solution (2). The test is not valid unless the chromatogram obtained with solution (3) shows two clearly separated spots.

B. Shake a quantity of the veterinary oral powder containing the equivalent of 0.5 g of amoxicillin with 5 ml of *water* for 5 minutes, filter, wash the residue first with *absolute ethanol* and then with *ether* and dry at a pressure not exceeding 0.7 kPa for 1 hour. Suspend 10 mg of the residue in 1 ml of *water* and add 2 ml of a mixture of 2 ml of *cupri-tartaric solution R1* and 6 ml of *water*. A magenta colour is produced immediately.

C. Dissolve 0.1 ml of *aniline* in a mixture of 1 ml of *hydrochloric acid* and 3 ml of *water*. Cool the solution in ice and add 1 ml of a freshly prepared 20% w/v solution of *sodium nitrite*. Add the resulting mixture drop wise to a cold solution of 0.1 g of the residue obtained in test B in 2 ml of 5M *sodium hydroxide*. The solution becomes deep cherry-red and a copious dark brown precipitate is produced.

ASSAY

Carry out the method for *liquid chromatography*, Appendix III D, injecting 50 µl of each of the following solutions. For solution (1) add 80 ml of mobile phase A to a quantity of the veterinary oral powder containing the equivalent of 60 mg of amoxicillin and shake for 15 minutes. Mix with the aid of ultrasound for 1 minute, add sufficient mobile phase A to produce 100 ml, mix and filter (Whatman GF/C filter paper is suitable). Solution (2) contains 0.070% w/v of *amoxicillin trihydrate EPCRS* in mobile phase A. Solution (3) contains 0.0004% w/v of *cefadroxil EPCRS* and 0.003% w/v of *amoxicillin trihydrate EPCRS* in mobile phase A.

The chromatographic conditions described under Amoxicillin Oily Injections may be used.

The test is not valid unless, in the chromatogram obtained with solution (3), the *resolution factor* between the peaks due to amoxicillin and cefadroxil is at least 2.0. If necessary, adjust the composition of the mobile phase to achieve the required resolution.

Calculate the content of $C_{16}H_{19}N_3O_5S$ in the veterinary oral powder from the chromatograms obtained and from the declared content of $C_{16}H_{19}N_3O_5S$ in *amoxicillin trihydrate EPCRS*.

LABELLING

The quantity of active ingredient is stated in terms of the equivalent amount of amoxicillin.

Amoxicillin Tablets

Action and use
Penicillin antibacterial.

DEFINITION

Amoxicillin Tablets contain Amoxicillin Trihydrate.

The tablets comply with the requirements stated under Tablets and with the following requirements.

Content of amoxicillin, $C_{16}H_{19}N_3O_5S$
90.0 to 110.0% of the stated amount.

IDENTIFICATION

A. Carry out the method for *thin-layer chromatography*, Appendix III A, using a *TLC silica gel silanised plate* (Merck silanised silica gel 60 F_{254s} (RP-18) plates are suitable) and a mixture of 10 volumes of *acetone* and 90 volumes of a 15.4% w/v solution of *ammonium acetate* adjusted to pH 5.0 with *glacial acetic acid* as the mobile phase. Apply separately to the plate 1 µl of each of the following solutions. For solution (1) dissolve a quantity of the powdered tablets containing the equivalent of 0.25 g of amoxicillin in sufficient *sodium hydrogen carbonate solution* to produce 100 ml. Solution (2) contains 0.25% w/v of *amoxicillin trihydrate EPCRS* in *sodium hydrogen carbonate solution*. Solution (3) contains 0.25% w/v of each of *amoxicillin trihydrate EPCRS* and *ampicillin trihydrate EPCRS* in *sodium hydrogen carbonate solution*. After removal of the plate, allow it to dry in air, expose it to iodine vapour until spots appear and examine in daylight. The principal spot in the chromatogram obtained with solution (1) is similar in position, colour and size to that in the chromatogram obtained with solution (2). The test is not valid unless the chromatogram obtained with solution (3) shows two clearly separated spots.

B. Shake a quantity of the powdered tablets containing the equivalent of 0.5 g of amoxicillin with 5 ml of *water* for 5 minutes, filter, wash the residue first with *absolute ethanol* and then with *ether* and dry at a pressure not exceeding 0.7 kPa for 1 hour. Suspend 10 mg of the residue in 1 ml of *water* and add 2 ml of a mixture of 2 ml of *cupri-tartaric solution R1* and 6 ml of *water*. A magenta colour is produced immediately.

C. Dissolve 0.1 ml of *aniline* in a mixture of 1 ml of *hydrochloric acid* and 3 ml of *water*. Cool the solution in ice and add 1 ml of a freshly prepared 20% w/v solution of *sodium nitrite.* Add the resulting mixture drop wise to a cold solution of 0.1 g of the residue obtained in test B in 2 ml of 5M *sodium hydroxide.* The solution becomes deep cherry-red and a copious dark brown precipitate is produced.

ASSAY

Weigh and powder 20 tablets. Carry out the method for *liquid chromatography,* Appendix III D, injecting 50 µl of each of the following solutions. For solution (1) add 80 ml of mobile phase A to a quantity of the powdered tablets containing the equivalent of 60 mg of amoxicillin and shake for 15 minutes. Mix with the aid of ultrasound for 1 minute, add sufficient mobile phase A to produce 100 ml, mix and filter (Whatman GF/C filter paper is suitable). Solution (2) contains 0.070% w/v of *amoxicillin trihydrate EPCRS* in mobile phase A. Solution (3) contains 0.0004% w/v of *cefadroxil EPCRS* and 0.003% w/v of *amoxicillin trihydrate EPCRS* in mobile phase A.

The chromatographic conditions described under Amoxicillin Oily Injections may be used.

The test is not valid unless, in the chromatogram obtained with solution (3), the *resolution factor* between the peaks due to amoxicillin and cefadroxil is at least 2.0. If necessary, adjust the composition of the mobile phase to achieve the required resolution.

Calculate the content of $C_{16}H_{19}N_3O_5S$ in the tablets from the chromatograms obtained and from the declared content of $C_{16}H_{19}N_3O_5S$ in *amoxicillin trihydrate EPCRS.*

LABELLING

The quantity of active ingredient is stated in terms of the equivalent amount of amoxicillin.

Ampicillin Sodium and Cloxacillin Sodium Intramammary Infusion (Lactating Cow)

Ampicillin and Cloxacillin Intramammary Infusion (LC)

Action and use
Penicillin antibacterial.

DEFINITION

Ampicillin Sodium and Cloxacillin Sodium Intramammary Infusion (Lactating Cow) is a sterile suspension of Ampicillin Sodium and Cloxacillin Sodium in a suitable vehicle containing suitable suspending agents.

The intramammary infusion complies with the requirements stated under Intramammary Infusions and with the following requirements.

Content of ampicillin, $C_{16}H_{19}N_3O_4S$
90.0 to 110.0% of the stated amount.

Content of cloxacillin, $C_{19}H_{18}ClN_3O_5S$
90.0 to 110.0% of the stated amount.

IDENTIFICATION

A. Carry out the method for *thin-layer chromatography,* Appendix III A, using a *TLC silica gel plate* (Merck silica gel 60 plates are suitable). Impregnate the plate by spraying it with a 0.1% w/v solution of *disodium edetate* in a 5% w/v solution of *sodium dihydrogen orthophosphate,* allow the plate to dry in air and heat at 105° for 1 hour. Use as the mobile phase a mixture of 5 volumes of *butan-1-ol,* 10 volumes of a 0.1% w/v solution of *disodium edetate* in a 5% w/v solution of *sodium dihydrogen orthophosphate,* 30 volumes of *glacial acetic acid* and 50 volumes of *butyl acetate.* Apply separately to the plate 1 µl of each of the following solutions. For solution (1) extract a quantity of the infusion containing the equivalent of 50 mg of ampicillin with three 15 ml quantities of *petroleum spirit (boiling range, 120° to 160°).* Discard the extracts, wash the residue with 10 ml of *ether* and dry in a current of air. Dissolve the residue in 50 ml of *phosphate buffer pH 7.0,* shake well, filter and use the filtrate. Solution (2) contains 0.1% w/v of *anhydrous ampicillin EPCRS* in *phosphate buffer pH 7.0.* After removal of the plate, allow it to dry, heat at 105° for 10 to 15 minutes and spray with a mixture of 100 volumes of *starch mucilage,* 6 volumes of *glacial acetic acid* and 2 volumes of a 1% w/v solution of *iodine* in a 4% w/v solution of *potassium iodide.* The principal spot in the chromatogram obtained with solution (1) corresponds to that in the chromatogram obtained with solution (2).

B. Carry out the method for *thin-layer chromatography,* Appendix III A, using a *TLC silica gel F_{254} silanised plate* (Merck plates are suitable) and, as the mobile phase, a mixture of 1 volume of *formic acid,* 30 volumes of *acetone* and 70 volumes of 0.05M *potassium hydrogen phthalate* that has been adjusted first to pH 6.0 with 5M *sodium hydroxide* and then to pH 9.0 with 0.1M *sodium hydroxide.* Apply separately to the plate 1 µl of each of the following solutions. Solution (1) is prepared as described in test A but using an amount of the infusion containing the equivalent of 0.130 g of cloxacillin. Solution (2) contains 0.28% w/v of *cloxacillin sodium EPCRS* in *phosphate buffer pH 7.0.* After removal of the plate, allow it to dry, heat at 105° for 10 to 15 minutes and spray with a mixture of 100 volumes of *starch mucilage,* 6 volumes of *glacial acetic acid* and 2 volumes of a 1% w/v solution of *iodine* in a 4% w/v solution of *potassium iodide.* The principal spot in the chromatogram obtained with solution (1) corresponds to that in the chromatogram obtained with solution (2).

C. Extract a quantity containing the equivalent of 50 mg of ampicillin with three 15 ml quantities of *petroleum spirit (boiling range, 120° to 160°).* Discard the extracts, wash the residue with 10 ml of *ether* and dry the residue at 55°. The residue produces an intense, persistent yellowish orange colour when introduced into a non-luminous Bunsen burner flame on a platinum wire moistened with *hydrochloric acid.*

TESTS
Water

Not more than 1.0% w/w, Appendix IX C. Use 1.5 g and a mixture of 70 volumes of *chloroform* and 30 volumes of *anhydrous methanol* as the solvent.

ASSAY

Express, as far as possible, weigh and mix the contents of 10 containers. Extract a quantity of the mixed contents containing the equivalent of 50 mg of ampicillin with three 15 ml quantities of *petroleum spirit (boiling range, 120° to 160°)* previously saturated with *ampicillin sodium* and *cloxacillin sodium.* Discard the extract, wash the residue with *ether* previously saturated with *ampicillin sodium* and *cloxacillin sodium,* dry in a current of air, dissolve in *water* and dilute to 100 ml with *water.* Centrifuge and use the clear supernatant liquid (solution A).

For ampicillin

Dilute 2 ml of solution A to 50 ml with *buffered copper sulphate solution pH 5.2,* transfer 10 ml to a stoppered test tube and heat in a water bath at 75° for 30 minutes. Rapidly cool to room temperature, dilute to 20 ml with *buffered copper sulphate solution pH 5.2* and measure the *absorbance* of the resulting solution at the maximum at 320 nm, Appendix II B, using in the reference cell a solution prepared by diluting 2 ml of solution A to 100 ml with *buffered copper sulphate solution pH 5.2*. Calculate the content of $C_{16}H_{19}N_3O_4S$ in a container of average content from the *absorbance* obtained by carrying out the operation at the same time using 2 ml of a solution prepared by dissolving 50 mg of *anhydrous ampicillin EPCRS* in 100 ml of *water*, diluting to 50 ml with *buffered copper sulphate solution pH 5.2* and beginning at the words 'transfer 10 ml...' and from the declared content of $C_{16}H_{19}N_3O_4S$ in *anhydrous ampicillin EPCRS*.

For cloxacillin

Dilute 2 ml of solution A to 100 ml with 1M *hydrochloric acid*. Measure the *absorbance* of the resulting solution at the maximum at 350 nm, Appendix II B, at 20° after exactly 12 minutes using 1M *hydrochloric acid* in the reference cell. Calculate the content of $C_{19}H_{18}ClN_3O_5S$ in a container of average content from the *absorbance* obtained by carrying out the operation at the same time using 2 ml of a solution prepared by dissolving 0.14 g of *cloxacillin sodium EPCRS* in 100 ml of *water* and from the declared content of $C_{19}H_{17}ClN_3NaO_5S$ in *cloxacillin sodium EPCRS*. Each mg of $C_{19}H_{17}ClN_3NaO_5S$ is equivalent to 0.9520 mg of $C_{19}H_{18}ClN_3O_5S$.

LABELLING

The label states the quantity of Ampicillin Sodium in terms of the equivalent amount of ampicillin, and the quantity of Cloxacillin Sodium in terms of the equivalent amount of cloxacillin.

Ampicillin Trihydrate and Cloxacillin Benzathine Intramammary Infusion (Dry Cow)

Ampicillin and Cloxacillin Intramammary Infusion (DC)

DEFINITION

Ampicillin Trihydrate and Cloxacillin Benzathine Intramammary Infusion (Dry Cow) is a sterile suspension of Ampicillin Trihydrate and Cloxacillin Benzathine in a suitable vehicle, containing suitable suspending agents.

The intramammary infusion complies with the requirements stated under Intramammary Infusions and with the following requirements.

Content of ampicillin, $C_{16}H_{19}N_3O_4S$
90.0 to 110.0% of the stated amount.

Content of cloxacillin, $C_{19}H_{18}ClN_3O_5S$
90.0 to 110.0% of the stated amount.

IDENTIFICATION

A. Extract a quantity containing the equivalent of 0.25 g of ampicillin with three 15 ml quantities of *petroleum spirit (boiling range, 120° to 160°)*. Discard the extracts, wash the residue with 10 ml of *ether* and dry in a current of air. Shake with 10 ml of *chloroform* and filter. Retain the filtrate. Wash the residue with two 5 ml quantities of *chloroform* and dry at room temperature at a pressure of 2 kPa. The *infrared absorption spectrum* of the residue, Appendix II A, is concordant with the *reference spectrum* of ampicillin trihydrate *(RSV 06)*.

B. Wash the filtrate obtained in test A with two 5 ml quantities of *water*, dry the chloroform layer with *anhydrous*

sodium sulphate, filter and dilute the filtrate to 20 ml with *chloroform*. The *infrared absorption spectrum* of the resulting solution, Appendix II A, is concordant with the *reference spectrum* of cloxacillin benzathine *(RSV 12)*.

TESTS
Water

Not more than 3.0% w/w, Appendix IX C. Use 1.5 g and a mixture of 70 volumes of *chloroform* and 30 volumes of *anhydrous methanol* as the solvent.

ASSAY

Express, as far as possible, weigh and mix the contents of 10 containers. Extract a quantity of the mixed contents containing the equivalent of 60 mg of ampicillin with three 15 ml quantities of *petroleum spirit (boiling range, 120° to 160°)* previously saturated with *ampicillin trihydrate* and *cloxacillin benzathine*. Discard the extracts, wash the residue with *ether* previously saturated with *ampicillin trihydrate* and *cloxacillin benzathine*, dry in a current of air, dissolve in 50 ml of *methanol* and dilute to 100 ml with *water*. Centrifuge and use the clear supernatant liquid (solution A).

For ampicillin

Dilute 2 ml of solution A to 50 ml with *buffered copper sulphate solution pH 5.2*, transfer 10 ml to a stoppered test tube and heat in a water bath at 75° for 30 minutes. Rapidly cool to room temperature, dilute to 20 ml with *buffered copper sulphate solution pH 5.2* and measure the *absorbance* of the resulting solution at the maximum at 320 nm, Appendix II B, using in the reference cell the unheated buffered solution of the infusion. Calculate the content of $C_{16}H_{19}N_3O_4S$ in a container of average content from the *absorbance* obtained by carrying out the operation at the same time using 2 ml of a solution prepared by dissolving 60 mg of *anhydrous ampicillin EPCRS* in 100 ml of a 50% v/v solution of *methanol*, diluting to 50 ml with *buffered copper sulphate solution pH 5.2*, and beginning at the words 'transfer 10 ml...' and from the declared content of $C_{16}H_{19}N_3O_4S$ in *anhydrous ampicillin EPCRS*.

For cloxacillin

Dilute 2 ml of solution A to 100 ml with 1M *hydrochloric acid*. Measure the *absorbance* of the resulting solution at the maximum at 350 nm, Appendix II B, at 20° after exactly 12 minutes, using 1M *hydrochloric acid* in the reference cell. Calculate the content of $C_{19}H_{18}ClN_3O_5S$ in a container of average content from the *absorbance* obtained by carrying out the operation at the same time using 2 ml of a solution prepared by dissolving 0.165 g of *cloxacillin benzathine BPCRS* in 100 ml of a 50% v/v solution of *methanol* and from the declared content of $C_{19}H_{18}ClN_3O_5S$ in *cloxacillin benzathine BPCRS*.

LABELLING

The label states the quantity of Ampicillin Trihydrate in terms of the equivalent amount of ampicillin and the quantity of Cloxacillin Benzathine in terms of the equivalent amount of cloxacillin.

Ampicillin Tablets

Action and use
Penicillin antibacterial.

DEFINITION
Ampicillin Tablets contain Ampicillin Trihydrate.

The tablets comply with the requirements stated under Tablets and with the following requirements.

Content of ampicillin, $C_{16}H_{19}N_3O_4S$
90.0 to 110.0% of the stated amount.

IDENTIFICATION
A. Carry out the method for *thin-layer chromatography*, Appendix III A, using a *TLC silica gel silanised plate* (Merck silanised silica gel 60 F_{254s} (RP-18) plates are suitable) and a mixture of 10 volumes of *acetone* and 90 volumes of a 15.4% w/v solution of *ammonium acetate* adjusted to pH 5.0 with *glacial acetic acid* as the mobile phase. Apply separately to the plate 1 µl of each of the following solutions. For solution (1) shake a quantity of the powdered tablets containing the equivalent of 0.125 g of ampicillin with sufficient *sodium hydrogen carbonate solution* to produce 50 ml and filter. Solution (2) contains 0.25% w/v of *ampicillin trihydrate EPCRS* in *sodium hydrogen carbonate solution*. Solution (3) contains 0.25% w/v of each of *ampicillin trihydrate EPCRS* and *amoxicillin trihydrate EPCRS* in *sodium hydrogen carbonate solution*. After removal of the plate, allow it to dry in air, expose it to iodine vapour until spots appear and examine in daylight. The principal spot in the chromatogram obtained with solution (1) is similar in position, colour and size to that in the chromatogram obtained with solution (2). The test is not valid unless the chromatogram obtained with solution (3) shows two clearly separated spots.

B. To a quantity of the powdered tablets containing the equivalent of 10 mg of ampicillin add sufficient *water* to produce 10 ml, shake for 15 minutes and filter. Place 0.1 ml of a 0.1% w/v solution of *ninhydrin* on a filter paper, dry at 105°, superimpose 0.1 ml of the solution of the preparation being examined, heat for 5 minutes at 105° and allow to cool. A mauve colour is produced.

C. Suspend a quantity of the powdered tablets containing the equivalent of 10 mg of ampicillin in 1 ml of *water* and add 2 ml of a mixture of 2 ml of *cupri-tartaric solution R1* and 6 ml of *water*. A magenta-violet colour is produced immediately.

TESTS
Disintegration
Maximum time, 45 minutes, Appendix XII A1.

ASSAY
Weigh and powder 20 tablets. Carry out the method for *liquid chromatography*, Appendix III D, injecting 50 µl of each of the following solutions. For solution (1) shake a quantity of the powdered tablets containing the equivalent of 60 mg of ampicillin with 80 ml of mobile phase A for 15 minutes, dilute to 100 ml with the same solvent, filter and dilute 5 ml of the resulting solution to 50 ml with mobile phase A. Solution (2) contains 0.006% w/v of *anhydrous ampicillin EPCRS* in mobile phase A. Solution (3) contains 0.025% w/v of *anhydrous ampicillin EPCRS* and 0.002% w/v of *cefradine EPCRS* in mobile phase A.

The chromatographic procedure may be carried out using (a) a stainless steel column (25 cm × 4.6 mm) packed with *octadecylsilyl silica gel for chromatography* (5 µm) (Hypersil 5

ODS is suitable), (b) as the mobile phase with a flow rate of 1 ml per minute a mixture of 15 volumes of mobile phase B and 85 volumes of mobile phase A described below and (c) a detection wavelength of 254 nm.

Mobile phase A   Dilute a mixture of 1 volume of *dilute acetic acid*, 100 volumes of 0.2M *potassium dihydrogen orthophosphate* and 100 volumes of *acetonitrile* to 2000 volumes with *water*.

Mobile phase B   Dilute a mixture of 1 volume of *dilute acetic acid*, 100 volumes of 0.2M *potassium dihydrogen orthophosphate* and 800 volumes of *acetonitrile* to 2000 volumes with *water*.

The assay is not valid unless, in the chromatogram obtained with solution (3), the *resolution factor* between the peaks due to ampicillin and cefradine is at least 3.0. If necessary, adjust the composition of the mobile phase to achieve the required resolution.

Calculate the content of $C_{16}H_{19}N_3O_4S$ in the tablets using the declared content of $C_{16}H_{19}N_3O_4S$ in *anhydrous ampicillin EPCRS*.

STORAGE
Ampicillin Tablets should be stored at a temperature not exceeding 20°.

LABELLING
The quantity of the active ingredient is stated in terms of the equivalent amount of ampicillin.

Apramycin Injection

Action and use
Aminoglycoside antibacterial.

DEFINITION
Apramycin Injection is a sterile solution of Apramycin Sulphate in Water for Injections.

The injection complies with the requirements stated under Parenteral Preparations and with the following requirements.

CHARACTERISTICS
An amber-coloured solution.

IDENTIFICATION
A. Carry out the method for *thin-layer chromatography*, Appendix III A, using a silica gel F_{254} precoated plate (Merck silica gel 60 F_{254} plates are suitable) and as the mobile phase a mixture of 20 volumes of *chloroform*, 40 volumes of 13.5M *ammonia* and 60 volumes of *methanol*, equilibrated for 1 hour before use. Allow the solvent front to ascend 10 cm above the line of application. Apply separately to the plate 5 µl of each of three solutions in *water* containing (1) a volume of the injection diluted to contain the equivalent of 0.6 mg of apramycin per ml, (2) 0.06% w/v of *apramycin BPCRS* and (3) 0.06% w/v each of *apramycin BPCRS* and *tobramycin EPCRS*. After removal of the plate, allow it to dry in air for 10 minutes, heat at 100° for 10 minutes, spray with *sodium hypochlorite solution* whilst hot and cool for 5 minutes. Spray with *absolute ethanol*, heat at 100° for 5 to 10 minutes, or until an area of the plate below the line of application gives at most a faint blue colour with one drop of a 1% w/v solution of *potassium iodide* containing 1% w/v *soluble starch*, and spray with the potassium iodide-starch solution. The principal spot in the chromatogram obtained with solution (1) corresponds to that in the chromatogram obtained with solution (2). The test is not valid unless the chromatogram obtained with solution (3) shows two clearly separated principal spots.

B. In the test for Related substances, the retention time of the principal peak in the chromatogram obtained with solution (1) corresponds to that of the principal peak in the chromatogram obtained with solution (2).

C. Yields reaction A characteristic of *sulphates*, Appendix VI.

TESTS

Acidity or alkalinity
pH, 4.5 to 7.5, Appendix V L.

Related substances
Carry out the method for *liquid chromatography*, Appendix III D, using the following solutions. Solution (1) contains a volume of the injection, diluted to contain the equivalent of 3 mg of apramycin per ml. Solution (2) contains 0.30% w/v of *apramycin BPCRS*. For solution (3) dilute 1 volume of solution (1) to 20 volumes.

The chromatographic procedure may be carried out using a column (25 cm × 4 mm) packed with fast cation-exchange polymeric beads (13 μm) with sulphonic acid functional groups (Dionex Fast Cation-1^R is suitable) and a stainless steel post-column reaction coil (380 cm × 0.4 mm) with internal baffles, maintained at 130°. Use in the reaction coil *ninhydrin reagent I* at a flow rate approximately the same as that for the mobile phase. For mobile phase A use a solution containing 1.961% w/v of *sodium citrate*, 0.08% v/v of *liquefied phenol* and 0.5% v/v of *thiodiglycol*, adjusted to pH 4.25 using *hydrochloric acid*. Mobile phase B is a solution containing 4.09% w/v of *sodium chloride* and 3.922% w/v of *sodium citrate* with 0.08% v/v of *liquefied phenol*, adjusted to pH 7.4 with *hydrochloric acid*. Degas both mobile phases using *helium* and use a flow rate of 0.8 ml per minute. Equilibrate the column using a mixture containing 75% of mobile phase A and 25% of mobile phase B. After each injection elute for 3 minutes using the same mixture and then carry out a linear gradient elution for 6 minutes to 100% of mobile phase B. Elute for a further 21 minutes using 100% of mobile phase B, then step-wise, re-equilibrate to a mixture of 75% of mobile phase A and 25% of mobile phase B and elute for at least 10 minutes. Use a detection wavelength of 568 nm.

The test is not valid unless, in the chromatogram obtained with solution (2), the *resolution factor* between compound A and 3-hydroxyapramycin, identified as indicated in the reference chromatogram supplied with *apramycin BPCRS*, is at least 0.8.

In the chromatogram obtained with solution (1) the areas of any peaks corresponding to 3-hydroxyapramycin, lividamine/2-deoxystreptamine (combined) and compound A (identified as indicated in the reference chromatogram supplied with *apramycin BPCRS*) are not greater than twice the area of the principal peak in the chromatogram obtained with solution (3) (5% each), the area of any peak corresponding to compound B is not greater than 0.8 times the area of the principal peak in the chromatogram obtained with solution (3) (2%), the area of any other *secondary peak* is not greater than 0.8 times the area of the principal peak in the chromatogram obtained with solution (3) (2%) and the sum of the areas of all the *secondary peaks* is not greater than 4.8 times the area of the principal peak in the chromatogram obtained with solution (3) (12%). Disregard any peak with an area less than 0.04 times the area of the principal peak in the chromatogram obtained with solution (3) (0.1%).

Pyrogens
Complies with the *test for pyrogens*, Appendix XIV D. Use per kg of the rabbit's weight 2 ml of a solution prepared from the

injection by dilution with *sodium chloride injection* to contain the equivalent of 10 mg of apramycin per ml.

ASSAY
Carry out the *biological assay of antibiotics*, Appendix XIV A, Method B. The precision of the assay is such that the fiducial limits of error are not less than 95% and not more than 105% of the estimated potency.

Calculate the content of apramycin in the injection taking each 1000 Units found to be equivalent to 1 mg of apramycin. The upper fiducial limit of error is not less than 97.0% and the lower fiducial limit of error is not more than 110.0% of the stated content.

LABELLING
The strength is stated in terms of the equivalent amount of apramycin in a suitable dose-volume.

Apramycin Veterinary Oral Powder

Action and use
Aminoglycoside antibacterial.

DEFINITION
Apramycin Veterinary Oral Powder contains Apramycin Sulphate.

The veterinary oral powder complies with the requirements stated under Veterinary Oral Powders and with the following requirements.

CHARACTERISTICS
Light brown, granular powder.

IDENTIFICATION
A. Carry out the method for *thin-layer chromatography*, Appendix III A, using a silica gel F$_{254}$ precoated plate (Merck silica gel 60 F$_{254}$ plates are suitable) and as the mobile phase a mixture of 20 volumes of *chloroform*, 40 volumes of 13.5M *ammonia* and 60 volumes of *methanol*, equilibrated for 1 hour before use. Allow the solvent front to ascend 10 cm above the line of application. Apply separately to the plate 5 μl of each of the following solutions. For solution (1) dissolve a quantity of the veterinary oral powder containing the equivalent of 60 mg of apramycin in *water* and dilute to 100 ml. Solution (2) contains 0.06% w/v of *apramycin BPCRS* in *water*. Solution (3) contains 0.06% w/v each of *apramycin BPCRS* and *tobramycin EPCRS* in *water*. After removal of the plate, allow it to dry in air for 10 minutes, heat at 100° for 10 minutes, spray with *sodium hypochlorite solution* whilst hot and cool for 5 minutes. Spray with *absolute ethanol*, heat at 100° for 5 to 10 minutes, or until an area of the plate below the line of application gives at most a faint blue colour with one drop of a 1% w/v solution of *potassium iodide* containing 1% w/v *soluble starch*, and spray with the potassium iodide-starch solution. The principal spot in the chromatogram obtained with solution (1) corresponds to that in the chromatogram obtained with solution (2). The test is not valid unless the chromatogram obtained with solution (3) shows two clearly separated principal spots.

B. In the test for Related substances, the retention time of the principal peak in the chromatogram obtained with solution (1) corresponds to that of the principal peak in the chromatogram obtained with solution (2).

C. Yields reaction A characteristic of *sulphates*, Appendix VI.

TESTS
Related substances
Carry out the method for *liquid chromatography*, Appendix III D, using the following solutions. For solution (1) dissolve a quantity of the oral powder containing the equivalent of 0.3 g of apramycin in *water* and dilute to 100 ml. Solution (2) contains 0.30% w/v of *apramycin BPCRS*. For solution (3) dilute 1 volume of solution (1) to 20 volumes.

The chromatographic conditions described under Apramycin Injection may be used.

The test is not valid unless, in the chromatogram obtained with solution (2), the *resolution factor* between compound A and 3-hydroxyapramycin, identified as indicated in the reference chromatogram supplied with *apramycin BPCRS*, is at least 0.8.

In the chromatogram obtained with solution (1) the areas of any peaks corresponding to 3-hydroxyapramycin, lividamine/2-deoxystreptamine (combined), compound A and compound B (identified as indicated in the reference chromatogram supplied with *apramycin BPCRS*) are not greater than 2.8, 2.0, 0.8 and 0.8 times respectively the area of the principal peak in the chromatogram obtained with solution (3) (7%, 5%, 2% and 2% respectively), the area of any other *secondary peak* is not greater than 0.8 times the area of the principal peak in the chromatogram obtained with solution (3) (2%) and the sum of the areas of all the *secondary peaks* is not greater than 6 times the area of the principal peak in the chromatogram obtained with solution (3) (15%). Disregard any peak with an area less than 0.04 times the area of the principal peak in the chromatogram obtained with solution (3) (0.1%).

ASSAY
Carry out the *biological assay of antibiotics*, Appendix XIV A, Method B. The precision of the assay is such that the fiducial limits of error are not less than 95% and not more than 105% of the estimated potency.

Calculate the content of apramycin in the veterinary oral powder taking each 1000 Units found to be equivalent to 1 mg of apramycin. The upper fiducial limit of error is not less than 97.0% and the lower fiducial limit of error is not more than 110.0% of the stated content.

LABELLING
The quantity of active ingredient is stated in terms of the equivalent amount of apramycin.

Apramycin Premix

Action and use
Aminoglycoside antibacterial.

DEFINITION
Apramycin Premix contains Apramycin Sulphate.

The premix complies with the requirements stated under Premixes and with the following requirements.

CHARACTERISTICS
Light brown granules.

IDENTIFICATION
A. Carry out the method for *thin-layer chromatography*, Appendix III A, using a silica gel F_{254} precoated plate (Merck silica gel 60 F_{254} plates are suitable) and as the mobile phase a mixture of 20 volumes of *chloroform*, 40 volumes of 13.5M *ammonia* and 60 volumes of *methanol*, equilibrated for 1 hour before use. Allow the solvent front to ascend 10 cm above the line of application. Apply separately to the plate 5 µl of each of the following solutions. For solution (1) shake a quantity of the premix containing the equivalent of 60 mg of apramycin with 60 ml of 0.1M *sodium hydrogen carbonate* at 60°, cool, dilute to 100 ml, filter and use the filtrate. Solution (2) contains 0.06% w/v of *apramycin BPCRS* in *water*. Solution (3) contains 0.06% w/v each of *apramycin BPCRS* and *tobramycin EPCRS* in *water*. After removal of the plate, allow it to dry in air for 10 minutes, heat at 100° for 10 minutes, spray with *sodium hypochlorite solution* whilst hot and cool for 5 minutes. Spray with *absolute ethanol*, heat at 100° for 5 to 10 minutes, or until an area of the plate below the line of application gives at most a faint blue colour with one drop of a 1% w/v solution of *potassium iodide* containing 1% w/v *soluble starch*, and spray with the potassium iodide-starch solution. The principal spot in the chromatogram obtained with solution (1) corresponds to that in the chromatogram obtained with solution (2). The test is not valid unless the chromatogram obtained with solution (3) shows two clearly separated principal spots.

B. In the test for Related substances, the retention time of the principal peak in the chromatogram obtained with solution (1) corresponds to that of the principal peak in the chromatogram obtained with solution (2).

C. Yields reaction A characteristic of *sulphates*, Appendix VI.

TESTS
Related substances
Carry out the method for *liquid chromatography*, Appendix III D, using the following solutions. For solution (1) shake a quantity of the premix containing the equivalent of 3 mg of apramycin per ml with 5% w/v of *sodium chloride* and centrifuge for 5 minutes at 4000 revolutions per minute. Filter the supernatant liquid using filters of nominal pore size of 5 µm and 0.45 µm. Solution (2) contains 0.30% w/v of *apramycin BPCRS*. For solution (3) dilute 1 volume of solution (1) to 20 volumes.

The chromatographic conditions described under Apramycin Injection may be used.

The test is not valid unless, in the chromatogram obtained with solution (2), the *resolution factor* between compound A and 3-hydroxyapramycin, identified as indicated in the reference chromatogram supplied with the *apramycin BPCRS*, is at least 0.8.

In the chromatogram obtained with solution (1) the areas of any peaks corresponding to 3-hydroxyapramycin, lividamine/2-deoxystreptamine (combined), compound A and compound B (identified as indicated in the reference chromatogram supplied with *apramycin BPCRS*) are not greater than 2.8, 2.0, 0.8 and 0.8 times respectively the area of the principal peak in the chromatogram obtained with solution (3) (7%, 5%, 2% and 2% respectively), the area of any other *secondary peak* is not greater than 0.8 times the area of the principal peak in the chromatogram obtained with solution (3) (2%) and the sum of the areas of all the *secondary peaks* is not greater than 6 times the area of the principal peak in the chromatogram obtained with solution (3) (15%). Disregard any peak with an area less than 0.04 times the area of the principal peak in the chromatogram obtained with solution (3) (0.1%).

ASSAY

To about 5 g of the premix, accurately weighed, add 250 ml of a solution containing 0.6% w/v of *sodium hydroxide* and 0.745% w/v of *ethylenediaminetetra-acetic acid* in *water*. Shake for 1 hour and allow to stand for 15 minutes. Decant the supernatant liquid and dilute to concentrations equivalent to the solutions of the Standard Preparation with the pH 8.0 buffer and carry out the *biological assay of antibiotics*, Appendix XIV A, Method B. The precision of the assay is such that the fiducial limits of error are not less than 95% and not more than 105% of the estimated potency.

Calculate the content of apramycin in the premix taking each 1000 Units found to be equivalent to 1 mg of apramycin. The upper fiducial limit of error is not less than 97.0% and the lower fiducial limit of error is not more than 110.0% of the stated content.

STORAGE

Apramycin Premix should be stored in a dry place.

LABELLING

The quantity of active ingredient is stated in terms of the equivalent amount of apramycin.

Azaperone Injection

Action and use

Dopamine receptor antagonist; neuroleptic (veterinary).

DEFINITION

Azaperone Injection is a sterile solution of Azaperone in Water for Injections.

The injection complies with the requirements stated under Parenteral Preparations and with the following requirements.

Content of azaperone, $C_{19}H_{22}FN_3O$
90.0 to 110.0% of the stated amount.

CHARACTERISTICS

A clear, yellow solution.

IDENTIFICATION

A. To a volume containing 80 mg of Azaperone add 5 ml of 0.5M *sulphuric acid* and 20 ml of *water*. Extract the solution with 50 ml of *ether*, make the aqueous phase alkaline with 1M *sodium hydroxide* and extract with 50 ml of *ether*. Wash the ether extracts with two 10 ml-quantities of *water*, shake with *anhydrous sodium sulphate*, filter and evaporate to dryness. The *infrared absorption spectrum* of the residue, Appendix II A, is concordant with the *reference spectrum* of azaperone *(RSV 08)*.

B. The *light absorption*, Appendix II B, in the range 230 to 350 nm of a 2-cm layer of the solution obtained in the Assay exhibits maxima at 242 nm and at 312 nm. The *absorbances* at the maxima are about 1.1 and about 0.38, respectively.

TESTS
Acidity
pH, 3.5 to 5.0, Appendix V L.

Related substances
Carry out in subdued light the method for *thin-layer chromatography*, Appendix III A, using a silica gel F_{254} precoated plate (Merck silica gel 60 F_{254} plates are suitable) and a mixture of 1 volume of *ethanol (96%)* and 9 volumes of *chloroform* as the mobile phase. Apply separately to the plate 10 μl of each of the following two solutions. For solution (1) dissolve the extracted residue obtained in

Identification test A in sufficient *chloroform* to produce a solution containing 1% w/v of Azaperone. For solution (2) dilute 1 volume of solution (1) to 100 volumes with *chloroform*. After removal of the plate allow it to dry in air and examine under *ultraviolet light (254 nm)*. Any *secondary spot* in the chromatogram obtained with solution (1) is not more intense than the spot in the chromatogram obtained with solution (2) (1%).

ASSAY

To a volume containing 0.4 g of Azaperone add 25 ml of 0.5M *sulphuric acid* and sufficient *water* to produce 250 ml. Mix, transfer 10 ml of the solution to a separating funnel containing 10 ml of 0.05M *sulphuric acid* and shake with 20 ml of *ether*. Wash the ether layer with two 10 ml quantities of 0.05M *sulphuric acid*. Make the combined acid extract and washings alkaline with 5 ml of 1M *sodium hydroxide*, add 50 ml of *ether*, shake and allow to separate. Extract the aqueous layer with 50 ml of *ether*. Wash the two ether solutions, in succession, with a 20 ml quantity of *water* and extract each of the two ether solutions, in succession, with two 20 ml quantities and one 5 ml quantity of 0.25M *sulphuric acid*. Combine the acid extracts and add sufficient 0.25M *sulphuric acid* to produce 100 ml. To 5 ml of the resulting solution add 5 ml of *methanol* and sufficient 0.25M *sulphuric acid* to produce 100 ml. Measure the *absorbance* of the resulting solution at the maximum at 242 nm, Appendix II B. Dissolve 40 mg of *azaperone BPCRS* in sufficient *methanol* to produce 250 ml, dilute 5 ml of the resulting solution to 100 ml with 0.25M *sulphuric acid* and measure the *absorbance* at 242 nm. Calculate the content of $C_{19}H_{22}FN_3O$ in the injection from the absorbances obtained using the declared content of $C_{19}H_{22}FN_3O$ in *azaperone BPCRS*.

STORAGE

Azaperone Injection should be protected from light.

Calcium Borogluconate Injection

DEFINITION

Calcium Borogluconate Injection is a sterile solution of Calcium Gluconate and Boric Acid in Water for Injections.

The injection complies with the requirements stated under Parenteral Preparations and with the following requirements.

Content of calcium, Ca
95.0 to 105.0% of the stated amount.

Content of boric acid, H_3BO_3
Not more than 2.3 times the stated content of calcium.

IDENTIFICATION

A. To 1 ml add sufficient *water* to produce a solution containing about 0.75% w/v of calcium and add 0.05 ml of *iron(III) chloride solution R1*. An intense yellow or yellowish green colour is produced.

B. Yields the reactions characteristic of *calcium salts*, Appendix VI.

C. To 1 ml add 0.15 ml of *sulphuric acid* and 5 ml of *methanol* and ignite. The mixture burns with a flame tinged with green.

Acidity
pH of the injection, diluted if necessary with *carbon dioxide-free water* to contain 1.5% w/v of calcium, 3.0 to 4.0, Appendix V L.

ASSAY

For calcium

Dilute a quantity containing the equivalent of 45 mg of calcium to about 50 ml with *water*. Titrate with 0.05M *disodium edetate VS* to within a few ml of the expected end point, add 4 ml of a 40% w/v solution of *sodium hydroxide* and 10 mg of *solochrome dark blue mixture* and continue the titration until the colour changes from pink to blue. Each ml of 0.05M *disodium edetate VS* is equivalent to 2.004 mg of Ca.

For boric acid

Dilute a quantity containing 0.1 g of Boric Acid to 50 ml with *water*, add 3 g of D-*mannitol* and titrate with 0.1M *sodium hydroxide VS* using *phenolphthalein solution R1* as indicator. Each ml of 0.1M *sodium hydroxide VS* is equivalent to 6.183 mg of H_3BO_3.

STORAGE

Calcium Borogluconate Injection should be protected from light. It may be supplied in containers of *glass type III*, Appendix XIX B.

LABELLING

The strength is stated as the amount of calcium in a suitable dose-volume. The label also states the proportion of boric acid present.

Calcium Copperedetate Injection

Action and use

Used in the treatment of copper deficiency.

DEFINITION

Calcium Copperedetate Injection is a sterile suspension of Calcium Copperedetate, with suitable stabilising and dispersing agents, in an oil-in-water emulsion.

The injection complies with the requirements stated under Parenteral Preparations and with the following requirements.

Content of copper, Cu

92.0 to 108.0% of the stated amount.

CHARACTERISTICS

Macroscopical   A blue, opaque, viscous suspension.

Microscopical   When diluted with *glycerol* and examined microscopically, cubic crystals 10 to 30 μm in diameter are visible, but large plate-like crystals are absent.

IDENTIFICATION

Ignite 1 g and dissolve the residue by warming in 10 ml of a mixture of equal volumes of *hydrochloric acid* and *water*; filter if necessary. The solution complies with the following tests.

A. Neutralise 2 ml of the solution with 5M *ammonia*, and add 1 ml of 6M *acetic acid* and 2 ml of *potassium iodide solution*. A white precipitate is produced and iodine is liberated, colouring the supernatant liquid brown.

B. To 5 ml of the solution add 25 ml of a 10% v/v solution of *mercaptoacetic acid* and filter. Make the filtrate alkaline with 5M *ammonia* and add 5 ml of a 2.5% w/v solution of *ammonium oxalate*. A white precipitate is produced which is soluble in *hydrochloric acid* but only sparingly soluble in 6M *acetic acid*.

ASSAY

Evaporate a quantity containing the equivalent of 0.13 g of copper to dryness, ignite at 600° to 700°, cool and heat the residue with 5 ml of a mixture of equal volumes of *hydrochloric acid* and *water* on a water bath for 15 minutes. Add 5 ml of *water*, filter and wash the residue with about 20 ml of *water*. Combine the filtrate and the washings, add 10 ml of *bromine water*, boil to remove the bromine, cool and add *dilute sodium carbonate solution* until a faint permanent precipitate is produced. Add 3 g of *potassium iodide* and 5 ml of 6M *acetic acid* and titrate the liberated iodine with 0.1M *sodium thiosulphate VS*, using *starch mucilage* as indicator, until only a faint blue colour remains; add 2 g of *potassium thiocyanate* and continue the titration until the blue colour disappears. Each ml of 0.1M *sodium thiosulphate VS* is equivalent to 6.354 mg of Cu.

LABELLING

The strength is stated as the equivalent amount of copper in a suitable dose-volume.

Catechu Tincture

DEFINITION

Catechu	Crushed 200 g
Cinnamon	Bruised 50 g
Ethanol (45 per cent)	1000 ml

Extemporaneous preparation

The following directions apply.

Prepare by maceration, Appendix XI F.

The tincture complies with the requirements for Tinctures stated under Extracts and with the following requirements.

TESTS

Ethanol content

36 to 40% v/v, Appendix VIII F, Method III.

Dry residue

12 to 17% w/v.

Relative density

0.990 to 1.010, Appendix V G.

Cefalonium Eye Ointment

Action and use

Cephalosporin antibacterial.

DEFINITION

Cefalonium Eye Ointment is a sterile preparation containing Cefalonium in a suitable non-aqueous basis.

The eye ointment complies with the requirements stated under Eye Preparations and with the following requirements.

Content of anhydrous cefalonium, $C_{20}H_{18}N_4O_5S_2$

90.0 to 112.0% of the stated amount.

IDENTIFICATION

A. In the Assay, the retention time of the principal peak in the chromatogram obtained with solution (1) corresponds to that of the principal peak in the chromatogram obtained with solution (2).

B. To a quantity of the eye ointment containing the equivalent of 20 mg of anhydrous cefalonium add a few drops of *sulphuric acid (80% v/v)* containing 1% v/v of *nitric acid* and mix. A pale green colour is produced which immediately changes to dark green.

TESTS
Related substances

Carry out the method for *liquid chromatography*, Appendix III D, using the following solutions. The solutions should be prepared immediately before use and stored in a refrigerator between injections. For solution (1) disperse a quantity of the eye ointment containing the equivalent of 0.10 g of anhydrous cefalonium in 50 ml of *petroleum spirit (boiling range, 60° to 80°)*, add 100 ml of 0.1M *hydrochloric acid* and shake vigorously by hand for 5 minutes and then mechanically for 30 minutes, filter and use the lower layer. For solution (2) dilute 2 volumes of solution (1) to 100 volumes with 0.1M *hydrochloric acid*. Solution (3) contains 0.0020% w/v of *isonicotinamide* in 0.1M *hydrochloric acid*. Solution (4) contains 0.0050% w/v of each of *cefalonium BPCRS* and *isonicotinamide* in 0.1M *hydrochloric acid*.

The chromatographic procedure may be carried out using (a) a stainless steel column (10 cm × 4.6 mm) packed with particles of silica the surface of which has been modified with chemically-bonded hexylsilyl groups (Spherisorb S5 C6 is suitable), (b) as the mobile phase with a flow rate of 2 ml per minute a mixture of 3 volumes of *acetonitrile* and 97 volumes of a solution of pH 3.4 containing 5 volumes of 0.1M *sodium acetate* and 95 volumes of 0.1M *acetic acid* and (c) a detection wavelength of 262 nm.

Inject 10 μl of each solution. For solution (1), allow the chromatography to proceed for at least 3.5 times the retention time of the principal peak. The test is not valid unless in the chromatogram obtained with solution (4) the *resolution factor* between the two principal peaks is at least 10.

In the chromatogram obtained with solution (1) the area of any peak corresponding to isonicotinamide is not greater than the area of the principal peak in the chromatogram obtained with solution (3) (2%) and the area of any other *secondary peak* is not greater than half the area of the principal peak in the chromatogram obtained with solution (2) (1%).

ASSAY

Carry out the method for *liquid chromatography*, Appendix III D, using the following solutions. The solutions should be prepared immediately before use and stored in a refrigerator between injections. For solution (1) disperse a quantity of the eye ointment containing the equivalent of 75 mg of anhydrous cefalonium in 50 ml of *petroleum spirit (boiling range, 60° to 80°)*, add 100 ml of 0.1M *hydrochloric acid* and shake vigorously by hand for 5 minutes and then mechanically for 30 minutes. Filter the lower layer and dilute 10 ml of the filtrate to 100 ml with 0.1M *hydrochloric acid*. Solution (2) contains 0.0075% w/v of *cefalonium BPCRS* in 0.1M *hydrochloric acid*.

The chromatographic procedure may be carried out using (a) a stainless steel column (10 cm × 4.6 mm) packed with particles of silica the surface of which has been modified with chemically-bonded hexylsilyl groups (Spherisorb S5 C6 is suitable), (b) as the mobile phase with a flow rate of 2 ml per minute a mixture of 3 volumes of *acetonitrile* and 97 volumes of a solution of pH 3.4 containing 5 volumes of 0.1M *sodium acetate* and 95 volumes of 0.1M *acetic acid* and (c) a detection wavelength of 262 nm. Inject 10 μl of each solution.

Calculate the content of $C_{20}H_{18}N_4O_5S_2$ using the declared content of $C_{20}H_{18}N_4O_5S_2$ in *cefalonium BPCRS*.

STORAGE

Cefalonium Eye Ointment should be stored at a temperature not exceeding 30°. It should not be allowed to freeze.

LABELLING

The quantity of active ingredient is stated in terms of the equivalent amount of anhydrous cefalonium.

Cefalonium Intramammary Infusion (Dry Cow)

Action and use
Cephalosporin antibacterial.

DEFINITION

Cefalonium Intramammary Infusion (Dry Cow) is a sterile suspension of Cefalonium in a suitable non-aqueous vehicle, containing suitable suspending agents.

The intramammary infusion complies with the requirements stated under Intramammary Infusions and with the following requirements.

Content of anhydrous cefalonium, $C_{20}H_{18}N_4O_5S_2$
90.0 to 112.0% of the stated amount.

IDENTIFICATION

A. In the Assay, the retention time of the principal peak in the chromatogram obtained with solution (1) corresponds to that of the principal peak in the chromatogram obtained with solution (2).

B. To a quantity of the intramammary infusion containing the equivalent of 20 mg of anhydrous cefalonium add a few drops of *sulphuric acid (80% v/v)* containing 1% v/v of *nitric acid* and mix. A pale green colour is produced which immediately changes to dark green.

TESTS
Related substances

Complies with the test described under Cefalonium Eye Ointment but using the solution described below as solution (1). The solutions should be prepared immediately before use and stored in a refrigerator between injections. Disperse a quantity of the intramammary infusion containing the equivalent of 0.10 g of anhydrous cefalonium in 50 ml of *petroleum spirit (boiling range, 60° to 80°)*, add 100 ml of 0.1M *hydrochloric acid* and shake vigorously by hand for 5 minutes and then mechanically for 30 minutes, filter and use the lower layer.

ASSAY

Express, as far as possible, weigh and mix the contents of 10 containers. Carry out the method for *liquid chromatography*, Appendix III D, using the following solutions. The solutions should be prepared immediately before use and stored in a refrigerator between injections. For solution (1) disperse a quantity of the mixed contents of the 10 containers containing the equivalent of 75 mg of anhydrous cefalonium in 50 ml of *petroleum spirit (boiling range, 60° to 80°)*, add 100 ml of 0.1M *hydrochloric acid* and shake vigorously by hand for 5 minutes and then mechanically for 30 minutes. Filter the lower layer and dilute 10 ml of the filtrate to 100 ml with 0.1M *hydrochloric acid*. Solution (2) contains 0.0075% w/v of *cefalonium BPCRS* in 0.1M *hydrochloric acid*.

The chromatographic procedure may be carried out using (a) a stainless steel column (10 cm × 4.6 mm) packed with particles of silica the surface of which has been modified with chemically-bonded hexylsilyl groups (Spherisorb S5 C6 is suitable), (b) as the mobile phase with a flow rate of 2 ml per minute a mixture of 3 volumes of *acetonitrile* and 97 volumes of a solution of pH 3.4 containing 5 volumes of 0.1M *sodium acetate* and 95 volumes of 0.1M *acetic acid* and (c) a detection wavelength of 262 nm. Inject 10 µl of each solution.

Calculate the content of $C_{20}H_{18}N_4O_5S_2$ in a container of average content using the declared content of $C_{20}H_{18}N_4O_5S_2$ in *cefalonium BPCRS*.

STORAGE

Cefalonium Intramammary Infusion (Dry Cow) should be stored at a temperature not exceeding 30°. It should not be allowed to freeze.

LABELLING

The quantity of active ingredient is stated in terms of the equivalent amount of anhydrous cefalonium.

Chlortetracycline Veterinary Oral Powder

Chlortetracycline Soluble Powder

Action and use
Tetracycline antibacterial.

DEFINITION

Chlortetracycline Veterinary Oral Powder is a mixture of Chlortetracycline Hydrochloride and Lactose or other suitable diluent.

The veterinary oral powder complies with the requirements stated under Veterinary Oral Powders and with the following requirements.

Content of chlortetracycline hydrochloride, $C_{22}H_{23}ClN_2O_8$,HCl
90.0 to 110.0% of the stated amount.

IDENTIFICATION

A. Complies with test A for Identification described under Chlortetracycline Tablets but using the following solutions. For solution (1) extract a quantity of the oral powder containing 10 mg of Chlortetracycline Hydrochloride with 20 ml of *methanol* and centrifuge. Solution (2) contains 0.05% w/v of *chlortetracycline hydrochloride EPCRS* in *methanol*. Solution (3) contains 0.05% w/v each of *chlortetracycline hydrochloride EPCRS*, *tetracycline hydrochloride EPCRS* and *metacycline hydrochloride EPCRS* in *methanol*.

B. To a quantity of the oral powder containing 10 mg of Chlortetracycline Hydrochloride add 20 ml of warm *ethanol (96%)*, allow to stand for 20 minutes, filter and evaporate to dryness on a water bath. A 0.1% w/v solution of the residue in *phosphate buffer pH 7.6* when heated at 100° for 1 minute exhibits a strong blue fluorescence in ultraviolet light.

Tetracycline hydrochloride and 4-epichlortetracycline hydrochloride
Not more than 8.0% and 6.0% respectively, determined as described under the Assay. Inject separately solutions (1) and (4).

ASSAY

Complies with the Assay described under Chlortetracycline Tablets but using the following solutions. For solution (1) mix a quantity of the oral powder containing 25 mg of Chlortetracycline Hydrochloride with 50 ml of 0.01M *hydrochloric acid*, shake for 10 minutes, dilute to 100 ml with 0.01M *hydrochloric acid* and filter (GF/C paper is suitable). Solution (2) contains 0.025% w/v of *chlortetracycline hydrochloride EPCRS* in 0.01M *hydrochloric acid*. Solution (3) contains 0.025% w/v each of *chlortetracycline*

hydrochloride EPCRS and *4-epichlortetracycline hydrochloride EPCRS* in 0.01M *hydrochloric acid*. Solution (4) contains 0.002% w/v of *tetracycline hydrochloride EPCRS* and 0.0015% w/v of *4-epichlortetracycline hydrochloride EPCRS* in 0.01M *hydrochloric acid*.

The assay is not valid unless the *resolution factor* between the two principal peaks in the chromatogram obtained with solution (3) is at least 1.5.

Calculate the content of $C_{22}H_{23}ClN_2O_8$,HCl in the oral powder using the declared content of $C_{22}H_{23}ClN_2O_8$,HCl in *chlortetracycline hydrochloride EPCRS*.

LABELLING

The label states the strength of the powder in terms of the concentration of Chlortetracycline Hydrochloride.

Chlortetracycline Tablets

Action and use
Tetracycline antibacterial.

DEFINITION

Chlortetracycline Tablets contain Chlortetracycline Hydrochloride.

The tablets comply with the requirements stated under Tablets and with the following requirements.

Content of chlortetracycline hydrochloride, $C_{22}H_{23}ClN_2O_8$,HCl
95.0 to 110.0% of the stated amount.

IDENTIFICATION

A. Carry out the method for *thin-layer chromatography*, Appendix III A, using *silica gel H* as the coating substance and a mixture of 6 volumes of *water*, 35 volumes of *methanol* and 59 volumes of *dichloromethane* as the mobile phase. Adjust the pH of a 10% w/v solution of *disodium edetate* to 8.0 with 10M *sodium hydroxide* and spray the solution evenly onto the plate (about 10 ml for a plate 100 mm × 200 mm). Allow the plate to dry in a horizontal position for at least 1 hour. At the time of use, dry the plate in an oven at 110° for 1 hour. Apply separately to the plate 1 µl of each of the following solutions. For solution (1) extract a quantity of the powdered tablets containing 10 mg of Chlortetracycline Hydrochloride with 20 ml of *methanol* and centrifuge. Solution (2) contains 0.05% w/v of *chlortetracycline hydrochloride EPCRS* in *methanol*. Solution (3) contains 0.05% w/v each of *chlortetracycline hydrochloride EPCRS*, *tetracycline hydrochloride EPCRS* and *metacycline hydrochloride EPCRS* in *methanol*. Allow the plate to dry in a stream of air and examine under *ultraviolet light (365 nm)*. The principal spot in the chromatogram obtained with solution (1) corresponds to that in the chromatogram obtained with solution (2). The test is not valid unless the chromatogram obtained with solution (3) shows three clearly separated spots.

B. To a quantity of the powdered tablets containing 10 mg of Chlortetracycline Hydrochloride add 20 ml of warm *ethanol (96%)*, allow to stand for 20 minutes, filter and evaporate to dryness on a water bath. A 0.1% w/v solution of the residue in *phosphate buffer pH 7.6* when heated at 100° for 1 minute exhibits a strong blue fluorescence in ultraviolet light.

TESTS

Tetracycline hydrochloride and 4-epichlortetracycline hydrochloride

Not more than 8.0% and 6.0% respectively, determined as described under Assay. Inject separately solutions (1) and (4).

Dissolution

Comply with the requirements for Monographs of the British Pharmacopoeia in the *dissolution test for tablets and capsules*, Appendix XII B1, using Apparatus 2. Use as the medium 900 ml of 0.1M *hydrochloric acid* and rotate the paddle at 50 revolutions per minute. Withdraw a sample of 10 ml of the medium and filter. Measure the *absorbance* of the filtered sample, suitably diluted if necessary, at the maximum at 266 nm, Appendix II B. Calculate the total content of chlortetracycline hydrochloride, $C_{22}H_{23}ClN_2O_8,HCl$, in the medium taking 346 as the value of A(1%, 1 cm) at the maximum at 266 nm.

ASSAY

Weigh and powder 20 tablets. Carry out the method for *liquid chromatography*, Appendix III D, using the following solutions. For solution (1) mix a quantity of the powdered tablets containing 25 mg of Chlortetracycline Hydrochloride with 50 ml of 0.01M *hydrochloric acid*, shake for 10 minutes, dilute to 100 ml with 0.01M *hydrochloric acid* and filter (GF/C paper is suitable). Solution (2) contains 0.025% w/v of *chlortetracycline hydrochloride EPCRS* in 0.01M *hydrochloric acid*. Solution (3) contains 0.025% w/v each of *chlortetracycline hydrochloride EPCRS* and *4-epichlortetracycline hydrochloride EPCRS* in 0.01M *hydrochloric acid*. Solution (4) contains 0.002% w/v of *tetracycline hydrochloride EPCRS* and 0.0015% w/v of *4-epichlortetracycline hydrochloride EPCRS* in 0.01M *hydrochloric acid*.

The chromatographic procedure may be carried out using (a) a stainless steel column (25 cm × 4.6 mm) packed with *octadecylsilyl silica gel for chromatography* (10 μm) (Nucleosil C18 is suitable) and maintained at 40°, (b) as the mobile phase with a flow rate of 2 ml per minute a mixture of 20 volumes of *dimethylformamide* and 80 volumes of 0.1M *oxalic acid* the mixture being adjusted to pH 2.2 with *triethylamine* and (c) a detection wavelength of 355 nm.

The assay is not valid unless the *resolution factor* between the two principal peaks in the chromatogram obtained with solution (3) is at least 1.5.

Calculate the content of $C_{22}H_{23}ClN_2O_8,HCl$ in the tablets using the declared content of $C_{22}H_{23}ClN_2O_8,HCl$ in *chlortetracycline hydrochloride EPCRS*.

Cloprostenol Injection

Action and use

Prostaglandin (PGF$_{2\alpha}$) analogue.

DEFINITION

Cloprostenol Injection is a sterile solution of Cloprostenol Sodium in Water for Injections.

The injection complies with the requirements stated under Parenteral Preparations and with the following requirements.

Content of cloprostenol, $C_{22}H_{29}ClO_6$

90.0 to 110.0% of the stated amount.

IDENTIFICATION

In the Assay, the chromatogram obtained with solution (2) shows a peak with the same retention time as the peak due to cloprostenol in the chromatogram obtained with solution (1).

Related substances

Carry out the method for *liquid chromatography*, Appendix III D, using the following solutions. Solution (1) is the injection being examined diluted, if necessary, to contain the equivalent of 0.009% w/v of cloprostenol. Solution (2) contains 0.00018% w/v of *cloprostenol sodium BPCRS* in *absolute ethanol*. For solution (3) dissolve 5 mg of *hydrocortisone acetate EPCRS* and 2.5 mg of *cloprostenol sodium BPCRS* in *absolute ethanol* and dilute to 10 ml with the mobile phase.

The chromatographic procedure may be carried out using (a) a stainless steel column (25 cm × 5 mm) packed with *base-deactivated octadecylsilyl silica gel for chromatography* (Waters Symmetry ODS is suitable), (b) as the mobile phase with a flow rate of 1.8 ml per minute a mixture of 270 volumes of *acetonitrile* and 730 volumes of a solution containing 0.24% w/v of *sodium dihydrogen orthophosphate* the pH of which has been adjusted to 2.5 with *orthophosphoric acid* and (c) a detection wavelength of 220 nm.

Inject 20 μl of solution (3) and adjust the sensitivity of the detector so that the two principal peaks in the chromatogram obtained are at least 50% of full-scale deflection of the recorder. The test is not valid unless the *resolution factor* between the peak due to hydrocortisone acetate (retention time about 25 minutes) and that of cloprostenol (retention time about 35 minutes) is at least 6.

Inject 20 μl of solution (2) and adjust the sensitivity of the detector to obtain a principal peak with a height corresponding to at least 50% of full-scale deflection of the recorder.

Inject separately 20 μl of solutions (1) and (2) and continue the chromatography for 1.5 times the retention time of the principal peak.

In the chromatogram obtained with solution (1) the sum of the areas of any *secondary peaks* is not more than 1.25 times the area of the principal peak in the chromatogram obtained with solution (2) (2.5%).

ASSAY

Carry out the method for *liquid chromatography*, Appendix III D, using the following solutions. Solution (1) is the injection being examined, diluted, if necessary, to contain the equivalent of 0.009% w/v of cloprostenol. Solution (2) contains 0.009% w/v of *cloprostenol sodium BPCRS* in *absolute ethanol*.

The chromatographic procedure described under Related substances may be used.

Inject separately 20 μl of solutions (1) and (2). Calculate the content of $C_{22}H_{29}ClO_6$ in the injection from the chromatograms obtained and using the declared content of $C_{22}H_{29}ClO_6$ in *cloprostenol sodium BPCRS*.

LABELLING

The strength is stated as the equivalent amount of cloprostenol in a suitable dose-volume.

STORAGE

Cloprostenol Sodium Injection should be protected from light.

Cloxacillin Benzathine Intramammary Infusion (Dry Cow)

Cloxacillin Intramammary Infusion (DC)

Action and use
Penicillin antibacterial.

DEFINITION

Cloxacillin Benzathine Intramammary Infusion (Dry Cow) is a sterile suspension of Cloxacillin Benzathine in a suitable non-aqueous vehicle containing suitable suspending agents.

The intramammary infusion complies with the requirements stated under Intramammary Infusions and with the following requirements.

Content of cloxacillin, $C_{19}H_{18}ClN_3O_5S$
90.0 to 110.0% of the stated amount.

IDENTIFICATION

Extract a quantity of the infusion containing the equivalent of 75 mg of cloxacillin with three 15 ml quantities of *petroleum spirit (boiling range, 120° to 160°)*, discard the extracts, wash the residue with *ether* and dry in a current of air. The residue obtained complies with the following tests.

A. The *infrared absorption spectrum*, Appendix II A, is concordant with the *reference spectrum* of cloxacillin benzathine *(RSV 12)*.

B. Shake 50 mg with 1 ml of 1M *sodium hydroxide* for 2 minutes, add 2 ml of *ether*, shake for 1 minute and allow to separate. Evaporate 1 ml of the ether layer to dryness, dissolve the residue in 2 ml of *glacial acetic acid* and add 1 ml of *dilute potassium dichromate solution*. A golden yellow precipitate is produced.

Water

Not more than 2.0% w/w, Appendix IX C. Use 3 g and a mixture of 70 volumes of *chloroform* and 30 volumes of *anhydrous methanol* as solvent.

ASSAY

Express, as far as possible, weigh and mix the contents of 10 containers. Extract a quantity of the mixed contents containing the equivalent of 80 mg of cloxacillin, with three 15 ml quantities of *petroleum spirit (boiling range, 120° to 160°)* previously saturated with *cloxacillin benzathine*. Discard the extract, wash the residue with *ether* previously saturated with *cloxacillin benzathine*, dry in a current of air, dissolve in 25 ml of *methanol* and dilute to 50 ml with *water*. Dilute 2 ml to 100 ml with *buffered copper sulphate solution pH 2.0*, transfer 10 ml to a stoppered test tube and heat in a water bath at 70° for 20 minutes. Rapidly cool to room temperature, dilute to 20 ml with *absolute ethanol* and measure the *absorbance* of the resulting solution at the maximum at 338 nm, Appendix II B, using in the reference cell 10 ml of the unheated buffered solution of the substance being examined, diluted to 20 ml with *absolute ethanol*.

Calculate the content of $C_{19}H_{18}ClN_3O_5S$ in a container of average content from the *absorbance* obtained by carrying out the procedure simultaneously using 2 ml of a solution prepared by dissolving 105 mg of *cloxacillin benzathine BPCRS* in 50 ml of a mixture of equal volumes of *methanol* and *water* and from the declared content of $C_{19}H_{18}ClN_3O_5S$ in *cloxacillin benzathine BPCRS*.

LABELLING

The label states the quantity of Cloxacillin Benzathine in terms of the equivalent amount of cloxacillin.

Cloxacillin Sodium Intramammary Infusion (Lactating Cow)

Cloxacillin Intramammary Infusion (LC)

Action and use
Penicillin antibacterial.

DEFINITION

Cloxacillin Sodium Intramammary Infusion (Lactating Cow) is a sterile suspension of Cloxacillin Sodium in a suitable non-aqueous vehicle containing suitable suspending and dispersing agents.

The intramammary infusion complies with the requirements stated under Intramammary Infusions and with the following requirements.

Content of cloxacillin, $C_{19}H_{18}ClN_3O_5S$
90.0 to 110.0% of the stated amount.

IDENTIFICATION

Extract a quantity containing the equivalent of 75 mg of cloxacillin with three 15 ml quantities of *petroleum spirit (boiling range, 120° to 160°)*. Discard the extracts, wash the residue with *ether* and dry in a current of air. The residue obtained complies with the following tests.

A. The *infrared absorption spectrum*, Appendix II A, is concordant with the *reference spectrum* of cloxacillin sodium *(RSV 13)*.

B. Yields the reactions characteristic of *sodium*, Appendix VI.

Water

Not more than 1.0% w/w, Appendix IX C. Use 3 g and as solvent a mixture of 70 volumes of *chloroform* and 30 volumes of *anhydrous methanol*.

ASSAY

Express, as far as possible, weigh and mix the contents of 10 containers. Carry out the method for *liquid chromatography*, Appendix III D, using the following solutions. For solution (1) extract a quantity of the mixed contents of the 10 containers containing the equivalent of 50 mg of cloxacillin with 15 ml of *petroleum spirit (boiling range, 120° to 160°)*, centrifuge and discard the supernatant liquid. Repeat the extraction with a further two 15 ml quantities of *petroleum spirit (boiling range, 120° to 160°)*. Shake the residue with 20 ml of *ether*, centrifuge and dry in a current of air until the solvents have evaporated. Dissolve the final residue in sufficient of the mobile phase to produce 50 ml and dilute 5 volumes of the resulting solution to 50 volumes with the mobile phase. Solution (2) contains 0.011% w/v of *cloxacillin sodium EPCRS* in the mobile phase. Solution (3) contains 0.01% w/v of each of *cloxacillin sodium EPCRS* and *flucloxacillin sodium EPCRS* in the mobile phase.

The chromatographic procedure may be carried out using (a) a stainless steel column (25 cm × 4.6 mm) packed with *octadecylsilyl silica gel for chromatography* (5 μm) (Hypersil 5 ODS is suitable), (b) as the mobile phase with a flow rate of 1 ml per minute a mixture of 25 volumes of *acetonitrile* and 75 volumes of a 0.27% w/v solution of *potassium dihydrogen orthophosphate* adjusted to pH 5.0 with 2M *sodium hydroxide* and (c) a detection wavelength of 225 nm.

The test is not valid unless, in the chromatogram obtained with solution (3), the *resolution factor* between the first peak (cloxacillin) and the second peak (flucloxacillin) is at least 2.5.

Calculate the content of $C_{19}H_{18}ClN_3O_5S$ in a container of average content weight using the declared content of $C_{19}H_{17}ClN_3NaO_5S$ in *cloxacillin sodium EPCRS*. Each mg of $C_{19}H_{17}ClN_3NaO_5S$ is equivalent to 0.9520 mg of $C_{19}H_{18}ClN_3O_5S$.

LABELLING

The label states the quantity of Cloxacillin Sodium in terms of the equivalent amount of cloxacillin.

Cobalt Depot-tablets

DEFINITION

Cobalt Depot-tablets are prepared from a mixture of approximately 57% of Cobalt Oxide, 40% of powdered iron and 3% of sodium silicate.

The tablets comply with the requirements stated under Tablets and with the following requirements.

Content of cobalt, Co

90.0 to 110.0% of the stated amount.

IDENTIFICATION

A. Boil 0.1 g of a crushed depot-tablet with 5 ml of *hydrochloric acid* and 2.5 ml of *water* for 10 minutes. Add 1.5 ml of *nitric acid*, continue boiling gently for a further 5 minutes, add 5 ml of *water* and boil again. To 1 ml of the cooled solution add an excess of 13.5M *ammonia*, mix well and centrifuge; reserve the precipitate for use in test B. Acidify the filtrate with 2M *hydrochloric acid*, add 1 ml of *isoamyl alcohol* and about 0.1 g of *ammonium thiocyanate*, shake and allow to separate. The upper layer is deep blue.

B. Wash the precipitate reserved in test A in *water* and dissolve it in 2M *hydrochloric acid*. The resulting solution yields reactions B and C characteristic of *iron salts*, Appendix VI.

Dissolution

Remove any loose powder from the surface of a depot-tablet before immersing it completely in *citro-phosphate buffer pH 6.5*, using 25 ml for a tablet containing 4 g of cobalt and 50 ml for a tablet containing 12 g of cobalt, and allow to stand at 37° for 24 hours. Remove the tablet, wash with *water* and determine the content of Co in the combined solution and washings by the method described in the Assay, beginning at the words 'add 5 ml of *triethanolamine* ...'. Repeat the test on a further 4 tablets. The content of Co dissolved from each tablet is not less than 0.6% and not more than 1.2% of the stated content.

ASSAY

Weigh and powder 5 depot-tablets. Dissolve a quantity of the powder containing 0.1 g of cobalt in 20 ml of *hydrochloric acid*, by repeated evaporation if necessary. Dilute with 50 ml of *water*, add 5 ml of *triethanolamine*, mix thoroughly and dilute to 300 ml with *water*. Add 4 g of *hydroxylamine hydrochloride* and 25 ml of 13.5M *ammonia*, warm to 80° and titrate with 0.05M *disodium edetate VS*, using *methyl thymol blue mixture* as indicator, until the colour changes from blue to purple. Each ml of 0.05M *disodium edetate VS* is equivalent to 2.946 mg of Co.

LABELLING

The label states the quantity of cobalt contained in each depot-tablet.

Co-trimazine Injection

Trimethoprim and Sulfadiazine Injection

Action and use

Dihydrofolate reductase inhibitor + sulfonamide antibacterial.

DEFINITION

Co-trimazine Injection is a sterile suspension in Water for Injections containing Trimethoprim and Sulfadiazine in the proportion one part to five parts.

PRODUCTION

Co-trimazine Injection is prepared by the addition, with aseptic precautions, of sterile Trimethoprim to a solution of sulfadiazine sodium previously sterilised by *filtration*. The solution of sulfadiazine sodium is prepared by the interaction of Sulfadiazine and Sodium Hydroxide.

The injection complies with the requirements stated under Parenteral Preparations and with the following requirements.

Content of trimethoprim, $C_{14}H_{18}N_4O_3$

90.0 to 110.0% of the stated amount.

Content of sulfadiazine, $C_{10}H_{10}N_4O_2S$

90.0 to 110.0% of the stated amount.

CHARACTERISTICS

A suspension of an almost white solid in a pale straw-coloured solution.

IDENTIFICATION

A. The *light absorption*, Appendix II B, in the range 250 to 325 nm of the solution obtained in the Assay for trimethoprim exhibits a maximum only at 271 nm.

B. Carry out the method for *thin-layer chromatography*, Appendix III A, using *silica gel GF$_{254}$* as the coating substance and a mixture of 5 volumes of *water*, 15 volumes of *dimethylformamide* and 75 volumes of *ethyl acetate* as the mobile phase. Apply separately to the plate 1 μl of each of the following solutions. For solution (1) ensure that the injection is homogeneous by gently inverting the container several times. To 2.5 ml of the well mixed injection add 4 ml of *hydrochloric acid* and dilute to 50 ml with 1.4M *methanolic ammonia*. Solution (2) contains 2.0% w/v of *sulfadiazine BPCRS* in 1.4M *methanolic ammonia*. Solution (3) contains 0.4% w/v of *trimethoprim BPCRS* in 1.4M *methanolic ammonia*. After removal of the plate, allow it to dry in air and examine under *ultraviolet light (254 nm)*. One of the principal spots in the chromatogram obtained with solution (1) corresponds to the principal spot in the chromatogram obtained with solution (2) and the other corresponds to the principal spot in the chromatogram obtained with solution (3).

C. To 5 ml of the filtrate obtained in the Assay for sulfadiazine add 10 ml of *water* and 5 ml of *thiobarbituric acid-citrate buffer*, mix and heat on a water bath for 30 minutes. A pink colour is produced.

Alkalinity

pH, 10.0 to 10.5, Appendix V L.

ASSAY

For trimethoprim

Extract the chloroform solution reserved in the Assay for sulfadiazine with three quantities, of 100, 50 and 50 ml, of 1M *acetic acid* and dilute the combined extracts to 500 ml with 1M *acetic acid*. To 5 ml add 35 ml of 1M *acetic acid* and sufficient *water* to produce 200 ml and measure the *absorbance* of the resulting solution at the maximum at 271 nm, Appendix II B. Calculate the content of

$C_{14}H_{18}N_4O_3$ taking 204 as the value of A(1%, 1 cm) at the maximum at 271 nm.

For sulfadiazine

Disperse the trimethoprim evenly throughout the injection by gently inverting the container several times, avoiding the formation of foam. Transfer a quantity of the injection containing the equivalent of 2 g of Sulfadiazine to a separating funnel containing 50 ml of 0.1M *sodium hydroxide* and extract with two quantities, of 100 ml and 50 ml, of *chloroform*, washing the extract with the same 25 ml quantity of 0.1M *sodium hydroxide*. Reserve the combined chloroform extracts for the Assay for trimethoprim.

Dilute the combined aqueous solutions and washings to 250 ml with *water*, filter and dilute 5 ml of the filtrate to 200 ml with *water*. Dilute 10 ml of this solution to 100 ml with *water*. To 3 ml of the resulting solution add 1 ml of 2M *hydrochloric acid* and 1 ml of a 0.1% w/v solution of *sodium nitrite* and allow to stand for 2 minutes. Add 1 ml of a 0.5% w/v solution of *ammonium sulphamate* and allow to stand for 3 minutes. Add 1 ml of a 0.1% w/v solution of *N-(1-naphthyl)ethylenediamine dihydrochloride*, allow to stand for 10 minutes, add sufficient *water* to produce 25 ml and measure the *absorbance* of the resulting solution at 538 nm, Appendix II B. Repeat the operation using 3 ml of a solution prepared by dissolving 0.2 g of *sulfadiazine BPCRS* in 50 ml of 0.1M *sodium hydroxide*, adding sufficient *water* to produce 200 ml, diluting 5.0 ml of the resulting solution to 250 ml with *water* and beginning at the words 'add 1 ml of 2M *hydrochloric acid* ...'. Calculate the content of $C_{10}H_{10}N_4O_2S$ in the injection from the absorbances obtained using the declared content of $C_{10}H_{10}N_4O_2S$ in *sulfadiazine BPCRS*.

LABELLING

The strength is stated as the amount of Trimethoprim and the equivalent amount of Sulfadiazine in a suitable dose-volume.

When trimethoprim and sulphadiazine injection is prescribed or demanded, Co-trimazine Injection shall be dispensed or supplied.

Co-trimazine Veterinary Oral Powder

Trimethoprim and Sulfadiazine Veterinary Oral Powder

Action and use

Dihydrofolate reductase inhibitor + sulfonamide antibacterial.

DEFINITION

Co-trimazine Veterinary Oral Powder consists of Trimethoprim and Sulfadiazine in the proportion of one part to five parts mixed with suitable wetting, dispersing and suspending agents.

The veterinary oral powder complies with the requirements stated under Veterinary Oral Powders and with the following requirements.

Content of trimethoprim, $C_{14}H_{18}N_4O_3$
92.5 to 107.5% of the stated amount.

Content of sulfadiazine, $C_{10}H_{10}N_4O_2S$
92.5 to 107.5% of the stated amount.

IDENTIFICATION

Carry out the method described under Co-trimazine Oral Suspension using solutions prepared in the following manner as solutions (1) and (2). For solution (1) shake a quantity of

the powder containing 0.2 g of Sulfadiazine with sufficient 1.4M *methanolic ammonia* to produce 100 ml, centrifuge and use the supernatant liquid. For solution (2) shake a quantity of the powder containing 0.2 g of Trimethoprim with sufficient 1.4M *methanolic ammonia* to produce 100 ml, centrifuge and use the supernatant liquid.

ASSAY

For trimethoprim

Extract the combined chloroform extracts from the Assay for sulfadiazine with four 50 ml quantities of a 5% v/v solution of 6M *acetic acid*. Wash the combined aqueous extracts with 5 ml of *chloroform*, discard the chloroform layer and dilute to 250 ml with a 5% v/v solution of 6M *acetic acid*. Dilute 20 ml to 100 ml with *water*. Determine the *absorbance* of the resulting solution at the maximum at 271 nm, Appendix II B, and calculate the content of $C_{14}H_{18}N_4O_3$ taking 204 as the value of A(1%, 1 cm) at the maximum at 271 nm.

For sulfadiazine

Transfer a quantity of the powder containing 0.125 g of Sulfadiazine to a separating funnel containing 20 ml of 0.1M *sodium hydroxide* and extract with four 50 ml quantities of *chloroform*. Wash each chloroform extract with the same two 10 ml quantities of 0.1M *sodium hydroxide*. Combine the aqueous washings and the aqueous layer from the separating funnel and reserve the combined chloroform extracts for the Assay for trimethoprim. Dilute the combined aqueous solutions to 250 ml with *water*, filter and dilute 10 ml of the filtrate to 200 ml with *water*. To 2 ml of the resulting solution add 0.5 ml of 4M *hydrochloric acid* and 1 ml of a 0.1% w/v solution of *sodium nitrite* and allow to stand for 2 minutes. Add 1 ml of a 0.5% w/v solution of *ammonium sulphamate* and allow to stand for 3 minutes. Add 1 ml of a 0.1% w/v solution of *N-(1-naphthyl)-ethylenediamine dihydrochloride*, allow to stand for 10 minutes and dilute to 25 ml with *water*. Measure the *absorbance* of the resulting solution at the maximum at 538 nm, Appendix II B, using in the reference cell a solution prepared at the same time and in the same manner using 2 ml of *water* and beginning at the words 'add 0.5 ml of 4M *hydrochloric acid*...'. Calculate the content of $C_{10}H_{10}N_4O_2S$ from the *absorbance* obtained by repeating the operation with 2 ml of a 0.0025% w/v solution of *sulfadiazine BPCRS* in 0.0005M *sodium hydroxide* and beginning at the words 'add 0.5 ml of 4M *hydrochloric acid* ...'.

When trimethoprim and sulphadiazine veterinary oral powder is prescribed or demanded, Co-trimazine Veterinary Oral Powder shall be dispensed or supplied.

Co-trimazine Oral Suspension

Trimethoprim and Sulfadiazine Oral Suspension

Action and use

Dihydrofolate reductase inhibitor + sulfonamide antibacterial.

DEFINITION

Co-trimazine Oral Suspension is a suspension of Trimethoprim and Sulfadiazine in the proportion of one part to five parts containing suitable suspending and dispersing agents. It may contain suitable antimicrobial preservatives.

The oral suspension complies with the requirements stated under Oral Liquids and with the following requirements.

Content of trimethoprim, $C_{14}H_{18}N_4O_3$

90.0 to 110.0% of the stated amount.

Content of sulfadiazine, $C_{10}H_{10}N_4O_2S$

90.0 to 110.0% of the stated amount.

IDENTIFICATION

Carry out the method for *thin-layer chromatography*, Appendix III A, using *silica gel GF_{254}* as the coating substance and a mixture of 75 volumes of *ethyl acetate*, 15 volumes of *dimethylformamide* and 5 volumes of *water* as the mobile phase. Apply separately to the plate 5 μl of each of the following solutions. Solution (1) is a dilution of the oral suspension in 1.4M *methanolic ammonia* containing 0.2% w/v of Sulfadiazine. Solution (2) is a dilution of the oral suspension in 1.4M *methanolic ammonia* containing 0.2% w/v of Trimethoprim. Solution (3) is a 0.2% w/v solution of *sulfadiazine BPCRS* in 1.4M *methanolic ammonia*. Solution (4) is a 0.2% w/v solution of *trimethoprim BPCRS* in 1.4M *methanolic ammonia*. After removal of the plate, allow it to dry in a current of air, spray with a 0.1% w/v solution of *4-dimethylaminobenzaldehyde* in a mixture of 1 ml of *hydrochloric acid* and 100 ml of *ethanol (96%)*, allow to dry and spray with *dilute potassium iodobismuthate solution*. The spot in the chromatogram obtained with solution (1) with an Rf value of about 0.7 corresponds to the principal spot in the chromatogram obtained with solution (3) and the spot in the chromatogram obtained with solution (2) with an Rf value of about 0.3 corresponds to the principal spot in the chromatogram obtained with solution (4).

ASSAY

For trimethoprim

Carry out the Assay for trimethoprim described under Co-trimazine Veterinary Oral Powder. Calculate the content of $C_{14}H_{18}N_4O_3$ taking 204 as the value of A(1%, 1cm) at the maximum at 271 nm.

For sulfadiazine

Carry out the Assay for sulfadiazine described under Co-trimazine Veterinary Oral Powder using a volume of the oral suspension containing 0.125 g of Sulfadiazine. Repeat the operation using 2 ml of a 0.0025% w/v solution of *sulfadiazine BPCRS* in 0.0005M *sodium hydroxide* beginning at the words 'add 0.5 ml of 4M *hydrochloric acid* ...'. Calculate the content of $C_{10}H_{10}N_4O_2S$ in the oral suspension from the absorbances obtained using the declared content of $C_{10}H_{10}N_4O_2S$ in *sulfadiazine BPCRS*.

LABELLING

The strength is stated as the amount of Trimethoprim and Sulfadiazine.

When trimethoprim and sulphadiazine oral suspension is prescribed or demanded, Co-trimazine Oral Suspension shall be dispensed or supplied.

Co-trimazine Tablets

Trimethoprim and Sulfadiazine Tablets

Action and use

Dihydrofolate reductase inhibitor + sulfonamide antibacterial.

DEFINITION

Co-trimazine Tablets contain Trimethoprim and Sulfadiazine in the proportion one part to five parts.

With the exception of the requirements for shape, the tablets comply with the requirements stated under Tablets and with the following requirements.

Content of trimethoprim, $C_{14}H_{18}N_4O_3$

92.5 to 107.5% of the stated amount.

Content of sulfadiazine, $C_{10}H_{10}N_4O_2S$

92.5 to 107.5% of the stated amount.

IDENTIFICATION

Comply with the test described under Co-trimazine Oral Suspension using solutions prepared in the following manner as solutions (1) and (2). For solution (1) shake a quantity of the finely powdered tablets containing 0.2 g of Sulfadiazine with sufficient 1.4M *methanolic ammonia* to produce 100 ml, centrifuge and use the supernatant liquid. For solution (2) shake a quantity of the finely powdered tablets containing 0.2 g of Trimethoprim with sufficient 1.4M *methanolic ammonia* to produce 100 ml, centrifuge and use the supernatant liquid.

ASSAY

Weigh and finely powder 20 tablets.

For trimethoprim

Carry out the Assay for trimethoprim described under Co-trimazine Veterinary Oral Powder.

For sulfadiazine

Carry out the Assay for sulfadiazine described under Co-trimazine Veterinary Oral Powder using a quantity of the powdered tablets containing 0.125 g of Sulfadiazine. Repeat the operation using 2 ml of a 0.0025% w/v solution of *sulfadiazine BPCRS* in 0.0005M *sodium hydroxide* beginning at the words 'add 0.5 ml of 4M *hydrochloric acid* ...'. Calculate the content of $C_{10}H_{10}N_4O_2S$ in the oral suspension from the absorbances obtained using the declared content of $C_{10}H_{10}N_4O_2S$ in *sulfadiazine BPCRS*.

LABELLING

The label states the quantity of Trimethoprim and of Sulfadiazine in each tablet.

When trimethoprim and sulphadiazine tablets are prescribed or demanded, Co-trimazine Tablets shall be dispensed or supplied.

Decoquinate Premix

Action and use

Antiprotozoal (veterinary).

DEFINITION

Decoquinate Premix contains Decoquinate.

The premix complies with the requirements stated under Premixes and with the following requirements.

Content of decoquinate, $C_{24}H_{35}NO_5$

95.0 to 105.0% of the stated amount.

IDENTIFICATION

Carry out the method for *thin-layer chromatography*, Appendix III A, using *silica gel GF_{254}* as the coating substance and a mixture of 30 volumes of *ethanol (96%)* and 70 volumes of *chloroform* as the mobile phase. Apply separately to the plate 10 μl of each of the following solutions. For solution (1) heat a quantity containing 0.1 g of Decoquinate with 40 ml of *chloroform* for 20 minutes on a water bath under a reflux condenser, cool and filter. Solution (2) contains 0.25% w/v of *decoquinate BPCRS* in *chloroform*. After removal of the plate, allow it to dry in a current of air and examine under *ultraviolet light (254 nm)*. The principal spot in the chromatogram obtained with solution (1) corresponds to that in the chromatogram obtained with solution (2).

ASSAY

Heat a quantity containing 0.2 g of Decoquinate with 50 ml of *chloroform* in an apparatus for the *continuous extraction of drugs*, Appendix XI F, for eight reflux cycles. Cool and add sufficient *chloroform* to produce 100 ml. Dilute 5 ml to 100 ml with *absolute ethanol*. To 5 ml add 10 ml of 0.1M *hydrochloric acid* and dilute to 100 ml with *absolute ethanol*. Measure the *absorbance* of the resulting solution at the maximum at 265 nm, Appendix II B. Dissolve 50 mg of *decoquinate BPCRS* in 10 ml of hot *chloroform* and, keeping the solution warm, add slowly 70 ml of *absolute ethanol*. Cool, dilute to 100 ml with *absolute ethanol* and immediately dilute 10 ml to 100 ml with *absolute ethanol*. To 10 ml of the resulting solution add 10 ml of 0.1M *hydrochloric acid* and dilute to 100 ml with *absolute ethanol*. Calculate the content of $C_{24}H_{35}NO_5$ in the premix from the absorbances obtained using the declared content of $C_{24}H_{35}NO_5$ in *decoquinate BPCRS*.

Deltamethrin Pour-on

Action and use
Insecticide (veterinary)

DEFINITION
Deltamethrin Pour-on is a *pour-on solution*. It contains Deltamethrin in a suitable, oily vehicle.

The pour-on complies with the requirements stated under Veterinary Liquid Preparations for Cutaneous Application and with the following requirements.

Content of deltamethrin, $C_{22}H_{19}Br_2NO_3$
90.0 to 110.0% of the stated amount.

IDENTIFICATION
In the Assay, the chromatogram obtained with solution (1) shows a peak with the same retention time as the peak in the chromatogram obtained with solution (2).

ASSAY
Carry out the method for *liquid chromatography*, Appendix III D, using the following solutions.
For solution (1) mix a weighed quantity of the preparation being examined containing 30 mg of Deltamethrin with sufficient *hexane* to produce 100 ml. Dilute 1 volume to 4 volumes with *hexane*. Solution (2) contains 0.0075% w/v of *deltamethrin BPCRS* in *hexane*. Solution (3) contains 0.0075% w/v of *deltamethrin impurity standard BPCRS* in *hexane*.

The chromatographic procedure may be carried out using (a) a stainless steel column (25 cm × 4.6 mm) packed with particles of silica the surface of which has been modified with chemically-bonded nitro-phenyl groups (5 μm) (Nucleosil-NO$_2$ is suitable), (b) *hexane* containing 0.25% v/v of *propan-2-ol* as the mobile phase with a flow rate of 2 ml per minute and (c) a detection wavelength of 230 nm.

The assay is not valid unless, in the chromatogram obtained with solution (3), a peak due to (*R*)-deltamethrin appears immediately before the principal peak, as indicated in the reference chromatogram supplied with *deltamethrin impurity standard BPCRS*.

Determine the *weight per ml* of the preparation, Appendix V G, and calculate the content of $C_{22}H_{19}Br_2NO_3$, weight in volume, using the declared content of $C_{22}H_{19}Br_2NO_3$ in *deltamethrin BPCRS*.

Dimetridazole Veterinary Oral Powder

Action and use
Antiprotozoal (veterinary).

DEFINITION
Dimetridazole Veterinary Oral Powder is a mixture of Dimetridazole and a suitable water-soluble diluent.

The veterinary oral powder complies with the requirements stated under Veterinary Oral Powders and with the following requirements.

Content of dimetridazole, $C_5H_7N_3O_2$
95.0 to 105.0% of the stated amount.

IDENTIFICATION
Mix a quantity containing 0.1 g of Dimetridazole with 20 ml of *ether*, shake, filter, add to the filtrate 10 ml of a 1% w/v solution of *picric acid* in *ether*, stir to induce crystallisation and allow to stand. The precipitate, after washing with *ether* and drying at 105°, has a *melting point* of about 160°, Appendix V A.

ASSAY
Transfer a quantity containing 0.4 g of Dimetridazole to a sintered glass funnel (ISO 4793, porosity grade 4, is suitable), add 10 ml of *chloroform*, stir for 1 minute and then apply gentle suction. Repeat the extraction with four further 10 ml quantities of *chloroform*. To the combined chloroform extracts add 50 ml of *anhydrous acetic acid* previously neutralised to *crystal violet solution* by the drop wise addition of 0.1M *perchloric acid VS* and carry out Method I for *non-aqueous titration*, Appendix VIII A, using *crystal violet solution* as indicator. Each ml of 0.1M *perchloric acid VS* is equivalent to 14.11 mg of $C_5H_7N_3O_2$.

Dimetridazole Premix

Action and use
Antiprotozoal (veterinary).

DEFINITION
Dimetridazole Premix contains Dimetridazole.

The premix complies with the requirements stated under Premixes and with the following requirements.

Content of dimetridazole, $C_5H_7N_3O_2$
95.0 to 105.0% of the stated amount.

IDENTIFICATION
Mix a quantity containing 0.1 g of Dimetridazole with 20 ml of *ether*, shake, filter, add to the filtrate 10 ml of a 1% w/v solution of *picric acid* in *ether*, stir to induce crystallisation and allow to stand. The precipitate, after washing with *ether* and drying at 105°, has a *melting point* of about 160°, Appendix V A.

ASSAY
Transfer a quantity containing 0.45 g of Dimetridazole to a sintered glass funnel (ISO 4793, porosity grade 4, is suitable), add 10 ml of *chloroform*, stir for 1 minute and then

apply gentle suction. Repeat the extraction with four further 10 ml quantities of *chloroform*. To the combined chloroform extracts add 50 ml of *anhydrous acetic acid* previously neutralised to *crystal violet solution* by the drop wise addition of 0.1M *perchloric acid VS* and carry out Method I for *non-aqueous titration*, Appendix VIII A, using *crystal violet solution* as indicator. Each ml of 0.1M *perchloric acid VS* is equivalent to 14.11 mg of $C_5H_7N_3O_2$.

STORAGE

Dimetridazole Premix should be protected from light.

Diprenorphine Injection

Action and use

Opioid receptor antagonist.

DEFINITION

Diprenorphine Injection is a sterile solution of Diprenorphine Hydrochloride in Water for Injections containing Methylthioninium Chloride (methylene blue). The pH is adjusted to about 4.

The injection complies with the requirements stated under Parenteral Preparations and with the following requirements.

Content of diprenorphine, $C_{26}H_{35}NO_4$

90.0 to 110.0% of the stated amount.

IDENTIFICATION

Carry out the method for *thin-layer chromatography*, Appendix III A, in subdued light using *silica gel GF_{254}* as the coating substance and a mixture of 10 volumes of *diethylamine*, 20 volumes of *ethyl acetate* and 70 volumes of *toluene* as the mobile phase. Apply separately to each half of the plate 10 µl of each of the following solutions. For solution (1) add 3 ml of 5M *ammonia* to a volume containing the equivalent of 0.5 mg of diprenorphine, mix and extract with two 5 ml quantities of *chloroform*. Combine the chloroform extracts, shake with 1 g of *anhydrous sodium sulphate*, filter, evaporate to dryness using a rotary evaporator and dissolve the residue in 0.4 ml of *chloroform*. Solution (2) contains 0.115% w/v of *diprenorphine BPCRS* in *chloroform*. Add to each point of application of solution (2) 10 µl of a mixture of 4 volumes of *methanol* and 1 volume of 13.5M *ammonia*. After removal of the plate, allow it to dry in air and examine under *ultraviolet light (254 nm)*. Spray one half of the plate with a mixture of 5 volumes of *chloroplatinic acid solution*, 35 volumes of *dilute potassium iodide solution* and 60 volumes of *acetone*. Spray the other half of the plate with a mixture of 1 volume of *iron(III) chloride solution R1* and 1 volume of *dilute potassium hexacyanoferrate(III) solution*. The spot in the chromatogram obtained with solution (1) corresponds in position, quenching and colour to that in the chromatogram obtained with solution (2).

TESTS

Acidity

pH, 3.5 to 4.5, Appendix V L.

ASSAY

For an injection containing the equivalent of more than 0.1% w/v of diprenorphine Dissolve 50 mg of *phenolphthalein* (internal standard) in sufficient *methanol* to produce 20 ml (solution A). Carry out the method for *gas chromatography*, Appendix III B, using the following solutions. For solution (1) add 2 ml of solution A to 2 ml of a 0.30% w/v solution of *diprenorphine BPCRS* in *methanol* and

evaporate the solvent using a rotary evaporator. To the dried residue add 1 ml of a mixture of 8 volumes of *dimethylformamide*, 2 volumes of N,O-*bis(trimethylsilyl) acetamide* and 1 volume of *trimethylchlorosilane* and allow to stand for 30 minutes. Prepare solution (2) in a similar manner to solution (3) but omitting the addition of solution A. For solution (3) add 2 ml of 5M *ammonia* to a volume containing the equivalent of 6 mg of diprenorphine and extract with three 7 ml quantities of *chloroform*. To the combined extracts add 2 ml of solution A, shake with 2 g of *anhydrous sodium sulphate*, filter and evaporate the filtrate to dryness using a rotary evaporator; treat the dried residue as described for solution (1).

The chromatographic procedure may be carried out using a glass column (1.5 m × 4 mm) packed with *acid-washed, silanised, diatomaceous support* (80 to 100 mesh) coated with 2% w/w of *methyl silicone gum* (SE 30 is suitable) and maintained at 245°.

Calculate the content of $C_{26}H_{35}NO_4$ using the declared content of $C_{26}H_{35}NO_4$ in *diprenorphine BPCRS*.

For an injection containing the equivalent of 0.1% w/v or less of diprenorphine Carry out the Assay described above, but dissolving 50 mg of *phenolphthalein* (internal standard) in sufficient *methanol* to produce 100 ml (solution A) and using the following solutions. For solution (1) add 2 ml of solution A to 5 ml of a 0.027% w/v solution of *diprenorphine BPCRS* in *methanol* and evaporate the solvent using a rotary evaporator; to the dried residue add 1 ml of a mixture of 8 volumes of *dimethylformamide*, 2 volumes of N,O-*bis(trimethylsilyl)acetamide* and 1 volume of *trimethylchlorosilane* and allow to stand for 30 minutes. Prepare solution (2) in a similar manner to solution (3) but omitting the addition of solution A. For solution (3) add 2 ml of 5M *ammonia* to a volume containing the equivalent of 1.36 mg of diprenorphine and extract with three 10 ml quantities of *chloroform*; to the combined extracts add 2 ml of solution A, shake with 3 g of *anhydrous sodium sulphate*, filter and evaporate the filtrate to dryness; treat the dried residue as described for solution (1).

LABELLING

The strength is stated as the equivalent amount of diprenorphine in a suitable dose-volume.

STORAGE

Diprenorphine Injection should be protected from light.

Etamiphylline Injection

Action and use

Non-selective phosphodiesterase inhibitor (xanthine); treatment of reversible airways obstruction.

DEFINITION

Etamiphylline Injection is a sterile solution of Etamiphylline Camsilate in Water for Injections.

The injection complies with the requirements stated under Parenteral Preparations and with the following requirements.

Content of etamiphylline camsilate, $C_{13}H_{21}N_5O_2,C_{10}H_{16}O_4S$

95.0 to 105.0% of the stated amount.

IDENTIFICATION

Prepare a quantity of the residue as described in the Assay. The residue complies with the following tests.

A. The *infrared absorption spectrum*, Appendix II A, is concordant with the *reference spectrum* of etamiphylline (*RSV 19*).

B. Yields the reactions characteristic of *xanthines*, Appendix VI.

TESTS

Acidity
pH, 3.9 to 5.4, Appendix V L.

Related substances
Carry out the method for *thin-layer chromatography*, Appendix III A, using *silica gel HF$_{254}$* as the coating substance and a mixture of 80 volumes of *chloroform*, 20 volumes of *ethanol (96%)* and 1 volume of 13.5M *ammonia* as the mobile phase. Apply separately to the plate 10 µl of each of the following solutions. For solution (1) dilute the injection with sufficient *water* to produce a solution containing 3.5% w/v of Etamiphylline Camsilate. For solution (2) dilute 1 volume of solution (1) to 500 volumes with *water*. After removal of the plate, allow it to dry in air and examine under *ultraviolet light (254 nm)*. Any *secondary spot* in the chromatogram obtained with solution (1) is not more intense than the spot in the chromatogram obtained with solution (2).

ASSAY

To a volume containing 0.7 g of Etamiphylline Camsilate add 15 ml of *water*, make alkaline with 5M *ammonia* and extract with three 25-ml quantities of *chloroform*, washing each extract with the same 5-ml quantity of *water*. Evaporate the combined extracts to dryness, dissolve the residue in 25 ml of *water* and titrate with 0.05M *sulphuric acid VS* using *bromocresol green solution* as indicator. Each ml of 0.05M *sulphuric acid VS* is equivalent to 51.16 mg of $C_{13}H_{21}N_5O_2,C_{10}H_{16}O_4S$.

Etamiphylline Veterinary Oral Powder

Action and use
Non-selective phosphodiesterase inhibitor (xanthine); treatment of reversible airways obstruction.

DEFINITION

Etamiphylline Veterinary Oral Powder is a mixture of Etamiphylline Camsilate and Glucose or other suitable diluent.

The veterinary oral powder complies with the requirements stated under Veterinary Oral Powders and with the following requirements.

Content of etamiphylline camsilate, $C_{13}H_{21}N_5O_2,C_{10}H_{16}O_4S$
95.0 to 105.0% of the stated amount.

IDENTIFICATION

Complies with the tests described under Etamiphylline Tablets using a quantity of the residue prepared as described in the Assay.

Related substances
Complies with the test described under Etamiphylline Tablets but using the following solutions. For solution (1) shake a quantity of the powder containing 0.2 g of Etamiphylline Camsilate with 20 ml of *chloroform*, filter, evaporate the filtrate to dryness and dissolve the residue in sufficient *water* to produce a solution containing 4% w/v of

Etamiphylline Camsilate. For solution (2) dilute 1 volume of solution (1) to 500 volumes with *water*.

ASSAY

Dissolve a quantity of the powder containing 0.5 g of Etamiphylline Camsilate in 25 ml of *water*, make alkaline with 5M *ammonia* and extract with three 25 ml quantities of *chloroform*, washing each extract with the same 5 ml quantity of *water*. Evaporate the combined chloroform extracts to dryness, dissolve the residue in 25 ml of *water* and titrate with 0.05M *sulphuric acid VS* using *bromocresol green solution* as indicator. Each ml of 0.05M *sulphuric acid VS* is equivalent to 51.16 mg of $C_{13}H_{21}N_5O_2,C_{10}H_{16}O_4S$.

Etamiphylline Tablets

Action and use
Non-selective phosphodiesterase inhibitor (xanthine); treatment of reversible airways obstruction.

DEFINITION

Etamiphylline Tablets contain Etamiphylline Camsilate. They are coated.

The tablets comply with the requirements stated under Tablets and with the following requirements.

Content of etamiphylline camsilate, $C_{13}H_{21}N_5O_2,C_{10}H_{16}O_4S$
95.0 to 105.0% of the stated amount.

IDENTIFICATION

Prepare a quantity of the residue as described in the Assay. The residue complies with the following tests.

A. The *infrared absorption spectrum*, Appendix II A, is concordant with the *reference spectrum* of etamiphylline (*RSV 19*).

B. Yields the reactions characteristic of *xanthines*, Appendix VI.

Related substances
Carry out the method for *thin-layer chromatography*, Appendix III A, using *silica gel HF$_{254}$* as the coating substance and a mixture of 1 volume of 13.5M *ammonia*, 20 volumes of *ethanol (96%)* and 80 volumes of *chloroform* as the mobile phase. Apply separately to the plate 10 µl of each of the following solutions. For solution (1) shake a quantity of the powdered tablets containing 0.2 g of Etamiphylline Camsilate with 5 ml of *methanol* and centrifuge. For solution (2) dilute 1 volume of solution (1) to 500 volumes with *methanol*. After removal of the plate, allow it to dry in air and examine under *ultraviolet light (254 nm)*. Any *secondary spot* in the chromatogram obtained with solution (1) is not more intense than the spot in the chromatogram obtained with solution (2) (0.2%).

ASSAY

Weigh and powder 20 tablets. Dissolve a quantity of the powder containing 0.5 g of Etamiphylline Camsilate in 30 ml of *water*, make alkaline with 5M *ammonia* and extract with three 25 ml quantities of *chloroform*, washing each chloroform extract with the same 5 ml quantity of *water*. Evaporate the combined chloroform extracts to dryness, dissolve the residue in 25 ml of *water* and titrate with 0.05M *sulphuric acid VS* using *bromocresol green solution* as indicator. Each ml of 0.05M *sulphuric acid VS* is equivalent to 51.16 mg of $C_{13}H_{21}N_5O_2,C_{10}H_{16}O_4S$.

Etorphine and Acepromazine Injection

Action and use
Opioid receptor agonist; analgesic.

DEFINITION
Etorphine and Acepromazine Injection is a sterile solution of Etorphine Hydrochloride and Acepromazine Maleate in Water for Injections containing a suitable antimicrobial preservative. The pH is adjusted to about 4.

The injection complies with the requirements stated under Parenteral Preparations and with the following requirements.

Content of etorphine hydrochloride, $C_{25}H_{33}NO_4,HCl$
0.22 to 0.27% w/v.

Content of acepromazine maleate, $C_{19}H_{22}N_2OS,C_4H_4O_4$
0.90 to 1.10% w/v.

CHARACTERISTICS
A clear, yellow solution.

IDENTIFICATION
A. The *light absorption*, Appendix II B, in the range 230 to 350 nm of a solution prepared by diluting a volume of the injection containing 10 mg of Acepromazine Maleate to 500 ml with *water* exhibits well-defined maxima at 242 nm and at 280 nm. The *absorbances* at the maxima are about 1.1 and about 0.85, respectively.

B. Carry out the method for *thin-layer chromatography*, Appendix III A, in subdued light using *silica gel GF_{254}* as the coating substance and *ethyl acetate* as the mobile phase and applying separately to each half of the plate 10 µl of each of two solutions containing (1) the injection being examined and (2) 0.09% w/v of *diprenorphine BPCRS* in *chloroform*. Add to each point of application 10 µl of a mixture of 4 volumes of *methanol* and 1 volume of 13.5M *ammonia*. After removal of the plate, allow it to dry in air and examine under *ultraviolet light (254 nm)*. Spray one half of the plate with a mixture of 5 volumes of *chloroplatinic acid solution*, 35 volumes of *dilute potassium iodide solution* and 60 volumes of *acetone*. Spray the other half of the plate with a mixture of 1 volume of *iron(III) chloride solution R1* and 1 volume of *dilute potassium hexacyanoferrate(III) solution*. The principal spot in the chromatogram obtained with solution (1) has an Rf value of about 1.15 relative to that of the spot in the chromatogram obtained with solution (2), absorbs ultraviolet light and yields a reddish violet colour with the iodoplatinate spray reagent and a blue colour with the iron-hexacyanoferrate spray reagent.

TESTS
Acidity
pH, 3.5 to 4.5, Appendix V L.

ASSAY
For etorphine hydrochloride
Dissolve 46 mg of *diprenorphine BPCRS* (internal standard) in sufficient *methanol* to produce 10 ml (solution A). Carry out the method for *gas chromatography*, Appendix III B, using the following solutions. For solution (1) add 1 ml of solution A to 2 ml of the injection and 2 ml of 5M *ammonia*, extract with three 7 ml quantities of *chloroform*, shake the combined extracts with 2 g of *anhydrous sodium sulphate*, filter and evaporate the filtrate to a small volume using a rotary evaporator. Transfer the contents to a stoppered test tube with the aid of 2 ml of *chloroform* and evaporate to dryness. To the residue add 1 ml of a mixture of 8 volumes of *dimethylformamide*, 2 volumes of N,O-*bis(trimethylsilyl)-*

acetamide and 1 volume of *trimethylchlorosilane* and allow to stand for 15 minutes. For solution (2) treat a volume of the injection containing 4.9 mg of Etorphine Hydrochloride in a similar manner but omitting the addition of solution A. Protect the solutions from light during preparation and subsequent use.

The chromatographic procedure may be carried out using a glass column (1.5 m × 4 mm) packed with *acid-washed, silanised diatomaceous support* (80 to 100 mesh) coated with 2% w/w of methyl silicone gum (SE 30 is suitable) and maintained at 245°.

Calculate the content of $C_{25}H_{33}NO_4$ using the declared content of $C_{26}H_{35}NO_4$ in *diprenorphine BPCRS* assuming that the trimethylsilyl derivatives of equal weights of etorphine and diprenorphine have the same response in the flame ionisation detector and hence calculate the content of $C_{25}H_{33}NO_4,HCl$ taking each mg of $C_{25}H_{33}NO_4$ to be equivalent to 1.089 mg of $C_{25}H_{33}NO_4,HCl$.

For acepromazine maleate
Protect the solutions from light throughout the Assay. To 1 ml add sufficient *ethanol (96%)* to produce 100 ml. Measure the *absorbance*, Appendix II B, of the resulting solution at the maximum at 370 nm. Calculate the content of $C_{19}H_{22}N_2OS,C_4H_4O_4$ taking 46.1 as the value of A(1%, 1 cm) at the maximum at 370 nm.

STORAGE
Etorphine and Acepromazine Injection should be protected from light.

Etorphine and Levomepromazine Injection

Action and use
Opioid receptor agonist; analgesic.

DEFINITION
Etorphine and Levomepromazine Injection is a sterile solution of Etorphine Hydrochloride and Levomepromazine in Water for Injections containing suitable stabilising agents. The pH is adjusted to about 4.

The injection complies with the requirements stated under Parenteral Preparations and with the following requirements.

Content of etorphine hydrochloride, $C_{25}H_{33}NO_4,HCl$
0.0066 to 0.0082% w/v.

Content of levomepromazine, $C_{19}H_{24}N_2OS$
1.6 to 2.0% w/v.

CHARACTERISTICS
A clear, colourless or pale yellow solution.

IDENTIFICATION
A. To 2 ml add 2 ml of 5M *sodium hydroxide*, extract the mixture with two 5 ml quantities of *cyclohexane* and evaporate the combined extracts to dryness. The *infrared absorption spectrum* of the residue, Appendix II A, is concordant with the *reference spectrum* of levomepromazine (*RSV 25*).

B. Carry out the method for *thin-layer chromatography*, Appendix III A, in subdued light using *silica gel GF_{254}* as the coating substance and *ethyl acetate* as the mobile phase applying separately to each half of the plate 10 µl of each of the following solutions. For solution (1) add 2 ml of 5M *ammonia* to 2 ml of the injection, extract with two 5 ml quantities of *chloroform*, shake the combined chloroform extracts with *anhydrous sodium sulphate*, filter, evaporate the filtrate and dissolve the residue in 0.4 ml of *chloroform*. Solution (2) contains 0.032% w/v of *diprenorphine BPCRS* in *chloroform*. Add to each point of application 10 µl of a mixture of 4 volumes of *methanol* and 1 volume of 13.5M ammonia. After removal of the plate, allow it to dry in air and examine under *ultraviolet light (254 nm)*. Spray one half of the plate with a mixture of 5 volumes of *chloroplatinic acid solution*, 35 volumes of *dilute potassium iodide solution* and 60 volumes of *acetone*. Spray the other half of the plate with a mixture of 1 volume of *iron(III) chloride solution R1* and 1 volume of *dilute potassium hexacyanoferrate(III) solution*. The principal spot in the chromatogram obtained with solution (1) has an Rf value of about 1.15 relative to that of the spot in the chromatogram obtained with solution (2), absorbs ultraviolet light and yields a reddish violet colour with the iodoplatinate spray reagent and a blue colour with the iron-hexacyanoferrate spray reagent.

TESTS

Acidity
pH, 3.5 to 4.5, Appendix V L.

ASSAY

For etorphine hydrochloride
Dissolve 46 mg of *diprenorphine BPCRS* (internal standard) in sufficient *methanol* to produce 50 ml (solution A). Carry out the method for *gas chromatography*, Appendix III B, using the following solutions. For solution (1) add 1 ml of solution A and 2 ml of 5M ammonia to 10 ml of the injection, extract with three 15 ml quantities of *chloroform*, shake the combined extracts with 5 g of *anhydrous sodium sulphate*, filter and evaporate the filtrate to a small volume using a rotary evaporator. Transfer the contents to a stoppered test tube with the aid of 2 ml of *chloroform* and evaporate to dryness. To the residue add 1 ml of a mixture of 8 volumes of *dimethylformamide*, 2 volumes of *N,O-bis(trimethylsilyl)-acetamide* and 1 volume of *trimethylchlorosilane* and allow to stand for 15 minutes. For solution (2) treat a volume of the Injection in the same manner but omitting the addition of solution A. Protect the solutions from light during preparation and subsequent use.

The chromatographic procedure may be carried out using a glass column (1.5 m × 4 mm) packed with *acid-washed, silanised diatomaceous support* (80 to 100 mesh) coated with 1% w/w of *phenyl methyl silicone fluid (50% phenyl)* (OV 17 is suitable) and maintained at 245°.

Calculate the content of $C_{25}H_{33}NO_4$ using the declared content of $C_{26}H_{35}NO_4$ in *diprenorphine BPCRS* assuming that the trimethylsilyl derivatives of equal weights of etorphine and diprenorphine have the same response in the flame ionisation detector and hence calculate the content of $C_{25}H_{33}NO_4$,HCl taking each mg of $C_{25}H_{33}NO_4$ to be equivalent to 1.089 mg of $C_{25}H_{33}NO_4$,HCl.

For levomepromazine
Protect the solutions from light throughout the assay. To 1 ml add sufficient 0.1M *hydrochloric acid* to produce 500 ml. Measure the *absorbance*, Appendix II B, of the resulting solution at the maximum at 302 nm. Calculate the content of $C_{19}H_{24}N_2OS$ taking 125 as the value of A(1%, 1 cm) at the maximum at 302 nm.

STORAGE
Etorphine and Levomepromazine Injection should be protected from light.

Fenbendazole Granules

Action and use
Antihelminthic.

DEFINITION
Fenbendazole Granules contain Fenbendazole mixed with suitable diluents.
The granules comply with the requirements stated under Granules and with the following requirements.

Content of fenbendazole, $C_{15}H_{13}N_3O_2S$
95.0 to 105.0% of the stated amount.

IDENTIFICATION
A. In the Assay, the retention time of the principal peak in the chromatogram obtained with solution (1) is the same as that of the principal peak in the chromatogram obtained with solution (2).

B. Carry out the method for *thin-layer chromatography*, Appendix III A, using a *TLC silica gel F_{254} plate* (Merck silica gel F_{254} plates are suitable) and as the mobile phase a mixture of 2.5 volumes of *water*, 6.5 volumes of *acetone*, 26 volumes of 13.5M ammonia and 65 volumes of *toluene*. Allow the solvent front to ascend 10 cm above the line of application. Apply separately to the plate 5 µl of each of the following solutions. For solution (1) mix with the aid of ultrasound a quantity of the powdered granules containing 80 mg of Fenbendazole with 80 ml of 0.1M *methanolic hydrochloric acid* for 90 minutes, cool, dilute to 100 ml with 0.1M *methanolic hydrochloric acid*, mix, filter through a 0.4-µm filter (Whatman GF/C is suitable) and use the filtrate. Solution (2) contains 0.08% w/v of *fenbendazole BPCRS* in 0.1M *methanolic hydrochloric acid*. After removal of the plate, allow it to dry in air for 10 minutes, heat at 100° for 5 minutes and examine under *ultraviolet light (254 nm and 365 nm)*. By each method of visualisation the principal spot in the chromatogram obtained with solution (1) corresponds to that in the chromatogram obtained with (2).

TESTS

Related impurities A, B and 1
Carry out the method for *liquid chromatography*, Appendix III D, using the following solutions. For solution (1) mix, with the aid of ultrasound, a quantity of the powdered granules containing 0.1 g of Fenbendazole with 50 ml of 0.1M *methanolic hydrochloric acid* for 30 minutes, cool, dilute to 100 ml with *methanol (65%)*, mix and filter through a glass-fibre filter (Whatman GF/C is suitable). For solution (2) dilute 1 volume of a 0.001% w/v solution of *fenbendazole impurity A EPCRS* (methyl (1H-benzimidazol-2-yl)carbamate) in 0.1M *methanolic hydrochloric acid* to 2 volumes with *methanol (65%)*. For solution (3) dilute 1 volume of a 0.001% w/v solution of *fenbendazole impurity B EPCRS* (methyl (5-chloro-1H-benzimidazol-2-yl)carbamate) in 0.1M *methanolic hydrochloric acid* to 2 volumes with *methanol (65%)*. For solution (4) dilute 1 volume of a 0.0010% w/v solution of *fenbendazole impurity 1 BPCRS* (5-phenylthio)-2-aminobenzimidazole) in 0.1M *methanolic hydrochloric acid* to 2 volumes with *methanol (65%)*. For solution (5) dilute 1 volume of a solution containing 0.002% w/v each of *fenbendazole impurity A EPCRS*, *fenbendazole impurity B EPCRS*, *fenbendazole impurity 1 BPCRS* and 0.20% w/v of *fenbendazole BPCRS* in 0.1M *methanolic hydrochloric acid* to 2 volumes with *methanol (65%)*.

The chromatographic procedure may be carried out using (a) a stainless steel column (25 cm × 4.6 mm) packed with *octadecylsilyl silica gel for chromatography* (5 μm) (Nucleosil C18 is suitable), (b) as the mobile phase with a flow rate of 1 ml per minute a mixture of 350 volumes of a 0.5% w/v solution of *sodium dihydrogen orthophosphate* and 650 volumes of *methanol* containing 1.88 g of *sodium hexanesulphonate*, the pH of which has been adjusted to 3.5 with *orthophosphoric acid* and (c) a detection wavelength of 280 nm.

Inject separately 20 μl of each solution. The test is not valid unless the chromatogram obtained with solution (5) closely resembles the reference chromatogram supplied with *fenbendazole BPCRS*.

In the chromatogram obtained with solution (1) the areas of any peaks corresponding to fenbendazole impurity A, fenbendazole impurity B and fenbendazole impurity 1 (5-(phenylthio)-2-aminobenzimidazole) are not greater than the areas of the corresponding peaks in the chromatograms obtained with solutions (2), (3) and (4) respectively (0.5% each).

ASSAY

Carry out the method for *liquid chromatography*, Appendix III D, using the following solutions.

For solution (1) mix with the aid of ultrasound a quantity of the powdered granules containing 0.1 g of Fenbendazole with 50 ml of 0.1M *methanolic hydrochloric acid* for 30 minutes, cool, dilute to 100 ml with *methanol (65%)*, mix, filter through a glass-fibre filter (Whatman GF/C is suitable). Dilute 5 volumes of the resulting solution to 50 volumes with 0.1M *hydrochloric acid* in *methanol (85%)*. Solution (2) contains a 0.01% w/v of *fenbendazole BPCRS* in a mixture of 1 volume of 0.1M *hydrochloric acid* and 1 volume of *methanol (85%)*.

The chromatographic procedure described under Related substances may be used.

Calculate the total content of $C_{15}H_{13}N_3O_2S$ in the granules from the chromatogram obtained using the declared content of $C_{15}H_{13}N_3O_2S$ in *fenbendazole BPCRS*.

IMPURITIES

The impurities limited by the requirements of this monograph include impurities A and B listed under Fenbendazole and the following:

1. (5-phenylthio)-2-aminobenzimidazole.

Fenbendazole Oral Suspension

Action and use
Anthelminthic.

DEFINITION
Fenbendazole Oral Suspension is an aqueous suspension of Fenbendazole.

The oral suspension complies with the requirements stated under Oral Liquids and with the following requirements.

Content of fenbendazole, $C_{15}H_{13}N_3O_2S$
95.0 to 105.0% of the stated amount.

IDENTIFICATION
In the Assay, the retention time of the principal peak in the chromatogram obtained with solution (1) is the same as that of the principal peak in the chromatogram obtained with solution (2).

TESTS
Related impurities A, B and 1
Carry out the method for *liquid chromatography*, Appendix III D, using the following solutions.
For solution (1), mix with the aid of ultrasound, a quantity of the oral suspension containing 0.1 g of Fenbendazole with 50 ml of 0.1M *methanolic hydrochloric acid* for 30 minutes, cool, dilute to 100 ml with *methanol (65%)*, mix, filter through a glass-fibre filter (Whatman GF/C is suitable).
For solution (2), dilute 1 volume of a 0.001% w/v solution of *fenbendazole impurity A EPCRS* (methyl (1*H*-benzimidazol-2-yl)carbamate) in 0.1M *methanolic hydrochloric acid* to 2 volumes with *methanol (65%)*. For solution (3) dilute 1 volume of a 0.001% w/v solution of *fenbendazole impurity B EPCRS* (methyl(5-chloro-1*H*-benzimidazol-2-yl)carbamate in 0.1M *methanolic hydrochloric acid* to 2 volumes with *methanol (65%)*. For solution (4) dilute 1 volume of a 0.001% w/v solution of *fenbendazole impurity 1 BPCRS* (5-phenylthio)-2-aminobenzimidazole) in 0.1M *methanolic hydrochloric acid* to 2 volumes with *methanol (65%)*. For solution (5) dilute 1 volume of a solution containing 0.002% w/v each of *fenbendazole impurity A EPCRS*, *fenbendazole impurity B EPCRS*, *fenbendazole impurity 1 BPCRS* and 0.20% w/v of *fenbendazole BPCRS* in 0.1M *methanolic hydrochloric acid* to 2 volumes with *methanol (65%)*.

The chromatographic procedure may be carried out using (a) a stainless steel column (25 cm × 4.6 mm) packed with *octadecylsilyl silica gel for chromatography* (5 μm) (Nucleosil C18 is suitable), (b) as the mobile phase with a flow rate of 1 ml per minute a mixture of 350 volumes of a 0.5% w/v solution of *sodium dihydrogen orthophosphate* and 650 volumes of *methanol* containing 1.88 g of *sodium hexanesulphonate*, the pH of which has been adjusted to 3.5 with *orthophosphoric acid* and (c) a detection wavelength of 280 nm.

Inject separately 20 μl of each solution. The test is not valid unless the chromatogram obtained with solution (5) closely resembles the reference chromatogram supplied with *fenbendazole BPCRS*.

In the chromatogram obtained with solution (1) the areas of any peaks corresponding to fenbendazole impurity A (methyl (1*H*-benzimidazol-2-yl)carbamate), fenbendazole impurity B (methyl (5-chloro-1*H*-benzimidazol-2-yl)carbamate) and fenbendazole impurity 1 (5-(phenylthio)-2-aminobenzimidazole) are not greater than the areas of the corresponding peaks in the chromatograms obtained with solutions (2), (3) and (4) respectively (0.5% each).

ASSAY
Carry out the method for *liquid chromatography*, Appendix III D, using the following solutions.
For solution (1) mix with the aid of ultrasound a quantity of the oral suspension containing 0.1 g of Fenbendazole with 50 ml of 0.1M *methanolic hydrochloric acid* for 30 minutes, cool, dilute to 100 ml with *methanol (65%)*, mix, filter through a glass-fibre filter (Whatman GF/C is suitable). Dilute 5 volumes of the resulting solution to 50 volumes with 0.1M *hydrochloric acid* in *methanol (85%)*. Solution (2) contains 0.01% w/v of *fenbendazole BPCRS* in a mixture of 1 volume of 0.1M *hydrochloric acid* and 1 volume of *methanol (85%)*.

The chromatographic procedure described under Related substances may be used.

Calculate the total content of $C_{15}H_{13}N_3O_2S$ in the oral suspension from the chromatogram obtained and using the declared content of $C_{15}H_{13}N_3O_2S$ in *fenbendazole BPCRS*.

IMPURITIES

The impurities limited by the requirements of this monograph include impurities A and B listed under Fenbendazole and the following:

1. (5-phenylthio)-2-aminobenzimidazole.

Fenbendazole Veterinary Oral Paste

Fenbendazole Veterinary Paste

Action and use
Anthelminthic.

DEFINITION

Fenbendazole Veterinary Oral Paste contains Fenbendazole finely dispersed in a suitable basis.

The veterinary oral paste complies with the requirements stated under Veterinary Oral Pastes and with the following requirements.

Content of fenbendazole, $C_{15}H_{13}N_3O_2S$
95.0 to 105.0% of the stated amount.

IDENTIFICATION

In the Assay, the retention time of the principal peak in the chromatogram obtained with solution (1) is the same as that of the principal peak in the chromatogram obtained with solution (2).

TESTS

Related impurities A, B and 1
Carry out the method for *liquid chromatography*, Appendix III D, using the following solutions.
For solution (1), mix with the aid of ultrasound, a quantity of the oral paste containing 0.1 g of Fenbendazole with 50 ml of 0.1M *methanolic hydrochloric acid* for 30 minutes, cool, dilute to 100 ml with *methanol (65%)*, mix, filter through a glass-fibre filter (Whatman GF/C is suitable).
For solution (2) dilute 1 volume of a 0.001% w/v solution of *fenbendazole impurity A EPCRS* (methyl (1*H*-benzimidazole-2-yl)carbamate) in 0.1M *methanolic hydrochloric acid* to 2 volumes with *methanol (65%)*. For solution (3) dilute 1 volume of a 0.001% w/v solution of *fenbendazole impurity B EPCRS* (methyl (5-chloro-1*H*-benzimidazole-2-yl)carbamate in 0.1M *methanolic hydrochloric acid* to 2 volumes with *methanol (65%)*. For solution (4) dilute 1 volume of a 0.001% w/v solution of *fenbendazole impurity 1 BPCRS* (5- phenylthio)-2-aminobenzimidazole in 0.1M *methanolic hydrochloric acid* to 2 volumes with *methanol (65%)*.
For solution (5) dilute 1 volume of a solution containing 0.002% w/v each of *fenbendazole impurity A EPCRS*, *fenbendazole impurity B EPCRS*, *fenbendazole impurity 1 BPCRS* and 0.20% w/v of *fenbendazole BPCRS* in 0.1M *methanolic hydrochloric acid* to 2 volumes with *methanol (65%)*.

The chromatographic procedure may be carried out using (a) a stainless steel column (25 cm × 4.6 mm) packed with *octadecylsilyl silica gel for chromatography* (5 µm) (Nucleosil C18 5µ is suitable), (b) as the mobile phase with a flow rate of 1 ml per minute a mixture of 350 volumes of a 0.5% w/v solution of *sodium dihydrogen orthophosphate* and 650 volumes of *methanol* containing 1.88 g of *sodium hexanesulphonate*, the pH of which has been adjusted to 3.5 with *orthophosphoric acid* and (c) a detection wavelength of 280 nm.

Inject separately 20 µl of each solution. The test is not valid unless the chromatogram obtained with solution (5) closely resembles the reference chromatogram supplied with *fenbendazole BPCRS*.

In the chromatogram obtained with solution (1) the areas of any peaks corresponding to fenbendazole impurity A (methyl (1*H*-benzimidazol-2-yl)carbamate), fenbendazole impurity B (methyl (5-chloro-1*H*-benzimidazol-2-yl)carbamate) and fenbendazole impurity 1 (5-(phenylthio)-2-aminobenzimidazole) are not greater than the areas of the corresponding peaks in the chromatograms obtained with solutions (2), (3) and (4) respectively (0.5% each).

ASSAY

Carry out the method for *liquid chromatography*, Appendix III D, using the following solutions.
For solution (1) mix with the aid of ultrasound a quantity of the oral paste containing 0.1 g of Fenbendazole with 50 ml of 0.1M *methanolic hydrochloric acid* for 30 minutes, cool, dilute to 100 ml with *methanol (65%)*, mix, filter through a glass-fibre filter (Whatman GF/C is suitable). Dilute 5 volumes of the resulting solution to 50 volumes with 0.1M *hydrochloric acid* in *methanol (85%)*. Solution (2) contains a 0.01% w/v solution of *fenbendazole BPCRS* in a mixture of 1 volume of 0.1M *hydrochloric acid* and 1 volume of *methanol (85%)*.

The chromatographic procedure described under Related substances may be used.

Calculate the content of $C_{15}H_{13}N_3O_2S$ in the veterinary oral paste from the chromatogram obtained and using the declared content of $C_{15}H_{13}N_3O_2S$ in *fenbendazole BPCRS*.

IMPURITIES

The impurities limited by the requirements of this monograph include impurities A and B listed under Fenbendazole and the following:

1. (5-phenylthio)-2-aminobenzimidazole.

Fenbendazole Veterinary Oral Powder

Action and use
Antihelminthic.

DEFINITION

Fenbendazole Veterinary Oral Powder contains Fenbendazole mixed with suitable diluents.

The veterinary oral powder complies with the requirements stated under Veterinary Oral Powders and with the following requirements.

Content of fenbendazole, $C_{15}H_{13}N_3O_2S$
95.0 to 105.0% of the stated amount.

IDENTIFICATION

A. In the Assay, the retention time of the principal peak in the chromatogram obtained with solution (1) is the same as that of the principal peak in the chromatogram obtained with solution (2).

B. Carry out the method for *thin-layer chromatography*, Appendix III A, using a *TLC silica gel F$_{254}$ plate* (Merck silica gel F$_{254}$ plates are suitable) and as the mobile phase a mixture of 2.5 volumes of *water*, 6.5 volumes of *acetone*, 26 volumes of *13.5M ammonia* and 65 volumes of *toluene*. Allow the solvent front to ascend 10 cm above the line of application. Apply separately to the plate 5 µl of each of the following solutions. For solution (1) mix, with the aid of ultrasound, a quantity of the powder containing 80 mg of Fenbendazole with 80 ml of 0.1M *methanolic hydrochloric acid* for 90 minutes, cool, dilute to 100 ml with 0.1M *methanolic hydrochloric acid*, mix, filter through a 0.4-µm filter (Whatman GF/C is suitable) and use the filtrate. Solution (2) contains 0.08% w/v of *fenbendazole BPCRS* in 0.1M *methanolic hydrochloric acid*. After removal of the plate, allow it to dry in air for 10 minutes, heat at 100° for 5 minutes and examine under *ultraviolet light (254 nm and 365 nm)*. By each method of visualisation the principal spot in the chromatogram obtained with solution (1) corresponds to that in the chromatogram obtained with (2).

TESTS

Related impurities A, B and 1

Carry out the method for *liquid chromatography*, Appendix III D, using the following solutions. For solution (1) mix with the aid of ultrasound a quantity of the powder containing 0.1 g of Fenbendazole with 25 ml each of *dimethylformamide* and *methanol* and 1 ml of 5M *hydrochloric acid* until a clear solution is produced, cool, dilute to 100 ml with *methanol (65%)*. For solution (2) dilute 1 volume of a 0.001% w/v solution of *fenbendazole impurity A EPCRS* in 0.1M *methanolic hydrochloric acid* to 2 volumes with *methanol (65%)*. For solution (3) dilute 1 volume of a 0.001% w/v solution of *fenbendazole impurity B EPCRS* in 0.1M *methanolic hydrochloric acid* to 2 volumes with *methanol (65%)*. For solution (4) dilute 1 volume of a 0.001% w/v solution of *fenbendazole impurity 1 BPCRS* in 0.1M *methanolic hydrochloric acid* to 2 volumes with *methanol (65%)*. For solution (5) dilute 1 volume of a solution containing 0.002% w/v each of *fenbendazole impurity A EPCRS, fenbendazole impurity B EPCRS, fenbendazole impurity 1 BPCRS* and 0.20% w/v of *fenbendazole BPCRS* in 0.1M *methanolic hydrochloric acid* to 2 volumes with *methanol (65%)*.

The chromatographic procedure may be carried out using (a) a stainless steel column (25 cm × 4.6 mm) packed with *octadecylsilyl silica gel for chromatography* (5 µm) (Nucleosil C18 is suitable), (b) as the mobile phase with a flow rate of 1 ml per minute a mixture of 350 volumes of a 0.5% w/v solution of *sodium dihydrogen orthophosphate* and 650 volumes of *methanol* containing 1.88 g of *sodium hexanesulphonate*, the pH of which has been adjusted to 3.5 with *orthophosphoric acid* and (c) a detection wavelength of 280 nm.

Inject separately 20 µl of each solution. The test is not valid unless the chromatogram obtained with solution (5) closely resembles the reference chromatogram supplied with *fenbendazole BPCRS*.

In the chromatogram obtained with solution (1) the areas of any peaks corresponding to fenbendazole impurity A (methyl (1*H*-benzimidazol-2-yl)carbamate), fenbendazole impurity B (methyl 5-chloro-1*H*-benzimidazol-2-yl)carbamate) and

fenbendazole impurity 1 (5-(phenylthio)-2-aminobenzimidazole) are not greater than the areas of the corresponding peaks in the chromatograms obtained with solutions (2), (3) and (4) respectively (0.5% each). Disregard any peaks due to preservatives.

ASSAY

Carry out the method for *liquid chromatography*, Appendix III D, using the following solutions. For solution (1) mix with the aid of ultrasound a quantity of the powder containing 0.1 g of Fenbendazole with 25 ml each of *dimethylformamide* and *methanol* and 1 ml of 5M *hydrochloric acid* until a clear solution is produced, cool, dilute to 100 ml with *methanol (85%)*. Dilute 5 volumes of the resulting solution to 50 volumes with 0.1M *hydrochloric acid* in *methanol (85%)*. Solution (2) is a 0.01% w/v solution of *fenbendazole BPCRS* in a mixture of 1 volume of 0.1M *hydrochloric acid* in 1 volume of *methanol (65%)*.

The chromatographic procedure described under Related substances may be used.

Calculate the content of $C_{15}H_{13}N_3O_2S$ in the oral powder from the chromatogram obtained using the declared content of $C_{15}H_{13}N_3O_2S$ in *fenbendazole BPCRS*.

IMPURITIES

The impurities limited by the requirements of this monograph include impurities A and B listed under Fenbendazole and the following:

1. (5-phenylthio)-2-aminobenzimidazole.

Serum Gonadotrophin Injection

Action and use

Equine serum gonadotrophin.

DEFINITION

Serum Gonadotrophin Injection is a sterile solution of Serum Gonadotrophin in Water for Injections. It is prepared by dissolving Serum Gonadotrophin for Injection in the requisite amount of Water for Injections immediately before use.

The injection complies with the requirements stated under Parenteral Preparations.

STORAGE

Serum Gonadotrophin Injection should be used immediately after preparation.

SERUM GONADOTROPHIN FOR INJECTION

DEFINITION

Serum Gonadotrophin for Injection is a sterile material consisting of Serum Gonadotrophin with or without excipients. It is supplied in a sealed container.

The contents of the sealed container comply with the requirements for Powders for Injections stated under Parenteral Preparations and with the following requirements.

CHARACTERISTICS

A white or pale grey, amorphous powder.

Soluble in *water*.

IDENTIFICATION

Causes enlargement of the ovaries of immature female rats when administered as directed in the Assay.

TESTS

Clarity, colour and acidity or alkalinity of solution

A solution containing 5000 IU per ml is *clear*, Appendix IV A, Method I, and *colourless*, Appendix IV B, Method I, and has a pH of 6.0 to 8.0, Appendix V L.

Water

Not more than 10.0% w/w, Appendix IX C. Use 80 mg.

Bacterial endotoxins

Carry out the *test for bacterial endotoxins*, Appendix XIV C, using Method C. Dissolve the contents of the sealed container in *water BET* to give a solution containing 1000 IU of serum gonadotrophin per ml (solution A). The endotoxin limit concentration of solution A is 35 IU of endotoxin per ml. Carry out the test using a suitable dilution of solution A as described under Method C.

ASSAY

Carry out the Assay described under Serum Gonadotrophin. For each container tested, the estimated potency is not less than 80% and not more than 125% of the stated potency. The fiducial limits of error are not less than 64% and not more than 156% of the stated potency.

STORAGE

The sealed container should be protected from light and stored at a temperature not exceeding 8°. Under these conditions the contents may be expected to retain their potency for not less than 2 years.

LABELLING

The label of the sealed container states the number of IU (Units) contained in it.

Griseofulvin Premix

Action and use

Antifungal.

DEFINITION

Griseofulvin Premix contains Griseofulvin. The particles of Griseofulvin are generally up to 5 µm in maximum dimension, although larger particles, which may occasionally exceed 30 µm, may be present.

The premix complies with requirements stated under Premixes and with the following requirements.

Content of griseofulvin, $C_{17}H_{17}ClO_6$

90.0 to 110.0% of the stated amount.

IDENTIFICATION

A. Shake a quantity of the premix containing 100 mg of Griseofulvin with 10 ml of *chloroform*. Centrifuge, decant the supernatant liquid, dry with *anhydrous sodium sulphate* and evaporate the chloroform. The *infrared absorption spectrum* of the residue, Appendix II A, is concordant with the *reference spectrum* of griseofulvin (*RSV 24*).

B. Shake a quantity of the premix containing 80 mg of Griseofulvin with 150 ml of *ethanol (96%)*. Dilute to 200 ml with *ethanol (96%)* and centrifuge. Dilute 2 ml of the supernatant liquid to 100 ml with *ethanol (96%)*. The *light absorption* of the resulting solution, Appendix II B, in the range 240 to 350 nm, exhibits two maxima at 291 nm and at 325 nm and a shoulder at 250 nm.

C. Dissolve 5 mg of the residue obtained in test A in 1 ml of *sulphuric acid* and add 5 mg of powdered *potassium dichromate*. A wine red colour is produced.

Related substances

Dissolve 50 mg of *9,10-diphenylanthracene* (internal standard) in sufficient *chloroform* to produce 50 ml (solution A). Carry out the method for *gas chromatography*, Appendix III B, using the following solutions. For solution (1) dissolve 5 mg of *griseofulvin BPCRS* in *chloroform* and add 2 ml of solution A and sufficient *chloroform* to produce 200 ml. Evaporate 20 ml of the solution to about 1 ml. For solution (2) add 60 ml of *chloroform* to a quantity of the premix containing 50 mg of Griseofulvin, heat at 60° with shaking for 20 minutes, cool and dilute to 100 ml with *chloroform*. Centrifuge and evaporate 20 ml of the supernatant liquid to about 1 ml. Prepare solution (3) in the same manner as solution (2) but adding 1 ml of solution A before diluting to 100 ml with *chloroform*.

The chromatographic procedure may be carried out using a glass column (1 m × 4 mm) packed with *acid-washed, silanised diatomaceous support* (100 to 120 mesh) coated with 1% w/w of cyanopropylmethyl phenylmethyl silicone fluid (OV 225 is suitable) and maintained at 250°.

In the chromatogram obtained with solution (3) the ratios of the areas of any peak corresponding to dechlorogriseofulvin (retention time about 0.6 times that of griseofulvin) and of any peak corresponding to dehydrogriseofulvin (retention time about 1.4 times that of griseofulvin) to the area of the peak due to the internal standard are, respectively, not greater than 0.6 times and 0.15 times the ratio of the area of the peak due to griseofulvin to that of the internal standard in the chromatogram obtained with solution (1).

ASSAY

To a quantity containing 35 mg of Griseofulvin add 60 ml of *ethyl acetate*, mix, heat to 60° and shake for 15 minutes. Allow to cool and dilute to 100 ml with *ethyl acetate*. Centrifuge and transfer two 5 ml aliquots of the clear supernatant liquid into separate 100 ml graduated flasks. To the first flask add 5.0 ml of a 13% v/v solution of *methanesulphonic acid* in *methanol*, allow to stand at 20° for 30 minutes and dilute to 100 ml with *methanol* (solution A). Dilute the contents of the second flask to 100 ml with *methanol* (solution B). To a third flask add 5.0 ml of the methanolic methanesulphonic acid solution and dilute to 100 ml with *methanol* (solution C). Measure the *absorbance* of each solution at 266 nm, Appendix II B. Calculate the content of $C_{17}H_{17}ClO_6$ from the difference between the absorbance obtained with solution A and the sum of the absorbances obtained with solutions B and C and from the difference obtained by repeating the operation using 35 mg of *griseofulvin BPCRS* in place of the preparation being examined and from the declared content of $C_{17}H_{17}ClO_6$ in *griseofulvin BPCRS*.

Iron Dextran Injection (10 per cent)

Action and use
Used in the prevention and treatment of iron deficiency anaemias.

DEFINITION
Iron Dextran Injection (10 per cent) is a sterile colloidal solution containing a complex of iron(III) hydroxide with dextrans of weight average molecular weight between 5000 and 7500.

PRODUCTION
Iron Dextran Injection (10 per cent) is produced by a method of manufacture designed to provide an iron-dextran complex with appropriate iron absorption characteristics. This may be confirmed for routine control purposes by the use of an appropriate combination of physico-chemical tests, subject to the agreement of the competent authority.

The method of manufacture is validated to demonstrate that, if tested, the injection would comply with the following test.

Undue toxicity Inject 0.10 ml into a tail vein of each of 10 mice; not more than three mice die within 5 days of injection. If more than three mice die within 5 days, repeat the test on another group of 20 mice. Not more than 10 of the 30 mice used in the combined tests die within 5 days of injection.

The injection complies with the requirements stated under Parenteral Preparations and with the following requirements.

Content of iron, Fe
9.5 to 10.5% w/v.

Content of dextrans
17.0 to 23.0% w/v.

CHARACTERISTICS
A dark brown, slightly viscous solution.

IDENTIFICATION
A. Add 5M *ammonia* to 0.15 ml of the injection previously diluted to 5 ml with *water*. No precipitate is produced.

B. To 1 ml add 20 ml of *water* and 5 ml of *hydrochloric acid* and boil for 5 minutes. Cool, add an excess of 13.5M *ammonia* and filter. Wash the precipitate with *water*, dissolve in the minimum volume of 2M *hydrochloric acid* and add sufficient *water* to produce 20 ml. The resulting solution yields reaction B characteristic of *iron salts*, Appendix VI.

C. Mix 1 ml with 100 ml of *water*. To 5 ml of this solution add 0.2 ml of *hydrochloric acid*, boil for 30 seconds, cool rapidly, add 4 ml of 13.5M *ammonia* and 10 ml of *hydrogen sulphide solution*, boil to remove hydrogen sulphide, cool and filter. Boil 5 ml of the filtrate with 5 ml of *cupri-tartaric solution R1*. The solution remains greenish and no precipitate is produced. Boil a further 5 ml of the filtrate with 0.5 ml of *hydrochloric acid* for 5 minutes, cool, add 2.5 ml of 5M *sodium hydroxide* and 5 ml of *cupri-tartaric solution R1* and again boil. A reddish precipitate is produced.

TESTS
Acidity
pH, 5.2 to 6.5, Appendix V L.

Chloride
To 5.0 ml add 75 ml of *water* and 0.05 ml of *nitric acid* and titrate immediately with 0.1M *silver nitrate VS*, determining the end point potentiometrically. Not less than 8.5 ml and not more than 17.0 ml of 0.1M *silver nitrate VS* is required.

Copper
To 2.5 ml add 5 ml of *nitric acid* and heat until the vigorous evolution of brown fumes ceases. Cool, add 2 ml of *sulphuric acid* and heat again until fumes are evolved, adding *nitric acid* dropwise from time to time until oxidation is complete. Cool, add 25 ml of *hydrochloric acid*, warm to dissolve, cool and extract with four 25 ml quantities of *isobutyl acetate*, discarding the extracts. Evaporate the acid solution to dryness, adding *nitric acid* dropwise if charring occurs. Dissolve the residue in 10 ml of 1M *hydrochloric acid*, reserving a portion of the solution for the test for Zinc. To 1 ml add 25 ml of *water* and 1 g of *citric acid*, make alkaline to *litmus paper* with 5M *ammonia*, dilute to 50 ml with *water*, add 1 ml of *sodium diethyldithiocarbamate solution* and allow to stand for 5 minutes. Any colour produced is not more intense than that produced by treating in the same manner a mixture of 3 ml of *copper standard solution (3 ppm Cu)* and 1 ml of 1M *hydrochloric acid*, beginning at the words 'add 25 ml of *water*' (120 µg per ml).

Lead
To 2.5 ml in a Kjeldahl flask add 10 ml of *water* and 10 ml of *nitric acid* and heat until the vigorous evolution of brown fumes ceases. Cool, add 10 ml of *sulphuric acid* and heat again until fumes are evolved, adding *nitric acid* dropwise from time to time until oxidation is complete. Cool, add 30 ml of *water*, bring to the boil and continue boiling until the volume of liquid is reduced to about 20 ml; cool and dilute to 50 ml with *water*. To 16 ml of the solution add 50 ml of *hydrochloric acid* and extract with four 20 ml quantities of *isobutyl acetate*, discarding the extracts. Evaporate the acid solution to dryness and dissolve the residue in 20 ml of *water*. 12 ml of the resulting solution complies with *limit test A for heavy metals*, Appendix VII. Use *lead standard solution (2 ppm Pb)* to prepare the standard (50 µg per ml).

Zinc
To 5 ml of the solution reserved in the test for Copper add 15 ml of 1M *sodium hydroxide*, boil, filter, wash the residue with *water* and dilute the combined filtrate and washings to 25 ml with *water*. To 5 ml of the resulting solution add 5 ml of 1M *hydrochloric acid* and 2 g of *ammonium chloride*, dilute to 50 ml with *water*, add 1 ml of freshly prepared *potassium hexacyanoferrate(II) solution* and allow to stand for 20 minutes. Any opalescence produced is not greater than that produced when 1 ml of freshly prepared *potassium hexacyanoferrate(II) solution* is added to a solution prepared from 3 ml of *zinc standard solution (25 ppm Zn)*, 3 ml of 1M *sodium hydroxide*, 6 ml of 1M *hydrochloric acid* and 2 g of *ammonium chloride* diluted to 50 ml with *water* and allowed to stand for 20 minutes (300 µg per ml).

Iron absorption
Dilute 1 volume of the injection with an equal volume of *water for injections*. Determine the iron absorption of the resulting solution using the following method. Using at least two rabbits, each weighing between 1.5 and 2.5 kg, clip the right hind leg free from hair over the injection site and swab the area with a bactericidal solution. Inject into each rabbit 0.4 ml of the injection per kg of the rabbit's weight using a 2 ml syringe fitted with a No. 12 hypodermic needle [22 gauge × 1.25 inch (0.7 × 32 mm approx.)]. Insert the needle at the distal end of the semitendinosus muscle, passing through the sartorius and entering the vastus medialis; the angle of the needle must be such that the full length is used. After 7 days, kill the rabbits and remove the legs into which the injections were made. Carefully cut open the muscles and examine the site of injection. It should be

only very lightly stained and should show no dark brown deposits or evidence of leakage along fascial planes. Skin the leg, dissect the flesh from the bone and cut it into small pieces. Transfer the pieces to a 1000 ml beaker, add 75 ml of 2M *sodium hydroxide* and sufficient *water* to cover the flesh, cover the beaker with a watch glass and boil until most of the solid matter has disintegrated. Cool, cautiously add 50 ml of *sulphuric acid*, heat the mixture almost to boiling and add carefully in 1 ml quantities, 10 ml of *fuming nitric acid*. Boil the mixture until charring commences and add further quantities of *fuming nitric acid* until no charring occurs when the excess of nitric acid has been boiled off. Cool, add 170 ml of *water*, boil until solution is complete, cool and dilute to 250 ml with *water*. To 5 ml of this solution add 3 ml of *sulphuric acid*, heat to fuming and complete the oxidation by the addition of small quantities of *nitric acid* until the solution is colourless. Cool, add 20 ml of *water*, boil for 3 minutes and add 10 ml of *ammonium citrate solution*, 10 ml of *ammonium mercaptoacetate solution*, 5M *ammonia* dropwise until the iron colour is fully developed, 1 ml of 5M *ammonia* in excess and sufficient *water* to produce 100 ml. Measure the *absorbance* of the resulting solution at 530 nm, Appendix II B. Prepare a solution by adding to 20 ml of *water* the same quantities of *ammonium citrate solution*, *ammonium mercaptoacetate solution* and 5M *ammonia* as used above, dilute to 100 ml with *water* and measure the *absorbance* at 530 nm. From the difference between the absorbances, calculate the amount of Fe present in the legs from a reference curve prepared by treating suitable aliquots of a solution of *ammonium iron(III) sulphate* containing 0.1 mg of Fe in 1 ml by the procedure described above beginning at the words 'add 10 ml of *ammonium citrate solution ...*'. Repeat the determination of Fe on the corresponding legs into which no injection was made, beginning at the words 'Carefully cut open the muscles...'. From the difference between the two amounts of iron, calculate the proportion of injected iron, as Fe, remaining in the leg tissues. Not more than 20% of the injected iron remains.

ASSAY

For iron

To 2 g add 10 ml of *water* and 5 ml of *sulphuric acid*, and stir for several minutes. Allow to stand for 5 minutes, cool and dilute to 50 ml with *water*. Prepare a suitable zinc amalgam by covering 300 g of *zinc shot* with a 2% w/v solution of *mercury(II) chloride* and stir for 10 minutes. Decant the solution, wash the residue three times with *water* and transfer it to a column (30 cm × 18 mm) fitted with a sintered-glass disc (ISO 4793, porosity grade 0, is suitable). Activate the zinc amalgam by passing through the column 200 ml of *sulphuric acid (5%)*. Pass the prepared solution slowly through the activated column and wash successively with 50 ml of *water*, four 25 ml quantities of *sulphuric acid (5% w/v)* and 50 ml of *water*. Titrate the combined eluates with 0.1M *ammonium cerium(IV) sulphate VS* using *ferroin solution* as indicator. Each ml of 0.1M *ammonium cerium(IV) sulphate VS* is equivalent to 5.585 mg of Fe. Determine the *weight per ml* of the injection, Appendix V G, and calculate the percentage w/v of Fe.

For dextrans

Dilute 1 g to 1000 ml with *water*, dilute 15 ml of this solution to 100 ml with *water*, transfer 3 ml of the second solution to a test tube and cool to 0°. Add, to form a lower layer, 6 ml of a solution, prepared and maintained at 0°, containing 0.2% w/v of *anthrone* in a mixture of 19 volumes of *sulphuric acid* and 1 volume of *water*, mix and immediately heat in a water bath for 5 minutes. Cool and measure the *absorbance* of the resulting solution at the maximum at 625 nm, Appendix II B. Repeat the operation using 3 ml of *water* in place of the dilution of the injection. From the difference between the absorbances calculate the content of glucose present from a reference curve prepared by treating suitable amounts of D-*glucose* by the same process. Each g of D-*glucose* is equivalent to 0.94 g of dextrans. Determine the *weight per ml* of the injection, Appendix V G, and calculate the percentage w/v of dextrans.

LABELLING

The label states that the contents are for animal treatment only.

When Iron Dextran Injection is prescribed or demanded for veterinary purposes, no strength being stated, Iron Dextran Injection (10 per cent) shall be dispensed or supplied. Iron Dextran Injection (10 per cent) contains, in 1 ml, 100 mg of iron.

Ivermectin Injection

Action and use
Antihelminthic.

DEFINITION

Ivermectin Injection is a sterile solution of Ivermectin in a suitable non-aqueous vehicle.

The injection complies with the requirements stated under Parenteral Preparations and with the following requirements.

Content of ivermectin, calculated as the sum of component H_2B_{1a} ($C_{48}H_{74}O_{14}$) and component H_2B_{1b} ($C_{47}H_{72}O_{14}$)

95.0 to 105.0% of the stated amount.

The ratio of the contents H_2B_{1a} / (H_2B_{1a} + H_2B_{1b}) is at least 90.0%.

IDENTIFICATION

A. Carry out the method for *thin-layer chromatography*, Appendix III A, using a silica gel 60 F_{254} precoated plate (Merck silica gel 60 F_{254} plates are suitable) and a mixture of 1 volume of *concentrated ammonia R1*, 9 volumes of *methanol* and 90 volumes of *dichloromethane* as the mobile phase. Apply separately to the plate 2 µl of each of the following solutions. For solution (1) dissolve a volume of the injection in sufficient *methanol* to produce a solution containing 0.05% w/v of Ivermectin; filter if necessary. Solution (2) contains 0.05% w/v of *ivermectin EPCRS* in *methanol*. After removal of the plate, allow it to dry in air and examine under *ultraviolet light (254 nm and 366 nm)*. The principal spot in the chromatogram obtained with solution (1) is similar in position, colour and size to that in the chromatogram obtained with solution (2).

B. In the Assay, the chromatogram obtained with solution (1) shows two principal peaks with retention times similar to those of the two principal peaks in the chromatogram obtained with solution (2).

TESTS

Clarity and colour of solution

The injection is *clear*, Appendix IV A, and not more intensely coloured than *reference solution* Y_4, Appendix IV B, Method II.

Related substances

Carry out the method for *liquid chromatography*, Appendix III D, using the following solutions. For solution (1) dissolve a volume of the injection in sufficient *methanol* to produce a solution containing 0.04% w/v of Ivermectin. Solutions (2), (3) and (4) contain 0.04% w/v, 0.0004% w/v and 0.00002% w/v respectively of *ivermectin EPCRS* in *methanol*. Inject 20 µl of each solution.

The chromatographic procedure may be carried out using (a) a stainless steel column (25 cm × 4.6 mm) packed with *octadecylsilyl silica gel for chromatography* (5 µm) (Apex ODS 1 is suitable), (b) as the mobile phase at a flow rate of 1.5 ml per minute a mixture of 39 volumes of *water*, 55 volumes of *methanol* and 106 volumes of *acetonitrile* and (c) a detection wavelength of 245 nm.

The test is not valid unless, in the chromatogram obtained with solution (2), the *resolution factor* between the first peak (component H_2B_{1b}) and the second peak (component H_2B_{1a}) is at least 3.0.

In the chromatogram obtained with solution (1) the area of any peak with a retention time of 1.3 to 1.5 relative to that of the principal peak is not greater than 2.7 times the area of the principal peak in the chromatogram obtained with solution (3) (2.7%), the area of any other *secondary peak* is not greater than the area of the principal peak in the chromatogram obtained with solution (3) (1%) and the sum of the areas of any such peaks is not greater than 6 times the area of the principal peak in the chromatogram obtained with solution (3) (6%). Disregard any peak with an area less than the area of the principal peak in the chromatogram obtained with solution (4) (0.05%).

ASSAY

Carry out the method for *liquid chromatography*, Appendix III D, using the following solutions. For solution (1) dissolve a volume of the injection in sufficient *methanol* to produce a solution containing 0.04% w/v of Ivermectin. Solution (2) contains 0.04% w/v of *ivermectin EPCRS* in *methanol*. Inject 20 µl of each solution.

The chromatographic conditions described under Related substances may be used.

Calculate the content of ivermectin ($H_2B_{1a} + H_2B_{1b}$) in the injection and the ratio $H_2B_{1a} / (H_2B_{1a} + H_2B_{1b})$ using as the declared content the contents of $C_{48}H_{74}O_{14}$ (H_2B_{1a}) and $C_{47}H_{72}O_{14}$ (H_2B_{1b}) in *ivermectin EPCRS*.

Ivermectin Veterinary Oral Paste

Ivermectin Veterinary Paste

Action and use
Anthelminthic.

DEFINITION

Ivermectin Veterinary Oral Paste contains Ivermectin in a suitable basis.

The veterinary oral paste complies with the requirements stated under Veterinary Oral Pastes and with the following requirements.

Content of ivermectin, calculated as the sum of component H_2B_{1a} ($C_{48}H_{74}O_{14}$) and component H_2B_{1b} ($C_{47}H_{72}O_{14}$)
95.0 to 110.0% of the stated amount.

The ratio of the contents $H_2B_{1a} / (H_2B_{1a} + H_2B_{1b})$ is at least 90.0%.

IDENTIFICATION

A. Carry out the method for *thin-layer chromatography*, Appendix III A, using a silica gel 60 F_{254} precoated plate (Merck silica gel 60 F_{254} plates are suitable) and a mixture of 1 volume of *concentrated ammonia R1*, 9 volumes of *methanol* and 90 volumes of *dichloromethane* as the mobile phase. Apply separately to the plate 2 µl of each of the following solutions. For solution (1) add 10 ml of *methanol* to a quantity of the oral paste containing 5 mg of Ivermectin and mix with the aid of ultrasound until completely dispersed. Solution (2) contains 0.05% w/v of *ivermectin EPCRS* in *methanol*. After removal of the plate, allow it to dry in air and examine under *ultraviolet light (254 nm and 366 nm)*. The principal spot in the chromatogram obtained with solution (1) is similar in position, colour and size to that in the chromatogram obtained with solution (2).

B. In the Assay, the chromatogram obtained with solution (1) shows two principal peaks with retention times similar to those of the two principal peaks in the chromatogram obtained with solution (2).

TESTS
Related substances

Carry out the method for *liquid chromatography*, Appendix III D, using the following solutions. For solution (1) disperse a quantity of the oral paste in *methanol* with the aid of ultrasound and add sufficient *methanol* to produce a solution containing 0.04% w/v of Ivermectin. Solutions (2), (3) and (4) contain 0.04% w/v, 0.0004% w/v and 0.00002% w/v respectively of *ivermectin EPCRS* in *methanol*. Inject 20 µl of each solution.

The chromatographic procedure may be carried out using (a) a stainless steel column (25 cm × 4.6 mm) packed with *octadecylsilyl silica gel for chromatography* (5 µm) (Apex ODS 1 is suitable), (b) as the mobile phase at a flow rate of 1.5 ml per minute a mixture of 39 volumes of *water*, 55 volumes of *methanol* and 106 volumes of *acetonitrile* and (c) a detection wavelength of 245 nm.

The test is not valid unless, in the chromatogram obtained with solution (2), the *resolution factor* between the first peak (component H_2B_{1b}) and the second peak (component H_2B_{1a}) is at least 3.0.

In the chromatogram obtained with solution (1) the area of any peak with a retention time of 1.3 to 1.5 relative to that of the principal peak is not greater than 3 times the area of the principal peak in the chromatogram obtained with solution (3) (3%), the area of any other *secondary peak* is not greater than the area of the principal peak in the chromatogram obtained with solution (3) (1%) and the sum of the areas of any such peaks is not greater than 6 times the area of the principal peak in the chromatogram obtained with solution (3) (6%). Disregard any peak with an area less than the area of the principal peak in the chromatogram obtained with solution (4) (0.05%).

ASSAY

Carry out the method for *liquid chromatography*, Appendix III D, using the following solutions. For solution (1) disperse a quantity of the oral paste in *methanol* with the aid of ultrasound and add sufficient *methanol* to produce a solution containing 0.04% w/v of Ivermectin. Solution (2) contains 0.04% w/v of *ivermectin EPCRS* in *methanol*. Inject 20 µl of each solution.

The chromatographic conditions described under Related substances may be used.

Calculate the content of ivermectin $(H_2B_{1a} + H_2B_{1b})$ in the oral paste and the ratio $H_2B_{1a} / (H_2B_{1a} + H_2B_{1b})$ using as the declared content the contents of $C_{48}H_{74}O_{14}$ (H_2B_{1a}) and $C_{47}H_{72}O_{14}$ (H_2B_{1b}) in *ivermectin EPCRS*.

Ivermectin Pour-on

Action and use
Antihelminthic.

DEFINITION

Ivermectin Pour-on is a *pour-on solution*. It contains Ivermectin in a suitable non-aqueous vehicle.

The pour-on complies with the requirements stated under Veterinary Liquid Preparations for Cutaneous Application and with the following requirements.

Content of ivermectin, calculated as the sum of component H_2B_{1a} ($C_{48}H_{74}O_{14}$) and component H_2B_{1b} ($C_{47}H_{72}O_{14}$)
95.0 to 105.0% of the stated amount.
The ratio of the contents $H_2B_{1a} / (H_2B_{1a} + H_2B_{1b})$ is at least 90.0%.

IDENTIFICATION

A. Carry out the method for *thin-layer chromatography*, Appendix III A, using a silica gel 60 F_{254} precoated plate (Merck silica gel 60 F_{254} plates are suitable) and a mixture of 1 volume of *concentrated ammonia R1*, 9 volumes of *methanol* and 90 volumes of *dichloromethane* as the mobile phase. Apply separately to the plate 2 µl of each of the following solutions. For solution (1) dissolve a quantity of the preparation being examined in sufficient *methanol* to produce a solution containing 0.05% w/v of Ivermectin. Solution (2) contains 0.05% w/v of *ivermectin EPCRS* in *methanol*. After removal of the plate, allow it to dry in air and examine under *ultraviolet light (254 nm and 366 nm)*. The principal spot in the chromatogram obtained with solution (1) is similar in position, colour and size to that in the chromatogram obtained with solution (2).

B. In the Assay, the chromatogram obtained with solution (1) shows two principal peaks with retention times similar to those of the two principal peaks in the chromatogram obtained with solution (2).

TESTS
Related substances
Carry out the method for *liquid chromatography*, Appendix III D, using the following solutions.
For solution (1) dissolve a quantity of the preparation being examined in sufficient *methanol* to produce a solution containing 0.04% w/v of Ivermectin. Solutions (2), (3) and (4) contain 0.04% w/v, 0.0004% w/v and 0.00002% w/v respectively of *ivermectin EPCRS* in *methanol*. Inject 20 µl of each solution.

The chromatographic procedure may be carried out using (a) a stainless steel column (25 cm × 4.6 mm) packed with *octadecylsilyl silica gel for chromatography* (5 µm) (Apex ODS 1 is suitable), (b) as the mobile phase at a flow rate of 1.5 ml per minute a mixture of 39 volumes of *water*, 55 volumes of *methanol* and 106 volumes of *acetonitrile* and (c) a detection wavelength of 245 nm.

The test is not valid unless, in the chromatogram obtained with solution (2), the *resolution factor* between the first peak

(component H_2B_{1b}) and the second peak (component H_2B_{1a}) is at least 3.0.

In the chromatogram obtained with solution (1) the area of any peak with a retention time of 1.3 to 1.5 relative to that of the principal peak is not greater than 2.7 times the area of the principal peak in the chromatogram obtained with solution (3) (2.7%), the area of any other *secondary peak* is not greater than the area of the principal peak in the chromatogram obtained with solution (3) (1%) and the sum of the areas of any such peaks is not greater than 6 times the area of the principal peak in the chromatogram obtained with solution (3) (6%). Disregard any peak with an area less than the area of the principal peak in the chromatogram obtained with solution (4) (0.05%).

ASSAY
Carry out the method for *liquid chromatography*, Appendix III D, using the following solutions.
For solution (1) dissolve a quantity of the preparation being examined in sufficient *methanol* to produce a solution containing 0.04% w/v of Ivermectin. Solution (2) contains 0.04% w/v of *ivermectin EPCRS* in *methanol*. Inject 20 µl of each solution.

The chromatographic conditions described under Related substances may be used.

Calculate the content of ivermectin $(H_2B_{1a} + H_2B_{1b})$ in the preparation being examined and the ratio $H_2B_{1a} / (H_2B_{1a} + H_2B_{1b})$ using as the declared content the contents of $C_{48}H_{74}O_{14}$ (H_2B_{1a}) and $C_{47}H_{72}O_{14}$ (H_2B_{1b}) in *ivermectin EPCRS*.

Kaolin Veterinary Oral Suspension

DEFINITION
Kaolin Veterinary Oral Suspension is a suspension containing 20% w/v of Light Kaolin or Light Kaolin (Natural) and 5% w/v each of Light Magnesium Carbonate and Sodium Bicarbonate in a suitable basis.

It should be freshly prepared unless the kaolin has been sterilised in which case it may be recently prepared.

Extemporaneous preparation
The following formula and directions apply.

Light Kaolin or Light Kaolin (Natural)	200 g
Light Magnesium Carbonate	50 g
Sodium Bicarbonate	50 g
Water	Sufficient to produce 1000 ml

The oral suspension complies with the requirements stated under Oral Liquids *and with the following requirements.*

Content of magnesium, Mg
1.04 to 1.25% w/w.

Content of sodium bicarbonate, $NaHCO_3$
4.05 to 4.65% w/w.

TESTS
Acid-insoluble matter
13.8 to 18.4% w/w, when determined by the following method. To 3 g add 15 ml of *water* and make acid to *blue litmus paper* by the cautious addition of 2M *hydrochloric acid*. Boil for 5 minutes, replacing water lost by evaporation, cool and decant the supernatant layer through a suitable filter. Boil the residue with 20 ml of *water* and 10 ml of 2M *hydrochloric acid*, cool, filter through the same filter and wash the residue with *water* until the washings are free from

chloride, reserving the filtrate and washings for the Assay for magnesium. Dry and ignite the residue to constant weight at red heat.

ASSAY

For magnesium

Dilute the combined filtrate and washings reserved in the determination of Acid-insoluble matter to 100 ml with *water*. To 20 ml of the resulting solution add 0.1 g of L-*ascorbic acid*, make slightly alkaline to *red litmus paper* with 5M *ammonia* and add 10 ml of *triethanolamine*, 10 ml of *ammonia buffer pH 10.9* and 1 ml of *potassium cyanide solution*. Titrate with 0.05M *disodium edetate VS* to a full blue colour using *mordant black 11 solution* as indicator. Each ml of 0.05M *disodium edetate VS* is equivalent to 1.215 mg of Mg.

For sodium bicarbonate

Boil 10 g with 100 ml of *water* for 5 minutes and filter. Boil the residue with 100 ml of *water* for 5 minutes and filter. Cool the combined filtrates and titrate with 0.5M *hydrochloric acid VS* using *methyl orange-xylene cyanol FF solution* as indicator. Add 10 ml of *ammonia buffer pH 10.9* and titrate with 0.05M *disodium edetate VS* using *mordant black 11 solution* as indicator. Each ml of 0.5M *hydrochloric acid VS*, after subtracting one fifth of the volume of 0.05M *disodium edetate VS*, is equivalent to 42.00 mg of $NaHCO_3$.

Kaolin Veterinary Oral Suspension contains, in 1 ml, 200 mg of Light Kaolin or Light Kaolin (Natural).

Levamisole Injection

Action and use

Immunostimulant; antihelminthic.

DEFINITION

Levamisole Injection is a sterile solution of Levamisole Hydrochloride in Water for Injections. It may contain suitable colouring matter.

The injection complies with the requirements stated under Parenteral Preparations and with the following requirements.

Content of levamisole hydrochloride, $C_{11}H_{12}N_2S,HCl$

92.5 to 107.5% of the stated amount.

IDENTIFICATION

A. Carry out the method for *thin-layer chromatography*, Appendix III A, using *silica gel G* as the coating substance and a mixture of 100 volumes of *ethyl acetate*, 10 volumes of *methanol* and 1 volume of 13.5M *ammonia* as the mobile phase. Apply separately to the plate 1 μl of each of the following solutions in *methanol*. For solution (1) dilute a volume of the injection to produce a solution containing 1% w/v of Levamisole Hydrochloride. Solution (2) contains 1% w/v of *levamisole hydrochloride BPCRS*. After removal of the plate, allow it to dry in air and spray with *potassium iodoplatinate solution*. The principal spot in the chromatogram obtained with solution (1) corresponds to that in the chromatogram obtained with solution (2).

B. Dilute a volume of the injection containing 0.75 g of Levamisole Hydrochloride to 20 ml with *water* and add 6 ml of 1M *sodium hydroxide*. Extract with 20 ml of *dichloromethane*, discard the aqueous layer and wash the dichloromethane layer with 10 ml of *water*. Shake with *anhydrous sodium sulphate*, filter and evaporate the dichloromethane at room temperature. The *melting point* of the residue, after drying

over *phosphorus pentoxide* at a pressure of 1.5 to 2.5 kPa at a temperature not exceeding 40°, is about 59°, Appendix V A.

C. The injection is laevorotatory.

D. Yields reaction B characteristic of *chlorides*, Appendix VI.

TESTS

Acidity

pH, 3.0 to 4.0, Appendix V L.

2,3-Dihydro-6-phenylimidazo[2,1-*b*]thiazole hydrochloride

Carry out the method for *thin-layer chromatography*, Appendix III A, using *silica gel G* as the coating substance and a mixture of 8 volumes of *glacial acetic acid*, 16 volumes of *methanol* and 90 volumes of *toluene* as the mobile phase. Apply separately to the plate 10 μl of each of the following two solutions. For solution (1) dilute a volume of the injection with *methanol* to produce a solution containing 5.0% w/v of Levamisole Hydrochloride. Solution (2) contains 0.021% w/v of *2,3-dihydro-6-phenylimidazo[2,1-b]thiazole BPCRS* in *methanol*. After removal of the plate, allow it to dry in air and spray with *potassium iodoplatinate solution*. Any spot in the chromatogram obtained with solution (1) corresponding to 2,3-dihydro-6-phenylimidazo[2,1-*b*]thiazole is not more intense than the spot in the chromatogram obtained with solution (2) (0.5%).

ASSAY

To a volume of the injection containing 0.75 g of Levamisole Hydrochloride add 50 ml of *water* and 15 ml of 2M *sodium hydroxide*, extract with three quantities, of 25, 20 and 15 ml, of *chloroform* and wash the combined extracts with two 10 ml quantities of *water*. To the combined extracts add 50 ml of *anhydrous acetic acid* and carry out Method I for *non-aqueous titration*, Appendix VIII A, using *1-naphtholbenzein solution* as indicator. Each ml of 0.1M *perchloric acid VS* is equivalent to 24.08 mg of $C_{11}H_{12}N_2S,HCl$.

STORAGE

Levamisole Injection should be protected from light.

Levamisole Oral Solution

Action and use

Immunostimulant; antihelminthic.

DEFINITION

Levamisole Oral Solution is an aqueous solution of Levamisole Hydrochloride.

The oral solution complies with the requirements stated under Oral Liquids and with the following requirements.

Content of levamisole hydrochloride, $C_{11}H_{12}N_2S,HCl$

92.5 to 107.5% of the stated amount.

IDENTIFICATION

A. Carry out the method for *thin-layer chromatography*, Appendix III A, using *silica gel G* as the coating substance and a mixture of 1 volume of 13.5M *ammonia*, 10 volumes of *methanol* and 100 volumes of *ethyl acetate* as the mobile phase. Apply separately to the plate 1 μl of each of the following solutions. For solution (1) dilute a volume of the oral solution with *methanol* to produce a solution containing 1% w/v of Levamisole Hydrochloride. Solution (2) contains 1% w/v of *levamisole hydrochloride BPCRS* in *methanol*. After removal of the plate, allow it to dry in air and spray with *potassium iodoplatinate solution*. The principal spot in the chromatogram obtained with solution (1) corresponds to that in the chromatogram obtained with solution (2).

B. To a quantity of the oral solution containing 0.3 g of Levamisole Hydrochloride add 10 ml of *water* and 6 ml of 1M *sodium hydroxide*. Extract with 20 ml of *dichloromethane*, discard the aqueous layer and wash the dichloromethane layer with 10 ml of *water*. Shake with *anhydrous sodium sulphate*, filter and evaporate the dichloromethane at room temperature. The *melting point* of the residue, after drying over *phosphorus pentoxide* at a pressure of 1.5 to 2.5 kPa at a temperature not exceeding 40°, is about 59°, Appendix V A.

C. The oral solution is laevorotatory.

2,3-Dihydro-6-phenylimidazo[2,1-*b*]thiazole hydrochloride

Carry out the method for *thin-layer chromatography*, Appendix III A, using *silica gel G* as the coating substance and a mixture of 8 volumes of *glacial acetic acid*, 16 volumes of *methanol* and 90 volumes of *toluene* as the mobile phase. Apply separately to the plate 50 μl of solution (1) and 10 μl of solution (2). For solution (1) dilute a volume of the oral solution to produce a solution containing 1.0% w/v of Levamisole Hydrochloride. Solution (2) contains 0.021% w/v of *2,3-dihydro-6-phenylimidazo[2,1-b]thiazole BPCRS* in *methanol*. After removal of the plate, allow it to dry in air and spray with *potassium iodoplatinate solution*. Any spot in the chromatogram obtained with solution (1) corresponding to 2,3-dihydro-6-phenylimidazo[2,1-*b*]thiazole is not more intense than the spot in the chromatogram obtained with solution (2) (0.5%).

ASSAY

To a volume of the oral solution containing 0.75 g of Levamisole Hydrochloride add 15 ml of 2M *sodium hydroxide*, extract with three quantities, of 25 ml, 20 ml and 15 ml, of *chloroform*, wash the combined extracts with two 10 ml quantities of *water* and discard the washings. To the clear chloroform solution, after drying with *anhydrous sodium sulphate* if necessary, add 50 ml of *anhydrous acetic acid*. Carry out Method I for *non-aqueous titration*, Appendix VIII A, using *1-naphtholbenzein solution* as indicator. Each ml of 0.1M *perchloric acid VS* is equivalent to 24.08 mg of $C_{11}H_{12}N_2S,HCl$.

Lincomycin Premix

Action and use
Lincosamide antibacterial.

DEFINITION
Lincomycin Premix contains Lincomycin Hydrochloride.

The premix complies with the requirements stated under Premixes and with the following requirements.

Content of lincomycin, $C_{18}H_{34}N_2O_6S$
90.0 to 105.0% of the stated amount.

IDENTIFICATION
In the Assay the chromatogram obtained with solution (2) shows a peak with the same retention time as the peak due to the trimethylsilyl derivative of lincomycin in the chromatogram obtained with solution (1).

Lincomycin B
Examine solution (3) as described in the Assay but increasing the sensitivity by eight to ten times while recording the peak due to the trimethylsilyl derivative of lincomycin B, which is

eluted immediately before the trimethylsilyl derivative of lincomycin. The area of the peak due to the trimethylsilyl derivative of lincomycin B, when corrected for the sensitivity factor, is not more than 5% of the area of the peak due to the trimethylsilyl derivative of lincomycin.

ASSAY
Carry out the method for *gas chromatography*, Appendix III B, using the following solutions. For solution (1) add 10 ml of a 0.8% w/w solution of *dotriacontane* (internal standard) in *chloroform* to 0.1 g of *lincomycin hydrochloride EPCRS*, dilute to 100 ml with a 2% w/v solution of *imidazole* in *chloroform*, shake to dissolve and filter. Place 4 ml of the filtrate in a 15 ml ground-glass-stoppered centrifuge tube, add 1 ml of a mixture of 99 volumes of N,O-*bis(trimethylsilyl)acetamide* and 1 volume of *trimethylchlorosilane* and swirl gently. Loosen the glass stopper and heat at 65° for 30 minutes. Prepare solution (2) in the same manner as solution (1) but omitting the internal standard and using a quantity of the premix containing the equivalent of 90 mg of lincomycin in place of the *lincomycin hydrochloride EPCRS*. Prepare solution (3) in the same manner as solution (1) but using a quantity of the premix containing the equivalent of 90 mg of lincomycin in place of the lincomycin hydrochloride EPCRS.

The chromatographic procedure may be carried out using a glass column (1.5 m × 3 mm) packed with *acid-washed silanised diatomaceous support* impregnated with 3% w/w of phenyl methyl silicone fluid (50% phenyl) (OV-17 is suitable) and maintained at 260° with both the inlet port and the detector at 260° to 290° and using *helium* as the carrier gas with a flow rate of 45 ml per minute.

Calculate the content of $C_{18}H_{34}N_2O_6S$ using the declared content of $C_{18}H_{34}N_2O_6S$ in *lincomycin hydrochloride EPCRS*.

LABELLING
The quantity of the active ingredient is stated in terms of the equivalent amount of lincomycin.

Lincomycin Tablets

Action and use
Lincosamide antibacterial.

DEFINITION
Lincomycin Tablets contains Lincomycin Hydrochloride.

The tablets comply with the requirements stated under Tablets and with the following requirements.

Content of lincomycin, $C_{18}H_{34}N_2O_6S$
90.0 to 105.0% of the stated amount.

IDENTIFICATION
A. Mix a quantity of the powdered tablets containing the equivalent of 200 mg of lincomycin with 5 ml of a mixture of 4 volumes of *chloroform* and 1 volume of *methanol*, filter and evaporate the filtrate. Dissolve the oily residue in 1 ml of *water*, add *acetone* until precipitation begins and add a further 20 ml of *acetone*. Filter, wash with two 10-ml quantities of *acetone*, dissolve the residue in the chloroform-methanol mixture, evaporate to dryness and dry at 60° at a pressure of 2 kPa for 1 hour. The *infrared absorption spectrum* of the residue, Appendix II A, is concordant with the *reference spectrum* of lincomycin hydrochloride (*RSV 52*).

B. In the Assay, the chromatogram obtained with solution (2) shows a peak with the same retention time as the peak due to the trimethylsilyl derivative of lincomycin in the chromatogram obtained with solution (1).

Lincomycin B

Examine solution (3) as described under the Assay but increasing the sensitivity by eight to ten times while recording the peak due to the trimethylsilyl derivative of lincomycin B, which is eluted immediately before the trimethylsilyl derivative of lincomycin. The area of the peak due to the trimethylsilyl derivative of lincomycin B, when corrected for the sensitivity factor, is not more than 5% of the area of the peak due to the trimethylsilyl derivative of lincomycin.

ASSAY

Carry out the Assay described under Lincomycin Premix but using in the preparation of solutions (2) and (3) a quantity of powdered tablets containing the equivalent of 90 mg of lincomycin in place of a quantity of the premix containing the equivalent of 90 mg of lincomycin.

LABELLING

The quantity of the active ingredient is stated in terms of the equivalent amount of lincomycin.

Meclofenamic Acid Granules

Action and use

Cyclo-oxygenase inhibitor; analgesic; anti-inflammatory.

DEFINITION

Meclofenamic Acid Granules contain Meclofenamic Acid mixed with suitable diluents.

The granules comply with the requirements stated under Granules and with the following requirements.

Content of meclofenamic acid, $C_{14}H_{11}Cl_2NO_2$

95.0 to 105.0% of the stated amount.

IDENTIFICATION

A. Shake a quantity of the powdered granules containing 0.2 g of Meclofenamic Acid with 50 ml of *ether*, filter and evaporate the filtrate to dryness. The *infrared absorption spectrum* of the residue, Appendix II A, is concordant with the *reference spectrum* of meclofenamic acid *(RSV 26)*.

B. To 5 ml of the clear supernatant liquid obtained in the Assay add sufficient 0.1M *sodium hydroxide* to produce 50 ml and mix. The *light absorption* of the resulting solution, Appendix II B, in the range 230 to 350 nm exhibits two maxima, at 279 nm and 317 nm.

C. Dissolve about 25 mg of the residue obtained in test A in 15 ml of *chloroform*. The solution exhibits a strong blue fluorescence when examined under ultraviolet light.

D. Dissolve about 1 mg of the residue obtained in test A in 2 ml of *sulphuric acid* and add 0.05 ml of 0.02M *potassium dichromate*. An intense purple colour is produced which rapidly fades to purplish brown.

Related substances

Carry out the method for *liquid chromatography*, Appendix III D, using the following solutions. Solution (1) contains 0.0035% w/v of *ethyl meclofenamate BPCRS* (internal standard) in *absolute ethanol*. For solution (2) shake a quantity of the powdered granules containing 20 mg of Meclofenamic Acid with 40 ml of *ether* for 20 minutes, filter, evaporate the filtrate to dryness and dissolve the residue in 2.0 ml of *ethanol (96%)*, warming if necessary. Prepare solution (3) in a similar manner, but dissolve the residue in

2.0 ml of *ethanol (96%)* containing 0.0035% w/v of the internal standard.

The chromatographic procedure may be carried out using (a) a stainless steel column (20 cm × 4 mm) packed with *octadecylsilyl silica gel for chromatography* (10 μm) (Spherisorb ODS 1 is suitable), (b) a mixture of 1 volume of *glacial acetic acid*, 25 volumes of *water* and 75 volumes of *methanol* as the mobile phase with a flow rate of 2 ml per minute and (c) a detection wavelength of 254 nm.

The test is not valid unless the *column efficiency* is at least 4500 theoretical plates per metre, determined using the peak due to the internal standard in the chromatogram obtained with solution (1).

In the chromatogram obtained with solution (3) the area of the peak immediately preceding the peak due to meclofenamic acid is not greater than one-seventh of the area of the peak due to the internal standard (0.05% of 2,6-dichloro-3-methylaniline). The area of any other *secondary peak* is not greater than the area of the peak due to the internal standard (0.35%).

ASSAY

Shake a quantity of the powdered granules containing 25 mg of Meclofenamic Acid with 150 ml of a mixture of 1 volume of 1M *hydrochloric acid* and 100 volumes of *methanol* for 15 minutes, dilute to 200 ml with the same solvent mixture, centrifuge and dilute 10 ml of the clear supernatant liquid to 100 ml with the same solvent mixture. Measure the *absorbance* of the resulting solution at the maximum at 335 nm, Appendix II B. Calculate the content of $C_{14}H_{11}Cl_2NO_2$ taking 235 as the value of A(1%, 1 cm) at the maximum at 335 nm.

STORAGE

Meclofenamic Acid Granules should be stored in a dry place.

Meloxicam Oral Suspension

Action and use

Cyclo-oxygenase inhibitor; analgesic; anti-inflammatory.

DEFINITION

Meloxicam Oral Suspension is a suspension of Meloxicam in a suitable vehicle.

The oral suspension complies with the requirements stated under Oral Liquids and with the following requirements.

Content of meloxicam, $C_{14}H_{13}N_3O_4S_2$

95.0 to 105.0% of the stated amount.

IDENTIFICATION

A. Carry out the method for *thin-layer chromatography*, Appendix III A, using a silica gel F_{254} high-performance precoated plate (Merck silica gel 60 F_{254} HPTLC plates are suitable) and a mixture of 1 volume of 13.5M *ammonia*, 20 volumes of *methanol* and 80 volumes of *dichloromethane* as the mobile phase but allowing the solvent front to ascend 8 cm above the line of application. Apply separately to the plate 5 μl of each of the following solutions. For solution (1) dilute a quantity of the oral suspension containing 3 mg of Meloxicam to 10 ml with *acetone*, stir for 10 minutes, filter and use the filtrate. For solution (2) dissolve 3 mg of *meloxicam BPCRS* in about 5 ml of *acetone*, add 0.5 ml of *water* and dilute to 10 ml with *acetone*. After removal of the plate, allow it to dry in air and examine under *ultraviolet light (254 and 365 nm)*. By each method of visualisation the principal spot in the chromatogram obtained with solution (1) is similar in position, colour and size to that in the chromatogram obtained with solution (2).

B. Disperse a quantity of the oral suspension containing 1.5 mg of Meloxicam in 5 ml of 0.1M *sodium hydroxide*, dilute to 100 ml with *methanol* and filter. The *light absorption* of the filtrate, Appendix II B, in the range 340 to 450 nm exhibits a maximum at 362 nm.

ASSAY

Carry out the method for *liquid chromatography*, Appendix III D, using the following solutions.

For solution (1) mix a quantity of the oral suspension containing 15 mg of Meloxicam with sufficient of the mobile phase to produce 50 ml, stir for 30 minutes and filter. Solution (2) contains 0.03% w/v of *meloxicam BPCRS* in the mobile phase.

The chromatographic procedure may be carried out using (a) a stainless steel column (10 cm × 4 mm) packed with *octadecylsilyl silica gel for chromatography* (10 μm) (Nucleosil C18 is suitable) and a pre-column 1-cm long packed with the same material both maintained at 40°, (b) as the mobile phase a mixture of 35 volumes of a mixture containing 10 parts of *propan-2-ol* and 65 parts of *methanol* and 65 volumes of a 0.2% w/v solution of *diammonium hydrogen orthophosphate* previously adjusted to pH 7.0 with *orthophosphoric acid* with a flow rate of 0.8 ml per minute and (c) a detection wavelength of 254 nm. Inject 10 μl of each solution and continue the chromatography for twice the retention time of the principal peak.

Determine the *weight per ml* of the oral suspension, Appendix V G, and calculate the content of $C_{14}H_{13}N_3O_4S_2$, weight in volume, from the declared content of $C_{14}H_{13}N_3O_4S_2$ in *meloxicam BPCRS*.

Mepivacaine Injection

Action and use
Local anaesthetic.

DEFINITION
Mepivacaine Injection is a sterile solution of Mepivacaine Hydrochloride in Water for Injections.

The injection complies with the requirements stated under Parenteral Preparations and with the following requirements.

Content of mepivacaine hydrochloride, $C_{15}H_{22}N_2O_2$,HCl
95.0 to 105.0% of the stated amount.

IDENTIFICATION
A. Carry out the method for *thin-layer chromatography*, Appendix III A, using a *TLC silica gel F_{254} plate* and a mixture of 1 volume of 13.5M *ammonia*, 5 volumes of *methanol* and 100 volumes of *ether* as the mobile phase, but allowing the solvent front to ascend 12 cm above the line of application. Apply separately to the plate 10 μl of each of the following solutions. For solution (1) dilute a quantity of the injection with sufficient *ethanol (96%)* to produce a solution containing 0.4% w/v of Mepivacaine Hydrochloride. Solution (2) contains 0.4% w/v of *mepivacaine hydrochloride BPCRS* in *ethanol (96%)*. Solution (3) contains 0.4% w/v of each of *mepivacaine hydrochloride BPCRS* and *lidocaine hydrochloride EPCRS* in *ethanol (96%)*. After removal of the plate, allow it to dry in air and examine under

ultraviolet light (254 nm). The principal spot in the chromatogram obtained with solution (1) is similar in position and size to the principal spot in the chromatogram obtained with solution (2). The test is not valid unless the chromatogram obtained with solution (3) shows two clearly separated principal spots.

B. In the Assay, the chromatogram obtained with solution (1) shows a peak with the same retention time as the principal peak in the chromatogram obtained with solution (2).

TESTS
Acidity
pH, 4.5 to 6.0, Appendix V L.

2,6-Dimethylaniline
Carry out the method for *liquid chromatography*, Appendix III D, using the following solutions.

For solution (1) dilute a quantity of the injection containing 0.1 g of Mepivacaine Hydrochloride to 100 ml with the mobile phase. Solution (2) contains 0.0002% w/v of *2,6-dimethylaniline* in the mobile phase.

The chromatographic procedure described under Assay may be used.

In the chromatogram obtained with solution (1) the area of any peak corresponding to 2,6-dimethylaniline is not greater than the area of the principal peak in the chromatogram obtained with solution (2) (0.2% of the content of mepivacaine hydrochloride).

ASSAY
Carry out the method for *liquid chromatography*, Appendix III D, using the following solutions.

For solution (1) dilute a quantity of the injection containing 0.1 g of Mepivacaine Hydrochloride to 100 ml with the mobile phase and dilute 1 volume of this solution to 20 volumes with the mobile phase. Solution (2) contains 0.005% w/v of *mepivacaine hydrochloride BPCRS* in the mobile phase.

The chromatographic procedure may be carried out using (a) a stainless steel column (25 cm × 3.2 mm) packed with *octadecylsilyl silica gel for chromatography* (5 μm) (Spherisorb ODS 1 is suitable), (b) as the mobile phase with a flow rate of 0.5 ml per minute a mixture of 1 volume of *triethylamine*, 400 volumes of *acetonitrile* and 600 volumes of a 0.2% w/v solution of *potassium dihydrogen orthophosphate*, the mixture adjusted to pH 4.0 with *orthophosphoric acid* and (c) a detection wavelength of 212 nm.

Calculate the content of $C_{15}H_{22}N_2O_2$,HCl in the injection using the declared content of $C_{15}H_{22}N_2O_2$,HCl in *mepivacaine hydrochloride BPCRS*.

Methyltestosterone Tablets

Action and use
Anabolic steroid.

DEFINITION
Methyltestosterone Tablets contain Methyltestosterone.

The tablets comply with the requirements stated under Tablets and with the following requirements.

Content of methyltestosterone, $C_{20}H_{30}O_2$
90.0 to 110.0% of the stated amount.

IDENTIFICATION

Shake a quantity of the powdered tablets containing 25 mg of Methyltestosterone with 50 ml of *chloroform* for 20 minutes, filter and evaporate the filtrate to dryness. The residue complies with the following tests.

A. The *infrared absorption spectrum*, Appendix II A, is concordant with the *reference spectrum* of methyltestosterone (RSV 28).

B. Complies with the test for *identification of steroids*, Appendix III A, using *impregnating solvent II* and *mobile phase D*.

Disintegration

Maximum time, 60 minutes, Appendix XII A1.

ASSAY

Weigh and powder 20 tablets. To a quantity of the powdered tablets containing 5 mg of Methyltestosterone, add sufficient *chloroform* to produce 50 ml, shake for 20 minutes, allow to settle and centrifuge in a stoppered tube. Evaporate 5 ml of the supernatant liquid to dryness, dissolve the residue in 2 ml of *aldehyde-free ethanol (96%)*, add 10 ml of a hot, freshly prepared and filtered 0.25% w/v solution of 2,4-*dinitrophenylhydrazine* in 2M *hydrochloric acid*, mix gently and heat on a water bath for 30 minutes, taking precautions against loss of liquid by evaporation. Cool, allow to stand overnight, filter through a sintered glass filter (ISO 4793, porosity grade 4, is suitable), wash the precipitate in succession with 50 ml of 2M *hydrochloric acid* and 50 ml of *water*, dry at 105° for 30 minutes and dissolve in sufficient *chloroform* to produce 100 ml. Measure the *absorbance* of the resulting solution at the maximum at 390 nm, Appendix II B, using in the reference cell a solution obtained by treating 2 ml of *aldehyde-free ethanol (96%)* in the same manner beginning at the words 'add 10 ml...'. Calculate the content of $C_{20}H_{30}O_2$ from the *absorbance* obtained by repeating the operation using a suitable quantity of *methyltestosterone EPCRS*.

STORAGE

Methyltestosterone Tablets should be protected from light.

Metronidazole Sterile Solution

Action and use

Imidazole antibacterial.

DEFINITION

Metronidazole Sterile Solution is a sterile solution of Metronidazole in Water for Injections.

The sterile solution complies with the requirements stated under Parenteral Preparations and with the following requirements.

Content of metronidazole, $C_6H_9N_3O_3$

95.0 to 110.0% of the stated amount.

CHARACTERISTICS

An almost colourless to pale yellow solution.

IDENTIFICATION

Shake a volume of the sterile solution containing 0.1 g of Metronidazole with 9 g of *sodium chloride* for 5 minutes, add 20 ml of *acetone*, shake for a further 5 minutes and allow to separate. Evaporate the upper layer to dryness. The *infrared absorption spectrum* of the residue, Appendix II A, is concordant with the *reference spectrum* of metronidazole (RSV 29).

TESTS

Acidity

pH, 4.5 to 6.0, Appendix V L.

Related substances

Carry out the method for *liquid chromatography*, Appendix III D, using the following solutions. Solution (1) contains 0.00050% w/v of 2-*methyl-5-nitroimidazole BPCRS* in the mobile phase. For solution (2) dilute a suitable volume of the sterile solution with sufficient mobile phase to produce a solution containing 0.1% w/v of Metronidazole. Solution (3) contains 0.00050% w/v of 2-*methyl-5-nitroimidazole BPCRS* in solution (2).

The chromatographic procedure may be carried out using (a) a stainless steel column (20 cm × 4.6 mm) packed with *octadecylsilyl silica gel for chromatography* (10 μm) (Spherisorb ODS 1 is suitable), (b) a mixture of 30 volumes of *methanol* and 70 volumes of 0.01M *potassium dihydrogen orthophosphate* as the mobile phase with a flow rate of 1 ml per minute and (c) a detection wavelength of 315 nm. Record the chromatograms for 3 times the retention time of the principal peak in the chromatogram obtained with solution (2).

Adjust the sensitivity so that the height of the peak due to 2-methyl-5-nitroimidazole in the chromatogram obtained with solution (3) is about 50% of full-scale deflection. Measure the height (*a*) of the peak due to 2-methyl-5-nitroimidazole and the height (*b*) of the lowest part of the curve separating this peak from the principal peak. The test is not valid unless *a* is greater than 10*b*.

In the chromatogram obtained with solution (2) the area of any *secondary peak* is not greater than the area of the peak due to 2-methyl-5-nitroimidazole in the chromatogram obtained with solution (1) (0.5%).

Nitrite

To a volume of the sterile solution containing 2.5 mg of Metronidazole add 40 ml of *water*, 2 ml of *sulphanilic acid solution*, 2 ml of *aminonaphthalenesulphonic acid solution* and sufficient *water* to produce 50 ml. Allow to stand at room temperature for 1 hour. Measure the *absorbance* of the resulting solution at the maximum at 524 nm, Appendix II B, using in the reference cell a solution prepared by treating 1 ml of *water* in the same manner, beginning at the words 'add 40 ml of *water*...'. The *absorbance* is not greater than that obtained by repeating the procedure using 1 ml of *nitrite standard solution (20 ppm)* treated at the same time and in the same manner, beginning at the words 'add 40 ml of *water*...' (0.8%, calculated with reference to the content of metronidazole).

ASSAY

Dilute a volume of the solution containing 50 mg of Metronidazole to 100 ml with 0.1M *hydrochloric acid*. Dilute 10 ml of the resulting solution to 250 ml with 0.1M *hydrochloric acid* and measure the *absorbance* of the resulting solution at the maximum at 277 nm, Appendix II B. Calculate the content of $C_6H_9N_3O_3$ taking 375 as the value of A(1%, 1 cm) at the maximum at 277 nm.

STORAGE

Metronidazole Sterile Solution should be protected from light.

LABELLING

The label states that solutions containing visible solid particles must not be used.

Metronidazole Sterile Suspension

Action and use
Imidazole antibacterial.

DEFINITION
Metronidazole Sterile Suspension is a sterile suspension of Metronidazole in Water for Injections. It is prepared by suspending Metronidazole for Injection in the requisite amount of Water for Injections immediately before use.

The sterile suspension complies with the requirements stated under Parenteral Preparations.

STORAGE
Metronidazole Sterile Suspension should be used immediately after preparation but in any case within the period recommended by the manufacturer when prepared and stored strictly in accordance with the manufacturer's instructions.

METRONIDAZOLE FOR INJECTION

DEFINITION
Metronidazole for Injection is a sterile material consisting of Metronidazole with or without excipients. It is supplied in a sealed container.

The contents of the sealed container comply with the requirements for Powders for Injections stated under Parenteral Preparations and with the following requirements.

Content of metronidazole, $C_6H_9N_3O_3$
95.0 to 105.0% of the stated amount.

IDENTIFICATION
Shake a quantity of the contents of a sealed container containing 0.1 g of Metronidazole with 40 ml of *chloroform* for 15 minutes, filter and evaporate the filtrate to dryness. The *infrared absorption spectrum* of the residue, Appendix II A, is concordant with the *reference spectrum* of metronidazole (RSV 29).

Related substances
Complies with the test described under Metronidazole Sterile Solution but preparing solution (2) in the following manner. Shake a quantity of the contents of a sealed container containing 0.1 g of Metronidazole with 40 ml of *chloroform* for 15 minutes, filter, evaporate the filtrate to dryness and dissolve the residue in 100 ml of the mobile phase.

ASSAY
Dissolve a quantity of the contents of a sealed container containing 50 mg of Metronidazole in sufficient 0.1M *hydrochloric acid* to produce 100 ml. Dilute 10 ml of the resulting solution to 250 ml with 0.1M *hydrochloric acid* and measure the *absorbance* of the resulting solution at the maximum at 277 nm, Appendix II B. Calculate the content of $C_6H_9N_3O_3$ taking 375 as the value of A(1%, 1 cm) at the maximum at 277 nm.

STORAGE
The sealed container should be protected from light.

Nandrolone Laurate Injection

Action and use
Anabolic steroid; androgen.

DEFINITION
Nandrolone Laurate Injection is a sterile solution of Nandrolone Laurate in Ethyl Oleate, or other suitable ester, in a suitable fixed oil or in any mixture of these.

The injection complies with the requirements stated under Parenteral Preparations and with the following requirements.

Content of nandrolone laurate, $C_{30}H_{48}O_3$
92.5 to 107.5% of the stated amount.

IDENTIFICATION
Carry out the method for *thin-layer chromatography*, Appendix III A, using a silica gel F_{254} precoated plate the surface of which has been modified by chemically-bonded octadecylsilyl groups (Whatman KC 18F plates are suitable) and a mixture of 20 volumes of *water*, 40 volumes of *acetonitrile* and 60 volumes of *propan-2-ol* as the mobile phase. Apply separately to the plate 5 µl of each of the following solutions. For solution (1) dilute the injection with *chloroform* to produce a solution containing 0.5% w/v of Nandrolone Laurate. Solution (2) contains 0.5% w/v of *nandrolone laurate BPCRS* in chloroform. For solution (3) mix equal volumes of solutions (1) and (2). After removal of the plate, allow it to dry in air until the solvent has evaporated and heat at 100° for 10 minutes. Allow to cool and examine under *ultraviolet light (254 nm)*. The principal spot in the chromatogram obtained with solution (1) corresponds to that in the chromatogram obtained with solution (2). The principal spot in the chromatogram obtained with solution (3) appears as a single, compact spot.

ASSAY
To a volume containing 0.1 g of Nandrolone Laurate add sufficient *chloroform* to produce 100 ml. Dilute 3 ml to 50 ml with *chloroform*. To 5 ml add 10 ml of *isoniazid solution* and sufficient *methanol* to produce 20 ml. Allow to stand for 45 minutes and measure the *absorbance* of the resulting solution at the maximum at 380 nm, Appendix II B, using as the reference solution 5 ml of *chloroform* treated in the same manner. Calculate the content of $C_{30}H_{48}O_3$ from the absorbance obtained by repeating the operation using a suitable quantity of *nandrolone BPCRS* and from the declared content of $C_{18}H_{26}O_2$ in *nandrolone BPCRS*. Each mg of $C_{18}H_{26}O_2$ is equivalent to 1.664 mg of $C_{30}H_{48}O_3$.

STORAGE
Nandrolone Laurate Injection should be protected from light.

Nitroxinil Injection

Action and use
Antihelminthic.

DEFINITION
Nitroxinil Injection is a sterile solution of the N-ethylglucamine salt of Nitroxinil in Water for Injections.

The injection complies with the requirements stated under Parenteral Preparations and with the following requirements.

Content of nitroxinil, $C_7H_3IN_2O_3$
95.0 to 105.0% of the stated amount.

IDENTIFICATION

A. The *light absorption*, Appendix II B, in the range 240 to 350 nm of the solution obtained in the Assay exhibits a maximum only at 271 nm.

B. Heat 0.5 ml with 3 ml of *sulphuric acid*; iodine vapour is evolved.

TESTS

Acidity or alkalinity

pH, 5.0 to 7.0, Appendix V L, determined using a 20% w/v solution of N-*ethylglucamine hydrochloride BPCRS* in place of a saturated solution of *potassium chloride* as the liquid junction solution.

Inorganic iodide

Dilute a volume containing 0.4 g of Nitroxinil to 100 ml with *water*. To 10 ml add 4 ml of 1M *sulphuric acid* and extract with three 10 ml quantities of *chloroform*. Add to the aqueous extract 1 ml of *hydrogen peroxide solution (100 vol)* and 1 ml of *chloroform*, shake for 2 minutes and allow to separate. Any purple colour produced in the chloroform layer is not more intense than that obtained in a solution prepared in the following manner. Add 2 ml of a 0.0026% w/v solution of *potassium iodide* to a mixture of 4 ml of 1M *sulphuric acid* and 8 ml of *water*, add 10 ml of *chloroform*, shake for 2 minutes, add to the aqueous layer 1 ml of *hydrogen peroxide solution (100 vol)* and 1 ml of *chloroform*, shake for 2 minutes and allow to separate (0.1% w/v of iodide).

ASSAY

To a volume containing 1.7 g of Nitroxinil add sufficient 0.01M *sodium hydroxide* to produce 500 ml and dilute 20 ml of this solution to 500 ml with 0.01M *sodium hydroxide*. To 5 ml of this solution add sufficient 0.01M *sodium hydroxide* to produce 100 ml and measure the *absorbance* of the resulting solution at the maximum at 271 nm, Appendix II B. Calculate the content of $C_7H_3IN_2O_3$ taking 660 as the value of A(1%, 1 cm) at the maximum at 271 nm.

STORAGE

Nitroxinil Injection should be protected from light.

Oxfendazole Oral Suspension

Action and use

Antihelminthic.

DEFINITION

Oxfendazole Oral Suspension is an aqueous suspension of Oxfendazole.

The oral suspension complies with the requirements stated under Oral Liquids and with the following requirements.

Content of oxfendazole, $C_{15}H_{13}N_3O_3S$

90.0 to 110.0% of the stated amount.

IDENTIFICATION

Shake a quantity of the oral suspension containing 0.1 g of Oxfendazole with 50 ml of *methanol* for 15 minutes, centrifuge, evaporate the supernatant liquid to a volume of about 2 ml, cool and filter. Wash the residue with a little *water* and dry at 105° at a pressure not exceeding 2.7 kPa for 1 hour. The residue complies with the following tests.

A. The *infrared absorption spectrum*, Appendix II A, is concordant with the *reference spectrum* of oxfendazole *(RSV 32)*.

B. The *light absorption*, Appendix II B, in the range 220 to 350 nm of a 0.001% w/v solution in 1M *hydrochloric acid* exhibits three maxima, at 226, 284 and 291 nm.

TESTS

Acidity

pH, 4.3 to 5.3, Appendix V L.

Related substances

Carry out the method for *thin-layer chromatography*, Appendix III A, using *silica gel G* as the coating substance and a mixture of 5 volumes of *glacial acetic acid* and 95 volumes of *ethyl acetate* as the mobile phase. Apply separately to the plate 20 μl of each of the following solutions. For solution (1) shake a quantity of the oral suspension containing 0.1 g of Oxfendazole with 20 ml of a mixture of 4 volumes of *ethyl acetate* and 1 volume of *glacial acetic acid* and filter. For solution (2) dilute 1 volume of solution (1) to 50 volumes with the same solvent mixture. Solution (3) contains 0.005% w/v of *fenbendazole BPCRS*. After removal of the plate, allow it to dry in air and examine under *ultraviolet light (254 nm)*. Any spot in the chromatogram obtained with solution (1) corresponding to methyl 5-phenylthio-1*H*-benzimidazol-2-ylcarbamate is not more intense than the spot in the chromatogram obtained with solution (3) (1%) and any other *secondary spot* is not more intense than the spot in the chromatogram obtained with solution (2) (2%).

ASSAY

Disperse a quantity of the well-mixed oral suspension containing 0.1 g of Oxfendazole in 15 ml of *water*. Add 200 ml of *methanol* and mix with the aid of ultrasound for 15 minutes, cool, add sufficient *methanol* to produce 500 ml and filter. Dilute 4 ml of the filtrate to 100 ml with *methanol* and measure the *absorbance* of the resulting solution at the maximum at 296 nm, Appendix II B. Calculate the content of $C_{15}H_{13}N_3O_3S$ taking 550 as the value of A(1%, 1 cm) at the maximum at 296 nm.

Oxyclozanide Oral Suspension

Action and use

Antihelminthic.

DEFINITION

Oxyclozanide Oral Suspension is an aqueous suspension of Oxyclozanide containing suitable suspending and dispersing agents.

The oral suspension complies with the requirements stated under Oral Liquids and with the following requirements.

Content of oxyclozanide, $C_{13}H_6Cl_5NO_3$

95.0 to 105.0% of the stated amount.

IDENTIFICATION

In test A for Related substances the principal spot in the chromatogram obtained with 10 μl of solution (1) corresponds to that in the chromatogram obtained with solution (3).

Related substances

A. Carry out the method for *thin-layer chromatography*, Appendix III A, using *silica gel G* as the coating substance and a mixture of 5 volumes of *glacial acetic acid*, 20 volumes of *acetone* and 60 volumes of *petroleum spirit (boiling range, 60° to 80°)* as the mobile phase. Apply separately to the plate 40 μl and 10 μl of solution (1), 4 μl of solution (2) and 10 μl of solution (3). For solution (1) dilute the oral suspension with *acetone* to contain 1.0% w/v of Oxyclozanide, centrifuge and use the supernatant liquid. Solution (2) contains 0.050% w/v of *3,5,6-trichloro-2-hydroxybenzoic acid BPCRS* in *acetone*. Solution (3) contains 1.0% w/v of *oxyclozanide BPCRS* in *acetone*. After removal of the plate, allow it to dry in air and spray with a 3.0% w/v solution of *iron(III) chloride hexahydrate* in *methanol*. In the chromatogram obtained with 40 µl of solution (1) any spot corresponding to 3,5,6-trichloro-2-hydroxybenzoic acid is not more intense than the spot in the chromatogram obtained with solution (2) (0.5%).

B. Carry out the method for *thin-layer chromatography*, Appendix III A, using *silica gel G* as the coating substance and a mixture of 1 volume of 13.5M *ammonia* as the mobile phase, 10 volumes of *methanol* and 100 volumes of *ethyl acetate*. Apply separately to the plate 40 µl of solution (1) and 4 µl of solution (2). For solution (1) dilute the oral suspension with *acetone* to contain 1.0% w/v of Oxyclozanide, centrifuge and use the supernatant liquid. Solution (2) contains 0.050% w/v of *2-amino-4,6-dichlorophenol hydrochloride BPCRS* in *acetone*. After removal of the plate, allow it to dry in air and spray with *phosphomolybdotungstic reagent* . In the chromatogram obtained with solution (1) any spot corresponding to 2-amino-4,6-dichlorophenol is not more intense than the spot in the chromatogram obtained with solution (2) (0.4%).

ASSAY

Protect the solutions from light throughout the Assay. To a quantity of the oral suspension containing 60 mg of Oxyclozanide add 60 ml of *acidified methanol* and boil gently on a water bath. Shake continuously for 20 minutes, cool to 2° and dilute to 100 ml with *acidified methanol*. Filter, dilute 5 ml of the filtrate to 100 ml with *acidified methanol* and measure the *absorbance* of the resulting solution at the maximum at 300 nm, Appendix II B. Calculate the content of $C_{13}H_6Cl_5NO_3$ taking 254 as the value of A(1%, 1 cm) at the maximum at 300 nm.

Oxytetracycline Injection

Action and use
Tetracycline antibacterial.

DEFINITION
Oxytetracycline Injection is a sterile solution of Oxytetracycline Hydrochloride in Water for Injections. It is prepared by dissolving Oxytetracycline Hydrochloride for Injection in the requisite amount of Water for Injections.

The injection complies with the requirements stated under Parenteral Preparations.

STORAGE
Oxytetracycline Injection should be used immediately after preparation but in any case within the period recommended by the manufacturer when prepared and stored strictly in accordance with the manufacturer's instructions.

OXYTETRACYCLINE HYDROCHLORIDE FOR INJECTION

DEFINITION
Oxytetracycline Hydrochloride for Injection is a sterile material consisting of Oxytetracycline Hydrochloride with or without excipients. It is supplied in a sealed container.

Content of oxytetracycline hydrochloride, $C_{22}H_{24}N_2O_9,HCl$
90.0 to 110.0% of the stated amount.

The contents of the sealed container comply with the requirements for Powders for Injections stated under Parenteral Preparations and with the following requirements.

IDENTIFICATION
A. Carry out the method for *thin-layer chromatography*, Appendix III A, using a silica gel precoated plate (Merck silica gel 60 plates are suitable) and a mixture of 6 volumes of *water*, 35 volumes of *methanol* and 59 volumes of *dichloromethane* as the mobile phase. Adjust the pH of a 10% w/v solution of *disodium edetate* to 7.0 with 10M *sodium hydroxide* and spray the solution evenly onto the plate (about 10 ml for a plate 100 mm × 200 mm). Allow the plate to dry in a horizontal position for at least 1 hour. Before use, dry the plate at 110° for 1 hour. Apply separately to the plate 1 µl of each of the following solutions. For solution (1) dissolve a quantity of the contents of a sealed container in sufficient *methanol* to produce a solution containing 0.05% w/v of Oxytetracycline Hydrochloride. Solution (2) contains 0.05% w/v of *oxytetracycline hydrochloride EPCRS* in *methanol*. Solution (3) contains 0.05% w/v of each of *oxytetracycline hydrochloride EPCRS* and *demeclocycline hydrochloride EPCRS* in *methanol*. After removal of the plate, dry it in a current of air and examine under *ultraviolet light (365 nm)*. The principal spot in the chromatogram obtained with solution (1) is similar in position, colour and size to that in the chromatogram obtained with solution (2). The test is not valid unless the chromatogram obtained with solution (3) shows two clearly separated spots.

B. To 0.5 mg add 2 ml of *sulphuric acid*; a deep crimson colour is produced. Add the solution to 1 ml of *water*; the colour changes to yellow.

C. Yield the reactions characteristic of *chlorides*, Appendix VI.

TESTS
Acidity
pH of a solution containing 10% w/v of Oxytetracycline Hydrochloride, 2.0 to 3.0, Appendix V L.

Clarity and colour of solution
A solution containing 10.0% w/v of Oxytetracycline Hydrochloride is *clear*, Appendix IV A, and yellow.

Light-absorbing impurities
The *absorbance*, Appendix II B, at 430 nm of a solution in *methanol*, filtered if necessary, containing 0.2% w/v of Oxytetracycline Hydrochloride is not more than 0.75. The *absorbance* at 490 nm of a solution in *methanol* containing 1% w/v of Oxytetracycline Hydrochloride is not more than 0.40.

Pyrogens
Comply with the *test for pyrogens*, Appendix XIV D. Use per kg of the rabbit's weight 1 ml of a solution in *water for injections* containing 5 mg of Oxytetracycline Hydrochloride per ml.

ASSAY
Determine the weight of the contents of 10 containers as described in the test for Uniformity of weight under Parenteral Preparations, Powders for Injections.

Carry out the method for *liquid chromatography*, Appendix III D, using the following solutions.

For solution (1) dissolve a quantity of the mixed contents of the 10 containers in sufficient 0.01M *hydrochloric acid* to produce a solution containing 0.005% w/v of Oxytetracycline

Hydrochloride. Solution (2) contains 0.005% w/v of *oxytetracycline EPCRS* in the same solvent. Solution (3) contains 0.1% w/v of *4-epioxytetracycline EPCRS* in the same solvent. Solution (4) contains 0.1% w/v of *tetracycline hydrochloride EPCRS* in the same solvent. For solution (5) dilute a mixture containing 1.5 ml of a 0.1% w/v solution of *oxytetracycline EPCRS* in 0.01M *hydrochloric acid*, 1 ml of solution (3) and 3 ml of solution (4) to 25 ml with the same solvent.

The chromatographic procedure may be carried out using (a) a column (25 cm × 4.6 mm) packed with *styrene-divinylbenzene copolymer* (8 to 10 μm) (Polymer Laboratories, PLRP-S 100A, is suitable) and maintained at 60°, (b) as the mobile phase with a flow rate of 1 ml per minute a solution prepared as described below and (c) a detection wavelength of 254 nm. To 50.0 g of *2-methylpropan-2-ol* add 200 ml of *water*, 60 ml of *0.33M phosphate buffer pH 7.5*, 50 ml of a 1.0% w/v solution of *tetrabutylammonium hydrogen sulphate* previously adjusted to pH 7.5 with 2M *sodium hydroxide* and 10 ml of a 0.04% w/v solution of *disodium edetate* previously adjusted to pH 7.5 with 2M *sodium hydroxide* and dilute to 1 litre with *water*.

Inject solution (5). The assay is not valid unless (a) the *resolution factor* between the first peak (4-epioxytetracycline) and the second peak (oxytetracycline) is at least 4.0, (b) the *resolution factor* between the second peak and the third peak (tetracycline) is at least 5.0 (if necessary reduce the content of 2-methylpropan-2-ol in the mobile phase to increase the resolution) and (c) the *symmetry factor* of the peak due to oxytetracycline is not more than 1.25.

Calculate the content of $C_{22}H_{24}N_2O_9,HCl$ in a container of average content weight using the declared content of $C_{22}H_{24}N_2O_9$ in *oxytetracycline EPCRS*. Each mg of $C_{22}H_{24}N_2O_9$ is equivalent to 1.079 mg of $C_{22}H_{24}N_2O_9,HCl$.

STORAGE
The sealed container should be protected from light.

LABELLING
The label states that the contents are to be used for intravenous injection only, in a well-diluted solution.

Oxytetracycline Intramammary Infusion (Lactating Cow)

Action and use
Tetracycline antibacterial.

DEFINITION
Oxytetracycline Intramammary Infusion (Lactating Cow) is a sterile preparation containing Oxytetracycline Hydrochloride. It is presented either as a sterile solution of Oxytetracycline Hydrochloride complexed with magnesium in a suitable vehicle or as a sterile suspension of Oxytetracycline Hydrochloride in a suitable vehicle. The vehicle may contain suitable suspending and dispersing agents.

The intramammary infusion complies with the requirements stated under Intramammary Infusions and with the following requirements.

Content of oxytetracycline hydrochloride, $C_{22}H_{24}N_2O_9,HCl$
90.0 to 115.0% of the stated amount.

IDENTIFICATION
A. Complies with test A for Identification described under Oxytetracycline Injection using the following solution as solution (1).

For infusions that are solutions of Oxytetracycline Hydrochloride complexed with magnesium Dilute a quantity of the infusion with sufficient *methanol* to produce a solution containing 0.05% w/v of Oxytetracycline Hydrochloride.

For infusions that are suspensions of Oxytetracycline Hydrochloride Stir a quantity of the infusion containing 10 mg of Oxytetracycline Hydrochloride with 10 ml of *petroleum spirit (boiling range, 100° to 120°)*, allow to settle and remove the petroleum spirit by decantation. Dissolve the residue in 20 ml of *methanol*.

B. To 0.5 ml add 0.1 ml of *sulphuric acid*; a deep red colour is produced. Add the solution to 1 ml of *water*; the colour changes to yellow.

C. *For infusions that are solutions of Oxytetracycline Hydrochloride complexed with magnesium* Dilute the infusion with *water* to produce a solution containing 1.0% w/v of Oxytetracycline Hydrochloride. The solution yields reaction A characteristic of *chlorides*, Appendix VI.

For infusions that are suspensions of Oxytetracycline Hydrochloride Stir a quantity of the infusion containing 50 mg of Oxytetracycline Hydrochloride with 5 ml of *petroleum spirit (boiling range, 100° to 120°)*, allow to settle and remove the petroleum spirit by decantation. Dissolve the residue in 10 ml of *water* and filter. The filtrate yields reaction A characteristic of *chlorides*, Appendix VI.

ASSAY
Express, as far as possible, weigh and mix the contents of 10 containers. Carry out the method for *liquid chromatography*, Appendix III D, using the following solutions.

For infusions that are solutions of Oxytetracycline Hydrochloride complexed with magnesium Prepare solution (1) in the following manner. To a quantity of the mixed contents of the 10 containers containing 0.1 g of Oxytetracycline Hydrochloride add 20 ml of 0.1M methanolic hydrochloric acid, prepared by diluting 1 volume of 1M *hydrochloric acid* to 10 volumes with *methanol*, mix and dilute to 200 ml with the same solvent. Centrifuge and dilute 1 volume of the supernatant liquid to 10 volumes with the same solvent.

For infusions that are suspensions of Oxytetracycline Hydrochloride Prepare solution (1) in the following manner. Disperse a quantity of the mixed contents of the 10 containers containing 0.1 g of Oxytetracycline Hydrochloride in 10 ml of *petroleum spirit (boiling range, 60° to 80°)* and extract with two 10 ml quantities of 0.1M *hydrochloric acid*. Filter the extracts and add sufficient 0.1M methanolic hydrochloric acid, prepared by diluting 1 volume of 1M *hydrochloric acid* to 10 volumes with *methanol*, to produce 200 ml. Centrifuge and dilute 1 volume of the supernatant liquid to 10 volumes with the same solvent.

For solution (2) dissolve 50 mg of *oxytetracycline EPCRS* in 10 ml of 0.1M methanolic hydrochloric acid, prepared by diluting 1 volume of 1M *hydrochloric acid* to 10 volumes with *methanol*, and add sufficient of the same solvent to produce 100 ml. Dilute 1 volume to 10 volumes with the same solvent. Solution (3) contains 0.1% w/v of *4-epioxytetracycline EPCRS* in 0.1M methanolic hydrochloric acid. Solution (4) contains 0.1% w/v of *tetracycline hydrochloride EPCRS* in 0.1M methanolic hydrochloric acid. For solution (5) dilute a mixture containing 3 ml of a 0.05% w/v solution of *oxytetracycline EPCRS* in

0.1M methanolic hydrochloric acid, 1 ml of solution (3) and 3 ml of solution (4) to 25 ml with the same solvent.

The chromatographic procedure may be carried out using (a) a column (25 cm × 4.6 mm) packed with *styrene-divinylbenzene copolymer* (8 to 10 μm) (Polymer Laboratories, PLRP-S 100A, is suitable) and maintained at 60°, (b) as the mobile phase with a flow rate of 1 ml per minute a solution prepared as described below and (c) a detection wavelength of 254 nm. To 50.0 g of *2-methylpropan-2-ol* add 200 ml of *water*, 60 ml of *0.33M phosphate buffer pH 7.5*, 50 ml of a 1.0% w/v solution of *tetrabutylammonium hydrogen sulphate* previously adjusted to pH 7.5 with 2M *sodium hydroxide* and 10 ml of a 0.04% w/v solution of *disodium edetate* previously adjusted to pH 7.5 with 2M *sodium hydroxide* and dilute to 1 litre with *water*.

Inject solution (5). The assay is not valid unless (a) the *resolution factor* between the first peak (4-epioxytetracycline) and the second peak (oxytetracycline) is at least 4.0, (b) the *resolution factor* between the second peak and the third peak (tetracycline) is at least 5.0 (if necessary reduce the content of 2-methylpropan-2-ol in the mobile phase to increase the resolution) and (c) the *symmetry factor* of the peak due to oxytetracycline is not more than 1.25.

Calculate the content of $C_{22}H_{24}N_2O_9$,HCl using the declared content of $C_{22}H_{24}N_2O_9$ in *oxytetracycline EPCRS*. Each mg of $C_{22}H_{24}N_2O_9$ is equivalent to 1.079 mg of $C_{22}H_{24}N_2O_9$,HCl.

LABELLING

The label states whether the infusion is a solution of Oxytetracycline Hydrochloride complexed with magnesium or a suspension of Oxytetracycline Hydrochloride.

Oxytetracycline Veterinary Oral Powder

Action and use
Tetracycline antibacterial.

DEFINITION

Oxytetracycline Veterinary Oral Powder is a mixture of Oxytetracycline Hydrochloride and Lactose or other suitable diluent.

Content of oxytetracycline hydrochloride, $C_{22}H_{24}N_2O_9$,HCl
90.0 to 110.0% of the stated amount.

The veterinary oral powder complies with the requirements under Veterinary Oral Powders and with the following requirements.

IDENTIFICATION

A. Complies with test A for Identification described under Oxytetracycline Injection but using a solution prepared in the following manner as solution (1). Extract a quantity of the oral powder containing 10 mg of Oxytetracycline Hydrochloride with 20 ml of *methanol*, centrifuge and use the supernatant liquid.

B. To a quantity of the powder containing 0.4 mg of Oxytetracycline Hydrochloride add 5 ml of a 1% w/v solution of *sodium carbonate*, shake and add 2 ml of *diazobenzenesulphonic acid solution*. A light brown colour is produced.

C. Shake a quantity of the powder containing 0.1 g of Oxytetracycline Hydrochloride with 10 ml of 2M *nitric acid* and filter. Decolourise the filtrate with *activated charcoal* and

filter again. The filtrate yields the reactions characteristic of *chlorides*, Appendix VI.

ASSAY

Carry out the method for *liquid chromatography*, Appendix III D, using the following solutions. For solution (1) dissolve a quantity of the oral powder in sufficient 0.01M *hydrochloric acid* to produce a solution containing 0.005% w/v of Oxytetracycline Hydrochloride. Solution (2) contains 0.005% w/v of *oxytetracycline EPCRS* in 0.01M *hydrochloric acid*. Solution (3) contains 0.1% w/v of *4-epioxytetracycline EPCRS* in the same solvent. Solution (4) contains 0.1% w/v of *tetracycline hydrochloride EPCRS* in the same solvent. For solution (5) dilute a mixture containing 1.5 ml of a 0.1% w/v solution of *oxytetracycline EPCRS* in 0.01M *hydrochloric acid*, 1 ml of solution (3) and 3 ml of solution (4) to 25 ml with the same solvent.

The chromatographic procedure may be carried out using (a) a column (25 cm × 4.6 mm) packed with *styrene-divinylbenzene copolymer* (8 to 10 μm) (Polymer Laboratories, PLRP-S 100A, is suitable) and maintained at 60°, (b) as the mobile phase with a flow rate of 1 ml per minute a solution prepared as described below and (c) a detection wavelength of 254 nm. To 50.0 g of *2-methylpropan-2-ol* add 200 ml of *water*, 60 ml of *0.33M phosphate buffer pH 7.5*, 50 ml of a 1.0% w/v solution of *tetrabutylammonium hydrogen sulphate* previously adjusted to pH 7.5 with 2M *sodium hydroxide* and 10 ml of a 0.04% w/v solution of *disodium edetate* previously adjusted to pH 7.5 with 2M *sodium hydroxide* and dilute to 1 litre with *water*.

Inject solution (5). The assay is not valid unless (a) the *resolution factor* between the first peak (4-epioxytetracycline) and the second peak (oxytetracycline) is at least 4.0, (b) the *resolution factor* between the second peak and the third peak (tetracycline) is at least 5.0 (if necessary reduce the content of 2-methylpropan-2-ol in the mobile phase to increase the resolution) and (c) the *symmetry factor* of the peak due to oxytetracycline is not more than 1.25.

Calculate the content of $C_{22}H_{24}N_2O_9$,HCl using the declared content of $C_{22}H_{24}N_2O_9$ in *oxytetracycline EPCRS*. Each mg of $C_{22}H_{24}N_2O_9$ is equivalent to 1.079 mg of $C_{22}H_{24}N_2O_9$,HCl.

LABELLING

The label states the strength of the powder in terms of the concentration of Oxytetracycline Hydrochloride.

Pentobarbital Injection

Action and use
Barbiturate.

DEFINITION

Pentobarbital Injection is a sterile[1] solution of Pentobarbital Sodium in a suitable vehicle.

The injection complies with the requirements stated under Parenteral Preparations and with the following requirements.

Content of pentobarbital sodium, $C_{11}H_{17}N_2NaO_3$
95.0 to 105.0% of the stated amount.

CHARACTERISTICS

A clear, colourless or almost colourless solution.

IDENTIFICATION

A. The *infrared absorption spectrum* of the residue obtained in the Assay, Appendix II A, is concordant with the *reference spectrum* of pentobarbital *(RSV 34)*.

B. *Melting point* of the residue obtained in the Assay, about 128°, Appendix V A.

C. When introduced on a platinum wire into the flame of a Bunsen burner, imparts a yellow colour to the flame.

TESTS
Alkalinity
pH, 10.0 to 11.5, Appendix V L.

Isomer
To a volume containing 0.3 g of Pentobarbital Sodium diluted, if necessary, to 5 ml with *water*, add 0.3 g of *4-nitrobenzyl bromide* dissolved in 10 ml of *ethanol (96%)* and heat under a reflux condenser for 30 minutes. Cool to 25°, filter, wash the residue with four 5 ml quantities of *water* and transfer as completely as possible to a small flask. Add 25 ml of *ethanol (96%)* and heat under a reflux condenser for 10 minutes. The residue, after drying at 105° for 30 minutes, melts completely between 136° and 155°.

ASSAY
To a volume containing 0.5 g of Pentobarbital Sodium diluted to 15 ml with *water* add 5 ml of 2M *hydrochloric acid*, extract with 50 ml of *ether* and then with successive 25 ml quantities of *ether* until complete extraction is effected. Wash the combined extracts with two 5 ml quantities of *water* and wash the combined aqueous washings with 10 ml of *ether*. Add the ether to the main ether extract, evaporate to low volume, add 2 ml of *absolute ethanol*, evaporate to dryness and dry the residue to constant weight at 105°. Each g of residue is equivalent to 1.097 g of $C_{11}H_{17}N_2NaO_3$.

When pentobarbitone injection is prescribed or demanded, Pentobarbital Injection shall be dispensed or supplied.

---

[1] Solutions containing 20% w/v of Pentobarbital Sodium in 100 ml and 500 ml quantities are also available for purposes other than injection; such solutions are not necessarily sterile but comply with all the other requirements of the monograph; they may be coloured.

Phenylbutazone Tablets

Action and use
Cyclo-oxygenase inhibitor; pyrazolone analgesic.

DEFINITION
Phenylbutazone Tablets contain Phenylbutazone. They are coated.

The tablets comply with the requirements stated under Tablets and with the following requirements.

Content of phenylbutazone, $C_{19}H_{20}N_2O_2$
95.0 to 105.0% of the stated amount.

IDENTIFICATION
Extract a quantity of the powdered tablets containing 0.2 g of Phenylbutazone with 40 ml of warm *acetone*, filter and evaporate the filtrate to dryness. The residue complies with the following tests.

A. The *infrared absorption spectrum*, Appendix II A, is concordant with the *reference spectrum* of phenylbutazone *(RSV 35)*.

B. To 0.1 g of the residue add 1 ml of *glacial acetic acid* and 2 ml of *hydrochloric acid* and heat on a water bath for 30 minutes. Cool, add 10 ml of *water* and filter. Add to the filtrate 3 ml of 0.1M *sodium nitrite*; a yellow colour is produced. Add 1 ml of this solution to 5 ml of *2-naphthol solution*; a brownish red precipitate is produced which dissolves on the addition of *ethanol (96%)* yielding a red solution.

TESTS
Dissolution
Comply with the requirements for Monographs of the British Pharmacopoeia in the *dissolution test for tablets and capsules*, Appendix XII B1, using as the medium 900 ml of a 0.68% w/v solution of *potassium dihydrogen orthophosphate* adjusted to pH 7.5 by the addition of 1M *sodium hydroxide* and rotating the basket at 100 revolutions per minute. Withdraw a sample of 10 ml of the medium. Measure the *absorbance* of the filtered sample, if necessary suitably diluted, at the maximum at 264 nm using a layer of suitable thickness, Appendix II B.

Calculate the total content of phenylbutazone, $C_{19}H_{20}N_2O_2$, in the medium taking 653 as the value of A(1%, 1 cm) at the maximum at 264 nm.

Related substances
Carry out the method for *thin-layer chromatography*, Appendix III A, using a silica gel GF_{254} precoated plate (Machery Nagel plates are suitable) and as the mobile phase a mixture of 10 volumes of *glacial acetic acid*, 40 volumes of *cyclohexane* and 50 volumes of *chloroform* containing 0.02% v/v of *butylated hydroxytoluene*. Allow the solvent front to ascend 4 cm, remove the plate and dry it in a current of cold air. Without delay and in an atmosphere of carbon dioxide apply separately to the plate 3 µl of each of the following solutions. For solution (1) shake a quantity of the powdered tablets containing 0.1 g of Phenylbutazone with 3 ml of *chloroform* containing 0.02% w/v of *butylated hydroxytoluene*, centrifuge and use the supernatant liquid. For solution (2) dilute 1 volume of solution (1) with sufficient of the same solvent mixture to produce a solution containing of 0.5 mg Phenylbutazone per ml. Expose the plate to carbon dioxide for 2 minutes and develop, allowing the solvent front to ascend 10 cm above the line of application. After removal of the plate, allow it to dry in air and examine under *ultraviolet light (254 nm)*. Any *secondary spot* in the chromatogram obtained with solution (1) is not more intense than the spot in the chromatogram obtained with solution (2) (1.5%).

ASSAY
Weigh and powder 20 tablets. Extract a quantity of the powder containing 0.5 g of Phenylbutazone with successive 30-, 30-, 15- and 15 ml quantities of warm *acetone*. Filter the combined extracts, cool and titrate with 0.1M *sodium hydroxide VS* using *bromothymol blue solution R3* as indicator and continuing the titration until the blue colour persists for at least 30 seconds. Repeat the titration without the powdered tablets; the difference between the titrations represents the amount of alkali required by the phenylbutazone. Each ml of 0.1M *sodium hydroxide VS* is equivalent to 30.84 mg of $C_{19}H_{20}N_2O_2$.

Piperazine Adipate Tablets

Action and use
Antihelminthic.

DEFINITION
Piperazine Adipate Tablets contain Piperazine Adipate.

The tablets comply with the requirements stated under Tablets and with the following requirements.

Content of piperazine adipate, $C_4H_{10}N_2,C_6H_{10}O_4$
92.5 to 107.5% of the stated amount.

IDENTIFICATION
Extract a quantity of the powdered tablets containing 1 g of Piperazine Adipate with 20 ml of *water* and filter. The filtrate complies with the following tests.

A. Dilute 1 ml to 5 ml with *water*, add 0.5 g of *sodium hydrogen carbonate*, 0.5 ml of *potassium hexacyanoferrate(III) solution* and 0.1 ml of *mercury*, shake vigorously for 1 minute and allow to stand for 20 minutes. A reddish colour slowly develops.

B. To 10 ml add 5 ml of *hydrochloric acid* and extract with three 10 ml quantities of *ether*. Reserve the aqueous layer and evaporate the combined ether extracts to dryness. The *melting point* of the residue, after washing with a small volume of *water* and drying at 105°, is about 152°, Appendix V A.

C. Warm the aqueous layer reserved in test B to remove dissolved ether, cool in ice and add, with stirring, 2 ml of a 50% w/v solution of *sodium nitrite*. Cool in ice for 15 minutes, stirring if necessary to induce crystallisation. The *melting point* of the crystals, after washing with 10 ml of cold *water* and drying at 105°, is about 159°, Appendix V A, Method I.

Disintegration
Maximum time, 60 minutes, Appendix XII A1.

ASSAY
Weigh and powder 20 tablets. Shake a quantity of the powder containing 0.2 g of Piperazine Adipate for 1 hour with 10 ml of *water*, filter and wash the residue with two 10 ml quantities of *water*. To the combined extract and washings add 5 ml of 1M *sulphuric acid* and 50 ml of *picric acid solution R1*, bring to the boil, allow to stand for several hours, filter through a sintered-glass crucible and wash the residue with successive 10 ml quantities of a mixture of equal volumes of a saturated solution of *picric acid* and *water* until the washings are free from sulphate. Finally, wash with five 10 ml quantities, of *absolute ethanol* and dry the residue to constant weight at 105°. Each g of residue is equivalent to 0.4268 g of $C_4H_{10}N_2,C_6H_{10}O_4$.

Piperazine Citrate Tablets

Action and use
Antihelminthic.

DEFINITION
Piperazine Citrate Tablets contain Piperazine Citrate.

The tablets comply with the requirements stated under Tablets and with the following requirements.

Content of anhydrous piperazine citrate, $(C_4H_{10}N_2)_3,2C_6H_8O_7$
81.6 to 96.8% of the stated amount of Piperazine Citrate.

IDENTIFICATION
Extract a quantity of the powdered tablets containing 1 g of Piperazine Citrate with 20 ml of *water* and filter. The filtrate complies with the following tests.

A. Dilute 1 ml to 5 ml with *water*, add 0.5 g of *sodium hydrogen carbonate*, 0.5 ml of *potassium hexacyanoferrate(III) solution* and 0.1 ml of *mercury*, shake vigorously for 1 minute and allow to stand for 20 minutes; a reddish colour slowly develops.

B. Mix 4 ml with 1 ml of *hydrochloric acid*, add 0.5 g of *sodium nitrite*, heat to boiling, cool in ice for 15 minutes, scratching the side of the container with a glass rod to induce crystallisation and filter. The *melting point* of the crystals, after washing with 10 ml of iced *water* and drying at 100° to 105°, is about 159°, Appendix V A, Method I.

C. Yield the reactions characteristic of *citrates*, Appendix VI.

ASSAY
Weigh and powder 20 tablets. Dissolve as completely as possible a quantity of the powder containing 0.2 g of Piperazine Citrate in 10 ml of *water*, filter and wash the filter with three 5 ml quantities of *water*. To the combined filtrate and washings add 3.5 ml of 0.5M *sulphuric acid* and 100 ml of *picric acid solution R1*, heat on a water bath for 15 minutes, allow to stand for 1 hour, filter, wash the residue with *piperazine dipicrate solution* until the washings are free from sulphate and dry the residue to constant weight at 105°. Each g of residue is equivalent to 0.3935 g of $(C_4H_{10}N_2)_3,2C_6H_8O_7$.

STORAGE
Piperazine Citrate Tablets should be protected from light.

Procaine Benzylpenicillin Injection

Action and use
Penicillin antibacterial.

DEFINITION
Procaine Benzylpenicillin Injection is a sterile suspension of Procaine Benzylpenicillin in Water for Injections.

The injection complies with the requirements stated under Parenteral Preparations and with the following requirements.

Content of total penicillins, calculated as $C_{13}H_{20}N_2O_2,C_{16}H_{18}N_2O_4S, H_2O$
90.0 to 110.0% of the stated amount of Procaine Benzylpenicillin.

Content of procaine, $C_{13}H_{20}N_2O_2$
36.0 to 44.0% of the stated amount of Procaine Benzylpenicillin.

CHARACTERISTICS
A white suspension.

IDENTIFICATION
A. Dilute a volume of the well-shaken suspension containing 10 mg of Procaine Benzylpenicillin to 10 ml with *water* and add 0.5 ml of *neutral red solution*. Add sufficient 0.01M *sodium hydroxide* to produce a permanent orange colour and then add 1 ml of *penicillinase solution*. A red colour is produced rapidly.

B. Carry out the method for *thin-layer chromatography*, Appendix III A, using a *TLC silica gel silanised plate* (Merck silanised silica gel 60 plates are suitable) and a mixture of 30 volumes of *acetone* and 70 volumes of a 15.4% w/v solution of *ammonium acetate* adjusted to pH 7.0 with 10M *ammonia* as the mobile phase. Apply separately to the plate 1 μl of each of the following solutions. For solution (1) shake a volume of the well-shaken suspension containing 50 mg of Procaine Benzylpenicillin with 5 ml of *methanol*, add a small quantity of *water* to dissolve any residue and dilute to 10 ml with *water*. Solution (2) contains 0.5% w/v of *procaine benzylpenicillin BPCRS* in *acetone*. After removal of the plate, allow it to dry in air, expose to iodine vapour until spots appear and examine in daylight. The two principal spots in the chromatogram obtained with solution (1) are similar in position, colour and size to those in the chromatogram obtained with solution (2). The test is not valid unless the chromatogram obtained with solution (2) shows two clearly separated spots.

C. Yields the reaction characteristic of *primary aromatic amines*, Appendix VI, producing a bright orange-red precipitate.

TESTS

Related substances

Carry out the method for *liquid chromatography*, Appendix III D, using the following solutions. For solution (1) add to a quantity of the well-shaken suspension containing 70 mg of Procaine Benzylpenicillin sufficient mobile phase to produce 50 ml, mix, filter and use the filtrate. For solution (2) mix 1 ml of solution (1) and 1 ml of a 0.007% w/v solution of *4-aminobenzoic acid* and add sufficient mobile phase to produce 100 ml. For solution (3) dissolve 4 mg of *4-aminobenzoic acid* in 25 ml of a solution containing 0.070% w/v of *procaine benzylpenicillin BPCRS* in the mobile phase.

The chromatographic procedure may be carried out using (a) a stainless steel column (25 cm × 4.6 mm) packed with *octadecylsilylsilica gel for chromatography* (5 μm) (Lichrospher ODS is suitable), (b) as the mobile phase with a flow rate of 1.5 ml per minute a mixture prepared as described below and (c) a detection wavelength of 225 nm. Mix 250 volumes of *acetonitrile*, 250 volumes of water and 500 volumes of a freshly prepared solution containing 1.4% w/v of *potassium dihydrogen orthophosphate* and 0.65% w/v of *tetrabutylammonium hydroxide*, adjusted to pH 7.0 with 1M *potassium hydroxide*; adjust the pH of the mixture to 7.2 with 2M *orthophosphoric acid*, if necessary.

Inject solution (3). When the chromatogram is recorded in the prescribed conditions the substances elute in the following order: 4-aminobenzoic acid, procaine, benzylpenicillin. Adjust the sensitivity so that the height of the peak due to benzylpenicillin in the chromatogram obtained with solution (2) is at least 50% of the full scale of the recorder. For solution (1) allow the chromatography to proceed for 1.5 times the retention time of the peak due to benzylpenicillin.

The test is not valid unless, in the chromatogram obtained with solution (3), the *resolution factor* between the peaks due to 4-aminobenzoic acid and procaine is at least 2.0. If necessary, adjust the concentration of acetonitrile in the mobile phase.

In the chromatogram obtained with solution (1) the area of any peak due to 4-aminobenzoic acid is not greater than 10 times the area of the corresponding peak in the chromatogram obtained with solution (2) (0.5%) and the area of any other *secondary peak* is not greater than the area of the peak corresponding to benzylpenicillin in the chromatogram obtained with solution (2) (1%).

Bacterial endotoxins

Carry out the *test for bacterial endotoxins*, Appendix XIV C, Method C. Dilute a quantity of the well-shaken suspension, if necessary, with *water BET* to produce a solution containing 3 mg of Procaine Benzylpenicillin per ml (solution A). The endotoxin limit concentration of solution A is 0.3 IU per ml. Carry out the test using a suitable dilution of solution A as described under Method C.

ASSAY

Carry out the method for *liquid chromatography*, Appendix III D, using the following solutions. For solution (1) add to a quantity of the well-shaken suspension containing 70 mg of Procaine Benzylpenicillin sufficient mobile phase to produce 100 ml, mix, filter and use the filtrate. Solution (2) contains 0.07% w/v of *procaine benzylpenicillin BPCRS* in the mobile phase. For solution (3) dissolve 4 mg of *4-aminobenzoic acid* in 25 ml of solution (2).

The chromatographic procedure described under Related substances may be used.

Inject solution (3). When the chromatogram is recorded in the prescribed conditions the substances elute in the following order: 4-aminobenzoic acid, procaine, benzylpenicillin. Adjust the sensitivity so that the height of the peak corresponding to 4-aminobenzoic acid is at least 50% of the full scale of the recorder. The assay is not valid unless, in the chromatogram obtained, the *resolution factor* between the peaks due to 4-aminobenzoic acid and procaine is at least 2.0. If necessary, adjust the concentration of acetonitrile in the mobile phase.

Calculate the content of $C_{13}H_{20}N_2O_2$ and of $C_{13}H_{20}N_2O_2,C_{16}H_{18}N_2O_4S,H_2O$ in the injection from the chromatograms obtained and using the declared content of $C_{13}H_{20}N_2O_2$ and of $C_{13}H_{20}N_2O_2,C_{16}H_{18}N_2O_4S,H_2O$ in *procaine benzylpenicillin BPCRS*.

3 g of Procaine Benzylpenicillin is approximately equivalent to 2 g of benzylpenicillin.

Procaine Benzylpenicillin Intramammary Infusions

Action and use
Penicillin antibacterial.

DEFINITION
Procaine Benzylpenicillin Intramammary Infusions are sterile suspensions of Procaine Benzylpenicillin in suitable vehicles containing suitable suspending and dispersing agents appropriate to their use. Infusions intended for administration to lactating animals are described as Procaine Benzylpenicillin Intramammary Infusions (Lactating Cow) and infusions intended for administration to animals at the end of lactation to control infections during the dry period are described as Procaine Benzylpenicillin Intramammary Infusions (Dry Cow).

The intramammary infusions comply with the requirements stated under Intramammary Infusions and with the following requirements.

Content of total penicillins, calculated as $C_{13}H_{20}N_2O_2,C_{16}H_{18}N_2O_4S,H_2O$
90.0 to 120.0% of the stated amount of Procaine Benzylpenicillin.

IDENTIFICATION

Carry out the method for *thin-layer chromatography*, Appendix III A, using a *TLC silica gel silanised plate* (Merck silanised silica gel 60 plates are suitable) and a mixture of 30 volumes of *acetone* and 70 volumes of a 15.4% w/v solution of *ammonium acetate* adjusted to pH 7.0 with 10M *ammonia* as the mobile phase. Apply separately to the plate 1 µl of each of the following solutions. For solution (1) extract a quantity of the infusion containing the equivalent of 50 mg of Procaine Benzylpenicillin with three 15 ml quantities of *petroleum spirit (boiling range, 120° to 160°)*, discard the extracts, wash the residue with 5 ml of *ether* and dry in a current of air. Dissolve the residue in 10 ml of *acetone* and filter if necessary. Solution (2) contains 0.5% w/v of *procaine benzylpenicillin BPCRS* in *acetone*. After removal of the plate, allow it to dry in air, expose to iodine vapour until spots appear and examine in daylight. The two principal spots in the chromatogram obtained with solution (1) are similar in position, colour and size to those in the chromatogram obtained with solution (2). The test is not valid unless the chromatogram obtained with solution (2) shows two clearly separated spots.

TESTS

Related substances

Carry out the method for *liquid chromatography*, Appendix III D, using the following solutions. For solution (1) extract a quantity of the infusion containing 70 mg of Procaine Benzylpenicillin with three 15 ml quantities of *petroleum spirit (boiling range, 120° to 160°)*, discard the extracts, wash the residue with 5 ml of *ether* and dry in a current of air. Dissolve the residue in 50 ml of the mobile phase, mix, filter and use the filtrate. For solution (2) mix 1 ml of solution (1) and 1 ml of a 0.007% w/v solution of *4-aminobenzoic acid* and add sufficient mobile phase to produce 100 ml. For solution (3) dissolve 4 mg of *4-aminobenzoic acid* in 25 ml of a solution containing 0.070% w/v of *procaine benzylpenicillin BPCRS* in the mobile phase.

The chromatographic procedure may be carried out using (a) a stainless steel column (25 cm × 4.6 mm) packed with *octadecylsilyl silica gel for chromatography* (5 µm) (Lichrospher ODS is suitable), (b) as the mobile phase a mixture prepared as described below and (c) a detection wavelength of 225 nm. Mix 250 volumes of *acetonitrile*, 250 volumes of *water* and 500 volumes of a freshly prepared solution containing 1.4% w/v of *potassium dihydrogen orthophosphate* and 0.65% w/v of *tetrabutylammonium hydroxide*, adjusted to pH 7.0 with 1M *potassium hydroxide*; adjust the pH of the mixture to 7.2 with 2M *orthophosphoric acid* if necessary.

Adjust the sensitivity so that the height of the peak due to benzylpenicillin in the chromatogram obtained with solution (2) is at least 50% of the full scale of the recorder. Continue the chromatography for 1.5 times the retention time of the peak due to benzylpenicillin. The test is not valid unless, in the chromatogram obtained with solution (3), the *resolution factor* between the first peak (4-aminobenzoic acid) and the second peak (procaine) is at least 2.0. If necessary, adjust the concentration of acetonitrile in the mobile phase.

In the chromatogram obtained with solution (1) the area of any peak due to 4-aminobenzoic acid is not greater than 10 times the area of the corresponding peak in the chromatogram obtained with solution (2) (0.5%) and the area of any other *secondary peak* is not greater than the area

of the peak corresponding to benzylpenicillin in the chromatogram obtained with solution (2) (1%).

Water

Not more than 1.0% w/w, Appendix IX C. Use 3 g and a mixture of 70 volumes of *chloroform* and 30 volumes of *anhydrous methanol* as the solvent.

ASSAY

Express, as far as possible, weigh and mix the contents of 10 containers. Carry out the method for *liquid chromatography*, Appendix III D, using the following solutions. For solution (1) extract a quantity of the mixed contents of the 10 containers containing 70 mg of Procaine Benzylpenicillin with three 15 ml quantities of *petroleum spirit (boiling range, 120° to 160°)*, discard the extracts, wash the residue with 5 ml of *ether* and dry in a current of air. Dissolve the residue in 50 ml of the mobile phase, mix, filter and use the filtrate. Solution (2) contains 0.070% w/v of *procaine benzylpenicillin BPCRS* in the mobile phase. For solution (3) dissolve 4 mg of *4-aminobenzoic acid* in 25 ml of solution (2).

The chromatographic procedure described under Related substances may be used.

Inject solution (3). When the chromatogram is recorded in the prescribed conditions the substances elute in the following order: 4-aminobenzoic acid, procaine, benzylpenicillin. Adjust the sensitivity so that the height of the peak corresponding to 4-aminobenzoic acid is at least 50% of the full scale of the recorder. The Assay is not valid unless, in the chromatogram obtained, the *resolution factor* between 4-aminobenzoic acid and procaine is at least 2.0. If necessary, adjust the concentration of acetonitrile in the mobile phase.

Calculate the content of $C_{13}H_{20}N_2O_2,C_{16}H_{18}N_2O_4S,H_2O$ in the intramammary infusion using the declared content of $C_{13}H_{20}N_2O_2,C_{16}H_{18}N_2O_4S,H_2O$ in *procaine benzylpenicillin BPCRS*.

Pyrethrum Extract

DEFINITION

Pyrethrum Extract is prepared from Pyrethrum Flower.

Extemporaneous preparation

Exhaust Pyrethrum Flower, in *coarse powder*, by percolation with a suitable hydrocarbon solvent; remove the solvent and concentrate at a low temperature. The resulting product may be decolourised by a suitable procedure. Determine the proportion of pyrethrins in a portion of the extract by the Assay. To the remainder add, if necessary, sufficient Light Liquid Paraffin or deodorised kerosene of commerce to produce an extract of the required strength.

The extract complies with the requirements for Labelling stated under Extracts and with the following requirements.

Content of pyrethrins

24.5% to 25.5% w/w, of which not less than half consists of pyrethrin I.

CHARACTERISTICS

A dark olive green or brown viscous liquid or, if decolourised, a pale amber liquid.

ASSAY

Carry out the Assay described under Pyrethrum Dusting Powder using 0.5 g of the well-mixed extract and beginning at the words 'Add 20 ml of 0.5M *ethanolic potassium hydroxide* ...'.

If the pyrethrum extract is coloured, carry out the following preliminary treatment. Transfer 0.5 g of the well-mixed extract to a stoppered flask, add 50 ml of *aromatic-free petroleum spirit (boiling range, 40° to 60°)*, swirl, add 1 g of diatomaceous earth (Filtercel is suitable), swirl to mix completely, stopper the flask and allow to stand at 20° to 22° for 16 hours. Mix the contents of the flask thoroughly, filter with gentle suction through a sintered-glass filter (ISO 4793, porosity grade 4, is suitable) and wash the residue with five 10 ml quantities of *aromatic-free petroleum spirit (boiling range, 40° to 60°)*. Remove the solvent from the combined filtrate and washings and evaporate to a volume of 1 to 2 ml. Complete the Assay described under Pyrethrum Dusting Powder beginning at the words 'Add 20 ml of 0.5M *ethanolic potassium hydroxide*...'.

STORAGE

Pyrethrum Extract should be kept in a well-filled container, protected from light and should be thoroughly stirred before use.

Pyrethrum Dusting Powder

DEFINITION

Pyrethrum Dusting Powder contains 1.6% w/w of Pyrethrum Extract in a suitable diluent.

Extemporaneous preparation

The following formula and directions apply.

Pyrethrum Extract	16 g
Diatomite, of commerce, in *fine powder*	300 g
Purified Talc, in *fine powder*	684 g
Chloroform	A sufficient quantity

Dissolve the Pyrethrum Extract in the Chloroform and spray the solution on the diatomite and Purified Talc while mixing; sift and mix.

The dusting powder complies with the requirements stated under Topical Powders and with the following requirements.

Content of pyrethrins

0.36 to 0.44% w/w, of which not less than half consists of pyrethrin I.

Fineness

Complies with the requirement stated under Topical Powders using a sieve of nominal mesh aperture of 180 μm.

ASSAY

Extract 30 g with *petroleum spirit (boiling range, 40° to 60°)* in an apparatus for the *continuous extraction of drugs*, Appendix XI F, for 8 hours. Continue the extraction with a fresh quantity of the solvent for a further 4 hours. Combine the extracts and evaporate on a water bath until only the last traces of solvent remain. Add 20 ml of 0.5M *ethanolic potassium hydroxide* and boil under a reflux condenser for 45 minutes. Transfer the solution to a beaker and wash the flask with sufficient hot *water*, adding the washings to the beaker, to produce a total volume of 200 ml. Boil until the volume is reduced to 150 ml, cool rapidly and transfer the solution to a stoppered flask, washing the beaker with three 20 ml quantities of *water* and transferring any gummy residue to the flask. Add 1 g of diatomaceous earth (Filtercel is suitable) and 10 ml of *barium chloride solution*, swirl gently and add sufficient *water* to produce 250 ml. Stopper the flask, shake vigorously until the separating liquid is clear and

filter the suspension through a filter paper (Whatman No. 1 is suitable).

For pyrethrin I

Transfer 200 ml of the filtrate to a separating funnel, rinsing the measuring vessel with two 5 ml quantities of *water*, and add 0.05 ml of *phenolphthalein solution R1*. Neutralise the solution by the drop wise addition of *hydrochloric acid* and add 1 ml of *hydrochloric acid* in excess. Add 5 ml of a saturated solution of *sodium chloride* and 50 ml of *aromatic-free petroleum spirit (boiling range, 40° to 60°)*, shake vigorously for 1 minute, allow to separate, remove and retain the lower layer. Filter the petroleum spirit extract through absorbent cotton into a second separating funnel containing 10 ml of *water*. Return the aqueous layer to the first separating funnel and repeat the extraction with 50 ml and then with 25 ml of *aromatic-free petroleum spirit (boiling range, 40° to 60°)*, reserving the aqueous layer for the assay of pyrethrin II, and filtering the petroleum spirit extracts through the same absorbent cotton into the second separating funnel. Shake the combined petroleum spirit extracts and water for about 30 seconds and allow to separate; remove the lower layer and add it to the aqueous liquid reserved for the assay of pyrethrin II. Wash the combined petroleum spirit extracts with a further 10 ml of *water*, adding the washings to the reserved aqueous liquid.

To the petroleum spirit extracts add 5 ml of 0.1M *sodium hydroxide*, shake vigorously for 1 minute, allow to separate and remove the clear lower layer, washing the stem of the separating funnel with 1 ml of *water*. Repeat the extraction by shaking for about 30 seconds with two quantities of 2.5 ml and 1.5 ml of 0.1M *sodium hydroxide* and add the extracts to the alkaline extract. Add to the flask 10 ml of *mercury(II) sulphate solution*, stopper, swirl and allow to stand in the dark at 25° ± 0.5° for exactly 60 minutes after the addition of the mercury(II) sulphate solution. Add 20 ml of *acetone* and 3 ml of a saturated solution of *sodium chloride*, heat to boiling on a water bath, allow the precipitate to settle and decant the supernatant liquid through a filter paper (Whatman No. 1 is suitable), retaining most of the precipitate in the flask. Wash the precipitate with 10 ml of *acetone*, again boil, allow to settle and decant through the same filter paper. Repeat the washing and decanting with three 10 ml quantities of hot *chloroform*. Transfer the filter paper to the flask, add 50 ml of a cooled mixture of three volumes of *hydrochloric acid* and two volumes of *water*, 1 ml of *strong iodine monochloride reagent* and 6 ml of *chloroform*. Titrate with 0.01M *potassium iodate VS*, running almost all the required volume of titrant into the flask in one portion. Continue the titration, shaking the flask vigorously for 30 seconds after each addition of the titrant, until the chloroform is colourless. Repeat the operation without the extract; the difference between the titrations represents the amount of potassium iodate required. Each ml of 0.01M *potassium iodate VS* is equivalent to 5.7 mg of pyrethrin I.

For pyrethrin II

Transfer the combined aqueous liquids reserved in the Assay for pyrethrin I to a beaker, cover with a watch glass and evaporate to 50 ml within 35 to 45 minutes. Cool, washing the underside of the watch glass with not more than 5 ml of *water* and adding the washings to the beaker. Filter through absorbent cotton into a separating funnel, washing with successive quantities of 10, 7.5, 7.5, 5 and 5 ml of *water*. Saturate the aqueous liquid with *sodium chloride*, add 10 ml of *hydrochloric acid* and 50 ml of *ether*, shake for 1 minute, allow to separate, and remove the lower layer. Repeat the extraction successively with 50, 25 and 25 ml of *ether*. Wash the combined ether extracts with three 10 ml quantities of a saturated solution of *sodium chloride* and transfer the ether layer to a flask with the aid of 10 ml of *ether*. Remove the bulk of the ether by distillation and remove the remainder with a gentle current of air and dry the residue at 100° for 10 minutes, removing any residual acid fumes with a gentle current of air. Add 2 ml of *ethanol (96%)* previously neutralised to *phenolphthalein solution R1* and 0.05 ml of *phenolphthalein solution R1*, swirl to dissolve the residue, add 20 ml of *carbon dioxide-free water* and titrate rapidly with 0.02M *sodium hydroxide VS* until the colour changes to brownish pink and persists for 30 seconds, keeping the flask stoppered between additions of alkali. Repeat the operation using the aqueous liquid reserved for the repeat operation in the Assay for pyrethrin I. The difference between the titrations represents the volume of 0.02M *sodium hydroxide VS* required. Each ml of 0.02M *sodium hydroxide VS* is equivalent to 3.74 mg of pyrethrin II.

Compound Pyrethrum Spray

DEFINITION

Pyrethrum Extract	3.8 g
Piperonyl Butoxide	7.6 g
Deodorised kerosene of commerce	988.6 g

The spray complies with the requirements stated under Veterinary Liquid Preparations for Cutaneous Application and with the following requirements.

Content of piperonyl butoxide, $C_{19}H_{30}O_5$
0.57 to 0.72% w/w.

Content of pyrethrins
0.08 to 0.11% w/w, of which not less than half consists of pyrethrin I.

IDENTIFICATION
To 0.1 ml add 5 ml of *tannic acid reagent*, shake vigorously for 1 minute and heat on a water bath for 5 minutes. A blue colour is produced.

ASSAY
For piperonyl butoxide
Carry out the Assay described under Piperonyl Butoxide, using as solution (2) a mixture of 7 g of the spray in sufficient *chloroform* to produce 20 ml and as solution (3) 7 g of the spray and 40 mg of *tetraphenylethylene* (internal standard) dissolved in sufficient *chloroform* to produce 20 ml. Calculate the content of $C_{19}H_{30}O_5$ using the declared content of $C_{19}H_{30}O_5$ in *piperonyl butoxide CRS*.

For pyrethrins
Transfer 120 g to a conical flask, add 20 ml of 0.5M *ethanolic potassium hydroxide* and boil under a reflux condenser for 45 minutes. Transfer the contents of the flask to a beaker, rinse the flask with *water* and add the rinsings to the beaker. Dilute to about 200 ml with *water* and heat until the volume is reduced to about 150 ml, avoiding loss by frothing. Cool and transfer the contents of the beaker to a separating funnel, washing the beaker with three 20 ml quantities of *water* and adding the washings to the funnel. Allow to separate and transfer the lower aqueous layer to a stoppered flask. Wash the oil in the separating funnel with two 20 ml quantities of *water* and add the washings to the flask. Complete the Assay described under Pyrethrum Dusting Powder, beginning at the words 'Add 1 g of diatomaceous earth . . .'.

Sodium Calcium Edetate Intravenous Infusion for Veterinary Use

Action and use
Chelating agent.

DEFINITION
Sodium Calcium Edetate Intravenous Infusion for Veterinary Use is a sterile solution of Sodium Calcium Edetate. It is prepared immediately before use by diluting Sterile Sodium Calcium Edetate Concentrate for Veterinary Use with a suitable diluent in accordance with the manufacturer's instructions.

The intravenous infusion complies with the requirements stated under Parenteral Preparations and with the following requirement.

LABELLING
The strength is stated as the equivalent amount of anhydrous sodium calcium edetate in a suitable dose-volume.

STERILE SODIUM CALCIUM EDETATE CONCENTRATE FOR VETERINARY USE
DEFINITION
Sterile Sodium Calcium Edetate Concentrate for Veterinary Use is a sterile solution of Sodium Calcium Edetate in Water for Injections containing the equivalent of 25% w/v of anhydrous sodium calcium edetate.

The concentrate complies with the requirements for Concentrated Solutions for Injections stated under Parenteral Preparations and with the following requirements.

Content of anhydrous sodium calcium edetate, $C_{10}H_{12}CaN_2Na_2O_8$
22.5 to 27.5% w/v.

CHARACTERISTICS
A colourless solution.

IDENTIFICATION
A. Dilute 2.5 ml with 7.5 ml of *water*, make alkaline to *litmus paper* with 5M *ammonia* and add 5 ml of a 2.5% w/v solution of *ammonium oxalate*. Not more than a trace of precipitate is produced.

B. To 10 ml add 2 ml of a 10% w/v solution of *lead(II) nitrate*, shake and add 5 ml of *dilute potassium iodide solution*; no yellow precipitate is produced. Make alkaline to *litmus paper* with 5M *ammonia* and add 5 ml of a 2.5% w/v solution of *ammonium oxalate*; a white precipitate is produced.

C. Evaporate to dryness and ignite. The residue yields the reactions characteristic of *sodium salts* and of *calcium salts*, Appendix VI.

TESTS
Acidity or alkalinity
pH, 6.5 to 8.0, Appendix V L.

Pyrogens
Complies with the *test for pyrogens*, Appendix XIV D. Use 2 ml per kg of the rabbit's weight.

ASSAY
To 2.5 ml add 90 ml of *water*, 7 g of *hexamine* and 5 ml of 2M *hydrochloric acid* and titrate with 0.05M *lead nitrate VS* using *xylenol orange solution* as indicator. Each ml of 0.05M *lead nitrate VS* is equivalent to 18.71 mg of $C_{10}H_{12}CaN_2Na_2O_8$.

STORAGE
Sterile Sodium Calcium Edetate Concentrate for Veterinary Use should be kept in containers made from lead-free glass.

LABELLING
The label states (1) 'Sterile Sodium Calcium Edetate Concentrate for Veterinary Use'; (2) that the solution must be diluted with Sodium Chloride Intravenous Infusion or Glucose Intravenous Infusion before administration.

Sulfadimidine Injection

Action and use
Sulfonamide antibacterial.

DEFINITION
Sulfadimidine Injection is a sterile solution of sulfadimidine sodium in Water for Injections free from dissolved air. It is prepared by the interaction of Sulfadimidine and Sodium Hydroxide.

The injection complies with the requirements stated under Parenteral Preparations and with the following requirements.

Content of sulfadimidine sodium, $C_{12}H_{13}N_4NaO_2S$
95.0 to 105.0% of the stated amount.

IDENTIFICATION
A. Acidify a volume containing 0.1 g of sulfadimidine sodium with 6M *acetic acid*, filter, reserving the filtrate, wash the residue with *water* and dry at 105°. The *infrared absorption spectrum* of the residue, Appendix II A, is concordant with the *reference spectrum* of sulfadimidine *(RSV 50)*.

B. The residue obtained in test A yields the reaction characteristic of *primary aromatic amines*, Appendix VI, producing a bright orange-red precipitate.

TESTS
Alkalinity
pH, 10.0 to 11.0, Appendix V L.

Colour of solution
An injection containing 1 g of sulfadimidine sodium in 3 ml is not more intensely coloured than *reference solution Y_4*, Appendix IV B, Method I.

Related substances
Carry out the method for *thin-layer chromatography*, Appendix III A, using *silica gel H* as the coating substance and a mixture of 18 volumes of 10M *ammonia* and 90 volumes of *butan-1-ol* as the mobile phase. Apply separately to the plate 10 μl of each of the following solutions. For solution (1) use the injection being examined diluted with *water* to contain 0.20% w/v of sulfadimidine sodium. Solution (2) contains 0.0020% w/v of *sulfanilamide* in a mixture of 1 volume of 13.5M *ammonia* and 9 volumes of *ethanol (96%)*. After removal of the plate, heat it at 105° for 10 minutes and spray with a 0.1% w/v solution of *4-dimethylaminobenzaldehyde* in *ethanol (96%)* containing 1% v/v of *hydrochloric acid*. Any *secondary spot* in the chromatogram obtained with solution (1) is not more intense than the spot in the chromatogram obtained with solution (2) (1%).

ASSAY
Dilute a volume containing 0.5 g of sulfadimidine sodium to 75 ml with *water*, add 10 ml of *hydrochloric acid* and pass air slowly through the solution until the vapours do not turn moistened *starch iodate paper* blue. Add 3 g of *potassium bromide*, cool in ice and titrate slowly with 0.1M *sodium nitrite VS*, stirring constantly and determining the end point electrometrically. Each ml of 0.1M *sodium nitrite VS* is equivalent to 30.03 mg of $C_{12}H_{13}N_4NaO_2S$.

STORAGE
Sulfadimidine Injection should be protected from light.

LABELLING
The strength is stated as the amount of sulfadimidine sodium in a suitable dose-volume.

Sulfadimidine Tablets

Action and use
Sulfonamide antibacterial.

DEFINITION
Sulfadimidine Tablets contain Sulfadimidine.

The tablets comply with the requirements stated under Tablets and with the following requirements.

Content of sulfadimidine, $C_{12}H_{14}N_4O_2S$
95.0 to 105.0% of the stated amount.

IDENTIFICATION
A. Triturate a quantity of the powdered tablets containing 0.5 g of Sulfadimidine with two 5 ml quantities of *chloroform* and discard the chloroform. Triturate the residue with 10 ml of 5M *ammonia* for 5 minutes, add 10 ml of *water* and filter. Warm the filtrate until most of the ammonia has been removed, cool, acidify with 6M *acetic acid*, wash the precipitate with *water* and dry at 105°. The *infrared absorption spectrum* of the residue, Appendix II A, is concordant with the *reference spectrum* of sulfadimidine *(RSV 50)*.

B. In the test for Related substances, the principal spot in the chromatogram obtained with solution (2) corresponds to that in the chromatogram obtained with solution (4).

C. The residue obtained in test A yields the reaction characteristic of *primary aromatic amines*, Appendix VI, producing a bright orange-red precipitate.

Related substances
Carry out the method for *thin-layer chromatography*, Appendix III A, using *silica gel GF$_{254}$* as the coating substance and a mixture of 3 volumes of 6M *ammonia*, 5 volumes of *water*, 40 volumes of *nitromethane* and 50 volumes of *1,4-dioxan* as the mobile phase. Apply separately to the plate 5 μl of each of the following solutions. For solution (1) extract a quantity of the powdered tablets containing 0.5 g of Sulfadimidine with 25 ml of a mixture of 1 volume of 13.5M *ammonia* and 9 volumes of *methanol* by shaking for 10 minutes, filter and use the filtrate. For solution (2) dilute 1 volume of solution (1) to 5 volumes with a mixture of 1 volume of 13.5M *ammonia* and 24 volumes of *methanol*. For solution (3) dilute 1 volume of solution (1) to 200 volumes with a mixture of 1 volume of 13.5M *ammonia* and 24 volumes of *methanol*. Solution (4) contains 0.40% w/v of *sulfadimidine EPCRS* in a mixture of 1 volume of 13.5M *ammonia* and 24 volumes of *methanol*. After removal of the plate, dry it at 100° to 105° and examine under *ultraviolet light (254 nm)*. Any *secondary spot* in the chromatogram obtained with solution (1) is not more intense than the spot in the chromatogram obtained with solution (3) (0.5%).

ASSAY

Weigh and powder 20 tablets. Dissolve a quantity of the powder containing 0.5 g of Sulfadimidine as completely as possible in a mixture of 50 ml of *water* and 10 ml of *hydrochloric acid*, add 3 g of *potassium bromide*, cool in ice and titrate slowly with 0.1M *sodium nitrite VS*, stirring constantly and determining the end point electrometrically. Each ml of 0.1M *sodium nitrite VS* is equivalent to 27.83 mg of $C_{12}H_{14}N_4O_2S$.

STORAGE

Sulfadimidine Tablets should be protected from light.

Sulfadoxine and Trimethoprim Injection

Action and use

Sulfonamide antibacterial.

DEFINITION

Sulfadoxine and Trimethoprim Injection is a sterile solution, in a suitable aqueous vehicle, containing Sulfadoxine and Trimethoprim in the proportion five parts to one part. The pH is adjusted to about 10 by the addition of Sodium Hydroxide. It may contain 0.1% w/v of Lidocaine Hydrochloride.

The injection complies with the requirements stated under Parenteral Preparations and with the following requirements.

Content of sulfadoxine, $C_{12}H_{14}N_4O_4S$

92.5 to 107.5% of the stated amount.

Content of trimethoprim, $C_{14}H_{18}N_4O_3$

92.5 to 107.5% of the stated amount.

CHARACTERISTICS

A clear, yellow solution.

IDENTIFICATION

A. Evaporate 50 ml of solution B obtained in the Assay for trimethoprim to about 10 ml, neutralise with 5M *sodium hydroxide* and then acidify with 2M *acetic acid*. Dissolve the precipitate by warming and adding a small volume of *ethanol (25%)*. Cool, recrystallise the precipitate from *ethanol (25%)*, wash with *water* and dry at 105°. The *infrared absorption spectrum* of the residue, Appendix II A, is concordant with the *reference spectrum* of sulfadoxine *(RSV 37)*.

B. Evaporate 100 ml of solution A obtained in the Assay for trimethoprim to about 4 ml, transfer to a test tube with the aid of about 4 ml of hot *water* and allow to cool. Wash the resulting crystals with *water* and dry at 105°. The *infrared absorption spectrum* of the residue, Appendix II A, is concordant with the *reference spectrum* of trimethoprim *(RSV 45)*.

C. Carry out the method for *thin-layer chromatography*, Appendix III A, using *silica gel G* as the coating substance and a mixture of 19 volumes of *chloroform* and 1 volume of *methanol* as the mobile phase. Apply separately to the plate 5 µl of each of the following solutions. For solution (1) dilute the injection with *methanol* to contain 2.5% w/v of Sulfadoxine. Solution (2) is a 0.040% w/v solution of *lidocaine hydrochloride EPCRS* in 0.1M *sodium hydroxide* in *methanol*. After removal of the plate, allow it to dry in air and spray with *potassium iodobismuthate solution*. For an injection labelled as containing Lidocaine Hydrochloride the chromatogram obtained with solution (1) exhibits a spot corresponding to the spot in the chromatogram obtained with solution (2); an injection not so labelled exhibits no such spot.

Alkalinity

pH, 9.0 to 10.5, when diluted with an equal volume of *carbon dioxide-free water*, Appendix V L.

ASSAY

For trimethoprim

Prepare an anion exchange column (Dowex 1-X1 is suitable) pre-treated in the following manner. Wash with 100 ml of *water*, rinse with 50 ml of 1M *sodium hydroxide*, wash with *water* until the washings are neutral, rinse with 70 ml of 0.1M *hydrochloric acid in methanol (70%)* and again wash with *water*; activate the column with 50 ml of 1M *sodium hydroxide*, again wash with *water* and finally moisten with *methanol (70%)*.

Apply to the anion-exchange column 20 ml of a dilution of the injection in *methanol (70%)* containing 50 mg of Trimethoprim and elute with *methanol (70%)* to a final elution volume of 200 ml (solution A). Elute the material remaining on the column with 150 ml of 0.1M *hydrochloric acid in methanol (70%)* and add sufficient 0.1M *hydrochloric acid in methanol (70%)* to produce 200 ml (solution B). Reserve solution B for the Assay for sulfadoxine and Identification test A. To 10 ml of solution A add 1 ml of 1M *sodium hydroxide* and sufficient *methanol (70%)* to produce 100 ml. Measure the *absorbance* of the resulting solution at the maximum at 288 nm, Appendix II B. Calculate the content of $C_{14}H_{18}N_4O_3$ taking 250 as the value of A(1%, 1 cm) at the maximum at 288 nm.

For sulfadoxine

To 2 ml of solution B obtained in the Assay for Trimethoprim add sufficient 0.1M *hydrochloric acid in methanol (70%)* to produce 250 ml. Measure the *absorbance* of the resulting solution at the maximum at 267 nm, Appendix II B. Calculate the content of $C_{12}H_{14}N_4O_4S$ from the *absorbance* obtained by repeating the procedure using 2 ml of a 0.125% w/v solution of *sulfadoxine BPCRS* in 0.1M *hydrochloric acid in methanol (70%)* in place of solution B and using the declared content of $C_{12}H_{14}N_4O_4S$ in *sulfadoxine BPCRS*.

STORAGE

Sulfadoxine and Trimethoprim Injection should be protected from light.

LABELLING

The label states (1) the amount of Sulfadoxine and of Trimethoprim in a suitable dose-volume; (2) where applicable, that the injection contains Lidocaine Hydrochloride.

Sulfadoxine and Trimethoprim Tablets

Action and use

Sulfonamide antibacterial.

DEFINITION

Sulfadoxine and Trimethoprim Tablets contain Sulfadoxine and Trimethoprim in the proportion five parts to one part.

The tablets comply with the requirements stated under Tablets and with the following requirements.

Content of sulfadoxine, $C_{12}H_{14}N_4O_4S$
92.5 to 107.5% of the stated amount.

Content of trimethoprim, $C_{14}H_{18}N_4O_3$
92.5 to 107.5% of the stated amount.

IDENTIFICATION

A. Evaporate 50 ml of solution B prepared in the Assay for trimethoprim to about 10 ml, neutralise with 5M *sodium hydroxide* and then acidify with 2M *acetic acid*. Dissolve the precipitate by warming and adding a small volume of *ethanol (25%)*. Cool, recrystallise the precipitate from *ethanol (25%)*, wash with *water* and dry at 105°. The *infrared absorption spectrum* of the residue, Appendix II A, is concordant with the *reference spectrum* of sulfadoxine *(RSV 37)*.

B. Extract a quantity of the powdered tablets containing 50 mg of Trimethoprim with two 10 ml quantities of *methanol*, evaporate and dissolve the residue in 10 ml of 0.1M *sodium hydroxide*. Extract the resulting turbid solution by shaking with 20 ml of *dichloromethane*, dry the extract with *anhydrous sodium sulphate*, evaporate, cool and dissolve the residue in 8 ml of hot *water*. Wash the precipitate with *water* and dry at 105°. The *infrared absorption spectrum* of the residue, Appendix II A, is concordant with the *reference spectrum* of trimethoprim *(RSV 45)*.

ASSAY

For trimethoprim

Prepare an anion exchange column (Dowex 1-X1 is suitable) pre-treated in the following manner. Wash with 100 ml of *water*, rinse with 50 ml of 1M *sodium hydroxide*, wash with *water* until the washings are neutral, rinse with 70 ml of 0.1M *hydrochloric acid* in *methanol (70%)* and again wash with *water*; activate the column with 50 ml of 1M *sodium hydroxide*, again wash with *water* and finally moisten with *methanol (70%)*.

Weigh and powder 20 tablets. Extract a quantity of the powder containing 0.2 g of Trimethoprim with two 10 ml quantities of *dimethylformamide* and then with two 20 ml quantities of *methanol*. To the combined extracts add sufficient *methanol* to produce 100 ml. To 25 ml of this solution add 10 ml of *water* and add the resulting solution to the prepared anion exchange column; elute with *methanol (70%)* to a final elution volume of 200 ml (solution A). Elute the material remaining on the column with 150 ml of 0.1M *hydrochloric acid* in *methanol (70%)* and add sufficient 0.1M *hydrochloric acid* in *methanol (70%)* to produce 200 ml (solution B). Reserve solution B for the Assay for sulfadoxine and Identification test A. To 10 ml of solution A add 1 ml of 1M *sodium hydroxide* and sufficient *methanol (70%)* to produce 100 ml. Measure the *absorbance* of the resulting solution at the maximum at 288 nm, Appendix II B. Calculate the content of $C_{14}H_{18}N_4O_3$ taking 250 as the value of A(1%, 1 cm) at the maximum at 288 nm.

For sulfadoxine

To 2 ml of solution B obtained in the Assay for Trimethoprim add sufficient 0.1M *hydrochloric acid* in *methanol (70%)* to produce 250 ml. Measure the *absorbance* of the resulting solution at the maximum at 267 nm, Appendix II B. Calculate the content of $C_{12}H_{14}N_4O_4S$ from the *absorbance* obtained by repeating the procedure using 2 ml of a 0.125% w/v solution of *sulfadoxine BPCRS* in 0.1M *hydrochloric acid* in *methanol (70%)* in place of solution B and using the declared content of $C_{12}H_{14}N_4O_4S$ in *sulfadoxine BPCRS*.

STORAGE

Sulfadoxine and Trimethoprim Tablets should be protected from light.

LABELLING

The label states the quantity of Sulfadoxine and of Trimethoprim in each tablet.

Sulfametoxypyridazine Injection

Action and use
Sulfonamide antibacterial.

DEFINITION

Sulfametoxypyridazine Injection is a sterile solution of sulfametoxypryridazine sodium in Water for Injections prepared by the interaction of Sulfametoxypyridazine and Sodium Hydroxide and to which not more than 0.4% w/v of Sodium Thiosulphate is added.

The injection complies with the requirements stated under Parenteral Preparations and with the following requirements.

Content of sulfametoxypyridazine, $C_{11}H_{12}N_4O_3S$
95.0 to 105.0% of the stated amount.

IDENTIFICATION

Acidify the injection with 6M *acetic acid*, mix with the aid of ultrasound to disperse the precipitate and filter. The residue after washing with *water*, drying at 105° and recrystallising from *ethanol (96%)*, complies with the following tests.

A. The *infrared absorption spectrum*, Appendix II A, is concordant with the *reference spectrum* of sulfametoxypyridazine *(RSV 38)*.

B. Yields the reaction characteristic of *primary aromatic amines*, Appendix VI, giving a bright orange-red precipitate.

TESTS

Alkalinity

pH, 9.7 to 10.3, Appendix V L.

Colour of solution

An injection containing the equivalent of 1 g of Sulfametoxypyridazine in 4 ml is not more intensely coloured than *reference solution BY_1*, Appendix IV B, Method II.

Related substances

Carry out the method for *thin-layer chromatography*, Appendix III A, using *silica gel GF_{254}* as the coating substance and a mixture of 1 volume of 6M *ammonia*, 9 volumes of *water*, 30 volumes of *propan-2-ol* and 50 volumes of *ethyl acetate* as the mobile phase. Apply separately to the plate 5 μl of each of the following solutions. For solution (1) acidify a quantity of the injection containing 0.5 g of Sulfametoxypyridazine with 6M *acetic acid*, mix with the aid of ultrasound to disperse the precipitate and filter. Dry the residue at 100° and dissolve in 25 ml of *acetone*. For solution (2) dilute 1 volume of solution (1) to 200 volumes with *acetone*. After removal of the plate, dry it at 100° to 105° and examine under *ultraviolet light (254 nm)*. Any *secondary spot* in the chromatogram obtained with solution (1) is not more intense than the spot in the chromatogram obtained with solution (2) (0.5%).

ASSAY

Dilute a volume containing the equivalent of 0.5 g of Sulfametoxypyridazine with a mixture of 75 ml of *water* and 10 ml of *hydrochloric acid*, add 3 g of *potassium bromide*, cool in ice and titrate slowly with 0.1M *sodium nitrite VS*, stirring constantly and determining the end point electrometrically. Each ml of 0.1M *sodium nitrite VS* is equivalent to 28.03 mg of $C_{11}H_{12}N_4O_3S$.

STORAGE

Sulfametoxypyridazine Injection should be protected from light.

LABELLING

The strength is stated as the equivalent amount of Sulfametoxypyridazine in a suitable dose-volume.

Testosterone Phenylpropionate Injection

Action and use

Androgen.

DEFINITION

Testosterone Phenylpropionate Injection is a sterile solution of Testosterone Phenylpropionate in Ethyl Oleate or other suitable ester, in a suitable fixed oil or in any mixture of these.

The injection complies with the requirements stated under Parenteral Preparations and with the following requirements.

Content of testosterone phenylpropionate, $C_{28}H_{36}O_3$
92.5 to 107.5% of the stated amount.

IDENTIFICATION

Dissolve a volume of the injection containing 50 mg of Testosterone Phenylpropionate in 8 ml of *petroleum spirit (boiling range, 40° to 60°)* and extract with three 8 ml quantities of a mixture of 7 volumes of *glacial acetic acid* and 3 volumes of *water*. Wash the combined extracts with 10 ml of *petroleum spirit (boiling range, 40° to 60°)*, dilute with *water* until the solution becomes turbid, allow to stand for 2 hours in ice and filter. The precipitate, after washing with *water* and drying at 105°, complies with the following tests.

A. The *infrared absorption spectrum*, Appendix II A, is concordant with the *reference spectrum* of testosterone phenylpropionate *(RSV 43)*. If the spectra are not concordant, dissolve the substances in the minimum volume of *dichloromethane*, evaporate to dryness and prepare new spectra of the residues.

B. Complies with the test for *identification of steroids*, Appendix III A, using *impregnating solvent III* and *mobile phase F*.

C. Dissolve 25 mg in 1 ml of *methanol*, add 2 ml of *semi-carbazide acetate solution*, heat under a reflux condenser for 30 minutes and cool. The *melting point* of the precipitate is about 218°, Appendix V A.

ASSAY

To a volume containing 0.1 g of Testosterone Phenylpropionate add sufficient *chloroform* to produce 100 ml. Dilute 3 ml to 50 ml with *chloroform*. To 5 ml add 10 ml of *isoniazid solution* and sufficient *methanol* to produce 20 ml. Allow to stand for 45 minutes and measure the *absorbance* of the resulting solution at the maximum at 380 nm, Appendix II B, using as the reference solution 5 ml of *chloroform* treated in similar manner. Measure the absorbance obtained by repeating the operation using a 0.006% w/v solution of *testosterone phenylpropionate BPCRS* in *chloroform* and beginning at the words ' to 5 ml ...'. Calculate the content of $C_{28}H_{36}O_3$ from the values of the absorbances obtained using the declared content of $C_{28}H_{36}O_3$ in *testosterone phenylpropionate BPCRS*.

STORAGE

Testosterone Phenylpropionate Injection should be protected from light.

LABELLING

The label states (1) the composition of the vehicle; (2) that the preparation is for intramuscular injection only.

Tylosin Injection

Action and use

Macrolide antibacterial.

DEFINITION

Tylosin Injection is a sterile solution of Tylosin in a mixture of equal parts by volume of Propylene Glycol and Water for Injections.

The injection complies with the requirements stated under Parenteral Preparations and with the following requirements.

CHARACTERISTICS

A pale yellow to amber-coloured solution.

IDENTIFICATION

A. Dilute a volume containing 0.1 g of Tylosin with *water* to give a solution containing 0.02% w/v of Tylosin. To 5 ml of this solution add 10 ml of 0.1M *sodium hydroxide* and extract with 10 ml of *chloroform*. Separate the chloroform layer and extract it with 25 ml of 0.1M *hydrochloric acid*. Discard the chloroform, wash the aqueous layer with 3 ml of *chloroform*, discard the washings and filter. The *light absorption*, Appendix II B, in the range 230 to 350 nm, exhibits a maximum only at 290 nm. The *absorbance* at the maximum is about 0.94.

B. To 10 ml of the filtrate obtained in test A add 1 ml of 2M *sodium hydroxide*, heat on a water bath for 20 minutes and cool. The *light absorption*, Appendix II B, in the range 250 to 430 nm, exhibits a maximum at 332 nm.

TESTS

Composition

Carry out the method for *liquid chromatography*, Appendix III D, using the following freshly prepared solutions. Solution (1) contains 0.02% w/v of *tylosin BPCRS* in a mixture of equal volumes of *water* and *acetonitrile*. For solution (2) dilute the injection with sufficient of a mixture of equal volumes of *water* and *acetonitrile* to produce a solution containing 0.02% w/v of Tylosin.

The chromatographic procedure may be carried out using (a) a stainless steel column (20 cm × 5 mm) packed with *octadecylsilyl silica gel for chromatography* (5 μm) (Nucleosil C18 is suitable), (b) as the mobile phase with a flow rate of 1 ml per minute, 0.85M *sodium perchlorate* in a 40% v/v solution of *acetonitrile*, the solution being adjusted to pH 2.5 using 1M *hydrochloric acid* and (c) a detection wavelength of 290 nm.

The chromatogram obtained with solution (1) shows similar resolution to the reference chromatogram supplied with *tylosin BPCRS*. If necessary adjust the molarity of the sodium perchlorate or raise the temperature of the column to a maximum of 50°. The order of elution of the six major components of *tylosin BPCRS* in the chromatogram obtained with solution (1) is desmycinosyltylosin, tylosin C, tylosin B, tylosin D, an aldol impurity and tylosin A.

The *column efficiency*, determined using the peak due to tylosin A in solution (1), should be at least 22,000 theoretical plates per metre.

Calculate the percentage content of components by *normalisation*. In the chromatogram obtained with solution (2) the content of tylosin A is not less than 80% and the total content of tylosins A, B, C and D is not less than 90%.

Tyramine

Dilute a volume containing 0.1 g of Tylosin with 5 ml of 0.03M *orthophosphoric acid* in a 25 ml graduated flask, add 1 ml of *pyridine* and 2 ml of a saturated solution of *ninhydrin* (approximately 4% w/v). Close the flask by covering with a piece of aluminium foil and heat in a water bath at 85° for at least 20 minutes. Cool rapidly and add sufficient *water* to produce 25 ml. Measure the *absorbance* of the resulting solution without delay at 570 nm, Appendix II B, using in the reference cell a solution prepared in the same manner but omitting the injection being examined. The absorbance is not greater than that obtained by carrying out the procedure at the same time using 5 ml of a solution in 0.03M *orthophosphoric acid* containing 35 µg of *tyramine* per ml and beginning at the words 'add 1 ml...' (0.175%).

ASSAY

Carry out the *biological assay of antibiotics*, Appendix XIV A. The precision of the assay is such that the fiducial limits of error are not less than 95% and not more than 105% of the estimated potency.

Calculate the content of tylosin in the injection taking each 1000 IU found to be equivalent to 1 mg of tylosin.

The upper fiducial limit of error is not less than 97.0% and the lower fiducial limit of error is not more than 110.0% of the stated content.

STORAGE

Tylosin Injection should be kept in a cool place.

LABELLING

The label states that the preparation is intended only for intramuscular injection.

Tylosin Tartrate and Sulfathiazole Sodium Veterinary Oral Powder

Action and use

Macrolide antibacterial.

DEFINITION

Tylosin Tartrate and Sulfathiazole Sodium Veterinary Oral Powder is a mixture of Tylosin Tartrate and Sulfathiazole Sodium. The proportions of the mixture are such that the ratio of tylosin to Sulfathiazole Sodium is about one to three.

The veterinary oral powder complies with the requirements stated under Veterinary Oral Powders and with the following requirements.

Content of sulfathiazole sodium, $C_9H_8NaO_2S_2,1^{1}/_2H_2O$

90.0 to 110.0% of the stated amount, calculated as sulfathiaziole sodium sesquihydrate.

IDENTIFICATION

A. Triturate a quantity of the powder containing the equivalent of 0.25 g of tylosin with two 25 ml quantities of *chloroform* and filter. Reserve the chloroform-insoluble residue for test B. Wash the combined filtrates by shaking for

1 minute with 20 ml of 0.1M *sodium hydroxide* and filter the chloroform layer through *anhydrous sodium sulphate*. Evaporate the filtrate to dryness and dry the residue over *phosphorus pentoxide* at a pressure not exceeding 0.7 kPa for 1 hour. The *infrared absorption spectrum* of the dried residue, Appendix II A, is concordant with the *reference spectrum* of tylosin *(RSV 46)*.

B. Dry the chloroform-insoluble residue reserved in test A at 105° for 1 hour. The *infrared absorption spectrum* of the dried residue, Appendix II A, is concordant with the *reference spectrum* of sulfathiazole sodium *(RSV 42)*.

TESTS
Composition

Carry out the method for *liquid chromatography*, Appendix III D, using the following solutions prepared immediately before use. Solution (1) contains 0.02% w/v of *tylosin BPCRS* in a mixture of equal volumes of *water* and *acetonitrile*. For solution (2) dissolve the powder in a mixture of equal volumes of *water* and *acetonitrile* to produce a solution containing the equivalent of 0.02% of tylosin.

The chromatographic procedure may be carried out using (a) a stainless steel column (20 cm × 5 mm) packed with *octadecylsilyl silica gel for chromatography* (5 µm) (Nucleosil C18 is suitable), (b) as the mobile phase with a flow rate of 1 ml per minute 0.85M *sodium perchlorate* in a 40% v/v solution of *acetonitrile*, the pH of the solution being adjusted to 2.5 using 1M *hydrochloric acid* and (c) a detection wavelength of 290 nm.

The chromatogram obtained with solution (1) shows similar resolution to the reference chromatogram supplied with *tylosin BPCRS*. If necessary adjust the molarity of the sodium perchlorate or raise the temperature of the column to a maximum of 50°. The order of elution of the six major components of *tylosin BPCRS* in the chromatogram obtained with solution (1) is desmycinosyltylosin, tylosin C, tylosin B, tylosin D, an aldol impurity and tylosin A.

The *column efficiency*, determined using the peak due to tylosin A in solution (1), should be at least 22,000 theoretical plates per metre.

Calculate the percentage content of components by *normalisation*. In the chromatogram obtained with solution (2) the content of tylosin A is not less than 80% and the total content of tylosins A, B, C and D is not less than 95%. A peak due to sulphathiazole will be observed eluting immediately after the solvent peak and should be disregarded.

Related substances

Carry out the method for *thin-layer chromatography*, Appendix III A, using *silica gel H* as the coating substance and a mixture of 18 volumes of 10M *ammonia* and 90 volumes of *butan-1-ol* as the mobile phase. Apply separately to the plate 10 µl of each of the following solutions. For solution (1) shake a quantity of the powder containing 0.1 g of Sulfathiazole Sodium with 10 ml of a mixture of 1 volume of 13.5M *ammonia* and 9 volumes of *ethanol (96%)*, filter and use the filtrate. Solution (2) contains 0.0050% w/v of *sulfanilamide* in a mixture of 9 volumes of *ethanol (96%)* and 1 volume of 13.5M *ammonia*. After removal of the plate, heat it at 105° for 10 minutes and spray with a 0.1% w/v solution of *4-dimethylaminobenzaldehyde* in *ethanol (96%)* containing 1% v/v of *hydrochloric acid*. Any *secondary spot* in the chromatogram obtained with solution (1) is not more intense than the spot in the chromatogram obtained with solution (2) (0.5%).

ASSAY

For tylosin activity

Transfer a quantity of the powder containing the equivalent of 0.2 g of tylosin to a 100 ml graduated flask with the aid of three 10 ml quantities of *methanol*, swirl to dissolve and add sufficient sterile *phosphate buffer pH 7.0* to produce 100 ml. Filter and dilute 5 ml of the filtrate to 100 ml with sterile *phosphate buffer pH 7.0*. Carry out the *biological assay of antibiotics*, Appendix XIV A. The precision of the assay is such that the fiducial limits of error are not less than 95% and not more than 105% of the estimated potency. Calculate the content of tylosin taking each 1000 IU found to be equivalent to 1 mg of tylosin. The upper fiducial limit of error is not less than 90.0% and the lower fiducial limit of error is not more than 110.0% of the stated amount.

For sulfathiazole sodium

Dissolve a quantity of the powder containing the equivalent of 0.4 g of sulphathiazole sodium sesquihydrate in a mixture of 75 ml of *water* and 10 ml of *hydrochloric acid*, add 3 g of *potassium bromide*, cool in ice and titrate slowly with 0.1M *sodium nitrite VS*, stirring constantly and determining the end point electrometrically. Each ml of 0.1M *sodium nitrite VS* is equivalent to 30.43 mg of $C_9H_8N_3NaO_2S_2,1\frac{1}{2}H_2O$.

LABELLING

The label states the quantity of Tylosin Tartrate in terms of the equivalent amount of tylosin and the quantity of Sulfathiazole Sodium in terms of the equivalent amount of sulfathiazole sodium sesquihydrate.

Tylosin Tablets

Action and use

Macrolide antibacterial.

DEFINITION

Tylosin Tablets contain Tylosin.

The tablets comply with the requirements stated under Tablets and with the following requirements.

IDENTIFICATION

A. Triturate a quantity of the powdered tablets containing 0.2 g of Tylosin with 20 ml of *chloroform*, filter, dry the chloroform by shaking with *anhydrous sodium sulphate*, filter and evaporate the filtrate to dryness. Dry the residue over *phosphorus pentoxide* at a pressure not exceeding 0.7 kPa for 1 hour. The *infrared absorption spectrum* of the dried residue, Appendix II A, is concordant with the *reference spectrum* of tylosin *(RSV 46)*.

B. Triturate a quantity of the powdered tablets containing 0.2 g of Tylosin with two 10 ml quantities of 0.1M *hydrochloric acid*, filter and dilute the filtrate to 100 ml with 0.1M *hydrochloric acid*. Dilute 10 ml of the resulting solution to 50 ml with 0.1M *hydrochloric acid* and then dilute 5 ml of this solution to 50 ml with the same solvent. The *light absorption* of the resulting solution, Appendix II B, in the range 230 to 350 nm, exhibits a maximum only at 290 nm. The *absorbance* at the maximum is about 0.94.

C. To 10 ml of the solution obtained in test B add 1 ml of 2M *sodium hydroxide*, heat on a water bath for 20 minutes and cool. The *light absorption*, Appendix II B, in the range 250 to 430 nm, exhibits a maximum at 332 nm.

TESTS

Composition

Carry out the method for *liquid chromatography*, Appendix III D, using the following solutions prepared immediately before use. Solution (1) contains 0.02% w/v of *tylosin BPCRS* in a mixture of equal volumes of *water* and *acetonitrile*. For solution (2) shake a quantity of the powdered tablets taken for the Assay containing 0.2 g of Tylosin with 50 ml of *methanol*, filter and dilute 5 ml of the filtrate to 100 ml with a mixture of equal volumes of *water* and *acetonitrile*.

The chromatographic procedure may be carried out using (a) a stainless steel column (20 cm × 5 mm) packed with *octadecylsilyl silica gel for chromatography* (5 μm) (Nucleosil C18 is suitable), (b) as the mobile phase with a flow rate of 1 ml per minute 0.85M *sodium perchlorate* in a 40% v/v solution of *acetonitrile*, the pH of the solution being adjusted to 2.5 using 1M *hydrochloric acid* and (c) a detection wavelength of 290 nm.

The chromatogram obtained with solution (1) shows similar resolution to the reference chromatogram supplied with the *tylosin BPCRS*. If necessary adjust the molarity of the sodium perchlorate or raise the temperature of the column to a maximum of 50°. The order of elution of the six major components of *tylosin BPCRS* in the chromatogram obtained with solution (1) is desmycinosyltylosin, tylosin C, tylosin B, tylosin D, an aldol impurity and tylosin A.

The *column efficiency*, determined using the peak due to tylosin A in solution (1), should be at least 22,000 theoretical plates per metre.

Calculate the percentage content of components by *normalisation*. In the chromatogram obtained with solution (2) the content of tylosin A is not less than 80% and the total content of tylosins A, B, C and D is not less than 95%.

Tyramine

Shake a quantity of the powdered tablets containing 50 mg of Tylosin with 5 ml of 0.03M *orthophosphoric acid*. Filter into a 25 ml graduated flask, add 1 ml of *pyridine* and 2 ml of a saturated solution of *ninhydrin* (approximately 4% w/v). Close the flask by covering with a piece of aluminium foil and heat in a water bath at 85° for at least 20 minutes. Cool rapidly and add sufficient *water* to produce 25 ml. Measure the *absorbance* of the resulting solution without delay at 570 nm, Appendix II B, using in the reference cell a solution prepared in the same manner but omitting the preparation being examined. The absorbance is not greater than that obtained by carrying out the procedure at the same time using 5 ml of a solution in 0.03M *orthophosphoric acid* containing 35 μg of *tyramine* per ml and beginning at the words 'add 1 ml...' (0.35%).

Dissolution

Comply with the requirements for Monographs of the British Pharmacopoeia in the *dissolution test for tablets and capsules*, Appendix XII B1, using Apparatus 2. Use as the medium 900 ml of 0.01M *hydrochloric acid* and rotate the paddle at 50 revolutions per minute. Withdraw a sample of 10 ml of the medium, filter and dilute to 100 ml with 0.01M *hydrochloric acid*. Measure the *absorbance* of this solution at the maximum at 290 nm, Appendix II B, using 0.01M *hydrochloric acid* in the reference cell. Calculate the total content of tylosin, $C_{46}H_{77}NO_{17}$ in the medium taking 233 as the value of A(1%, 1 cm) at the maximum at 290 nm.

ASSAY

Weigh and powder 20 tablets. Transfer a quantity of the powdered tablets containing to 0.2 g of Tylosin to a 100 ml graduated flask with the aid of three 10 ml quantities of *methanol*, swirl to dissolve the tylosin and add sufficient sterile *phosphate buffer pH 7.0* to produce 100 ml. Filter and dilute 5 ml of the filtrate to 100 ml with sterile *phosphate buffer pH 7.0*. Carry out the *biological assay of antibiotics*, Appendix XIV A. The precision of the assay is such that the fiducial limits of error are not less than 95% and not more than 105% of the estimated potency. Calculate the content of tylosin in the tablets, taking each 1000 IU found to be equivalent to 1 mg of tylosin. The upper fiducial limit of error is not less than 97.0% and the lower fiducial limit of error is not more than 110.0% of the stated amount.

Monographs

Immunological Products

VETERINARY IMMUNOSERA

Veterinary Antisera

(*Immunosera for Veterinary Use, Ph Eur monograph 0030*)

Veterinary Immunosera comply with the requirements of the European Pharmacopoeia monograph for Immunosera for Veterinary Use. These requirements are reproduced below.

The provisions of this monograph apply to the following immunosera.

Antitoxic sera

Clostridium Novyi Alpha Antitoxin★

Clostridium Perfringens Antitoxins

(*incorporating* Clostridium Perfringens Beta Antitoxin★

and Clostridium Perfringens Epsilon Antitoxin★)

Clostridium Tetani Antitoxin★

★Monographs of the European Pharmacopoeia

Ph Eur _____

DEFINITION

Immunosera for veterinary use are preparations containing immunoglobulins, purified immunoglobulins or immunoglobulin fragments obtained from serum or plasma of immunised animals. They may be preparations of crude polyclonal antisera or purified preparations.

The immunoglobulins or immunoglobulin fragments have the power of specifically neutralising the antigen used for immunisation. The antigens include microbial or other toxins, bacterial and viral antigens, venoms of snakes and hormones. The preparation is intended for parenteral administration to provide passive immunity.

PRODUCTION

GENERAL PROVISIONS

Immunosera are obtained from the serum or plasma of healthy animals immunised by administration of one or more suitable antigens.

The production method shall have been shown to yield consistently batches of immunosera of acceptable safety (5.2.6) and efficacy (5.2.7).

DONOR ANIMALS

The animals used are exclusively reserved for production of immunoserum. They are maintained under conditions protecting them from the introduction of disease, as far as possible. The donor animals, and any animals in contact with them, are tested and shown to be free from a defined list of infectious agents and re-tested at suitable intervals. The list of agents for testing includes not only those agents that are relevant to the donor animal, but also those that are relevant to the recipient target species for the product. Where the donor animals have not been demonstrated to be free from a relevant pathogen, a justification must be provided and a validated inactivation or purification procedure must be included in the manufacturing procedure. The feed originates from a controlled source. Where the donor animals are chickens, use chickens from a flock free from specified pathogens (5.2.2). Where applicable for the species used, measures are taken to avoid contamination with agents of transmissible spongiform encephalopathies. As far as possible, animals being introduced into the herd are from a known source and have a known breeding and rearing history. The introduction of animals into the herd follows specified procedures, including defined quarantine measures. During the quarantine period the animals are observed and tested to establish that they are free from the list of agents relevant for the donor animals. It may be necessary to test the animals in quarantine for freedom from additional agents, depending on their known breeding and rearing history or any lack of information on their source.

Any routine or therapeutic medicinal treatment administered to the animals in quarantine or thereafter must be recorded.

IMMUNISING ANTIGEN

The principles described in the Production section of *Vaccines for veterinary use (0062)* are applied to the production of the immunogen. The antigen used is identified and characterised. The starting materials used for antigen preparation must be controlled to minimise the risk of contamination with extraneous agents. The antigen may be blended with a suitable adjuvant. The immunogen is produced on a batch basis. The batches must be prepared and tested in such a manner that assures that each batch will be equally safe and free from extraneous agents and will produce a satisfactory, consistent immune response.

IMMUNISATION

The donor animals are immunised according to a defined schedule. For each animal, the details of the dose of immunising antigen, route of administration and dates of administration are recorded. Animals are kept under general health surveillance and the development of specific antibodies are monitored at appropriate stages of the immunisation process.

COLLECTION OF BLOOD OR PLASMA

Animals are thoroughly examined before each collection. Only healthy animals may be used as a donor animal. Collection of blood is made by venepuncture or plasmapheresis. The puncture area is shaved, cleaned and disinfected. The method of collection and the volume to be collected on each occasion are specified. The blood or plasma is collected in such a manner as to maintain sterility of the product. If the serum or plasma is stored before further processing, precautions are taken to avoid microbial contamination.

The blood or plasma collection is conducted at a site separate from the area where the animals are kept or bred and the area where the immunoserum is further processed.

Clear criteria are established for determining the time between immunisation and first collection of blood or plasma as well as the time between subsequent collections and the length of time over which collections are made. The criteria applied must take into account the effect of the collections on the health and welfare of the animal as well as the effect on the consistency of production of batches of the finished product, over time.

The rate of clearance of any residues that may arise from the immunising antigen or medication given needs to be taken into account. In the case of the risk of residues from chemical substances, consideration could be given to the inclusion of a withdrawal period for the finished product. If the immunising agent consists of a live organism, the time between immunisation and collection may need to take into account the time required for the donor to eliminate the immunogen, particularly if any residual live organisms might be harmful to the recipient.

PREPARATION OF THE FINISHED PRODUCT

Several single plasma or serum collections from one or more animals may be pooled to form a bulk for preparation of a batch. The number of collections that may be used to produce a bulk and the size of the bulk are defined. Where pooling is not undertaken, the production procedure must be very carefully controlled to ensure that the consistency of the product is satisfactory.

The active substance is subjected to a purification and/or inactivation procedure unless omission of such a step has been justifed and agreed with the competent authority. The procedure applied must have been validated and be shown not to adversely impair the biological activity of the product. The validation studies must address the ability of the procedure to inactivate or remove any potential contaminants such as pathogens that could be transmitted from the donor to the recipient target species and infectious agents such as those that cause ubiquitous infections in the donor animals and cannot be readily eliminated from these donor animals.

For purified immunosera, the globulins containing the immune substances may be obtained from the crude immunoserum by enzyme treatment and fractional precipitation or by other suitable chemical or physical methods.

Antimicrobial preservatives
Antimicrobial preservatives are used to prevent spoilage or adverse effects caused by microbial contamination occurring during use of a product. Antimicrobial preservatives are not included in freeze-dried products but, if justified, taking into account the maximum recommended period of use after reconstitution, they may be included in the diluent for multidose freeze-dried products. For single-dose liquid preparations, inclusion of antimicrobial preservatives is not normally acceptable, but may be acceptable, for example where the same product is filled in single-dose and multidose containers and is for use in non-food producing species. For multidose liquid preparations, the need for effective antimicrobial preservation is evaluated taking into account likely contamination during use and the maximum recommended period of use after broaching of the container.

During development studies the effectiveness of the antimicrobial preservative throughout the period of validity shall be demonstrated to the satisfaction of the competent authority.

The efficacy of the antimicrobial preservative is evaluated as described in chapter 5.1.3; for a multidose preparation, additional samples are taken, to monitor the effect of the antimicrobial preservative over the proposed in-use shelf-life.

If neither the A criteria nor the B criteria can be met, then in justified cases the following criteria are applied to antisera for veterinary use: bacteria, no increase at 24 h and 7 days, 3 log reduction at 14 days, no increase at 28 days; fungi, no increase at 14 days and 28 days.

Addition of antibiotics as antimicrobial preservative is not acceptable.

Unless otherwise prescribed in the monograph, the final bulk is distributed aseptically into sterile, tamper-proof containers which are then closed so as to exclude contamination.

The preparation may be freeze-dried.

In-process tests   Suitable tests are carried out in-process, such as on samples from collections before pooling to form a bulk.

BATCH TESTS
The tests that are necessary to demonstrate the suitability of a batch of a product will vary and are influenced by a number of factors, including the detailed method of production. The tests to be conducted by the manufacturer on a particular product are agreed with the competent authority. If a product is treated by a validated procedure for inactivation of extraneous agents, the test for extraneous

agents can be omitted on that product with the agreement of the competent authority. If a product is treated by a validated procedure for inactivation of mycoplasmas, the test for mycoplasmas can be omitted on that product with the agreement of the competent authority.

Only a batch that complies with each of the relevant requirements given below under Identification, Tests and Potency and/or in the relevant specific monograph may be released for use. With the agreement of the competent authority, certain tests may be omitted where in-process tests give an equal or better guarantee that the batch would comply or where alternative tests validated with respect to the Pharmacopoeia method have been carried out.

Certain tests, e.g. for antimicrobial preservatives, for foreign proteins and for albumin, may be carried out by the manufacturer on the final bulk rather than on the batch, batches or sub-batches of finished product prepared from it. In some circumstances, e.g. when collections are made into plasmapheresis bags and each one is, essentially, a batch, pools of samples may be tested, with the agreement of the competent authority.

It is recognised that, in accordance with General Notices (1.1. General Statements), for an established antiserum the routine application of the safety test will be waived by the competent authority in the interests of animal welfare when a sufficient number of consecutive batches have been produced and found to comply with this test, thus demonstrating consistency of the manufacturing process. Significant changes to the manufacturing process may require resumption of routine testing to re-establish consistency. The number of consecutive batches to be tested depends on a number of factors such as the type of antiserum, the frequency of production of batches, and experience with the immunoserum during developmental safety testing and during application of the batch safety test. Without prejudice to the decision of the competent authority in the light of information available for a given antiserum, testing of 10 consecutive batches is likely to be sufficient for the majority of products. For products with an inherent safety risk, it may be necessary to continue to conduct the safety test on each batch.

Animal tests   In accordance with the provisions of the European Convention for the Protection of Vertebrate Animals Used for Experimental and Other Scientific Purposes, tests must be carried out in such a way as to use the minimum number of animals and to cause the least pain, suffering, distress or lasting harm. The criteria for judging tests in monographs must be applied in the light of this. For example, if it is indicated that an animal is considered to show positive, infected etc. when typical clinical signs occur then as soon as sufficient indication of a positive result is obtained the animal in question shall be either euthanised or given suitable treatment to prevent unnecessary suffering. In accordance with the General Notices, alternative test methods may be used to demonstrate compliance with the monograph and the use of such tests is particularly encouraged when this leads to replacement or reduction of animal use or reduction of suffering.

pH (*2.2.3*)
The pH of crude and purified immunosera is shown to be within the limits set for the products.

Formaldehyde
If formaldehyde is used for production of immunoserum, a test for free formaldehyde is carried out as prescribed under Tests.

Other inactivating agents

When other inactivation methods are used, appropriate tests are carried out to demonstrate that the inactivating agent has been removed or reduced to an acceptable residual level.

Batch potency test

If a specific monograph exists for the product, the test described under Potency is not necessarily carried out for routine testing of batches of antiserum. The type of batch potency test to be carried out will depend on the claims being made for the product. Wherever possible, *in vitro* tests must be used. The type of test required may include measurement of antibodies against specific infectious organisms, determination of the type of antibody (e.g. neutralising or opsonising). All tests must be validated. The criteria for acceptance must be set with reference to a batch that has been shown to comply with the requirements specified under Potency if a specific monograph exists for the product, and which has been shown to have satisfactory efficacy, in accordance with the claims being made for the product.

Total immunoglobulins

A test for the quantities of total immunoglobulins and/or total gammaglobulins and/or specific immunoglobulin classes is carried out. The results obtained must be within the limits set for the product and agreed with the competent authority. The batch contains not more than the level shown to be safe in the safety studies and, unless the batch potency test specifically covers all appropriate immunoglobulins, the level in the batch is not less than that in the batch or batches shown to be effective in the efficacy studies.

Total protein

For products where claims are being made which relate to the protein content, as well as demonstrating that the batch contains not more than the stated upper limit, the batch shall be shown to contain not less than that in the batch or batches shown to be effective in the efficacy studies.

Extraneous agents

In addition to the test described under Tests, specific tests may be required depending on the nature of the preparation, its risk of contamination and the use of the product.

In particular, specific tests for important potential pathogens may be required when the donor and recipient species are the same and when these agents would not be detected reliably by the general screening test described under Tests.

Water

Where applicable, the freeze-drying process is checked by a determination of water and shown to be within the limits set for the product.

IDENTIFICATION

The identity of the product is established by immunological tests and, where necessary, by determination of biological activity. The potency test may also serve for identification.

TESTS

The following requirements refer to liquid immunosera and reconstituted freeze-dried immunosera.

Foreign proteins

When examined by precipitation tests with specific antisera against plasma proteins of a suitable range of species, only protein from the declared animal species is shown to be present.

Albumin

Purified immunosera comply with a test for albumin. Unless otherwise prescribed in the monograph, when examined electrophoretically, purified immunosera show not more than a trace of albumin, and the content of albumin is in any case not greater than 30 g/l of the reconstituted preparation, where applicable.

Total protein

Dilute the preparation to be examined with a 9 g/l solution of *sodium chloride R* to obtain a solution containing about 15 mg of protein in 2 ml. To 2 ml of this solution in a round-bottomed centrifuge tube add 2 ml of a 75 g/l solution of *sodium molybdate R* and 2 ml of a mixture of 1 volume of *nitrogen-free sulphuric acid R* and 30 volumes of *water R*. Shake, centrifuge for 5 min, discard the supernatant liquid and allow the inverted tube to drain on filter paper. Determine the nitrogen in the residue by the method of sulphuric acid digestion (2.5.9) and calculate the content of protein by multiplying by 6.25. The results obtained are not greater than the upper limit stated on the label.

Antimicrobial preservative

Determine the amount of antimicrobial preservative by a suitable physicochemical method. The amount is not less than the minimum amount shown to be effective and is not greater than 115 per cent of that stated on the label.

Formaldehyde (2.4.18)

Where formaldehyde has been used in the preparation, the concentration of free formaldehyde is not greater than 0.5 g/l, unless a higher amount has been shown to be safe.

Sterility (2.6.1)

Immunosera for veterinary use comply with the test for sterility. When the volume of liquid in a container is greater than 100 ml, the method of membrane filtration is used wherever possible. If this method is used, incubate the media for not less than 14 days. Where the method of membrane filtration cannot be employed, the method of direct inoculation may be used. Where the volume of liquid in each container is at least 20 ml, the minimum volume to be used for each culture medium is 10 per cent of the contents of the container or 5 ml, whichever is the least. The appropriate number of items to be tested (2.6.1) is 1 per cent of the batch with a minimum of 4 and a maximum of 10.

Mycoplasmas (2.6.7)

Immunosera for veterinary use comply with the test for mycoplasmas.

Safety

A test is conducted in one of the species for which the product is recommended. Unless an overdose is specifically contraindicated on the label, twice the maximum recommended dose for the species used is administered by a recommended route. If there is a warning against administration of an overdose, a single dose is administered. For products to be used in mammals, use 2 animals of the minimum age for which the product is recommended. For avian products, use not fewer than 10 birds of the minimum age recommended. The birds are observed for 21 days. The other species are observed for 14 days. No abnormal local or systemic reaction occurs.

Extraneous agents

A test for extraneous agents is conducted by inoculation of cell cultures sensitive to pathogens of the species of the donor animal and into cells sensitive to pathogens of each of the recipient target species stated on the label (2.6.25). Observe the cells for 14 days. During this time, carry out at least one passage. The cells are checked daily for cytopathic effect and are checked at the end of 14 days for the presence of a haemadsorbing agent. The batch complies with the test if there is no evidence of the presence of an extraneous agent.

For immunosera of avian origin, if a test in cell culture is insufficient to detect potential extraneous agents, a test is conducted by inoculation of embryonated eggs from flocks free from specified pathogens (5.2.2) or by some other suitable method (polymerase chain reaction (PCR) for example).

POTENCY

Carry out a suitable test for potency.

Where a specific monograph exists, carry out the biological assay prescribed in the monograph and express the result in International Units per millilitre when such exist.

STORAGE

Protected from light, at a temperature of 5 ± 3 °C. Liquid immunosera must not be allowed to freeze.

LABELLING

The label states:
— that the preparation is for veterinary use;
— whether or not the preparation is purified;
— the minimum number of International Units per millilitre, where such exist;
— the volume of the preparation in the container;
— the indications for the product;
— the instructions for use including the interval between any repeat administrations and the maximum number of administrations that is recommended;
— the recipient target species for the immunoserum;
— the dose recommended for different species;
— the route(s) of administration;
— the name of the species of the donor animal;
— the maximum quantity of total protein;
— the name and amount of any antimicrobial preservative or other substance added to the immunoserum;
— any contra-indications to the use of the product including any required warning on the dangers of administration of an overdose;
— for freeze-dried immunosera:
  — the name or composition and the volume of the reconstituting liquid to be added;
  — the period within which the immunoserum is to be used after reconstitution.

Ph Eur

Clostridium Novyi Alpha Antitoxin

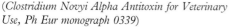

(*Clostridium Novyi Alpha Antitoxin for Veterinary Use, Ph Eur monograph 0339*)

Ph Eur

DEFINITION

Clostridium novyi alpha antitoxin for veterinary use is a preparation containing the globulins that have the power of specifically neutralising the alpha toxin formed by *Clostridium novyi*. It consists of the serum or a preparation obtained from the serum of animals immunised against *C. novyi* alpha toxin.

PRODUCTION

CHOICE OF COMPOSITION

The antitoxin is shown to be satisfactory with respect to safety (5.2.6) and efficacy (5.2.7). For the latter, it shall be demonstrated, for each target species, that the product, when administered at the minimum recommended dose and

according to the recommended schedule(s), provides a response or responses consistent with the claims made for the product.

Batch potency test

The test described under Potency is not necessarily carried out for routine testing of batches of antitoxin. It is carried out on 1 or more occasions as decided by or with the agreement of the competent authority. Where the test is not carried out, a suitable validated alternative test is carried out, the criteria for acceptance being set with reference to a batch of antitoxin that has given satisfactory results in the test described under Potency and that has been shown to be satisfactory with respect to immunogenicity in the target species. The following test may be used after a satisfactory correlation with the test described under Potency has been established.

Determine the level of antibodies against *C. novyi* alpha toxin in the batch of antitoxin using a suitable method such as an immunochemical method (2.7.1) or neutralisation in cell cultures. Use a homologous reference serum calibrated in International Units of clostridium novyi alpha antitoxin.

The International Unit is the specific neutralising activity for *C. novyi* alpha toxin contained in a stated amount of the International Standard, which consists of a quantity of dried immune horse serum. The equivalence in International Units of the International Standard is stated by the World Health Organisation.

The potency of the finished product is expressed in International Units per millilitre and is shown to be not less than the minimum number stated on the label.

IDENTIFICATION

The antitoxin is shown, by a suitable immunochemical method (2.7.1), to react specifically with the alpha toxin formed by *C. novyi*.

POTENCY

The potency of clostridium novyi alpha antitoxin is determined by comparing the dose necessary to protect mice or other suitable animals against the toxic effects of a fixed dose of *C. novyi* alpha toxin with the quantity of a reference preparation of clostridium novyi alpha antitoxin, calibrated in International Units, necessary to give the same protection. For this comparison, a suitable preparation of *C. novyi* alpha toxin for use as a test toxin is required. The dose of the test toxin is determined in relation to the reference preparation; the potency of the antitoxin to be examined is determined in relation to the reference preparation using the test toxin.

Preparation of test toxin

Prepare the test toxin from a sterile filtrate of an approximately 5-day culture in liquid medium of *C. novyi* type B and dry by a suitable method. Select the test toxin by determining for mice the L+/10 dose and the LD_{50}, the observation period being 72 h. A suitable alpha toxin contains not less than one L+/10 dose in 0.05 mg and not less than 10 LD_{50} in each L+/10 dose.

Determination of test dose of toxin

Prepare a solution of the reference preparation in a suitable liquid so that it contains 1 IU/ml. Prepare a solution of the test toxin in a suitable liquid so that 1 ml contains a precisely known amount such as 1 mg. Prepare mixtures of the solution of the reference preparation and the solution of the test toxin such that each mixture contains 1.0 ml of the solution of the reference preparation (1 IU), one of a series of graded volumes of the solution of the test toxin and sufficient of a suitable liquid to bring the total volume to

2.0 ml. Allow the mixtures to stand at room temperature for 60 min. Using not fewer than 2 mice, each weighing 17-22 g, for each mixture, inject a dose of 0.2 ml intramuscularly or subcutaneously into each mouse. Observe the mice for 72 h. If all the mice die, the amount of toxin present in 0.2 ml of the mixture is in excess of the test dose. If none of the mice die, the amount of toxin present in 0.2 ml of the mixture is less than the test dose. Prepare similar fresh mixtures such that 2.0 ml of each mixture contains 1.0 ml of the solution of the reference preparation (1 IU) and 1 of a series of graded volumes of the solution of the test toxin separated from each other by steps of not more than 20 per cent and covering the expected end-point. Allow the mixtures to stand at room temperature for 60 min. Using not fewer than 2 mice for each mixture, inject a dose of 0.2 ml intramuscularly or subcutaneously into each mouse. Observe the mice for 72 h. Repeat the determination at least once and combine the results of the separate tests that have been carried out with mixtures of the same composition so that a series of totals is obtained, each total representing the mortality due to a mixture of a given composition. The test dose of toxin is the amount present in 0.2 ml of that mixture which causes the death of one half of the total number of mice injected with it.

Determination of the potency of the antitoxin to be examined

Preliminary test Dissolve a quantity of the test toxin in a suitable liquid so that 1 ml contains 10 times the test dose (solution of the test toxin). Prepare mixtures of the solution of the test toxin and of the antitoxin to be examined such that each mixture contains 1.0 ml of the solution of the test toxin, one of a series of graded volumes of the antitoxin to be examined and sufficient of a suitable liquid to bring the final volume to 2.0 ml. Allow the mixtures to stand at room temperature for 60 min. Using not fewer than 2 mice for each mixture, inject a dose of 0.2 ml intramuscularly or subcutaneously into each mouse. Observe the mice for 72 h. If none of the mice die, 0.2 ml of the mixture contains more than 0.1 IU. If all the mice die, 0.2 ml of the mixture contains less than 0.1 IU.

Final test Prepare mixtures of the solution of the test toxin and of the antitoxin to be examined such that 2.0 ml of each mixture contains 1.0 ml of the solution of the test toxin and one of a series of graded volumes of the antitoxin to be examined, separated from each other by steps of not more than 20 per cent and covering the expected end-point as determined by the preliminary test. Prepare further mixtures such that 2.0 ml of each mixture contains 1.0 ml of the solution of the test toxin and one of a series of graded volumes of the solution of the reference preparation, in order to confirm the test dose of the toxin. Allow the mixtures to stand at room temperature for 60 min. Using not fewer than 2 mice for each mixture, proceed as described in the preliminary test. The test mixture which contains 0.1 IU in 0.2 ml is that mixture which kills the same or almost the same number of mice as the reference mixture containing 0.1 IU in 0.2 ml. Repeat the determination at least once and calculate the average of all valid estimates. Estimates are valid only if the reference preparation gives a result within 20 per cent of the expected value.

The confidence limits ($P = 0.95$) have been estimated to be:
— 85 per cent and 114 per cent when 2 animals per dose are used,
— 91.5 per cent and 109 per cent when 4 animals per dose are used,
— 93 per cent and 108 per cent when 6 animals per dose are used.

The potency of the finished product is expressed in International Units per millilitre and is shown to be not less than the minimum number stated on the label.

Ph Eur

Clostridium Perfringens Antitoxins

DEFINITION

Clostridium Perfringens Antitoxins are preparations containing either the individual antitoxic globulins or a combination of the antitoxic globulins that have the specific power of neutralising either the beta toxin or the beta and epsilon toxins produced by *Clostridium perfringens type B*, the beta toxin produced by *Cl. perfringens type C* or the epsilon toxin produced by *Cl. perfringens type D*.

The name Clostridium Perfringens Beta Antitoxin may be used for preparations stated to contain beta antitoxins only.

The names Clostridium Perfringens Epsilon Antitoxin or Clostridium Perfringens Type D Antitoxin may be used for preparations stated to contain epsilon antitoxins only.

The name Clostridium Perfringens Type B Antitoxin (synonym Lamb Dysentery Antiserum) may be used for preparations stated to contain both beta and epsilon antitoxin.

The antitoxins comply with the requirements stated under Veterinary Immunosera with the modifications below and with the requirements of one or both of the following two monographs according to the composition of the antitoxin as stated on the label.

LABELLING

The label states (1) whether the preparation contains beta or epsilon antitoxin or both; (2) the type or types of *Cl. perfringens* against which the antitoxin will provide protection.

Clostridium Perfringens Beta Antitoxin

(*Clostridium Perfringens Beta Antitoxin for Veterinary Use, Ph Eur monograph 0340*)

Ph Eur

DEFINITION

Clostridium perfringens beta antitoxin for veterinary use is a preparation containing principally the globulins that have the power of specifically neutralising the beta toxin formed by *Clostridium perfringens* (types B and C). It consists of the serum or a preparation obtained from the serum of animals immunised against *C. perfringens* beta toxin.

PRODUCTION

Choice of composition

The antitoxin is shown to be satisfactory with respect to safety (5.2.6) and efficacy (5.2.7). For the latter, it shall be demonstrated, for each target species, that the product, when administered at the minimum recommended dose and according to the recommended schedule(s), provides a response or responses consistent with the claims made for the product.

Batch potency test

The test described under Potency it not necessarily carried out for routine testing of batches of antitoxin. It is carried out on 1 or more occasions as decided by or with agreement of the competent authority. Where the test is not carried out, a suitable validated alternative test is carried out, the criteria for acceptance being set with reference to a batch of antitoxin that has given satisfactory results in the test described under Potency and that has been shown to be satisfactory with respect to immunogenicity in the target species.

The following test may be used after a satisfactory correlation with the test described under Potency has been established.

Determine the level of antibodies against *C. perfringens* beta toxin in the batch of antitoxin using a suitable method such as an immunochemical method (*2.7.1*) or a neutralisation in cell cultures. Use a homologous reference serum calibrated in International Units of clostridium perfringens beta antitoxin.

The International Unit is the specific neutralising activity for *C. perfringens* beta toxin contained in a stated amount of the International Standard, which consists of a quantity of dried immune horse serum. The equivalence in International Units of the International Standard is stated by the World Health Organisation.

The potency of the finished product is expressed in International Units per millilitre and is shown to be not less than the minimum number stated on the label.

IDENTIFICATION

The antitoxin is shown, by a suitable immunochemical method (*2.7.1*), to react specifically with the beta toxin formed by *C. perfringens*.

POTENCY

The potency of clostridium perfringens beta antitoxin is determined by comparing the dose necessary to protect mice or other suitable animals against the toxic effects of a fixed dose of *C. perfringens* beta toxin with the quantity of a reference preparation of clostridium perfringens beta antitoxin, calibrated in International Units, necessary to give the same protection. For this comparison, a suitable preparation of *C. perfringens* beta toxin for use as a test toxin is required. The dose of the test toxin is determined in relation to the reference preparation; the potency of the clostridium perfringens beta antitoxin to be examined is determined in relation to the reference preparation using the test toxin.

Preparation of test toxin

Prepare the test toxin from a sterile filtrate of an early culture in liquid medium of *C. perfringens* type B or type C and dry by a suitable method. Select the test toxin by determining for mice the L+ dose and the LD_{50}, the observation period being 72 h. A suitable beta toxin contains not less than one L+ dose in 0.2 mg and not less than 25 LD_{50} in each L+ dose.

Determination of test dose of toxin

Prepare a solution of the reference preparation in a suitable liquid so that it contains 5 IU/ml. Prepare a solution of the test toxin in a suitable liquid so that 1 ml contains a precisely known amount such as 10 mg. Prepare mixtures of the solution of the reference preparation and the solution of the test toxin such that each mixture contains 2.0 ml of the solution of the reference preparation (10 IU), one of a series of graded volumes of the solution of the test toxin and sufficient of a suitable liquid to bring the total volume to 5.0 ml. Allow the mixtures to stand at room temperature for 30 min. Using not fewer than two mice, each weighing 17-22 g, for each mixture, inject a dose of 0.5 ml intravenously or intraperitoneally into each mouse. Observe the mice for 72 h. If all the mice die, the amount of toxin present in 0.5 ml of the mixture is in excess of the test dose. If none of the mice die, the amount of toxin present in 0.5 ml of the

mixture is less than the test dose. Prepare similar fresh mixtures such that 5.0 ml of each mixture contains 2.0 ml of the solution of the reference preparation (10 IU) and 1 of a series of graded volumes of the solution of the test toxin separated from each other by steps of not more than 20 per cent and covering the expected end-point. Allow the mixtures to stand at room temperature for 30 min.

Using not fewer than 2 mice for each mixture, inject a dose of 0.5 ml intravenously or intraperitoneally into each mouse. Observe the mice for 72 h. Repeat the determination at least once and combine the results of the separate tests that have been made with mixtures of the same composition so that a series of totals is obtained, each total representing the mortality due to a mixture of a given composition. The test dose of toxin is the amount present in 0.5 ml of that mixture which causes the death of one half of the total number of mice injected with it.

Determination of the potency of the antitoxin to be examined

Preliminary test Dissolve a quantity of the test toxin in a suitable liquid so that 2.0 ml contains 10 times the test dose (solution of the test toxin). Prepare mixtures of the solution of the test toxin and the antitoxin to be examined such that each mixture contains 2.0 ml of the solution of the test toxin, one of a series of graded volumes of the antitoxin to be examined and sufficent of a suitable liquid to bring the final volume to 5.0 ml. Allow the mixtures to stand at room temperature for 30 min. Using not fewer than 2 mice for each mixture, inject a dose of 0.5 ml intravenously or intraperitoneally into each mouse. Observe the mice for 72 h. If none of the mice die, 0.5 ml of the mixture contains more than 1 IU. If all the mice die, 0.5 ml of the mixture contains less than 1 IU.

Final test Prepare mixtures of the solution of the test toxin and of the antitoxin to be examined such that 5.0 ml of each mixture contains 2.0 ml of the solution of the test toxin and one of a series of graded volumes of the antitoxin to be examined, separated from each other by steps of not more than 20 per cent and covering the expected end-point as determined by the preliminary test. Prepare further mixtures such that 5.0 ml of each mixture contains 2.0 ml of the solution of the test toxin and one of a series of graded volumes of the solution of the reference preparation, in order to confirm the test dose of the toxin. Allow the mixtures to stand at room temperature for 30 min. Using not fewer than 2 mice for each mixture, proceed as described in the preliminary test. The test mixture which contains 1 IU in 0.5 ml is that mixture which kills the same or almost the same number of mice as the reference mixture containing 1 IU in 0.5 ml. Repeat the determination at least once and calculate the average of all valid estimates. Estimates are valid only if the reference preparation gives a result within 20 per cent of the expected value.

The confidence limits ($P = 0.95$) have been estimated to be:
— 85 per cent and 114 per cent when 2 animals per dose are used,
— 91.5 per cent and 109 per cent when 4 animals per dose are used,
— 93 per cent and 108 per cent when 6 animals per dose are used.

The potency of the finished product is expressed in International Units per millilitre and is shown to be not less than the minimum number stated on the label.

Clostridium Perfringens Epsilon Antitoxin

(Clostridium Perfringens Epsilon Antitoxin for Veterinary Use, Ph Eur monograph 0341)

Ph Eur

DEFINITION

Clostridium perfringens epsilon antitoxin for veterinary use is a preparation containing the globulins that have the power of specifically neutralising the epsilon toxin formed by *Clostridium perfringens* type D. It consists of the serum or a preparation obtained from the serum of animals immunised against *C. perfringens* epsilon toxin.

PRODUCTION

CHOICE OF COMPOSITION

The antitoxin is shown to be satisfactory with respect to safety (*5.2.6*) and efficacy (*5.2.7*). For the latter, it shall be demonstrated, for each target species, that the product, when administered at the minimum recommended dose and according to the recommended schedule(s), provides a response or responses consistent with the claims made for the product.

Batch potency test

The test described under Potency is not necessarily carried out for routine testing of batches of antitoxin. It is carried out on one or more occasions as decided by or with the agreement of the competent authority. Where the test is not carried out, a suitable validated alternative test is carried out, the criteria for acceptance being set with reference to a batch of antitoxin that has given satisfactory results in the test described under Potency and that has been shown to be satisfactory with respect to immunogenicity in the target species. The following test may be used after a satisfactory correlation with the test described under Potency has been established.

Determine the level of antibodies against *C. perfringens* epsilon toxin in the batch of antitoxin using a suitable method such as an immunochemical method (*2.7.1*) or neutralisation in cell cultures. Use a homologous reference serum calibrated in International Units of clostridium perfringens epsilon antitoxin.

The International Unit is the specific neutralising activity for *C. perfringens* epsilon toxin contained in a stated amount of the International Standard, which consists of a quantity of dried immune horse serum. The equivalence in International Units of the International Standard is stated by the World Health Organisation.

The potency of the finished product is expressed in International Units per millilitre and is shown to be not less than the minimum number stated on the label.

IDENTIFICATION

The antitoxin is shown, by a suitable immunochemical method (*2.7.1*), to react specifically with the epsilon toxin formed by *C. perfringens*.

POTENCY

The potency of clostridium perfringens epsilon antitoxin is determined by comparing the dose necessary to protect mice or other suitable animals against the toxic effects of a fixed dose of *C. perfringens* epsilon toxin with the quantity of a reference preparation of clostridium perfringens epsilon antitoxin, calibrated in International Units, necessary to give the same protection. For this comparison, a suitable preparation of *C. perfringens* epsilon toxin for use as a test

toxin is required. The dose of the test toxin is determined in relation to the reference preparation, the potency of the antitoxin to be examined is determined in relation to the reference preparation using the test toxin.

Preparation of test toxin

Prepare the test toxin from a sterile filtrate of an early culture in liquid medium of *C. perfringens* type D and dry by a suitable method. Select the test toxin by determining for mice the L+/10 dose and the LD_{50}, the observation period being 72 h. A suitable epsilon toxin contains not less than one L+/10 dose in 0.005 mg and not less than 20 LD_{50} in each L+/10 dose.

Determination of test dose of toxin

Prepare a solution of the reference preparation in a suitable liquid so that it contains 0.5 IU/ml. Prepare a solution of the test toxin in a suitable liquid so that 1 ml contains a precisely known amount such as 1 mg. Prepare mixtures of the solution of the reference preparation and the solution of the test toxin such that each mixture contains 2.0 ml of the solution of the reference preparation (1 IU), one of a series of graded volumes of the solution of the test toxin and sufficient of a suitable liquid to bring the total volume to 5.0 ml. Allow the mixtures to stand at room temperature for 30 min. Using not fewer than 2 mice, each weighing 17-22 g, for each mixture, inject a dose of 0.5 ml intravenously or intraperitoneally into each mouse. Observe the mice for 72 h. If all the mice die, the amount of toxin present in 0.5 ml of the mixture is in excess of the test dose. If none of the mice die, the amount of toxin present in 0.5 ml of the mixture is less than the test dose. Prepare similar fresh mixtures such that 5.0 ml of each mixture contains 2.0 ml of the solution of the reference preparation (1 IU) and 1 of a series of graded volumes of the solution of the test toxin, separated from each other by steps of not more than 20 per cent and covering the expected end-point. Allow the mixtures to stand at room temperature for 30 min. Using not fewer than 2 mice for each mixture, inject a dose of 0.5 ml intravenously or intraperitoneally into each mouse. Observe the mice for 72 h. Repeat the determination at least once and combine the results of the separate tests that have been made with mixtures of the same composition so that a series of totals is obtained, each total representing the mortality due to a mixture of a given composition. The test dose of the toxin is the amount present in 0.5 ml of that mixture which causes the death of one half of the total number of mice injected with it.

Determination of the potency of the antitoxin to be examined

Preliminary test Dissolve a quantity of the test toxin in a suitable liquid so that 2.0 ml contains 10 times the test dose (solution of the test toxin). Prepare mixtures of the solution of the test toxin and of the antitoxin to be examined such that each mixture contains 2.0 ml of the solution of the test toxin, one of a series of graded volumes of the antitoxin to be examined and sufficient of a suitable liquid to bring the final volume to 5.0 ml. Allow the mixtures to stand at room temperature for 30 min. Using not fewer than 2 mice for each mixture, inject a dose of 0.5 ml intravenously or intraperitoneally into each mouse. Observe the mice for 72 h. If none of the mice die, 0.5 ml of the mixture contains more than 0.1 IU. If all the mice die, 0.5 ml of the mixture contains less than 0.1 IU.

Final test Prepare mixtures of the solution of the test toxin and of the antitoxin to be examined such that 5.0 ml of each mixture contains 2.0 ml of the solution of the test toxin and one of a series of graded volumes of the antitoxin to be examined, separated from each other by steps of not more than 20 per cent and covering the expected end-point as determined by the preliminary test. Prepare further mixtures such that 5.0 ml of each mixture contains 2.0 ml of the solution of the test toxin and one of a series of graded volumes of the solution of the reference preparation to confirm the test dose of the toxin. Allow the mixtures to stand at room temperature for 30 min. Using not fewer than 2 mice for each mixture proceed as described in the preliminary test. The test mixture which contains 0.1 IU in 0.5 ml is that mixture which kills the same or almost the same number of mice as the reference mixture containing 0.1 IU in 0.5 ml. Repeat the determination at least once and calculate the average of all valid estimates. Estimates are valid only if the reference preparation gives a result within 20 per cent of the expected value.

The confidence limits ($P = 0.95$) have been estimated to be:
— 85 per cent and 114 per cent when 2 animals per dose are used,
— 91.5 per cent and 109 per cent when 4 animals per dose are used,
— 93 per cent and 108 per cent when 6 animals per dose are used.

The potency of the finished product is expressed in International Units per millilitre and is shown to be not less than the minimum number stated on the label.

Ph Eur

Clostridium Tetani Antitoxin

Tetanus Antitoxin (Veterinary)

(*Tetanus Antitoxin for Veterinary Use, Ph Eur monograph 0343*)

Ph Eur

DEFINITION

Tetanus antitoxin for veterinary use is a preparation containing principally the globulins that have the power of specifically neutralising the neurotoxin formed by *Clostridium tetani*. It consists of the serum or a preparation obtained from the serum of animals immunised against tetanus toxin.

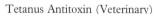

PRODUCTION
CHOICE OF COMPOSITION
The antitoxin is shown to be satisfactory with respect to safety (*5.2.6*) and efficacy (*5.2.7*). For the latter, it shall be demonstrated, for each target species, that the product, when administered at the minimum recommended dose and according to the recommended schedule(s), provides a response or responses consistent with the claims made for the product. The ability of the product to neutralise the neurotoxin formed by *C. tetani* must also be demonstrated, e.g. by conducting the test in mice as described below.

Demonstration of neurotoxin neutralisation
The ability of tetanus antitoxin to neutralise the neurotoxin of *C. tetani* is determined by establishing the dose necessary to protect mice (or guinea-pigs) against the toxic effects of a fixed dose of tetanus toxin. The test must be conducted in parallel with a test of a reference preparation of tetanus antitoxin, calibrated in International Units, using a quantity expected to give the same protection. The ability of the test antitoxin to neutralise the neurotoxin (potency) can then be expressed in International Units. For this study, a suitable preparation of tetanus toxin for use as a test toxin is

required. The dose of the test toxin is determined in relation to the reference preparation; the potency of the antitoxin to be examined is determined in relation to the reference preparation using the test toxin.

Preparation of test toxin Prepare the test toxin from a sterile filtrate of an 8-10 day culture in liquid medium of *C. tetani*. A test toxin may be prepared by adding this filtrate to *glycerol R* in the proportion of 1 volume of filtrate to 1 to 2 volumes of *glycerol R*. The solution of test toxin may be stored at or slightly below 0 °C. The toxin may also be dried by a suitable method. Select the test toxin by determining for mice the Lp/10 dose and the paralytic dose 50 per cent. A suitable toxin contains not less than 1000 times the paralytic dose 50 per cent in 1 Lp/10 dose.

Lp/10 dose (Limes paralyticum) This is the smallest quantity of toxin which when mixed with 0.1 IU of antitoxin and injected subcutaneously into mice (or guinea-pigs) causes tetanic paralysis in the animals on or before the 4th day after injection.

Paralytic dose 50 per cent This is the quantity of toxin which when injected subcutaneously into mice (or guinea-pigs) causes tetanic paralysis in one half of the animals on or before the 4th day after injection.

Determination of test dose of toxin Reconstitute or dilute the reference preparation with a suitable liquid so that it contains 0.5 IU/ml. Measure or weigh a quantity of the test toxin and dilute with or dissolve in a suitable liquid. Prepare mixtures of the solution of the reference preparation and the solution of the test toxin so that each mixture will contain 0.1 IU of antitoxin in the volume chosen for injection and one of a series of graded volumes of the solution of the test toxin, separated from each other by steps of not more than 20 per cent and covering the expected end-point. Adjust each mixture with a suitable liquid to the same final volume (0.4 ml to 0.6 ml if mice are used for the test or 4.0 ml if guinea-pigs are used). Allow the mixtures to stand at room temperature for 60 min. Using not fewer than 2 animals for each mixture, inject the chosen volume subcutaneously into each animal. Observe the animals for 96 h and make daily records of the degree of tetanus developing in each group of animals. Repeat the test at least once and calculate the test dose as the mean of the different tests. The test dose of the toxin is the amount present in that mixture which causes tetanic paralysis in one half of the total number of animals injected with it.

Determination of the neutralising ability of the antitoxin to be examined
Preliminary test Measure or weigh a quantity of the test toxin and dilute with or dissolve in a suitable liquid so that the solution contains 5 test doses per millilitre (solution of the test toxin). Prepare mixtures of the solution of the test toxin and of the antitoxin to be examined so that for each mixture the volume chosen for injection contains the test dose of toxin and one of a series of graded volumes of the antitoxin to be examined. Adjust each mixture to the same final volume with a suitable liquid. Allow the mixtures to stand at room temperature for 60 min. Using not fewer than 2 animals for each mixture, inject the chosen volume subcutaneously into each animal. Observe the animals for 96 h and make daily records of the degree of tetanus developing in each group of animals. Using the results, select suitable mixtures for the final test.

Final test Prepare mixtures of the solution of the test toxin and of the antitoxin to be examined so that for each mixture the volume chosen for the injection contains the test dose of toxin and one of a series of graded volumes of the antitoxin to be examined, separated from each other by steps of not more than 20 per cent and covering the expected end-point as determined in the preliminary test. Prepare further mixtures with the same amount of test toxin and graded volumes of the reference preparation, centred on 0.1 IU in the volume chosen for injection, to confirm the test dose of the toxin. Adjust each mixture to the same final volume with a suitable liquid. Allow the mixtures to stand at room temperature for 60 min. Using not fewer than 2 animals for each mixture, inject the chosen volume subcutaneously into each animal. Observe the animals for 96 h and make daily records of the degree of tetanus developing in each group of animals. The test mixture which contains 0.1 IU in the volume injected is that mixture which causes tetanic paralysis in the same, or almost the same, number of animals as the reference mixture containing 0.1 IU in the volume injected. Repeat the determination at least once and calculate the mean of all valid estimates. Estimates are valid only if the reference preparation gives a result within 20 per cent of the expected value.

The confidence limits ($P = 0.95$) have been estimated to be:
— 85 per cent and 114 per cent when 2 animals per dose are used,
— 91.5 per cent and 109 per cent when 3 animals per dose are used,
— 93 per cent and 108 per cent when 6 animals per dose are used.

IDENTIFICATION

The antitoxin is shown, by a suitable immunochemical method (2.7.1), to react specifically with the neurotoxin formed by *C. tetani*. The potency test may also serve for identification.

POTENCY

Determine the titre of antibodies against the neurotoxin formed by *C. tetani* using a suitable immunochemical method (2.7.1) such as a toxin-binding-inhibition test (ToBI test) and a homologous reference serum, calibrated in International Units per millilitre.

The International Unit is the specific neutralising activity for tetanus toxin contained in a stated amount of the International Standard which consists of a quantity of dried immune horse serum. The equivalence in International Units of the International Standard is stated by the World Health Organisation.

The potency of the finished product is expressed in International Units per millilitre and is shown to be not less than the minimum number stated on the label.

_____ *Ph Eur*

Veterinary Vaccines

*(Vaccines for Veterinary Use,
Ph Eur monograph 0062)*

Veterinary Vaccines comply with the requirements of the European Pharmacopoeia monograph for Vaccines for Veterinary Use. These requirements are reproduced below.

The provisions of this monograph apply to the following vaccines.

Inactivated Bacterial Vaccines

Bovine Leptospirosis Vaccine (Inactivated)★
Canine Leptospirosis Vaccine (Inactivated)★
Clostridium Botulinum Vaccine★
Clostridium Chauvoei Vaccine★
Clostridium Novyi Type B Vaccine★
Clostridium Perfringens Vaccines★
Clostridium Septicum Vaccine★
Clostridium Tetani Vaccines★
Fowl Cholera Vaccine (Inactivated)★
Furunculosis Vaccine for Salmonids, Inactivated★
Mannheimia Vaccine (Inactivated) for Cattle★
Mannheimia Vaccine (Inactivated) for Sheep★
Pasteurella Vaccine (Inactivated) for Sheep★
Porcine Actinobacillosis Vaccine, Inactivated★
Porcine E. Coli Vaccine, Inactivated★
Porcine Progressive Atrophic Rhinitis Vaccine, Inactivated★
Ruminant E. Coli Vaccine, Inactivated★
Swine Erysipelas Vaccine, Inactivated★
Vibriosis Vaccine for Salmonids, Inactivated, Cold-water★
Vibriosis Vaccine for Salmonids, Inactivated★

Living Bacterial Vaccines

Anthrax Vaccine, Living★
Brucella Melitensis (Strain Rev. 1) Vaccine, Living★
Salmonella Dublin Vaccine, Living

Inactivated Viral Vaccines

Aujesky's Disease Vaccine, Inactivated★
Avian Infectious Bronchitis Vaccine, Inactivated★
Avian Paramyxovirus 3 Vaccine, Inactivated★
Bovine Viral Diarrhoea Vaccine (Inactivated)
Calf Coronavirus Diarrhoea Vaccine (Inactivated)★
Calf Rotavirus Diarrhoea Vaccine (Inactivated)★
Canine Adenovirus Vaccine, Inactivated★
Canine Parvovirus Vaccine, Inactivated ★
Egg-drop Syndrome 76 (Adenovirus) Vaccine★
Equine Herpesvirus Vaccine, Inactivated★
Equine Influenza Vaccine★
Feline Calicivirus Vaccine, Inactivated★
Feline Infectious Enteritis Vaccine, Inactivated★
Feline Leukaemia Vaccine, Inactivated★
Feline Viral Rhinotracheitis Vaccine, Inactivated★
Foot and Mouth Disease (Ruminants) Vaccine★
Infectious Bursal Disease Vaccine, Inactivated★
Louping-ill Vaccine
Newcastle Disease Vaccine, Inactivated★
Ovine Enzootic Abortion Vaccine
Porcine Parvovirus Vaccine, Inactivated★

Rabies Veterinary Vaccine, Inactivated*

Swine Influenza Vaccine, Inactivated*

Living Viral Vaccines

Aujesky's Disease Vaccine, Living*

Avian Infectious Bronchitis Vaccine, Living*

Avian Viral Tenosynovitis Vaccine (Live)*

Bovine Parainfluenza Virus Vaccine, Living*

Bovine Respiratory Syncytial Virus Vaccine, Living*

Canine Adenovirus Vaccine, Living *

Canine Distemper Vaccine, Living*

Canine Parainfluenza Virus Vaccine (Live)

Canine Parvovirus Vaccine, Living*

Contagious Pustular Dermatitis Vaccine, Living

Duck Plague Vaccine (Live)

Duck Viral Hepatitis Type I Vaccine (Live)*

Feline Calicivirus Vaccine, Living*

Feline Infectious Enteritis Vaccine, Living*

Feline Viral Rhinotracheitis Vaccine, Living*

Ferret and Mink Distemper Vaccine, Living*

Fowl Pox Vaccine, Living*

Infectious Avian Encephalomyelitis Vaccine, Living*

Infectious Bovine Rhinotracheitis Vaccine, Living*

Infectious Bursal Disease Vaccine, Living*

Infectious Chicken Anaemia Vaccine (Live)*

Laryngotracheitis Vaccine, Living*

Marek's Disease Vaccine, Living*

Myxomatosis Vaccine (Live) for Rabbits*

Newcastle Disease and Avian Infectious Bronchitis Vaccine, Living

Newcastle Disease Vaccine, Living*

Rabies Vaccine for Foxes, Living*

Swine Fever Vaccine, Living*

Helminth Vaccine

Lungworm (Dictyocaulus Viviparus) Oral Vaccine, Living

---

*Monograph of the European Pharmacopoeia

Ph Eur _____

In the case of combined vaccines, for each component that is the subject of a monograph in the Pharmacopoeia, the provisions of that monograph apply to that component, modified where necessary as indicated (see Tests (Safety) below, Evaluation of safety of veterinary vaccines (5.2.6) and Evaluation of efficacy of veterinary vaccines (5.2.7)).

DEFINITION

Vaccines for veterinary use are preparations containing antigenic substances and are administered for the purpose of inducing a specific and active immunity against disease provoked by bacteria, toxins, viruses, fungi or parasites. The vaccines, live or inactivated, confer active immunity that may be transferred passively via maternal antibodies against the immunogens they contain and sometimes also against antigenically related organisms. Vaccines may contain bacteria, toxins, viruses or fungi, living or inactivated, parasites, or antigenic fractions or substances produced by these organisms and rendered harmless whilst retaining all or part of their antigenic properties; vaccines may also contain combinations of these constituents. The antigens may be produced by recombinant DNA technology. Suitable

adjuvants may be included to enhance the immunising properties of the vaccines.

Terminology used in monographs on vaccines for veterinary use is defined in chapter 5.2.1.

BACTERIAL VACCINES AND BACTERIAL TOXOIDS

Bacterial vaccines and bacterial toxoids are prepared from cultures grown on suitable solid or liquid media, or by other suitable means; the requirements of this section do not apply to bacterial vaccines prepared in cell cultures or in live animals. The strain of bacterium used may have been modified by genetic engineering. The identity, antigenic potency and purity of each bacterial culture used is carefully controlled.

Bacterial vaccines contain inactivated or live bacteria or their antigenic components; they are liquid preparations of various degrees of opacity or they may be freeze-dried.

Bacterial toxoids are prepared from toxins by diminishing their toxicity to a very low level or by completely eliminating it by physical or chemical means whilst retaining adequate immunising potency. The toxins are obtained from selected strains of specified micro-organisms grown in suitable media or are obtained by other suitable means, for example, chemical synthesis.

The toxoids may be:
— liquid,
— precipitated with alum or other suitable agent,
— purified and/or adsorbed on aluminium phosphate, aluminium hydroxide, calcium phosphate or other adsorbent prescribed in the monograph.

Bacterial toxoids are clear or slightly opalescent liquids. Adsorbed toxoids are suspensions or emulsions. Certain toxoids may be freeze-dried.

Unless otherwise indicated, statements and requirements given below for bacterial vaccines apply equally to bacterial vaccines, bacterial toxoids and products containing a combination of bacterial cells and toxoid.

VIRAL VACCINES

Viral vaccines are prepared by growth in suitable cell cultures (5.2.4), in tissues, in micro-organisms, in fertilised eggs or, where no other possibility is available, in live animals, or by other suitable means. The strain of virus used may have been modified by genetic engineering. They are liquid or freeze-dried preparations of one or more viruses or viral subunits or peptides.

Live viral vaccines are prepared from viruses of attenuated virulence or of natural low virulence for the target species.

Inactivated viral vaccines are treated by a validated procedure for inactivation of the virus and may be purified and concentrated.

VECTOR VACCINES

Vector vaccines are liquid or freeze-dried preparations of one or more types of live micro-organisms (bacteria or viruses) that are non-pathogenic or have low pathogenicity for the target species and in which have been inserted one or more genes encoding antigens that stimulate an immune response protective against other microorganisms.

PRODUCTION

The methods of preparation, which vary according to the type of vaccine, are such as to maintain the identity and immunogenicity of the antigen and to ensure freedom from contamination with extraneous agents.

Substances of animal origin used in the production of vaccines for veterinary use comply with the requirements of chapter *5.2.5.* Other substances used in the preparation of vaccines for veterinary use comply with requirements of the Pharmacopoeia (where a relevant monograph exists) and are prepared in a manner that avoids contamination of the vaccine.

SUBSTRATES FOR PRODUCTION

Cell cultures used in the production of vaccines for veterinary use comply with the requirements of chapter *5.2.4.*

Where a monograph refers to chicken flocks free from specified pathogens (SPF), these flocks comply with the requirements prescribed in chapter *5.2.2.*

For production of inactivated vaccines, where vaccine organisms are grown in poultry embryos, such embryos are derived either from SPF flocks (*5.2.2*) or from healthy non-SPF flocks free from the presence of certain agents and their antibodies, as specified in the monograph. It may be necessary to demonstrate that the inactivation process is effective against specified potential contaminants. For the production of a master seed lot and for all passages of a micro-organism up to and including the working seed lot, eggs from SPF flocks (*5.2.2*) are used.

Where it is unavoidable to use animals or animal tissues in the production of veterinary vaccines, such animals shall be free from specified pathogens, as appropriate to the source species and the target animal for the vaccine.

MEDIA

At least the qualitative composition must be recorded of media used for seed culture preparation and for production. The grade of each named ingredient is specified. Where media or ingredients are claimed as proprietary, this is indicated and an appropriate description recorded. Ingredients that are derived from animals are specified as to the source species and country of origin, and must comply with the criteria described in chapter *5.2.5.* Preparation processes for media used, including sterilisation procedures, are documented.

The addition of antibiotics during the manufacturing process is normally restricted to cell culture fluids and other media, egg inocula and material harvested from skin or other tissues.

BACTERIAL SEED LOTS
General requirements

The genus and species (and varieties where appropriate) of the bacteria used in the vaccine are stated. Bacteria used in manufacture are handled in a seed-lot system wherever possible. Each master seed lot is tested as described below. A record of the origin, date of isolation, passage history (including purification and characterisation procedures) and storage conditions is maintained for each master seed lot. Each master seed lot is assigned a specific code for identification purposes.

Propagation

The minimum and maximum number of subcultures of each master seed lot prior to the production stage are specified. The methods used for the preparation of seed cultures, preparation of suspensions for seeding, techniques for inoculation of seeds, titre and concentration of inocula and the media used, are documented. It shall be demonstrated that the characteristics of the seed material (for example, dissociation or antigenicity) are not changed by these subcultures. The conditions under which each seed lot is stored are documented.

Identity and purity

Each master seed lot is shown to contain only the species and strain of bacterium stated. A brief description of the method of identifying each strain by biochemical, serological and morphological characteristics and distinguishing it as far as possible from related strains is recorded, as is also the method of determining the purity of the strain. If the master seed lot is shown to contain living organisms of any kind other than the species and strain stated, then it is unsuitable for vaccine production.

VIRUS SEED LOTS
General requirements

Viruses used in manufacture are handled in a seed-lot system. Each master seed lot is tested as described below. A record of the origin, date of isolation, passage history (including purification and characterisation procedures) and storage conditions is maintained for each seed lot. Each master seed lot is assigned a specific code for identification purposes. Production of vaccine is not normally undertaken using virus more than 5 passages from the master seed lot. In the tests on the master seed lot described below, the organisms used are not normally more than 5 passages from the master seed lot at the start of the tests, unless otherwise indicated.

Where the master seed lot is contained within a permanently infected master cell seed, the following tests are carried out on an appropriate volume of virus from disrupted master cell seed. Where relevant tests have been carried out on disrupted cells to validate the suitability of the master cell seed, these tests need not be repeated.

Propagation

The master seed lot and all subsequent passages are propagated on cells, on embryonated eggs or in animals that have been shown to be suitable for vaccine production (see above), and, where applicable, using substances of animal origin that meet the requirements prescribed in chapter *5.2.5.*

Identification

A suitable method to identify the vaccine strain and to distinguish it as far as possible from related strains must be used.

Bacterial and fungal contamination

The master seed lot complies with the test for sterility (*2.6.1*).

Mycoplasmas (*2.6.7*)

The master seed lot complies with the test for mycoplasmas (culture method and indicator cell culture method).

Absence of extraneous viruses

Monographs may contain requirements for freedom from extraneous agents, otherwise the requirements stated below apply.

Preparations of monoclonal or polyclonal antibodies containing high levels of neutralising antibody to the virus of the seed lot are made on a batch basis, using antigen that is not derived from any passage level of the virus isolate giving rise to the master seed virus. Each batch of serum is maintained at 56 °C for 30 min to inactivate complement. Each batch is shown to be free of antibodies to potential contaminants of the seed virus and is shown to be free of any non-specific inhibiting effects on the ability of viruses to infect and propagate within cells (or eggs, where applicable). If such a serum cannot be obtained, other methods are used to remove or neutralise the seed virus specifically.

If the seed lot virus would interfere with the conduct and sensitivity of a test for extraneous viruses, a sample of the master seed lot is treated with a minimum amount of the monoclonal or polyclonal antibody so that the vaccine virus is neutralised as far as possible or removed. The final virus-serum mixture shall, if possible, contain at least the virus content of 10 doses of vaccine per 0.1 ml for avian vaccines and per millilitre for other vaccines. For avian vaccines, the testing to be carried out on seed lots is given in chapter 2.6.24. For mammalian vaccines, the seed lot or the mixture of seed lot and antiserum is tested for freedom from extraneous agents as follows.

The mixture is inoculated onto cultures of at least 70 cm^2 of the required cell types. The cultures may be inoculated at any suitable stage of growth up to 70 per cent confluency. At least 1 monolayer of each type must be retained as a control. The cultures must be monitored daily for a week. At the end of this period the cultures are freeze thawed 3 times, centrifuged to remove cell debris and re-inoculated onto the same cell type as above. This is repeated twice. The final passage must produce sufficient cells in appropriate vessels to carry out the tests below.

Cytopathic and haemadsorbing agents are tested for using the methods described in the relevant sections on testing cell cultures (5.2.4) and techniques such as immuno-fluorescence are used for detection of specific contaminants for the tests in cell cultures. The master seed lot is inoculated onto:

— primary cells of the species of origin of the virus,
— cells sensitive to viruses pathogenic for the species for which the vaccine is intended,
— cells sensitive to pestiviruses.

If the master seed lot is shown to contain living organisms of any kind, other than the virus of the species and strain stated, or foreign viral antigens, then it is unsuitable for vaccine production.

INACTIVATION

Inactivated vaccines are subjected to a validated inactivation procedure. The testing of the inactivation kinetics described below is carried out once for a given production process. The rest of this section applies to each production run. When conducting tests for inactivation, it is essential to take account of the possibility that under the conditions of manufacture, organisms may be physically protected from inactivant.

Inactivation kinetics

The inactivating agent and the inactivation procedure shall be shown, under conditions of manufacture, to inactivate the vaccine micro-organism. Adequate data on inactivation kinetics shall be obtained. Normally, the time required for inactivation shall be not more than 67 per cent of the duration of the inactivation process.

Aziridine

If an aziridine compound is used as the inactivating agent then it shall be shown that no inactivating agent remains at the end of the inactivation procedure. This may be accomplished by neutralising the inactivating agent with thiosulphate and demonstrating residual thiosulphate in the inactivated harvest at the completion of the inactivation procedure.

Formaldehyde

If formaldehyde is used as the inactivating agent, then a test for free formaldehyde is carried out as prescribed under Tests.

Other inactivating agents

When other inactivation methods are used, appropriate tests are carried out to demonstrate that the inactivating agent has been removed or reduced to an acceptable residual level.

Inactivation and/or detoxification testing

A test for complete inactivation and/or detoxification is performed immediately after the inactivation and/or detoxification procedure and, if applicable, the neutralisation or removal of the inactivating or detoxifying agent.

Bacterial vaccines The test selected shall be appropriate to the vaccine bacteria being used and shall consist of at least 2 passages in production medium or, if solid medium has been used for production, in a suitable liquid medium or in the medium prescribed in the monograph. The product complies with the test if no evidence of any live micro-organism is observed.

Bacterial toxoids The test selected shall be appropriate to the toxin or toxins present and shall be the most sensitive available.

Viral vaccines The test selected shall be appropriate to the vaccine virus being used and must consist of at least 2 passages in cells, embryonated eggs or, where no other suitably sensitive method is available, in animals. The quantity of cell samples, eggs or animals shall be sufficient to ensure appropriate sensitivity of the test. For tests in cell cultures, not less than 150 cm^2 of cell culture monolayer is inoculated with 1.0 ml of inactivated harvest. The product complies with the test if no evidence of the presence of any live virus or other micro-organism is observed.

CHOICE OF VACCINE COMPOSITION AND CHOICE OF VACCINE STRAIN

For the choice of vaccine composition and choice of vaccine strain, important aspects to be evaluated include safety, efficacy and stability. General requirements for evaluation of safety and efficacy are given in chapter 5.2.6 and chapter 5.2.7. These requirements may be made more explicit or supplemented by the requirements of specific monographs.

For live vaccines, a maximum virus titre or bacterial count acceptable from the point of view of safety is established during development studies. This is then used as the maximum acceptable titre for each batch of vaccine at release.

Potency and immunogenicity The tests given under the headings Potency and Immunogenicity in monographs serve 2 purposes:

— the Potency section establishes by a well-controlled test in experimental conditions, the minimum acceptable vaccinating capacity for all vaccines within the scope of the definition, which must be guaranteed throughout the period of validity;
— well-controlled experimental studies are normally a part of the overall demonstration of efficacy of a vaccine (see chapter 5.2.7); the test referred to in the section 'Immunogenicity' (which is usually a cross-reference to the Potency section) is suitable as a part of this testing.

For most vaccines, the tests cited under Potency or Immunogenicity are not suitable for the routine testing of batches.

For live vaccines, the minimum acceptable virus titre or bacterial count that gives satisfactory results in the Potency test and other efficacy studies is established during development. For routine testing it must be demonstrated for each batch that the titre or count at release is such that at the end of the period of validity, in the light of stability studies, the vaccine, stored in the recommended conditions, will contain not less than the minimum acceptable virus titre or bacterial count determined during development studies.

For inactivated vaccines, if the test described under Potency is not used for routine testing, a batch potency test is established during development. The aim of the batch potency test is to ensure that each batch of vaccine would, if tested, comply with the test described under Potency or Immunogenicity. The acceptance criteria for the batch potency test are therefore established by correlation with the test described under Potency. Where a batch potency test is described in a monograph, this is given as an example of a test that is considered suitable, after establishment of correlation with the potency test; other test models can also be used.

Route of administration During development of a vaccine, safety and immunogenicity are demonstrated for each route of administration to be recommended. The following is a non-exhaustive list of such routes of administration:
— intramuscular,
— subcutaneous,
— intravenous,
— ocular,
— oral,
— nasal,
— foot-stab,
— wing web,
— intradermal,
— intraperitoneal,
— *in ovo*.

Methods of administration During development of a vaccine, safety and immunogenicity are demonstrated for each method of administration to be recommended. The following is a non-exhaustive list of such methods of administration:
— injection,
— drinking water,
— spray,
— eye-drop,
— scarification,
— implantation,
— immersion.

Categories of animal Monographs may indicate that a given test is to be carried out for each category of animal of the target species for which the product is recommended or is to be recommended. The following is a non-exhaustive list of categories that are to be taken into account.
— *Mammals:*
    — pregnant animals/non-pregnant animals,
    — animals raised primarily for breeding/animals raised primarily for food production,
    — animals of the minimum age or size recommended for vaccination.
— *Avian species:*
    — birds raised primarily for egg production/birds raised primarily for production of meat,
    — birds before point of lay/birds after onset of lay.
— *Fish:*
    — broodstock fish/fish raised primarily for food production.

Stability Evidence of stability is obtained to justify the proposed period of validity. This evidence takes the form of the results of virus titrations, bacterial counts or potency tests carried out at regular intervals until 3 months beyond the end of the shelf life on not fewer than 3 representative consecutive batches of vaccine kept under recommended storage conditions together with results from studies of moisture content (for freeze-dried products), physical tests on the adjuvant, chemical tests on substances such as the adjuvant constituents and preservatives and pH, as appropriate.

Where applicable, studies on the stability of the reconstituted vaccine are carried out, using the product reconstituted in accordance with the proposed recommendations.

FINAL BULK VACCINE
The final bulk vaccine is prepared by combining one or more batches of antigen that comply with all the relevant requirements with any auxiliary substances, such as adjuvants, stabilisers, antimicrobial preservatives and diluents.

Antimicrobial preservatives
Antimicrobial preservatives are used to prevent spoilage or adverse effects caused by microbial contamination occurring during use of a vaccine which is expected to be no longer than 10 h after first broaching. Antimicrobial preservatives are not included in freeze-dried products but, if justified, taking into account the maximum recommended period of use after reconstitution, they may be included in the diluent for multi-dose freeze-dried products. For single-dose liquid preparations, inclusion of antimicrobial preservatives is not acceptable unless justified and authorised, but may be acceptable, for example where the same vaccine is filled in single-dose and multidose containers and is used in non-food-producing species. For multidose liquid preparations, the need for effective antimicrobial preservation is evaluated taking into account likely contamination during use and the maximum recommended period of use after broaching of the container.

During development studies the effectiveness of the antimicrobial preservative throughout the period of validity shall be demonstrated to the satisfaction of the competent authority.

The efficacy of the antimicrobial preservative is evaluated as described in chapter *5.1.3* and in addition samples are tested at suitable intervals over the proposed in use shelf-life.
If neither the A criteria nor the B criteria can be met, then in justified cases the following criteria are applied to vaccines for veterinary use: bacteria, no increase from 24 h to 7 days, 3 log reduction at 14 days, no increase at 28 days; fungi, no increase at 14 days and 28 days.

Addition of antibiotics as antimicrobial preservative is generally not acceptable.

Test for inactivation and/or detoxification
For inactivated vaccines, where the auxiliary substances would interfere with a test for inactivation and/or detoxification, a test for inactivation or detoxification is carried out during preparation of the final bulk, after the different batches of antigen have been combined but before addition of auxiliary substances; the test for inactivation or detoxification may then be omitted on the final bulk and the batch.

Where there is a risk of reversion to toxicity, the test for detoxification performed at the latest stage of the production process at which the sensitivity of the test is not compromised (e.g. after the different batches of antigen have been combined but before the addition of auxiliary substances) is important to demonstrate a lack of reversion to toxicity.

In-process tests
Certain tests may be carried out on the final bulk vaccine rather than on the batch or batches prepared from it; such tests include those for antimicrobial preservatives, free formaldehyde and the potency determination for inactivated vaccines.

BATCH

Unless otherwise prescribed in the monograph, the final bulk vaccine is distributed aseptically into sterile, tamper-proof containers which are then closed so as to exclude contamination.

Only a batch that complies with each of the requirements given below under Identification, Tests and Potency or in the relevant individual monograph may be released for use. With the agreement of the competent authority, certain of the batch tests may be omitted where in-process tests give an equal or better guarantee that the batch would comply or where alternative tests validated with respect to the Pharmacopoeia method have been carried out.

The identification test can often be conveniently combined with the batch potency test to avoid unnecessary use of animals. For a given vaccine, a validated *in vitro* test can be used to avoid the unnecessary use of animals.

It is recognised that, in accordance with General Notices *(1.1. General statements)*, for an established vaccine the routine application of the safety test will be waived by the competent authority in the interests of animal welfare when a sufficient number of consecutive production batches have been produced and found to comply with the test, thus demonstrating consistency of the manufacturing process. Significant changes to the manufacturing process may require resumption of routine testing to re-establish consistency. The number of consecutive batches to be tested depends on a number of factors such as the type of vaccine, the frequency of production of batches and experience with the vaccine during development safety testing and during application of the batch safety test. Without prejudice to the decision of the competent authority in the light of information available for a given vaccine, testing of 10 consecutive batches is likely to be sufficient for most products. For products with an inherent safety risk, it may be necessary to continue to conduct the safety test on each batch.

Animal tests In accordance with the provisions of the European Convention for the Protection of Vertebrate Animals Used for Experimental and Other Scientific Purposes, tests must be carried out in such a way as to use the minimum number of animals and to cause the least pain, suffering, distress or lasting harm. The criteria for judging tests in monographs must be applied in the light of this. For example, if it is indicated that an animal is considered to be positive, infected etc. when typical clinical signs occur then as soon as it is clear that the result will not be affected the animal in question shall be either humanely killed or given suitable treatment to prevent unnecessary suffering. In accordance with the General Notices, alternative test methods may be used to demonstrate compliance with the monograph and the use of such tests is particularly encouraged when this leads to replacement or reduction of animal use or reduction of suffering.

Physical tests

A vaccine with an oily adjuvant is tested for viscosity by a suitable method and shown to be within the limits set for the product. The stability of the emulsion shall be demonstrated.

Chemical tests

Tests for the concentrations of appropriate substances such as aluminium and preservatives are carried out to show that these are within the limits set for the product.

pH

The pH of liquid products and diluents is measured and shown to be within the limits set for the product.

Water

Where applicable, the freeze-drying process is checked by a determination of water and shown to be within the limits set for the product.

IDENTIFICATION

For inactivated vaccines, the identification prescribed in monographs is usually an antibody induction test since this is applicable to all vaccines.

TESTS

The monographs also indicate tests to be carried out on each particular vaccine.

All hen eggs, chickens and chicken cell cultures for use in quality control tests shall be derived from an SPF flock *(5.2.2)*.

Formaldehyde

(2.4.18; use Method B if sodium metabisulphite has been used to neutralise excess formaldehyde). Where formaldehyde has been used in the preparation, the concentration of free formaldehyde is not greater than 0.5 g/l, unless a higher amount has been shown to be safe.

Phenol *(2.5.15)*

When the vaccine contains phenol, the concentration is not greater than 5 g/l.

Sterility *(2.6.1)*

Where prescribed in the monograph, vaccines comply with the test for sterility. Where the volume of liquid in a container is greater than 100 ml, the method of membrane filtration is used wherever possible. Where the method of membrane filtration cannot be used, the method of direct inoculation may be used. Where the volume of liquid in each container is at least 20 ml, the minimum volume to be used for each culture medium is 10 per cent of the contents or 5 ml, whichever is less. The appropriate number of items to be tested *(2.6.1)* is 1 per cent of the batch with a minimum of 4 and a maximum of 10.

For avian live viral vaccines, for non-parenteral use only, the requirement for sterility is usually replaced by requirements for absence of pathogenic micro-organisms and for a maximum of 1 non-pathogenic micro-organism per dose.

Extraneous agents

Monographs prescribe a set of measures that taken together give an acceptable degree of assurance that the final product does not contain infectious extraneous agents. These measures include:

1) Production within a seed-lot system and a cell-seed system, wherever possible;

2) Extensive testing of seed lots and cell seed for extraneous agents;

3) Requirements for SPF flocks used for providing substrates for vaccine production;

4) Testing of substances of animal origin, which must, wherever possible, undergo an inactivation procedure;

5) For live vaccines, testing of the final product for infectious extraneous agents; such tests are less extensive than those carried out at earlier stages because of the guarantees given by in-process testing.

In cases of doubt, the tests intended for the seed lot of a live vaccine may also be applied to the final product. If an extraneous agent is found in such a test, the vaccine does not comply the monograph.

Avian live viral vaccines comply with the tests for extraneous agents in batches of finished products *(2.6.25)*.

Mycoplasmas (2.6.7)

Where prescribed in a monograph, the vaccine complies with the test for mycoplasmas (culture method).

Safety

In general, 2 doses of an inactivated vaccine and/or 10 doses of a live vaccine are injected by a recommended route.

It may be necessary to reduce the prescribed number of doses under certain circumstances or amend the method of re-constitution and injection, for example for a combined vaccine, where it is difficult to reconstitute 10 doses of the live component in 2 doses of the inactivated component. The animals are observed for the longest period stated in the monographs. No abnormal local or systemic reaction occurs. Where several batches are prepared from the same final bulk, the safety test is carried out on the first batch and then omitted for further batches prepared from the same final bulk.

During development studies, the type and degree of reactions expected with the vaccine are defined in the light of safety testing. This definition is then used as part of the operating procedure for the batch safety test to evaluate acceptable and unacceptable reactions.

The immune status of animals to be used for the safety test is specified in the individual monograph. For most monographs, one of the 3 following categories is specified:

1) the animals must be free from antibodies against the virus/bacterium/toxin etc. contained in the vaccine,

2) the animals are preferably free from antibodies but animals with a low level of antibody may be used as long as the animals have not been vaccinated and the administration of the vaccine does not cause an anamnestic response,

3) the animals must not have been vaccinated against the disease the vaccine is intended to prevent.

As a general rule, category 1 is specified for live vaccines. For other vaccines, category 2 is usually specified but where most animals available for use in tests would comply with category 1, this may be specified for inactivated vaccines also. Category 3 is specified for some inactivated vaccines where determination of antibodies prior to testing is unnecessary or impractical. For poultry vaccines, as a general rule the use of SPF birds is specified.

For avian vaccines, the safety test is generally carried out using 10 SPF chickens (5.2.2), except that for vaccines not recommended for use in chickens it is carried out using 10 birds of one of the species for which the vaccine is recommended, the birds being free from antibodies against the disease agent for which the vaccine is intended to provide protection.

POTENCY

See Choice of vaccine composition and choice of vaccine strain under Production.

STORAGE

Store protected from light at a temperature of $5 \pm 3 \,^{\circ}\text{C}$, unless otherwise indicated. Liquid preparations are not to be allowed to freeze, unless otherwise indicated.

LABELLING

The label states:

— that the preparation is for veterinary use,
— the volume of the preparation and the number of doses in the container,
— the route of administration,
— the type or types of bacteria or viruses used and for live vaccines the minimum and the maximum number of live bacteria or the minimum and the maximum virus titre,
— where applicable, for inactivated vaccines, the minimum potency in International Units,
— where applicable, the name and amount of antimicrobial preservative or other substance added to the vaccine,
— the name of any substance that may cause an adverse reaction,
— for freeze-dried vaccines:
  — the name or composition and the volume of the reconstituting liquid to be added,
  — the period within which the vaccine is to be used after reconstitution,
— for vaccines with an oily adjuvant, that if the vaccine is accidentally injected into man, urgent medical attention is necessary,
— the animal species for which the vaccine is intended,
— the indications for the vaccine,
— the instructions for use,
— any contra-indications to the use of the product including any required warning on the dangers of administration of an overdose,
— the doses recommended for different species.

Ph Eur

Anthrax Vaccine, Living

(Anthrax Spore Vaccine (Live) for Veterinary Use, Ph Eur monograph 0441)

Ph Eur

DEFINITION

Anthrax spore live vaccine for veterinary use consists of a suspension of live spores of an attenuated, non-capsulated strain of *Bacillus anthracis*.

PRODUCTION

The strain used is either: not lethal to the guinea-pig or the mouse; or lethal to the guinea-pig but not to the rabbit; or lethal to some rabbits. *B. anthracis* is grown in an appropriate medium. At the end of growth the spores are suspended in a stabilising solution and counted. The vaccine may contain an adjuvant.

IDENTIFICATION

B. anthracis present in the vaccine is identified by means of morphological and serological tests, culture and biochemical tests.

TESTS

Safety

Carry out the test on one of the species of animals for which the vaccine is intended. If the vaccine is intended for several species, including the goat, carry out the test on goats. Administer subcutaneously or intradermally to each of 2 animals, of the minimum age recommended for vaccination and having no antibodies against *B. anthracis*, twice the dose stated on the label for the species used and observe the animals for 14 days. No abnormal systemic reaction is produced but a local reaction may occur at the site of injection. The severity of the local reaction may vary according to the strain of the spores and the adjuvants used in the preparation, but necrosis does not occur.

Spore count

The number of live spores determined by plate count is not less than 80 per cent of that stated on the label.

Bacterial and fungal contamination

Carry out the test by microscopic examination and by inoculation of suitable media. The vaccine does not contain contaminating bacteria or fungi.

POTENCY

For a strain of *B. anthracis* which is not lethal to the guinea-pig or the mouse, the test may be carried out in guinea-pigs. For a strain which is lethal to the guinea-pig but not to the rabbit, the test may be carried out in rabbits. For a strain which is lethal to some rabbits, carry out the test in sheep.

If the test is carried out in guinea-pigs or in rabbits, use 10 healthy animals (group a). Inject subcutaneously or intradermally into each animal 1/10 of the smallest dose of the vaccine stated on the label for sheep. Observe the animals for 21 days. If more than 2 animals die from non-specific causes, repeat the test. Use as controls 3 animals of the same species and of the same origin.

If the test is carried out in sheep, use 5 healthy animals (group b). Inject subcutaneously or intradermally into each animal 1/10 of the smallest dose of the vaccine stated on the label for sheep. Observe the animals for 21 days. Use as controls 3 sheep of the same origin. Inject subcutaneously into each vaccinated animal of group (a) or group (b) at least 100 MLD and into each control animal 10 MLD of a strain of *B. anthracis* pathogenic for the species of animal used in the test. Observe all the animals for 10 days. All the vaccinated animals survive and all the controls die from anthrax during the observation period. If a vaccinated animal dies after the challenge, repeat the test. If in the second test a vaccinated animal dies, the vaccine fails the test.

LABELLING

The label states:
— the strain used for preparation of the vaccine,
— the number of viable spores per millilitre.

Ph Eur

Aujeszky's Disease Vaccine, Inactivated

(Aujeszky's Disease Vaccine (Inactivated) for Pigs, Ph Eur monograph 0744)

Ph Eur

DEFINITION

Aujeszky's disease vaccine (inactivated) for pigs consists of a suspension of an appropriate strain of Aujeszky's disease virus inactivated without affecting its immunogenic properties or a suspension of an inactivated fraction of the virus having adequate immunogenic properties.

PRODUCTION

The virus strain is grown in suitable cell cultures (5.2.4). The viral suspension is harvested and inactivated; it may be treated to fragment the virus and the viral fragments may be purified and concentrated.

The test for inactivation is carried out using two passages in the same type of cell culture as that used in the production of the vaccine or cells shown to be at least as sensitive. The quantity of inactivated virus used in the test is equivalent to not less than twenty-five doses of the vaccine. No live virus is detected.

Suitable adjuvants and antimicrobial preservatives may be added. The vaccine may be freeze-dried.

CHOICE OF VACCINE COMPOSITION

The vaccine is shown to be satisfactory with respect to safety and immunogenicity. The following tests may be used during demonstration of safety (5.2.6) and efficacy (5.2.7).

Safety

A. A test is carried out in each category of animals for which the vaccine is intended (sows, fattening pigs). The animals used do not have antibodies against Aujeszky's disease virus or against a fraction of the virus. Two doses of vaccine are injected by a recommended route into each of not fewer than ten animals. After 14 days, one dose of vaccine is injected into each of the animals. The animals are observed for a further 14 days. No abnormal local or systemic reaction is produced during the 28 days of the test. If the vaccine is intended for use in pregnant sows, for the test in this category of animal the observation period is prolonged up to farrowing and any effects on gestation or the offspring are noted.

B. The animals used in the test for immunogenicity are also used to evaluate safety. The rectal temperature of each vaccinated animal is measured at the time of vaccination and 6 h, 24 h and 48 h later. No animal shows a temperature rise greater than 1.5 °C and the number of animals showing a temperature greater than 41 °C does not exceed 10 per cent of the group. No other systemic reactions (for example, anorexia) are noted. At slaughter, the injection site is examined for local reactions. No abnormal local reactions attributable to the vaccine are produced.

C. The animals used for field trials are also used to evaluate safety. A test is carried out in each category of animals for which the vaccine is intended (sows, fattening pigs). Not fewer than three groups each of not fewer than twenty animals are used with corresponding groups of not fewer than ten controls. The rectal temperature of each vaccinated animal is measured at the time of vaccination and 6 h, 24 h and 48 h later. No animal shows a temperature rise greater than 1.5 °C and the number of animals showing a temperature greater than 41 °C does not exceed 25 per cent of the group. At slaughter, the injection site is examined for local reactions. No abnormal local reactions attributable to the vaccine are produced.

Immunogenicity Not fewer than ten fattening pigs of the age recommended for vaccination and which do not have antibodies against Aujeszky's disease virus or against a fraction of the virus are used. The body mass of none of the pigs differs from the average body mass of the group by more than 20 per cent. Each pig is vaccinated according to the recommended schedule and by a recommended route. Five similar pigs are used as controls. At the end of the fattening period (80 kg to 90 kg), each pig is weighed and then challenged by the intranasal route with a suitable quantity of a virulent strain of Aujeszky's disease virus (challenge with at least 10^6 CCID$_{50}$ of a virulent strain having undergone not more than three passages and administered in not less than 4 ml of diluent has been found to be satisfactory). The titre of challenge virus is determined in swabs taken from the nasal cavity of each animal daily from the day before challenge until virus is no longer detected. Each animal is weighed 7 days after challenge or at the time of death if this occurs earlier and the average daily gain is calculated as a percentage. For each group (vaccinated and controls), the

average of the average daily gains is calculated. The vaccine complies with the test if:
— all the vaccinated pigs survive and the difference between the averages of the daily gains for the two groups is not less than 1.5,
— the geometrical mean titres and the duration of excretion of the challenge virus are significantly lower in vaccinates than in controls.

The test is not valid unless all the control pigs display signs of Aujeszky's disease and the average of their daily gains is less than − 0.5.

If the vaccine is intended for use in sows for the passive protection of piglets, the suitability of the strain for this purpose may be demonstrated by the following method. Eight sows which do not have antibodies against Aujeszky's disease virus or against a fraction of the virus are vaccinated according to the recommended schedule and by a recommended route; four sows are kept as controls. The piglets from the sows are challenged with a suitable quantity of a virulent strain of Aujeszky's disease virus at 6 to 10 days of age. The piglets are observed for 21 days. The vaccine is satisfactory if not less than 80 per cent protection against mortality is found in the piglets from the vaccinated sows compared to those from the control sows. The test is not valid if the average number of piglets per litter for each group is less than six.

BATCH TESTING
The test described under Potency is not necessarily carried out for routine testing of batches of vaccine. It is carried out for a given vaccine, on one or more occasions, as decided by or with the agreement of the competent authority; where the test is not carried out a suitable, validated, alternative test is carried out, the criteria for acceptance being set with reference to a batch of vaccine that has given satisfactory results in the test described under Potency.

IDENTIFICATION
In animals having no antibodies against Aujeszky's disease virus or against a fraction of the virus, the vaccine stimulates the production of specific antibodies against Aujeszky's disease virus or the fraction of the virus used in the production of the vaccine.

TESTS
Safety
Inject two doses of the vaccine by a recommended route into each of not fewer than two pigs of the minimum age recommended for vaccination and having no antibodies against Aujeszky's disease virus or against a fraction of the virus. Observe the animals for 14 days and then inject one dose of the vaccine into each piglet. Observe the animals for a further 14 days. No abnormal local or systemic reaction occurs during the 28 days of the test.

Inactivation
Wherever possible, carry out a suitable test for residual infectious Aujeszky's disease virus using two passages in the same type of cell culture as used in the production of the vaccine or cells shown to be at least as sensitive. Otherwise, inject one dose of the vaccine subcutaneously into each of five healthy non-immunised rabbits. Observe the animals for 14 days after the injection. No abnormal reaction (in particular a local rash) occurs. If the vaccine strain is not pathogenic for the rabbit, carry out the test in two sheep.

Extraneous viruses
On the pigs used for the safety test carry out tests for antibodies. The vaccine does not stimulate the formation of antibodies, other than those against Aujeszky's disease virus, against viruses pathogenic for pigs or against viruses that could interfere with the diagnosis of infectious diseases of pigs (including the viruses of the pestivirus group).

Sterility
The vaccine complies with the test for sterility prescribed in the monograph on *Vaccines for veterinary use (0062)*.

POTENCY
Use not fewer than five pigs each weighing 15 kg to 35 kg and which do not have antibodies against Aujeszky's disease virus or against a fraction of the virus. The body mass of none of the pigs differs from the average body mass of the group by more than 25 per cent. Administer to each pig by a recommended route one dose of the vaccine. Use five similar pigs as controls. Three weeks later weigh each pig and then challenge by the intranasal route with a suitable quantity of a virulent strain of Aujeszky's disease virus. Weigh each animal 7 days after challenge or at the time of death if this occurs earlier and calculate the average daily gain as a percentage. For each group (vaccinated and controls), calculate the average of the average daily gains. The vaccine passes the test if the vaccinated pigs survive and the difference between the averages of the daily gains for the two groups is not less than 1.1. The test is not valid unless all the control pigs display signs of Aujeszky's disease and the average of their daily gains is less than − 0.5.

LABELLING
The label states:
— whether the vaccine strain is pathogenic for the rabbit,
— whether the vaccine is a whole-virus vaccine or a subunit vaccine.

_____ Ph Eur

Aujeszky's Disease Vaccine, Living

(Aujeszky's Disease Vaccine (Live) for Pigs for Parenteral Administration, Freeze-dried, Ph Eur monograph 0745)

Ph Eur _____

DEFINITION
Freeze-dried Aujeszky's disease vaccine (live) for pigs for parenteral administration is a preparation of an attenuated strain of Aujeszky's disease virus. It may be administered after mixing with an adjuvant.

PRODUCTION
The virus strain is grown in suitable cell cultures (5.2.4) or in fertilised hen eggs from flocks free from specified pathogens (5.2.2). The viral suspension is harvested, mixed with a suitable stabilising liquid and freeze-dried.

CHOICE OF VACCINE STRAIN
Only a virus strain shown to be satisfactory with respect to the following characteristics may be used in the preparation of the vaccine: safety; transmissibility, including transmission across the placenta and by semen; irreversibility of attenuation; immunogenicity. The strain may have a genetic marker. The following tests may be used during demonstration of safety (5.2.6) and efficacy (5.2.7).
Safety
A. 10 piglets, 3 to 4 weeks old and which do not have antibodies against Aujeszky's disease virus or against a

fraction of the virus, each receive by a recommended route a quantity of virus corresponding to 10 doses of vaccine. 10 piglets of the same origin and age and which do not have antibodies against Aujeszky's disease virus or against a fraction of the virus are kept as controls. The animals are observed for 21 days. The piglets remain in good health. The weight curve of the vaccinated piglets does not differ significantly from that of the controls.

B. The animals used in the test for immunogenicity are also used to evaluate safety. The rectal temperature of each vaccinated animal is measured at the time of vaccination and 6 h, 24 h and 48 h later. No animal shows a temperature rise greater than 1.5 °C and the number of animals showing a temperature greater than 41 °C does not exceed 10 per cent of the group. No other systemic reactions (for example, anorexia) are noted. At slaughter, the injection site is examined for local reactions. No abnormal local reactions attributable to the vaccine are produced.

C. The animals used for field trials are also used to evaluate safety. A test is carried out in each category of animals for which the vaccine is intended (sows, fattening pigs). Not fewer than 3 groups each of not fewer than 20 animals are used with corresponding groups of not fewer than 10 controls. The rectal temperature of each animal is measured at the time of vaccination and 6 h, 24 h and 48 h later. No animal shows a temperature rise greater than 1.5 °C and the number of animals showing a temperature greater than 41 °C does not exceed 25 per cent of the group. At slaughter, the injection site is examined for local reactions. No abnormal local reactions attributable to the vaccine are produced.

D. 10 piglets, 3 to 5 days old and which do not have antibodies against Aujeszky's disease virus or against a fraction of the virus, each receive by the intranasal route a quantity of virus corresponding to 10 doses of vaccine. The animals are observed for 21 days. None of the piglets dies or shows signs of neurological disorder attributable to the vaccine virus.

E. This test is not necessary for gE-negative strains. 5 piglets, 3 to 5 days old, each receive $10^{4.5}$ $CCID_{50}$ of vaccine virus intracerebrally. None of the piglets dies or shows signs of neurological disorder.

F. 10 piglets, 3 to 4 weeks old and which do not have antibodies against Aujeszky's disease virus or against a fraction of the virus, each receive a daily injection of 2 mg of prednisolone per kilogram of body mass for 5 consecutive days. On the third day each piglet receives a quantity of virus corresponding to 1 dose of vaccine by a recommended route. Antimicrobial agents may be administered to prevent aspecific signs. Observe the animals for 21 days following administration of the virus. The piglets remain in good health.

G. 15 pregnant sows which do not have antibodies against Aujeszky's disease virus or against a fraction of the virus are used. Each of 5 sows receive by a recommended route a quantity of virus corresponding to 10 doses of vaccine during the fourth or fifth week of gestation. 5 other sows each receive the same dose of virus by the same route during the tenth or eleventh week of gestation. The other 5 pregnant sows are kept as controls. The number of piglets born to the vaccinated sows, any abnormalities in the piglets and the duration of gestation do not differ significantly from those of the controls. For the piglets from vaccinated sows: carry out tests for serum antibodies against Aujeszky's disease virus; carry out tests for Aujeszky's disease virus antigen in the liver

and lungs of those piglets showing abnormalities and in a quarter of the remaining healthy piglets. No Aujeszky's disease virus antigen is found in piglets born to the vaccinated sows and no antibodies against Aujeszky's disease virus are found in the serum taken before ingestion of colostrum.

Virus excretion 18 pigs, 3 to 4 weeks old and which do not have antibodies against Aujeszky's disease virus or against a fraction of the virus are used. 14 of the pigs each receive 1 dose of vaccine by the recommended route and at the recommended site and the remaining 4 pigs are kept as contact controls. Suitably sensitive tests for the virus are carried out individually on the nasal and oral secretions as follows: nasal and oral swabs are collected daily from the day before vaccination until 10 days after vaccination. The vaccine is acceptable if the virus is not isolated from the secretions collected.

Transmissibility The test is carried out on 4 separate occasions. Each time 4 piglets, 3 to 4 weeks old and which do not have antibodies against Aujeszky's disease virus or against a fraction of the virus, each receive by a recommended route a quantity of virus corresponding to 1 dose of vaccine. 1 day after the administration, 2 other piglets of the same age which do not have antibodies against Aujeszky's disease virus or against a fraction of the virus are kept close together with them. After 5 weeks all the animals are tested for the presence of antibodies against Aujeszky's disease virus. Antibodies against Aujeszky's disease virus are not detected in any group of contact controls. All the treated piglets show an antibody response.

Reversion to virulence 2 piglets, 3 to 5 days old and which do not have antibodies against Aujeszky's disease virus or against a fraction of the virus, each receive by the intranasal route a quantity of virus corresponding to 1 dose of vaccine. 3 to 5 days later brain, lung, tonsils and local lymph glands are taken from each piglet and the samples are pooled. 1 ml of the pooled organ suspension is administered intranasally into each of 2 other piglets of the same age and susceptibility. This operation is then repeated not fewer than 4 times, the last time in not fewer than 5 piglets. The presence of the virus is verified at each passage by direct or indirect means. If the virus has disappeared, a second series of passages is carried out. The piglets do not die or show neurological disorders from causes attributable to the vaccine virus. There is no indication of an increase of virulence as compared with the non-passaged virus.

Immunogenicity Not fewer than 10 fattening pigs of the age recommended for vaccination and which do not have antibodies against Aujeszky's disease virus or against a fraction of the virus are used. The body mass of none of the pigs differs from the average body mass of the group by more than 20 per cent. Each pig is vaccinated according to the recommended schedule and by a recommended route. 5 similar pigs are used as controls. At the end of the fattening period (80 kg to 90 kg), each pig is weighed and then challenged by the intranasal route with a suitable quantity of a virulent strain of Aujeszky's disease virus (challenge with at least 10^6 $CCID_{50}$ of a virulent strain having undergone not more than 3 passages and administered in not less than 4 ml of diluent has been found to be satisfactory). The titre of virus is determined in swabs taken from the nasal cavity of each pig daily from the day before challenge until virus is no longer detected. Each pig is weighed 7 days after challenge or at the time of death if this occurs earlier and the average daily gain is calculated as a percentage. For each group

(vaccinated and controls), the average of the average daily gains is calculated. The vaccine complies with the test if:
— all the vaccinated pigs survive and the difference between the averages of the average daily gains for the 2 groups is not less than 1.5,
— the geometrical mean titres and the duration of excretion of the challenge virus are significantly lower in vaccinates than in controls.

The test is not valid unless all the control pigs display signs of Aujeszky's disease and the average of their average daily gains is less than − 0.5.

If the vaccine is intended for use in sows for the passive protection of piglets, the suitability of the strain for this purpose may be demonstrated by the following method. 8 sows which do not have antibodies against Aujeszky's disease virus or against a fraction of the virus are vaccinated according to the recommended schedule and by the recommended route; 4 sows are kept as controls. The piglets from the sows are challenged with a suitable quantity of a virulent strain of Aujeszky's disease virus at 6 to 10 days of age. The piglets are observed for 21 days. The vaccine is satisfactory if not less than 80 per cent protection against mortality is found in the piglets from the vaccinated sows compared to those from the control sows. The test is not valid if the average number of piglets per litter for each group is less than 6.

BATCH TESTING
The test described under Potency is not necessarily carried out for routine testing of batches of vaccine. It is carried out for a given vaccine, on one or more occasions, as decided by or with the agreement of the competent authority; where the test is not carried out a suitable, validated alternative test is carried out, the criteria for acceptance being set with reference to a batch of vaccine that has given satisfactory results in the test described under Potency.

IDENTIFICATION
In animals having no antibodies against Aujeszky's disease virus or against a fraction of the virus, the vaccine stimulates the production of specific neutralising antibodies.

TESTS
Safety
Administer 10 doses of the vaccine in a suitable volume by a recommended route to each of not fewer than 2 pigs of the minimum age recommended for vaccination and which do not have antibodies against Aujeszky's disease virus or against a fraction of the virus. Observe the animals for 14 days. No abnormal local or systemic reaction occurs.

Extraneous viruses
Neutralise the vaccine using a monospecific antiserum or monoclonal antibodies and inoculate into cell cultures known to be sensitive to viruses pathogenic for pigs and to pestiviruses. Maintain these cultures for 14 days and make at least 1 passage during this period. No cytopathic effect develops; the cells show no evidence of the presence of haemadsorbing agents. Carry out a specific test for pestiviruses.

Sterility
The vaccine complies with the test for sterility prescribed in the monograph on *Vaccines for veterinary use (0062)*.

Mycoplasmas (*2.6.7*)
The vaccine complies with the test for mycoplasmas.

Virus titre
Titrate the reconstituted vaccine on the same substrate as used for production (cell cultures or inoculation into the

allantoic cavity of fertilised hen eggs). 1 dose of the vaccine contains not less than the quantity of virus equivalent to the minimum virus titre stated on the label.

POTENCY
Use not fewer than 5 pigs weighing 15 kg to 35 kg and which do not have antibodies against Aujeszky's disease virus or against a fraction of the virus. The body mass of none of the pigs differs from the average body mass of the group by more than 25 per cent. Administer to each pig by a recommended route 1 dose of the vaccine. Use 5 similar pigs as controls. 3 weeks later weigh each pig and then challenge by the intranasal route with a suitable quantity of a virulent strain of Aujeszky's disease virus. Weigh each animal 7 days after challenge or at the time of death if this occurs earlier and calculate the average daily gain as a percentage. For each group (vaccinated and controls), calculate the average of the average daily gains. The vaccine complies with the test if all the vaccinated pigs survive and the difference between the averages of the average daily gains for the 2 groups is not less than 1.6. The test is not valid unless all the control pigs display signs of Aujeszky's disease and the average of their average daily gains is less than − 0.5.

LABELLING
The label states:
— the substrate used for production of the vaccine (cell cultures or eggs),
— the minimum virus titre.

Ph Eur

Avian Infectious Bronchitis Vaccine (Inactivated)

Infectious Bronchitis Vaccine, Inactivated

(*Ph Eur monograph 0959*)

CAUTION *Accidental injection of oily vaccine can cause serious local reactions in man. Expert medical advice should be sought immediately and the doctor should be informed that the vaccine is an oil emulsion.*

Ph Eur

DEFINITION
Avian infectious bronchitis vaccine (inactivated) consists of an emulsion or a suspension of one or more serotypes of avian infectious bronchitis virus which have been inactivated in such a manner that the immunogenic activity is retained. This monograph describes vaccines intended to protect against a drop in egg production or quality; for vaccines also intended to protect against respiratory symptoms, a demonstration of efficacy additional to that described under Potency is required.

PRODUCTION
The virus is propagated in fertilised hen eggs from healthy flocks or in suitable cell cultures (*5.2.4*).

An amplification test for residual live avian infectious bronchitis virus is carried out on each batch of antigen immediately after inactivation and on the final bulk vaccine or, if the vaccine contains an adjuvant, on the bulk antigen or mixture of bulk antigens immediately before the addition of adjuvant; the test is carried out in fertilised hen eggs from flocks free from specified pathogens (SPF) (*5.2.2*) or in suitable cell cultures (*5.2.4*) and the quantity of inactivated virus used is equivalent to not less than 10 doses of vaccine. No live virus is detected.

The vaccine may contain one or more suitable adjuvants.

CHOICE OF VACCINE COMPOSITION

The vaccine is shown to be satisfactory with respect to safety and immunogenicity for each category of chickens for which it is intended. The following test may be used during demonstration of efficacy (5.2.7).

Immunogenicity

The test described under Potency is suitable to demonstrate immunogenicity.

BATCH POTENCY TEST

The test described under Potency is not carried out for routine testing of batches of vaccine. It is carried out, for a given vaccine, on one or more occasions, as decided by or with the agreement of the competent authority; where the test is not carried out, a suitable validated test is carried out, the criteria for acceptance being set with reference to a batch of vaccine that has given satisfactory results in the test described under Potency.

The following test may be used after a satisfactory correlation with the test described under Potency has been established by a statistical evaluation.

Administer 1 dose of vaccine intramuscularly to each of 10 chickens, between 2 weeks of age and the minimum age stated for vaccination and from an SPF flock (5.2.2), and keep 5 hatch mates as unvaccinated controls. Collect serum samples from each chicken just before administration of the vaccine and after the period defined when testing the reference vaccine; determine the antibody titre of each serum, for each serotype in the vaccine, by a suitable serological method, for example, serum neutralisation. The antibody levels are not significantly less than those obtained with a batch that has given satisfactory results in the test described under Potency (reference vaccine). The test is not valid unless the sera collected from the unvaccinated controls and from the chickens just before the administration of the vaccine are free from detectable specific antibody.

IDENTIFICATION

In susceptible animals, the vaccine stimulates the production of specific antibodies against each of the virus serotypes in the vaccine, detectable by virus neutralisation.

TESTS

Safety

Inject a double dose of vaccine by a recommended route into each of ten 14- to 28-day-old chickens from an SPF flock (5.2.2). Observe the chickens for 21 days. No abnormal local or systemic reaction occurs.

Inactivation

A. For vaccine prepared with embryo-adapted strains of virus, inject 2/5 of a dose into the allantoic cavity of ten 9- to 11-day-old fertilised hen eggs from an SPF flock (5.2.2) and incubate. Observe for 5 to 6 days and pool separately the allantoic liquid from eggs containing live embryos and that from eggs containing dead embryos, excluding those that die within the first 24 h after injection. Examine for abnormalities all embryos which die after 24 h of injection or which survive 5 to 6 days. No death or abnormality attributable to the vaccine virus occurs.

Inject into the allantoic cavity of each of ten 9- to 11-day-old fertilised hen eggs from an SPF flock (5.2.2) 0.2 ml of the pooled allantoic liquid from the live embryos and into each of 10 similar eggs 0.2 ml of the pooled liquid from the dead embryos and incubate for 5 to 6 days. Examine for abnormalities all embryos which die after 24 h of injection

or which survive 5 to 6 days. No death or abnormality attributable to the vaccine virus occurs.

If more than 20 per cent of the embryos die at either stage repeat the test from that stage. The vaccine complies with the test if there is no death or abnormality attributable to the vaccine virus.

B. For vaccine prepared with cell-culture-adapted strains of virus, inoculate 10 doses of the vaccine into suitable cell cultures. If the vaccine contains an oil adjuvant, eliminate it by suitable means. Incubate at 38 ± 1 °C for 7 days. Make a passage on another set of cell cultures and incubate at 38 ± 1 °C for 7 days. None of the cultures show signs of infection.

Extraneous agents

Use the chickens from the test for safety. 21 days after injection of the double dose of vaccine, inject 1 dose by the same route into each chicken. Collect serum samples from each chicken 2 weeks later and carry out tests for antibodies to the following agents by the methods given in chapter 5.2.2: avian encephalomyelitis virus, avian leucosis viruses, haemagglutinating avian adenovirus, infectious bursal disease virus, infectious laryngotracheitis virus, influenza A virus, Marek's disease virus, Newcastle disease virus. The vaccine does not stimulate the formation of antibodies against these agents.

Sterility

The vaccine complies with the test for sterility prescribed in the monograph on *Vaccines for veterinary use (0062)*.

POTENCY

Carry out a potency test for each serotype in the vaccine. Use 4 groups of not fewer than 30 chickens from an SPF flock (5.2.2.), treated as follows.

Group A: unvaccinated controls.

Group B: vaccinated with inactivated avian infectious bronchitis vaccine.

Group C: vaccinated with live avian infectious bronchitis vaccine and inactivated avian infectious bronchitis vaccine according to the recommended schedule.

Group D: vaccinated with live avian infectious bronchitis vaccine.

Monitor egg production and quality in all birds from point of lay until at least 4 weeks after challenge. At the peak of lay, challenge all groups with a quantity of virulent avian infectious bronchitis virus sufficient to cause a drop in egg production or quality over 3 consecutive weeks during the 4 weeks following challenge. The vaccine complies with the test if egg production or quality is significantly better in group C than in group D and significantly better in group B than in group A. The test is not valid unless there is a drop in egg production in group A compared to the normal level noted before challenge of at least 35 per cent where challenge has been made with a Massachusetts-type strain; where it is necessary to carry out a challenge with a strain of another serotype for which there is documented evidence that the strain will not cause a 35 per cent drop in egg production, the challenge must produce a drop in egg production commensurate with the documented evidence and in any case not less than 15 per cent.

LABELLING

The label states:

— the category and age of the chickens for which the vaccine is intended;

— the strains and serotypes of virus used in the production of the vaccine and the serotypes against which the vaccine is intended to protect;

— whether the strain in the vaccine is embryo-adapted or cell-culture-adapted.

_____ Ph Eur

Avian Infectious Bronchitis Vaccine, Living

(Avian Infectious Bronchitis Vaccine (Live),
Ph Eur monograph 0442)

Ph Eur _____

1. DEFINITION

Avian infectious bronchitis vaccine (live) is a preparation of one or more suitable strains of different types of avian infectious bronchitis virus. This monograph applies to vaccines intended for administration to chickens for active immunisation against respiratory disease caused by avian infectious bronchitis virus.

2. PRODUCTION

2-1. PREPARATION OF THE VACCINE

The vaccine virus is grown in embryonated hens' eggs or in cell cultures.

2-2. SUBSTRATE FOR VIRUS PROPAGATION

2-2-1. Embryonated hens' eggs

If the vaccine virus is grown in embryonated hens' eggs, they are obtained from flocks free from specified pathogens (SPF) (5.2.2).

2-2-2. Cell cultures

If the vaccine virus is grown in cell cultures, they comply with the requirements for cell cultures for production of veterinary vaccines (5.2.4).

2-3. SEED LOTS

2-3-1. Extraneous agents

The master seed lot complies with the tests for extraneous agents in seed lots (2.6.24). In these tests on the master seed lot, the organisms used are not more that 5 passages from the master seed lot at the start of the test.

2-4. CHOICE OF VACCINE VIRUS

The vaccine virus shall be shown to be satisfactory with respect to safety (5.2.6) and efficacy (5.2.7) for the chickens for which it is intended.

The following tests for safety (section 2-4-1), increase in virulence (section 2-4-2) and immunogenicity (section 2-4-3) may be used during the demonstration of safety and immunogenicity.

2-4-1. Safety

2-4-1-1. Safety for the respiratory tract and kidneys   Carry out the test in chickens not older than the youngest age to be recommended for vaccination. Use vaccine virus at the least attenuated passage level that will be present between the master seed lot and a batch of the vaccine. Use not fewer than 15 chickens from an SPF flock (5.2.2) and from the same origin. Administer to each chicken by the oculonasal route a quantity of the vaccine virus equivalent to not less than 10 times the maximum virus titre likely to be contained in 1 dose of the vaccine. On each of days 5, 7 and 10 after administration of the virus, kill not fewer than 5 of the chickens, take samples of trachea and kidney. Fix kidney samples for histological examination. Remove the tracheas

and cut 10 rings from each trachea (3 from the top, 4 from the mid-part and 3 from the bottom); examine each ring under low magnification and score for ciliostasis on a scale from 0 (100 per cent ciliary activity) to 4 (no activity, complete ciliostasis); calculate the mean ciliostasis score (the maximum for each trachea being 40) for the 5 chickens killed on each of days 5, 7 and 10. The test is not valid if more than 10 per cent of the chickens die from causes not attributable to the vaccine virus. The vaccine virus complies with the test if:

— no chicken shows notable clinical signs of avian infectious bronchitis or dies from causes attributable to the vaccine virus,

— the average ciliostasis score is not more than 25,

— at most moderate inflammatory lesions are seen during kidney histological examination.

2-4-1-2. Safety for the reproductive tract   If the recommendations for use state or imply that the vaccine may be used in females of less than 3 weeks old that are subsequently kept to sexual maturity, it shall be demonstrated that there is no damage to development of the reproductive tract when the vaccine is given to chickens of the minimum age to be recommended for vaccination. The following test may be carried out: use not fewer than 40 female chickens not older than the minimum age recommended for vaccination and from an SPF flock (5.2.2); use the vaccine virus at the least attenuated passage level that will be present in a batch of vaccine; administer to each chicken by a recommended route a quantity of virus equivalent to not less than the maximum titre likely to be present in 1 dose of vaccine; at least 10 weeks after administration of the vaccine virus, kill the chickens and carry out macroscopic examination of the oviducts. The vaccine virus complies with the test if abnormalities are present in not more than 5 per cent of the oviducts.

2-4-2. Increase in virulence

The test for increase in virulence consists of the administration of the vaccine virus, at the least attenuated virus passage level that will be present between the master seed lot and a batch of the vaccine, to a group of five 2-week-old chickens from an SPF flock (5.2.2), sequential passages, 5 times where possible, to further similar groups and testing of the final recovered virus for increase in virulence. If the properties of the vaccine virus allow sequential passage to 5 groups via natural spreading, this method may be used, otherwise passage as described below is carried out and the maximally passaged virus that has been recovered is tested for increase in virulence. Care must be taken to avoid contamination by virus from previous passages. Administer by eye-drop a quantity of the vaccine virus that will allow recovery of virus for the passages described below. 2 to 4 days after administration of the vaccine virus, prepare a suspension from the mucosa of the trachea of each chicken and pool these samples. Administer 0.05 ml of the pooled samples by eye-drop to each of 5 other 2-week-old chickens from an SPF flock (5.2.2). Carry out this passage operation not fewer than 5 times; verify the presence of the virus at each passage. If the virus is not found at a passage level, carry out a second series of passages. Carry out the test for safety for the respiratory tract and kidney (section 2-4-1-1) and, where applicable, the test for safety for the reproductive tract (section 2-4-1-2) using the unpassaged vaccine virus and the maximally passaged virus that has been recovered. Administer the virus by the route to be recommended for vaccination likely to be the least safe. The vaccine virus complies with the test if no indication of increase in virulence of the maximally passaged virus compared with the unpassaged virus is observed. If virus is not recovered at any passage level in the first and second series of passages, the vaccine virus also complies with the test.

2-4-3. Immunogenicity

Immunogenicity is demonstrated for each strain of virus to be included in the vaccine. A test is carried out for each route and method of administration to be recommended using in each case chickens from an SPF flock (5.2.2) not older than the youngest age to be recommended for vaccination. The quantity of the vaccine virus administered to each chicken is not greater than the minimum virus titre to be stated on the label and the virus is at the most attenuated passage level that will be present in a batch of the vaccine. 1 or both of the tests below may be used during the demonstration of immunogenicity.

2-4-3-1. Ciliary activity of tracheal explants   Use not fewer than 25 chickens of the same origin and from an SPF flock (5.2.2). Vaccinate by a recommended route not fewer than 20 chickens. Maintain not fewer than 5 chickens as controls. Challenge each chicken after 21 days by eye-drop with a sufficient quantity of virulent avian infectious bronchitis virus of the same type as the vaccine virus to be tested. Kill the chickens 4 to 7 days after challenge and prepare transverse sections from the upper part (3), the middle part (4) and the lower part (3) of the trachea of each chicken. Examine all explants as soon as possible and at the latest 2 h after sampling by low-magnification microscopy for ciliary activity. For a given tracheal section, ciliary activity is considered as normal when at least 50 per cent of the internal ring shows vigorous ciliary movement. A chicken is considered not affected if not fewer than 9 out of 10 rings show normal ciliary activity.

The test is not valid if:

— fewer than 80 per cent of the control chickens show cessation or extreme loss of vigour of ciliary activity,

— and/or during the period between the vaccination and challenge more than 10 per cent of vaccinated or control chickens show abnormal clinical signs or die from causes not attributable to the vaccine.

The vaccine virus complies with the test if not fewer than 80 per cent of the vaccinated chickens show normal ciliary activity.

2-4-3-2. Virus recovery from tracheal swabs   Use not fewer than 30 chickens of the same origin and from an SPF flock (5.2.2). Vaccinate by a recommended route not fewer than 20 chickens. Maintain not fewer than 10 chickens as controls. Challenge each chicken after 21 days by eye-drop with a sufficient quantity of virulent avian infectious bronchitis virus of the same type as the vaccine virus to be tested. Kill the chickens 4 to 7 days after challenge and prepare a suspension from swabs of the tracheal mucosa of each chicken. Inoculate 0.2 ml of the suspension into the allantoic cavity of each of 5 embryonated hens' eggs, 9 to 11 days old, from an SPF flock (5.2.2). Incubate the eggs for 6-8 days after inoculation. Eggs that after 1 day of incubation do not contain a live embryo are eliminated and considered as non-specific deaths. Record the other eggs containing a dead embryo and after 6-8 days' incubation examine each egg containing a live embryo for lesions characteristic of avian infectious bronchitis. Make successively 3 such passages. If 1 embryo of a series of eggs dies or shows characteristic lesions, the inoculum is considered to be a carrier of avian infectious bronchitis virus. The examination of a series of eggs is

considered to be definitely negative if no inoculum concerned is a carrier. The test is not valid if:

— the challenge virus is re-isolated from fewer than 80 per cent of the control chickens,

— and/or during the period between vaccination and challenge more than 10 per cent of the vaccinated or control chickens show abnormal clinical signs or die from causes not attributable to the vaccine,

— and/or more than 1 egg in any group is eliminated because of non-specific embryo death.

The vaccine virus complies with the test if the challenge virus is re-isolated from not more than 20 per cent of the vaccinated chickens.

3. BATCH TESTS

3-1. Identification

3-1-1. Vaccines containing one type of virus   The vaccine, diluted if necessary and mixed with avian infectious bronchitis virus antiserum specific for the virus type, no longer infects embryonated hens' eggs from an SPF flock (5.2.2) or susceptible cell cultures (5.2.4) into which it is inoculated.

3-1-2. Vaccines containing more than one type of virus   The vaccine, diluted if necessary and mixed with type-specific antisera against each strain present in the vaccine except that to be identified, infects embryonated hens' eggs from an SPF flock (5.2.2) or susceptible cell cultures (5.2.4) into which it is inoculated whereas after further admixture with type-specific antiserum against the strain to be identified it no longer produces such infection.

3-2. Bacteria and fungi

Vaccines intended for administration by injection comply with the test for sterility prescribed in the monograph *Vaccines for veterinary use (0062)*.

Vaccines not intended for administration by injection either comply with the test for sterility prescribed in the monograph *Vaccines for veterinary use (0062)* or with the following test: carry out a quantitative test for bacterial and fungal contamination; carry out identification tests for microorganisms detected in the vaccine; the vaccine does not contain pathogenic microorganisms and contains not more than 1 non-pathogenic microorganism per dose.

Any liquid supplied with the vaccine complies with the test for sterility prescribed in the monograph *Vaccines for veterinary use (0062)*.

3-3. Mycoplasmas

The vaccine complies with the test for mycoplasmas (2.6.7).

3-4. Extraneous agents

The vaccine complies with the tests for extraneous agents in batches of finished product (2.6.25).

3-5. Safety

Use not fewer than 10 chickens from an SPF flock (5.2.2) and of the youngest age recommended for vaccination. Administer by a recommended route to each chicken, 10 doses of the vaccine. Observe the chickens at least daily for 21 days. The test is not valid if more than 20 per cent of the chickens show abnormal clinical signs or die from causes not attributable to the vaccine. The vaccine complies with the test if no chicken shows notable clinical signs of disease or dies from causes attributable to the vaccine.

3-6. Virus titre

Titrate the vaccine virus by inoculation into embryonated hens' eggs from an SPF flock (5.2.2) or into suitable cell cultures (5.2.4). If the vaccine contains more than 1 strain of virus, titrate each strain after having neutralised the others

with type-specific avian infectious bronchitis antisera.
The vaccine complies with the test if 1 dose contains for each vaccine virus not less than the minimum titre stated on the label.

3-7. Potency

The vaccine complies with the requirements of 1 of the tests prescribed under Immunogenicity (section 2-4-3) when administered according to the recommended schedule by a recommended route and method. It is not necessary to carry out the potency test for each batch of the vaccine if it has been carried out on a representative batch using a vaccinating dose containing not more than the minimum virus titre stated on the label.

_____ *Ph Eur*

Avian Paramyxovirus 3 Vaccine, Inactivated

*(Avian Paramyxovirus 3 Vaccine (Inactivated),
Ph Eur monograph 1392)*

Ph Eur _____

DEFINITION

Avian paramyxovirus 3 vaccine (inactivated) consists of an emulsion or a suspension of a suitable strain of avian paramyxovirus 3 that has been inactivated in such a manner that immunogenic activity is retained. The vaccine is used for protection against loss in egg production and egg quality in turkeys.

PRODUCTION

The virus is propagated in embryonated eggs from healthy flocks or in suitable cell cultures (*5.2.4*).

The test for inactivation is carried out in embryonated eggs or suitable cell cultures and the quantity of inactivated virus used is equivalent to not less than ten doses of vaccine. No live virus is detected.

The vaccine may contain an adjuvant.

CHOICE OF VACCINE COMPOSITION

The vaccine is shown to be satisfactory with respect to safety (*5.2.6*) and immunogenicity (*5.2.7*) for each category of turkeys for which it is intended. The following test may be used during demonstration of immunogenicity.

Immunogenicity The test described under Potency is suitable for demonstrating immunogenicity.

BATCH TESTING

Batch potency test

Carry out a suitable validated test for which satisfactory correlation with the test described under Potency has been established, the criteria for acceptance being set with reference to a batch that has given satisfactory results in the latter test.

IDENTIFICATION

When injected into animals free from antibodies against avian paramyxovirus 3, the vaccine stimulates the production of such antibodies.

TESTS

Safety

Inject twice the vaccinating dose by a recommended route into each of ten turkeys, 14 to 28 days old and free from antibodies against avian paramyxovirus 3. Observe the birds for 21 days. No abnormal local or systemic reaction occurs.

Inactivation

Inject two-fifths of a dose into the allantoic cavity of each of ten embryonated hen eggs, 9 to 11 days old, from flocks free from specified pathogens (*5.2.2*) (SPF eggs) and incubate. Observe for 6 days and pool separately the allantoic fluid from eggs containing live embryos, and that from eggs containing dead embryos, excluding those dying within 24 h of the injection. Examine embryos that die within 24 h of injection for the presence of avian paramyxovirus 3: the vaccine does not comply with the test if avian paramyxovirus 3 is found.

Inject into the allantoic cavity of each of ten SPF eggs, 9 to 11 days old, 0.2 ml of the pooled allantoic fluid from the live embryos and, into each of ten similar eggs, 0.2 ml of the pooled fluid from the dead embryos and incubate for 5 to 6 days. Test the allantoic fluid from each egg for the presence of haemagglutinins using chicken erythrocytes.

The vaccine complies with the test if there is no evidence of haemagglutinating activity and if not more than 20 per cent of the embryos die at either stage. If more than 20 per cent of the embryos die at one of the stages, repeat that stage; the vaccine complies with the test if there is no evidence of haemagglutinating activity and not more than 20 per cent of the embryos die at that stage.

Antibiotics may be used in the test to control extraneous bacterial infection.

Extraneous agents

Inject a double dose by a recommended route into each of ten chickens, 14 to 28 days old and from a flock free from specified pathogens (*5.2.2*). After 3 weeks, inject one dose by the same route. Collect serum samples from each chicken 2 weeks later and carry out tests for antibodies against the following agents by the methods prescribed for chicken flocks free from specified pathogens (*5.2.2*): avian encephalomyelitis virus, avian infectious bronchitis virus, avian leucosis viruses, egg-drop syndrome virus, avian bursal disease virus, avian infectious laryngotracheitis virus, influenza A virus, Marek's disease virus. The vaccine does not stimulate the formation of antibodies against these agents.

Sterility

The vaccine complies with the test for sterility prescribed in the monograph on *Vaccines for veterinary use (0062)*.

POTENCY

Use two groups each of not fewer than twenty turkeys free from antibodies against avian paramyxovirus 3. Vaccinate one group in accordance with the recommendations for use. Keep the other group as controls. The test is invalid if serological tests carried out on serum samples obtained at the time of first vaccination show the presence of antibodies against avian paramyxovirus 3 in either vaccinates or controls or if tests carried out at the time of challenge show such antibodies in controls. At the egg-production peak, challenge the two groups by the oculo-nasal route with a sufficient quantity of a virulent strain of avian paramyxovirus 3. For not less than 6 weeks after challenge, record the number of eggs laid weekly for each group, distinguishing between normal and abnormal eggs. The vaccine complies with the test if egg production and quality are significantly better in the vaccinated group than in the control group.

_____ *Ph Eur*

Avian Viral Tenosynovitis Vaccine (Live)

(Ph Eur monograph 1956)

Ph Eur _____

1. DEFINITION

Avian viral tenosynovitis vaccine (live) is a preparation of a suitable strain of avian tenosynovitis virus (avian orthoreovirus). This monograph applies to vaccines intended for administration to chickens for active immunisation.

2. PRODUCTION

2-1. PREPARATION OF THE VACCINE

The vaccine virus is grown in cell cultures.

2-2. SUBSTRATE FOR VIRUS PROPAGATION

2-2-1. Cell cultures

Cell cultures comply with the requirements for cell cultures for production of veterinary vaccines (*5.2.4*).

2-3. SEED LOTS

2-3-1. Extraneous agents

The master seed lot complies with the tests for extraneous agents in seed lots (*2.6.24*). In these tests on the master seed lot, the organisms used are not more than 5 passages from the master seed lot at the start of the tests.

2-4. CHOICE OF VACCINE VIRUS

The vaccine virus shall be shown to be satisfactory with respect to safety (*5.2.6*) and efficacy (*5.2.7*) for the chickens for which it is intended.

The following tests for safety (section 2-4-1), increase in virulence (section 2-4-2) and immunogenicity (section 2-4-3) may be used during the demonstration of safety and immunogenicity.

2-4-1. Safety

Carry out the test for each route and method of administration to be recommended for vaccination using in each case chickens not older than the youngest age to be recommended for vaccination. Use vaccine virus at the least attenuated passage level that will be present between the master seed lot and a batch of the vaccine. For each test use not fewer than 20 chickens, from an SPF flock (*5.2.2*). Administer to each chicken a quantity of the vaccine virus not less than 10 times the maximum virus titre likely to be contained in 1 dose of the vaccine. Observe the chickens at least daily for 21 days. Carry out histological examination of the joints and tendon sheaths of the legs and feet at the end of the observation period (as a basis for comparison in the test for increase in virulence). The test is not valid if more than 10 per cent of the chickens die from causes not attributable to the vaccine virus. The vaccine virus complies with the test if no chicken shows notable clinical signs of avian viral tenosynovitis or dies from causes attributable to the vaccine virus.

2-4-2. Increase in virulence

The test for increase in virulence consists of the administration of the vaccine virus at the least attenuated passage level that will be present between the master seed lot and a batch of the vaccine to a group of five 1-day-old chicks from an SPF flock (*5.2.2*), sequential passages, 5 times where possible, to further groups of 1-day-old chicks and testing of the final recovered virus for increase in virulence. If the properties of the vaccine virus allow sequential passage to 5 groups via natural spreading, this method may be used, otherwise passage as described below is carried out and the maximally passaged virus that has been recovered is tested for increase in virulence. Care must be taken to avoid contamination by virus from previous passages. Administer by a suitable route a quantity of the vaccine virus that will allow recovery of virus for the passages described below. Kill the chickens at the moment when the virus concentration in the most suitable material (for example, tendons, tendon sheaths and liquid exudates from the hock joints, spleen) is sufficient. Prepare a suspension from this material from each chicken and pool these samples. Administer 0.1 ml of the pooled samples by the route of administration most likely to lead to increase in virulence to each of 5 other chickens of the same age and origin. Carry out this passage operation not fewer than 5 times; verify the presence of the virus at each passage. If the virus is not found at a passage level, carry out a second series of passages. Carry out the test for safety (section 2-4-1) using the unpassaged vaccine virus and the maximally passaged vaccine virus that has been recovered. The vaccine virus complies with the test if no indication of increase in virulence of the maximally passaged virus compared with the unpassaged virus is observed. If the virus is not recovered at any passage level in the first and second series of passages, the vaccine virus also complies with the test.

2-4-3. Immunogenicity

A test is carried out for each route and method of administration to be recommended using in each case chickens not older than the youngest age to be recommended for vaccination. The quantity of the vaccine virus administered to each chicken is not greater than the minimum virus titre to be stated on the label and the virus is at the most attenuated passage level that will be present in a batch of the vaccine. Use not fewer than 30 chickens of the same origin and from an SPF flock (*5.2.2*). Administer the vaccine by a recommended route to not fewer than 20 chickens. Maintain not fewer than 10 chickens as controls. Challenge each chicken after 21 days by a suitable route with a sufficient quantity of virulent avian tenosynovitis virus. Observe the chickens at least daily for 21 days after challenge. Record the deaths and the surviving chickens that show clinical signs of disease. If the challenge is administered by the foot pad, any transient swelling of the foot pad during the first 5 days after challenge may be considered non-specific. At the end of the observation period, kill all the surviving chickens and carry out macroscopic and/or microscopic examination for lesions of the joints and tendon sheaths of the legs and feet, e.g. exudate and swelling. The test is not valid if:

— during the observation period after challenge fewer than 80 per cent of the control chickens die or show severe clinical signs of avian viral tenosynovitis or show macroscopical and/or microscopical lesions in the joints and tendon sheaths of the legs and feet,

— or if during the period between vaccination and challenge more than 10 per cent of the control or vaccinated chickens show abnormal clinical signs or die from causes not attributable to the vaccine.

The vaccine virus complies with the test if during the observation period after challenge not fewer than 90 per cent of the vaccinated chickens survive and show no notable clinical signs of disease or show macroscopical and/or microscopical lesions in the joints and tendon sheaths of the legs and feet.

3. BATCH TESTS

3-1. Identification
Carry out an immunostaining test in cell cultures to identify the vaccine virus.

3-2. Bacteria and fungi
Vaccines intended for administration by injection comply with the test for sterility prescribed in the monograph *Vaccines for veterinary use (0062)*.

Vaccines not intended for administration by injection either comply with the test for sterility prescribed in the monograph *Vaccines for veterinary use (0062)* or with the following test: carry out a quantitative test for bacterial and fungal contamination; carry out identification tests for microorganisms detected in the vaccine; the vaccine does not contain pathogenic microorganisms and contains not more than 1 non-pathogenic microorganism per dose.

Any liquid supplied with the vaccine complies with the test for sterility prescribed in the monograph *Vaccines for veterinary use (0062)*.

3-3. Mycoplasmas
The vaccine complies with the test for mycoplasmas (*2.6.7*).

3-4. Extraneous agents
The vaccine complies with the tests for extraneous agents in batches of finished product (*2.6.25*).

3-5. Safety
Use not fewer than 10 chickens from an SPF flock (*5.2.2*) and of the youngest age recommended for vaccination. Administer by a recommended route and method to each chicken 10 doses of the vaccine. Observe the chickens at least daily for 21 days. The test is not valid if more than 20 per cent of the chickens show abnormal clinical signs or die from causes not attributable to the vaccine. The vaccine complies with the test if no chicken shows notable clinical signs of disease or dies from causes attributable to the vaccine.

3-6. Virus titre
Titrate the vaccine virus by inoculation into suitable cell cultures (*5.2.4*). The vaccine complies with the test if 1 dose contains not less than the minimum virus titre stated on the label.

3-7. Potency
The vaccine complies with the requirements of the test prescribed under Immunogenicity (section 2-4-3) when administered by a recommended route and method. It is not necessary to carry out the potency test for each batch of the vaccine if it has been carried out on a representative batch using a vaccinating dose containing not more than the minimum virus titre stated on the label.

——————————————————————— *Ph Eur*

Bovine Parainfluenza Virus Vaccine, Living

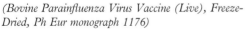

(Bovine Parainfluenza Virus Vaccine (Live), Freeze-Dried, Ph Eur monograph 1176)

Ph Eur _____

DEFINITION
Freeze-dried bovine parainfluenza virus vaccine (live) is a preparation of a suitable strain of bovine parainfluenza 3 virus.

PRODUCTION
The vaccine strain is grown in suitable cell cultures (*5.2.4*). The viral suspension is harvested, mixed with a suitable stabilising liquid and freeze-dried.

CHOICE OF VACCINE STRAIN
Only a virus strain shown to be satisfactory with respect to reversion to virulence, safety and immunogenicity may be used in the preparation of the vaccine. The following tests may be used during demonstration of safety (*5.2.6*) and efficacy (*5.2.7*).

Reversion to virulence   Administer by the intranasal route to 2 susceptible calves that do not have antibodies against bovine parainfluenza virus 3 a quantity of virus that will allow optimal re-isolation of the virus for subsequent passages. On each of days 3 to 7 after administration of the virus, take nasal swabs from each calf and collect in not more than 5 ml of a suitable medium which is then used to inoculate cell cultures to verify the presence of virus; use about 1 ml of the suspensions from swabs that contain the maximum amount of virus, as indicated by the titration in cell cultures, to inoculate 2 other calves of the same age and sensitivity; repeat these operations until 5 passages on calves have been carried out. No calf shows clinical signs attributable to the vaccinal virus. No indication of increase of virulence, compared to the original vaccinal virus is observed; account is taken of the titre of excreted virus in the nasal swabs.

Safety   The test is carried out for each recommended route of administration. Use calves of the minimum age recommended for vaccination and preferably having no antibodies against bovine parainfluenza 3 virus or, where justified, use calves with a very low level of such antibodies as long as they have not been vaccinated against bovine parainfluenza virus and administration of the vaccine does not cause an anamnestic response. Administer to 5 calves a quantity of virus corresponding to not less than 10 times the maximum virus titre that may be expected in a batch of vaccine. Observe the animals for 21 days. Measure the body temperature of each animal on the day before vaccination, at the time of vaccination and for the 4 subsequent days. No abnormal effect on body temperature and no abnormal local or systemic reactions occur.

Immunogenicity   The test described under Potency is suitable to demonstrate immunogenicity of the vaccine strain.

BATCH TESTING
If the test for potency has been carried out with satisfactory results on a representative batch of vaccine, this test may be omitted as a routine control on other batches of vaccine prepared from the same seed lot, subject to agreement by the competent authority.

IDENTIFICATION
Carry out an immunofluorescence test in suitable cell cultures, using a monospecific antiserum.

TESTS
Safety
Use calves of the minimum age recommended for vaccination and preferably having no antibodies against bovine parainfluenza 3 virus or, where justified, use calves with a very low level of such antibodies as long as they have not been vaccinated against bovine parainfluenza virus and administration of the vaccine does not cause an anamnestic response. Administer 10 doses of the vaccine by a recommended route to each of 2 calves. Observe the animals for 21 days. No abnormal local or systemic reaction occurs.

Extraneous viruses

Neutralise the vaccine using a monospecific antiserum against bovine parainfluenza 3 virus and inoculate into cell cultures known to be sensitive to viruses pathogenic for cattle. Maintain these cultures for 14 days and make at least one passage during this period. No cytopathic effect develops; the cells show no evidence of the presence of haemadsorbing agents. Carry out a specific test for pestiviruses.

Bacterial and fungal contamination

The vaccine complies with the test for sterility prescribed under *Vaccines for veterinary use (0062)*.

Mycoplasmas *(2.6.7)*

The vaccine complies with the test for mycoplasmas.

Virus titre

Titrate the vaccine in suitable cell cultures. One dose of the vaccine contains not less than the quantity of virus equivalent to the minimum virus titre stated on the label.

POTENCY

Use not fewer than 10 calves of the minimum age recommended for vaccination and that do not have antibodies against bovine parainfluenza 3 virus; calves having low levels of such antibodies may be used if it has been demonstrated that valid results are obtained in these conditions. Collect sera from the animals before vaccination, 7 days and 14 days after the time of vaccination and just before challenge. Vaccinate not fewer than 5 of the calves according to the instructions for use. Keep 5 calves as controls. Observe the animals for 21 days and then administer to each of them by a respiratory tract route a suitable quantity of a low-passage virulent strain of bovine parainfluenza 3 virus. Monitor each animal for clinical signs, in particular respiratory symptoms, and virus shedding (by nasal swabs or tracheobronchial washing) for 14 days after challenge. The vaccine complies with the test if in vaccinated animals compared to controls there is (a) a significant reduction in mean titre and in mean duration of virus excretion and (b) a notable reduction in general and local signs (if the challenge virus used produces such signs). The test is not valid if tests for antibodies against bovine parainfluenza 3 virus on the sera indicate that there was intercurrent infection with the virus during the test or if more than 2 of the 5 control animals show no excretion of the challenge virus, as shown by nasal swabs or samples harvested by tracheobronchial washing.

Ph Eur

Bovine Respiratory Syncytial Virus Vaccine, Living

(Bovine Respiratory Syncytial Virus Vaccine (Live), Freeze-dried, Ph Eur monograph 1177)

Ph Eur

DEFINITION

Freeze-dried bovine respiratory syncytial virus vaccine (live) is a preparation of a suitable strain of bovine respiratory syncytial virus.

PRODUCTION

The vaccine strain is grown in suitable cell cultures *(5.2.4)*. The viral suspension is harvested, mixed with a suitable stabilising solution and freeze-dried.

CHOICE OF VACCINE STRAIN

Only a virus strain shown to be satisfactory with respect to reversion to virulence, safety and immunogenicity may be used in the preparation of the vaccine. The following tests may be used during demonstration of safety *(5.2.6)* and efficacy *(5.2.7)*.

Reversion to virulence   Administer by the intranasal route to two susceptible calves that do not have antibodies against bovine respiratory syncytial virus a quantity of virus that will allow optimal re-isolation of the virus for subsequent passages. On each of days 3 to 7 after administration of the virus, take nasal swabs from each calf and collect in not more than 5 ml of a suitable medium which is then used to inoculate cell cultures to verify the presence of virus; use about 1 ml of the suspensions from swabs that contain the maximum amount of virus, as indicated by the titration in cell cultures, to inoculate two other calves of the same age and sensitivity; repeat these operations until five passages on calves have been carried out. No calf shows clinical signs attributable to the vaccinal virus. No indication of increase of virulence compared to the original vaccinal virus is observed; account is taken of the titre of excreted virus in the nasal swabs.

Safety   Safety studies are conducted in calves of the minimum age for which the vaccine is recommended and for each recommended route of administration.

A. Administer by a recommended route to five calves, without antibodies against bovine respiratory syncytial virus, a quantity of virus corresponding to not less than ten times the maximum virus titre that may be expected in a batch of vaccine. Observe the animals for 21 days. Measure the rectal temperature of each animal on the day before vaccination, at the time of vaccination and daily for the following 7 days. No abnormal effect on body temperature and no abnormal local or systemic reaction are noted.

B. The animals used for the field trials are also used to evaluate the incidence of hypersensitivity reactions in vaccinated animals following subsequent exposure to the vaccine or to wild virus. The vaccine is satisfactory if it is not associated with an abnormal incidence of immediate hypersensitivity reactions.

Immunogenicity   The test described under Potency is suitable to demonstrate immunogenicity of the vaccine strain.

BATCH TESTING

If the test for potency has been carried out with satisfactory results on a representative batch of vaccine, this test may be omitted as a routine control on other batches of vaccine prepared from the same seed lot, subject to agreement by the competent authority.

IDENTIFICATION

Identify the vaccine by an immunofluorescence test in suitable cell cultures using a monospecific antiserum.

TESTS

Safety

Administer ten doses of the vaccine by a recommended route to each of two calves of the minimum age recommended for vaccination and that do not have antibodies against bovine respiratory syncytial virus. Observe the animals for 21 days. No abnormal local or systemic reaction occurs.

Extraneous viruses

Neutralise the vaccine using a monospecific antiserum against bovine respiratory syncytial virus and inoculate into cell cultures known to be sensitive to viruses pathogenic for cattle. Maintain the cultures for 14 days and make at least one passage during this period. No cytopathic effect develops; the cells show no evidence of the presence of haemadsorbing agents. Carry out a specific test for pestiviruses.

Bacterial and fungal contamination
The vaccine complies with the test for sterility prescribed under *Vaccines for veterinary use (0062)*.

Mycoplasmas (*2.6.7*)
The vaccine complies with the test for mycoplasmas.

Virus titre
Titrate the vaccine in suitable cell cultures. One dose of the vaccine contains not less than the quantity of virus equivalent to the minimum titre stated on the label.

POTENCY

Use not fewer than ten calves of the minimum age recommended for vaccination and that do not have antibodies against bovine respiratory syncytial virus. Collect sera from the animals before the time of vaccination, 7 and 14 days after the time of vaccination and just before challenge. Vaccinate not fewer than five of the calves according to the instructions for use. Keep five calves as controls. Observe the animals for 21 days and then administer to each of them by a respiratory tract route a suitable quantity of a low-passage virulent strain of bovine respiratory syncytial virus. Monitor each animal for clinical signs, in particular respiratory symptoms, and virus shedding (by nasal swabs or tracheobronchial washing) for 14 days after challenge. The vaccine complies with the test if there is: (a) a significant reduction in mean titre and in mean duration of virus excretion in vaccinates compared to controls and (b) a notable reduction in general and local clinical signs in vaccinated animals (if the challenge virus used produces such signs). The test is not valid if antibodies to bovine respiratory syncytial virus are detected in any sample from control animals before challenge or if more than two of the five control animals show no excretion of the challenge virus, as shown by nasal swabs or samples harvested by tracheobronchial washing.

Ph Eur

Bovine Viral Diarrhoea Vaccine (Inactivated)

(*Ph Eur monograph 1952*)

Ph Eur

DEFINITION

Bovine viral diarrhoea vaccine (inactivated) is a preparation of one or more suitable strains of bovine diarrhoea virus inactivated by a suitable method. This monograph applies to vaccines intended for vaccination of heifers and cows to protect the foetus against transplacental infection.

PRODUCTION

The vaccine virus strain or strains are grown in suitable cell cultures (*5.2.4*).

The test for inactivation is carried out using a quantity of virus equivalent to not less than 25 doses of vaccine in cells of the same type as those used for production of the vaccine or cells shown to be at least as sensitive; the cells are passaged after 7 days and observed for a total of not less than 14 days. No infectious virus is detected.

CHOICE OF VACCINE COMPOSITION
The vaccine shall be shown to be satisfactory with respect to safety (*5.2.6*) and immunogenicity (*5.2.7*) in cattle.

The following tests may be used during the demonstration of safety and immunogenicity.

Safety Carry out a safety test for each recommended route and for each category of cattle for which the vaccine is intended. Use cattle of the minimum age recommended for vaccination and that are free from bovine diarrhoea virus and from antibodies against the virus. Inject a double dose of vaccine into each of not fewer than 10 animals. Observe the animals for 14 days. No abnormal local or systemic reaction occurs. If the vaccine is intended for administration to pregnant cattle, carry out the test in these animals at the beginning of each trimester for which use is not contra-indicated and extend the observation period to calving. No undesirable effect on gestation or the offspring occurs. If the vaccine is intended for administration shortly before or at insemination, absence of undesirable effects on conception rate must be demonstrated.

Immunogenicity The test for potency is suitable to demonstrate the immunogenicity of the vaccine with respect to bovine diarrhoea virus of genotype 1; if protection against bovine diarrhoea virus of genotype 2 is claimed, an additional test, similar to that described under Potency, but using bovine diarrhoea virus of genotype 2 for challenge, is carried out.

BATCH POTENCY TEST
The test described under Potency is not carried out for routine testing of batches of vaccine. It is carried out for a given vaccine on one or more occasions as decided by or with the agreement of the competent authority. Where the test is not carried out, a suitable validated test is carried out, the criteria for acceptance being set with reference to a batch of vaccine that has given satisfactory results in the test described under Potency.
The following test may be used after a satisfactory correlation with the test described under Potency has been established.

Inject subcutaneously a suitable dose of the vaccine into each of 5 suitable seronegative laboratory animals or calves. Keep 2 animals as controls. A second dose of vaccine may be administered after a suitable interval if this has been shown to provide a suitably discriminating test system. Collect blood samples before the first vaccination and at a given interval between 14 and 21 days after the last vaccination. Determine the antibody titres against bovine diarrhoea virus by seroneutralisation on suitable cell cultures. The test is invalid if the control animals show antibodies against bovine diarrhoea virus. The vaccine complies with the test if the level of antibodies is not lower than that found for a batch of vaccine that has given satisfactory results in the test described under Potency.

IDENTIFICATION
When administered to animals free from specific neutralising antibodies against bovine diarrhoea virus, the vaccine stimulates the production of such antibodies.

TESTS
Safety
Inject a double dose of the vaccine by a recommended route into each of 2 cattle not older than the minimum age recommended for vaccination and that are free from bovine diarrhoea virus and antibodies against the virus. Observe the animals for 14 days. No abnormal local or systemic reaction occurs.

Inactivation

Carry out a test for residual infectious bovine diarrhoea virus by inoculating not less than 10 doses onto cells known to be sensitive to bovine diarrhoea virus; passage the cells after 7 days and observe the second culture for not less than 7 days. No live virus is detected. If the vaccine contains an adjuvant, separate the adjuvant if possible from the liquid phase by a method that does not interfere with the detection of possible live virus.

Bacteria and fungi

The vaccine complies with the requirement for sterility prescribed in the monograph on *Vaccines for veterinary use (0062)*.

POTENCY

Use heifers free from bovine diarrhoea virus that do not have neutralising antibodies against bovine diarrhoea virus. Vaccinate not fewer than 13 animals using the recommended schedule. Keep not fewer than 7 heifers as non-vaccinated controls. Keep all the animals as one group. Inseminate the heifers. Take a blood sample from non-vaccinated heifers shortly before challenge. The test is discontinued if fewer than 10 vaccinated heifers or 5 non-vaccinated heifers are pregnant at the time of challenge. Between the 60th and 90th days of gestation, challenge the animals. For both test models described (observation until calving and harvest of foetuses at 28 days), challenge may be made by the intranasal inoculation of a suitable quantity of a non-cytopathic strain of bovine diarrhoea virus or alternatively, where the animals are observed until calving, challenge may be made by contact with a persistently viraemic animal. Observe the animals clinically from challenge either until the end of gestation or until harvest of foetuses after 28 days. If abortion occurs, examine the aborted foetus for bovine diarrhoea virus by suitable methods. If animals are observed until calving, immediately after birth and prior to ingestion of colostrum, examine all calves for viraemia and antibodies against bovine diarrhoea virus. If foetuses are harvested 28 days after challenge, examine the foetuses for bovine diarrhoea virus by suitable methods. Transplacental infection is considered to have occurred if virus is detected in foetal organs or in the blood of newborn calves or if antibodies are detected in precolostral sera of calves. The test is invalid if any of the non-vaccinated heifers have neutralising antibody before challenge or if transplacental infection fails to occur in more than 10 per cent of non-vaccinated heifers. The vaccine complies with the test if 90 per cent or more of the vaccinated animals are protected from transplacental infection.

Ph Eur

Brucella Melitensis (Strain Rev. 1) Vaccine, Living

(Brucellosis Vaccine (Live) (Brucella Melitensis Rev. 1 Strain), Freeze-dried, for Veterinary Use, Ph Eur monograph 0793)

Ph Eur

DEFINITION

Brucellosis vaccine (live) (Brucella melitensis Rev. 1 strain), freeze-dried, for veterinary use is a freeze-dried suspension of live *Brucella melitensis* Rev. 1 strain. The vaccine contains not fewer than 0.5×10^9 and not more than 4×10^9 live bacteria per dose.

PRODUCTION

Brucella melitensis Rev. 1 strain is cultured in a suitable medium. The method of culture is such as to avoid bacterial dissociation and thus maintain the smooth characteristic of the culture. The bacteria are suspended in a buffer solution which may contain a suitable stabiliser. The suspension is distributed into containers and freeze-dried.

CHOICE OF VACCINE STRAIN

Only a vaccine strain shown to be satisfactory with respect to safety and immunogenicity may be used in the production of the vaccine. The following test may be used during demonstration of efficacy (5.2.7).

Immunogenicity

40 ewe lambs, 4 to 5 months old, from a non-vaccinated flock free from brucellosis are used. For the challenge strain, a 24-hour culture of *Brucella melitensis* strain H38 in trypticase agar is used. A preliminary test using animals of the same breed and age as for the main test is carried out to determine the challenge dose, which is between 10^7 and 10^8 colony-forming units and is chosen so as to produce abortion in all non-vaccinated animals. Half the animals are vaccinated at 4 to 6 months of age, according to the recommended schedule and using the minimum recommended dose. Oestrus is synchronised in the 40 animals which are then inseminated at 10 to 12 months of age. A diagnosis of pregnancy is made on all animals 2 to 3 months after insemination and all non-gravid animals are excluded from the test. All gravid animals are challenged by conjunctival instillation of the challenge dose of *Brucella melitensis* strain H38. The occurrence of abortion is noted and aetiology confirmed by testing for the presence of the challenge strain in the aborted foetus and in the ewe (using selective media of Kuzdas and Morse or of Farrell). Tests for the presence of the challenge strain are carried out on each animal at lambing. Tests for the presence of the challenge strain in the prescapular and retromammary lymph nodes are carried out at slaughter of the animals 4 to 6 weeks after lambing. The test is not valid unless at least 70 per cent of non-vaccinated animals: show abortion caused by the challenge strain; show infection with the challenge strain at lambing; show infection of the prescapular and retromammary lymph nodes at slaughter. The vaccine complies with the test if: not more than 30 per cent of vaccinated animals show abortion caused by the challenge strain; the challenge strain is found in not more than 50 per cent of vaccinated animals at lambing; the challenge strain is found in not more than 40 per cent of vaccinated animals at slaughter.

IDENTIFICATION

Brucella melitensis present in the vaccine is identified by suitable morphological, serological and biochemical tests and by culture: Rev. 1 strain is inhibited by addition to the suitable culture medium of 3 µg of benzylpenicillin sodium per millilitre; the strain grows on agar containing 2.5 µg of streptomycin per millilitre.

TESTS

Safety

Use 2 sheep, 4 to 6 months old and having no antibodies against *B. melitensis*. Administer 1 dose of vaccine by a recommended route to each sheep. Observe the animals for 21 days. No abnormal local or systemic reaction occurs.

Determination of dissociation phase

Examine not fewer than 200 colonies by a suitable technique. The culture of the vaccine strain is seen to be in the smooth (S) phase. Not fewer than 95 per cent of the colonies are of the smooth type.

Extraneous micro-organisms

The reconstituted vaccine does not contain extraneous micro-organisms. Verify the absence of micro-organisms other than *Brucella melitensis* Rev. 1 strain as described in the test for sterility prescribed in the monograph on *Vaccines for veterinary use (0062)*.

Live bacteria

Make a count of live bacteria on a solid medium suitable for the culture of *Brucella melitensis* Rev. 1 strain. The vaccine contains not fewer than 0.5×10^9 and not more than 4×10^9 live bacteria per dose.

Fifty per cent persistence time

Inject subcutaneously a suspension containing 10^8 live bacteria of the vaccine to be examined into each of 32 female CD1 mice, aged 5 to 6 weeks. Kill the mice in groups of eight, selected at random, 3, 6, 9 and 12 weeks later. Remove the spleens and homogenise individually and aseptically in 10 volumes of *phosphate buffered saline pH 6.8 R*. Spread the suspension on plates containing a suitable culture medium, using 0.4 ml per plate and not fewer than 3 plates per spleen (lower limit of detection: 5 bacteria per spleen). Carry out in parallel a similar test using *Brucella melitensis Rev. 1 strain BRP* (reference strain). Calculate the 50 per cent persistence time by the usual statistical methods (*5.3*) for probit analysis. The 50 per cent persistence time for the vaccine strain does not differ significantly from that of the reference strain.

STORAGE

Store at a temperature of 2 °C to 8 °C.

LABELLING

The label states:
— the number of *Brucella melitensis* Rev. 1 strain per dose,
— that the vaccine is intended for sheep and goats 4 to 6 months old,
— that the vaccine may be dangerous for man,
— that the vaccine is not to be used in pregnant or lactating animals,
— that the vaccine may be dangerous for cattle and that they are not to be kept in contact with vaccinated animals.

_____ *Ph Eur*

Calf Coronavirus Diarrhoea Vaccine (Inactivated)

(*Ph Eur monograph 1953*)

Ph Eur _____

DEFINITION

Calf coronavirus diarrhoea vaccine (inactivated) is a preparation of one or more suitable strains of bovine coronavirus, inactivated in such a manner that immunogenic properties are maintained. The vaccine is administered to the dam to aid in the control of coronavirus diarrhoea in offspring during the first few weeks of life.

PRODUCTION

Each virus strain is grown separately in suitable cell cultures (*5.2.4*). The viral suspensions of each strain are harvested separately and inactivated by a method that maintains immunogenicity. The viral suspensions may be purified and concentrated.

The test for inactivation is carried out using 2 passages in cell cultures of the same type as those used for production or in cells shown to be at least as sensitive. The quantity of virus used in the test is equivalent to not less than 10 doses of vaccine. No live virus is detected.

The vaccine may contain an adjuvant.

CHOICE OF VACCINE COMPOSITION

The vaccine is shown to be satisfactory with respect to safety (*5.2.6*) and efficacy (*5.2.7*) in the pregnant cow. The following tests may be used during demonstration of safety and immunogenicity.

Safety Carry out the test for each proposed route of administration. Administer by a proposed route and at the proposed stage or stages of pregnancy, a double dose of vaccine to each of not fewer than 10 pregnant cows that have not been vaccinated against bovine coronavirus. After the proposed interval, inject 1 dose into each cow. After each injection, measure the body temperature on the day of the injection and on the 4 following days. Observe the cows until calving. No abnormal local or systemic reaction occurs; any effects on gestation and the offspring are noted.

Immunogenicity The test described under Potency is suitable to demonstrate immunogenicity of the strain.

BATCH TESTING

Batch potency test

The test described under Potency is not carried out for routine testing of batches of vaccine. It is carried out, for a given vaccine, on one or more occasions, as decided by or with the agreement of the competent authority; where the test is not carried out, a suitable validated test is carried out, the criteria for acceptance being set with reference to a batch of vaccine that has given satisfactory results in the test described under Potency. The following test may be used after a suitable correlation with the test described under Potency has been established.

To obtain a valid assay, it may be necessary to carry out a test using several groups of animals, each receiving a different dose. For each dose required, carry out the test as follows. Vaccinate not fewer than 5 animals of a suitable species, free from specific antibodies against bovine coronavirus, using 1 injection of a suitable dose. Maintain not fewer than 2 animals as unvaccinated controls. Where the recommended schedule requires a booster injection to be given, a booster vaccination may also be given in this test provided it has been demonstrated that this will still provide a suitably sensitive test system. At a given interval not less than 14 days after the last injection, collect blood from each animal and prepare serum samples. Use a suitable validated test to measure the antibody response. The antibody level is not significantly less than that obtained with a batch that has given satisfactory results in the test described under Potency and there is no significant increase in antibody titre in the controls.

IDENTIFICATION

Injected into animals free from specific antibodies against bovine coronavirus, the vaccine stimulates the formation of such antibodies.

TESTS

Safety

Use cattle not less than 6 months old and preferably having no antibodies against bovine coronavirus or, where justified, use cattle with a low level of such antibodies as long as they have not been vaccinated against bovine coronavirus and administration of the vaccine does not cause an anamnestic response. Administer to each of 2 animals a double dose of vaccine by a recommended route. After 14 days, administer 1 dose to each animal. Observe the animals for 14 days. No abnormal local or systemic reaction occurs.

Inactivation

Carry out a test for residual infectious virus using 10 doses of vaccine and 2 passages in cell cultures of the same type as those used for production of the vaccine or other cell cultures of suitable sensitivity. No live virus is detected. If the vaccine contains an adjuvant which interferes with the test, separate it if possible from the liquid phase of the vaccine by a method that does not inactivate virus nor interfere in any other way with detection of live viruses.

Extraneous viruses

Carry out tests for antibodies on the cattle used for the safety test. Take a blood sample at the end of the second observation period. The vaccine does not stimulate the formation of antibodies against bovine herpes virus 1 (BHV1), bovine leukaemia virus (BLV) and bovine viral diarrhoea virus (BVDV).

Sterility

The vaccine complies with the test for sterility prescribed in the monograph on *Vaccines for veterinary use (0062)*.

POTENCY

Use not fewer than 15 pregnant cows, where possible having no antibodies against bovine coronavirus. Where such cows are not available, use cows that: have not been vaccinated against bovine coronavirus; come from a farm where there is no recent history of infection with bovine coronavirus; and have a low level of antibodies against bovine coronavirus, the levels being comparable in all animals. Vaccinate not fewer than 10 pregnant cows according to the recommended schedule. Keep not fewer than 5 pregnant cows as unvaccinated controls. Starting at calving, take the colostrum and then milk from each cow and keep it in suitable conditions. Determine individually the protective activity of the colostrum and milk from each cow using calves born from healthy cows, and which may be born by Caesarean section, and maintained in an environment where they are not exposed to infection by bovine coronavirus. Feed colostrum and then milk to each calf every 6 h or according to the recommended schedule. At 5-7 days after birth, challenge each calf by the oral administration of a suitable quantity of a virulent strain of bovine coronavirus. Observe the calves for 7 days. Note the incidence, severity and duration of diarrhoea and the duration and quantity of virus excretion. The vaccine complies with the test if there is a significant reduction in diarrhoea and virus excretion in calves given colostrum and milk from vaccinated cows compared to those given colostrum and milk from controls.

LABELLING

The label states the recommended schedule for administering colostrum and milk, *post-partum*.

_____ *Ph Eur*

Calf Rotavirus Diarrhoea Vaccine (Inactivated)

(Ph Eur monograph 1954)

Ph Eur _____

DEFINITION

Calf rotavirus diarrhoea vaccine (inactivated) is a preparation of one or more suitable strains of bovine rotavirus, inactivated in such a manner that immunogenic properties are maintained. The vaccine is administered to the dam to aid in the control of rotavirus diarrhoea in offspring during the first few weeks of life.

PRODUCTION

Each virus strain is grown separately in suitable cell cultures *(5.2.4)*. The viral suspensions of each strain are harvested separately and inactivated by a method that maintains immunogenicity. The viral suspensions may be purified and concentrated.

The test for inactivation is carried out using 2 passages in cell cultures of the same type as those used for production or in cells shown to be at least as sensitive. The quantity of virus used in the test is equivalent to not less than 100 doses of vaccine. No live virus is detected.

The vaccine may contain an adjuvant.

CHOICE OF VACCINE COMPOSITION

The vaccine is shown to be satisfactory with respect to safety *(5.2.6)* and efficacy *(5.2.7)* in the pregnant cow. The following tests may be used during demonstration of safety and immunogenicity.

Safety   Carry out the test for each proposed route of administration. Administer by a proposed route and at the proposed stage or stages of pregnancy, a double dose of vaccine to each of not fewer than 10 pregnant cows that have not been vaccinated against bovine rotavirus. After the proposed interval, inject 1 dose into each cow. After each injection, measure the body temperature on the day of the injection and on the 4 following days. Observe the cows until calving. No abnormal local or systemic reaction occurs; any effects on gestation and the offspring are noted.

Immunogenicity   The test described under Potency is suitable to demonstrate immunogenicity of the strain.

BATCH TESTING

Batch potency test

The test described under Potency is not carried out for routine testing of batches of vaccine. It is carried out, for a given vaccine, on one or more occasions, as decided by or with the agreement of the competent authority; where the test is not carried out, a suitable validated test is carried out, the criteria for acceptance being set with reference to a batch of vaccine that has given satisfactory results in the test described under Potency. The following test may be used after a suitable correlation with the test described under Potency has been established.

To obtain a valid assay, it may be necessary to carry out a test using several groups of animals, each receiving a different dose. For each dose required, carry out the test as follows. Vaccinate not fewer than 5 animals of a suitable species, free from specific antibodies against bovine rotavirus, using 1 injection of a suitable dose. Maintain not fewer than 2 animals as unvaccinated controls. Where the recommended schedule requires a booster injection to be given, a booster vaccination may also be given in this test provided it has been demonstrated that this will still provide a suitably sensitive test system. At a given interval not less than 14 days after the last injection, collect blood from each animal and prepare serum samples. Use a suitable validated test to measure the antibody response. The antibody level is not significantly less than that obtained with a batch that has given satisfactory results in the test described under Potency and there is no significant increase in antibody titre in the controls.

IDENTIFICATION

Injected into animals free from specific antibodies against bovine rotavirus, the vaccine stimulates the formation of such antibodies.

TESTS

Safety

Use cattle not less than 6 months old and preferably having no antibodies against bovine rotavirus or, where justified, use cattle with a low level of such antibodies as long as they have not been vaccinated against bovine rotavirus and administration of the vaccine does not cause an anamnestic response. Administer to each of 2 animals a double dose of vaccine by a recommended route. After 14 days, administer 1 dose to each animal. Observe the animals for 14 days. No abnormal local or systemic reaction occurs.

Inactivation

Carry out a test for residual infectious virus using 10 doses of vaccine and 2 passages in cell cultures of the same type as those used for production of the vaccine or other cell cultures of suitable sensitivity. No live virus is detected. If the vaccine contains an adjuvant which interferes with the test, separate it if possible from the liquid phase of the vaccine by a method that does not inactivate virus nor interfere in any other way with detection of live viruses.

Extraneous viruses

Carry out tests for antibodies on the cattle used for the safety test. Take a blood sample at the end of the second observation period. The vaccine does not stimulate the formation of antibodies against bovine herpes virus 1 (BHV 1), bovine leukaemia virus (BLV) and bovine viral diarrhoea virus (BVDV).

Sterility

The vaccine complies with the test for sterility prescribed in the monograph on *Vaccines for veterinary use (0062)*.

POTENCY

Use not fewer than 15 pregnant cows, where possible having no antibodies against bovine rotavirus. Where such cows are not available, use cows that: have not been vaccinated against bovine rotavirus; come from a farm where there is no recent history of infection with bovine rotavirus; and have a low level of antibodies against bovine rotavirus, the levels being comparable in all animals. Vaccinate not fewer than 10 pregnant cows according to the recommended schedule. Keep not fewer than 5 pregnant cows as unvaccinated controls. Starting at calving, take the colostrum and then milk from each cow and keep it in suitable conditions. Determine individually the protective activity of the colostrum and milk from each cow using calves born from healthy cows, and which may be born by Caesarean section, and maintained in an environment where they are not exposed to infection by bovine rotavirus. Feed colostrum and then milk to each calf every 6 h or according to the recommended schedule. At 5-7 days after birth, challenge each calf by the oral administration of a suitable quantity of a virulent strain of bovine rotavirus. Observe the calves for 7 days. Note the incidence, severity and duration of diarrhoea

and the duration and quantity of virus excretion. The vaccine complies with the test if there is a significant reduction in diarrhoea and virus excretion in calves given colostrum and milk from vaccinated cows compared to those given colostrum and milk from controls.

LABELLING

The label states the recommended schedule for administering colostrum and milk, *post-partum*.

_____ *Ph Eur*

Canine Adenovirus Vaccine, Inactivated

(Canine Adenovirus Vaccine (Inactivated), Ph Eur monograph 1298)

Ph Eur _____

DEFINITION

Canine adenovirus vaccine (inactivated) is a suspension of one or more suitable strains of canine adenovirus 1 (canine contagious hepatitis virus) and/or canine adenovirus 2, inactivated in such a way that adequate immunogenicity is maintained.

PRODUCTION

The test for inactivation is carried out using a quantity of virus equivalent to at least 10 doses of vaccine with 2 passages in cell cultures of the same type as those used for production or in cell cultures shown to be at least as sensitive. No live virus is detected.

The vaccine may contain an adjuvant.

CHOICE OF VACCINE COMPOSITION

The vaccine is shown to be satisfactory with respect to safety (5.2.6) and efficacy (5.2.7). The following tests may be used during demonstration of safety and immunogenicity.

Safety Carry out the test for each recommended route of administration in animals of the minimum age recommended for vaccination. Use a batch of vaccine of the maximum potency likely to be attained.

Use for each test not fewer than 10 dogs that do not have antibodies against canine adenovirus 1 or 2. Administer to each dog a double dose of vaccine. If the recommended schedule requires a second dose, administer one dose after the recommended interval. Observe the dogs for 14 days after the last administration. No abnormal local or systemic reaction occurs.

If the vaccine is intended for use in pregnant bitches, vaccinate bitches at the stage of pregnancy or at different stages of pregnancy according to the recommended schedule. Prolong observation until 1 day after parturition. No abnormal local or systemic reaction occurs. No adverse effects on the pregnancy and offspring are noted.

Immunogenicity For vaccines intended to protect against hepatitis, the test described under Potency is suitable for demonstration of immunogenicity. If the vaccine is indicated for protection against respiratory signs, a further test to demonstrate immunogenicity for this indication is also necessary.

BATCH TESTING

Batch potency test

The test described under Potency is not carried out for routine testing of batches of vaccine. It is carried out for a given vaccine on one or more occasions as decided by or with the agreement of the competent authority. Where the test is not carried out, a suitable validated alternative test is carried out, the criteria for acceptance being set with reference to a batch of vaccine that has given satisfactory results in the test described under Potency.

IDENTIFICATION

When injected into susceptible animals, the vaccine stimulates the formation of specific antibodies against the type or types of canine adenovirus stated on the label.

TESTS

Safety

Use dogs of the minimum age recommended for vaccination and preferably having no canine adenovirus-neutralising antibodies or, where justified, use dogs with a low level of such antibodies as long as they have not been vaccinated against canine adenovirus and administration of the vaccine does not cause an anamnestic response. Administer a double dose of vaccine by a recommended route to each of 2 dogs. Observe the dogs for 14 days. No abnormal local or systemic reaction occurs.

Inactivation

Carry out a test for residual infectious canine adenovirus using 10 doses of vaccine by inoculation into sensitive cell cultures; make a passage after 6-8 days and maintain the cultures for 14 days. No live virus is detected. If the vaccine contains an adjuvant, separate the adjuvant from the liquid phase by a method that does not inactivate or otherwise interfere with the detection of live virus.

Sterility

The vaccine complies with the test for sterility prescribed in the monograph on *Vaccines for veterinary use (0062)*.

POTENCY

Use 7 dogs of the minimum age recommended for vaccination and that do not have antibodies against canine adenovirus. Vaccinate 5 of the animals by a recommended route and according to the recommended schedule. Keep the other 2 dogs as controls. 21 days later inject intravenously into each of the 7 animals a quantity of a virulent strain of canine adenovirus sufficient to cause death or typical signs of the disease in a susceptible dog. Observe the animals for a further 21 days. Dogs displaying typical signs of serious infection with canine adenovirus are killed humanely to avoid unnecessary suffering. The test is invalid and must be repeated if one or both of the controls do not die from or display typical signs of serious infection with canine adenovirus. The vaccine complies with the test if the vaccinated animals remain in good health.

LABELLING

The label states the type or types of canine adenovirus present in the vaccine.

Ph Eur

Canine Adenovirus Vaccine, Living

*(Canine Adenovirus Vaccine (Live),
Ph Eur monograph 1951)*

Ph Eur

DEFINITION

Canine adenovirus vaccine (live) is a preparation of 1 or more suitable strains of canine adenovirus 2. This monograph applies to vaccines intended for active immunisation of dogs against canine contagious hepatitis and/or respiratory disease caused by canine adenovirus.

PRODUCTION

The virus strain is propagated in suitable cell cultures (5.2.4). The viral suspension is harvested, titrated and may be mixed with a suitable stabilising solution. The vaccine may be freeze-dried.

CHOICE OF VACCINE STRAIN

The vaccine is shown to be satisfactory with respect to safety (5.2.6), absence of increase in virulence and immunogenicity (5.2.7). The following tests may be used during demonstration of safety, absence of increase in virulence and immunogenicity.

Safety The test is carried out for each route of administration to be stated on the label. Use not fewer than 5 puppies of the minimum age recommended for vaccination and that do not have antibodies to canine adenovirus. Administer to each puppy by a recommended route a quantity of virus corresponding to not less than 10 times the maximum titre that may be expected in a dose of vaccine. Observe the dogs for 14 days. The puppies remain in good health and no abnormal local or systemic reaction occurs.

If the vaccine is intended for use or may be used in pregnant bitches, administer the virus to 5 bitches at the recommended stage or at a range of stages of pregnancy according to the recommended schedule. Prolong the observation period until 1 day after parturition. The bitches remain in good health and there is no abnormal local or systemic reaction. No adverse effects on the pregnancy or the offspring are noted.

Increase in virulence Administer by a recommended route to each of 2 puppies, 5-7 weeks old and which do not have antibodies against canine adenovirus, a quantity of virus that will allow recovery of virus for the passages described below. Kill the puppies 4-6 days later. Remove from each puppy nasal and pharyngeal mucosa, tonsils, lung, spleen and, if they are likely to contain virus, liver and kidney. Pool the samples; administer by a suitable route, for example intranasally, 1 ml of the pooled organ suspension to each of 2 other puppies of the same age and susceptibility; carry out these operations at least 5 times; verify the presence of the virus at each passage by direct or indirect means. If the virus has disappeared, carry out a second series of passages. Inoculate virus from the highest recovered passage level to 5 puppies of the minimum age recommended for vaccination, observe for 14 days and compare the reactions that occur with those seen in the test for safety described above. There is no indication of an increase of virulence as compared with the non-passaged virus.

Immunogenicity For vaccines intended to protect against hepatitis, test A described under Potency is suitable for demonstration of Immunogenicity. For vaccines intended to protect against respiratory signs, test B described under Potency is suitable for demonstration of immunogenicity.

BATCH TESTING

If the test for Potency has been carried out with satisfactory results on a representative batch of vaccine, this test may be omitted as a routine control on other batches of vaccine prepared from the same seed lot.

IDENTIFICATION

The vaccine mixed with monospecific antiserum against canine adenovirus 2 no longer infects susceptible cell cultures.

TESTS

Safety

Use 2 puppies not older than the minimum age recommended for vaccination and which do not have antibodies against canine adenovirus. Administer 10 doses of the vaccine to each dog by a recommended route. Observe for 14 days. The dogs remain in good health and no abnormal local or systemic reaction occurs.

Extraneous viruses

Mix the vaccine with a suitable monospecific antiserum against canine adenovirus 2 and inoculate into cell cultures known for their susceptibility to viruses pathogenic for the dog. Carry out a passage after 6-8 days and maintain the cultures for a total of 14 days. No cytopathic effect develops and the cells show no evidence of the presence of haemadsorbing agents.

Bacterial and fungal contamination

The vaccine, reconstituted if necessary, complies with the test for sterility prescribed in the monograph on *Vaccines for veterinary use (0062)*.

Mycoplasmas *(2.6.7)*

The vaccine, reconstituted if necessary, complies with the test for mycoplasmas.

Virus titre

Reconstitute the vaccine, if necessary, and titrate in suitable cell cultures. 1 dose of the vaccine contains not less than the quantity of virus equivalent to the minimum virus titre stated on the label.

POTENCY

Depending on the indications for the vaccine, it complies with test A and/or B for potency.

A. Use 7 puppies of the minimum age recommended for vaccination and that do not have antibodies against canine adenovirus. Vaccinate 5 of the animals by a recommended route and according to the recommended schedule. Keep the other 2 dogs as controls. 21 days later, inject intravenously into each of the 7 animals a quantity of a virulent strain of canine adenovirus 1 (canine contagious hepatitis virus) sufficient to cause death or typical signs of the disease in a susceptible dog. Observe the animals for a further 21 days. Dogs displaying typical signs of serious infection with canine adenovirus are killed humanely to avoid unnecessary suffering. The test is invalid and must be repeated if 1 or both of the controls do not die from or display typical signs of serious infection with canine adenovirus. The vaccine complies with the test if the vaccinated animals remain in good health showing no clinical signs except for a possible transient elevated rectal temperature.

B. Use 20 dogs of the minimum age recommended for vaccination and that do not have antibodies against canine adenovirus. Vaccinate 10 of the dogs by a recommended route and according to the recommended schedule. Keep the other 10 dogs as controls. 21 days later, administer intranasally to each of the 20 animals a quantity of a virulent strain of canine adenovirus 2 sufficient to cause typical signs of respiratory disease in a susceptible dog. Observe the animals daily for a further 10 days. Record the incidence of signs of respiratory and general disease in each dog (for example, sneezing, coughing, nasal and lachrymal discharge, loss of appetite). Collect nasal swabs or washings from each dog daily from days 2 to 10 after challenge and test these samples to determine the presence and titre of excreted virus. The vaccine complies with the test if there is a notable decrease in the incidence and severity of clinical signs and in virus excretion in vaccinates compared to controls.

Ph Eur

Canine Distemper Vaccine, Living

(Canine Distemper Vaccine (Live), Freeze-dried, Ph Eur monograph 0448)

Ph Eur _____

DEFINITION

Freeze-dried canine distemper vaccine (live) is a preparation of a strain of distemper virus that is attenuated for dogs.

PRODUCTION

The virus is propagated in suitable cell cultures *(5.2.4)* or in fertilised hen eggs from flocks free from specified pathogens *(5.2.2)*. The viral suspension is harvested, titrated and may be mixed with a suitable stabilising solution. The vaccine is then freeze-dried.

CHOICE OF VACCINE STRAIN

The vaccine strain is shown to be satisfactory with respect to safety *(5.2.6)*, absence of increase in virulence and immunogenicity *(5.2.7)*. The following tests may be used during demonstration of safety, absence of increase in virulence and immunogenicity.

Safety The test is carried out for each recommended route of administration. Use five susceptible puppies of the minimum age recommended for vaccination and that do not have antibodies against canine distemper virus. Administer to each puppy by a recommended route a quantity of virus corresponding to not less than ten times the maximum titre that may be expected in a dose of vaccine. Observe the puppies for 42 days. The puppies remain in good health and there is no abnormal local or systemic reaction.

If the vaccine is intended for use in pregnant bitches, administer the virus to five bitches at the recommended stage of pregnancy or at a range of stages of pregnancy according to the recommended schedule. Prolong observation until 1 day after parturition. The dogs remain in good health and there is no abnormal local or systemic reaction. No adverse effects on the pregnancy or the offspring are noted.

Increase in virulence Administer by a recommended route to each of two puppies, 5 to 7 weeks old and which do not have antibodies against canine distemper virus a quantity of virus corresponding to one dose of vaccine. Kill the puppies 5 to 10 days later, remove nasal mucosa, tonsils, thymus, spleen and the lungs and their local lymph nodes from each puppy and pool the samples; administer intranasally 1 ml of the pooled organ suspension to each of two other puppies of the same age and susceptibility; carry out these operations at least five times; verify the presence of the virus at each passage by direct or indirect means. If the virus has disappeared, carry out a second series of passages. Inoculate virus from the highest recovered passage level to puppies, observe for 42 days and compare any reactions that occur with those seen in the test for safety described above. There is no indication of an increase of virulence as compared with the non-passaged virus.

Immunogenicity The test described under Potency may be used to demonstrate the immunogenicity of the strain.

BATCH TESTING

If the test for potency has been carried out with satisfactory results on a representative batch of vaccine, this test may be omitted as a routine control on other batches of vaccine prepared from the same seed lot.

IDENTIFICATION

The vaccine reconstituted as stated on the label and mixed with a monospecific distemper antiserum against canine distemper virus no longer provokes cytopathic effects in susceptible cell cultures.

TESTS

Safety

Use two puppies of the minimum age recommended for vaccination and which do not have antibodies against canine distemper virus. Administer ten doses of the vaccine to each dog by a recommended route. Observe for 14 days. The dogs remain in good health and no abnormal local or systemic reaction occurs.

Extraneous viruses

Mix the vaccine with a suitable monospecific antiserum against canine distemper virus and inoculate into cell cultures known for their susceptibility to viruses pathogenic for the dog. Carry out a passage after 6 to 8 days and maintain the cultures for 14 days. No cytopathic effect develops and the cells show no evidence of the presence of haemadsorbing agents.

Bacterial and fungal contamination

The reconstituted vaccine complies with the test for sterility prescribed under *Vaccines for veterinary use (0062)*.

Mycoplasmas (*2.6.7*)

The reconstituted vaccine complies with the test for mycoplasmas.

Virus titre

Titrate the reconstituted vaccine in suitable cell cultures. One dose of the vaccine contains not less than the quantity of virus equivalent to the minimum virus titre stated on the label.

POTENCY

Use seven susceptible puppies, 8 to 16 weeks old and free from antibodies against canine distemper virus. Vaccinate five puppies according to the instructions for use. Keep the two other animals as controls. Observe all the animals for 21 days. Inject intravenously into each animal a quantity of canine distemper virus sufficient to cause in a susceptible dog death or typical signs of the disease. Observe the animals for a further 21 days. Dogs displaying typical signs of serious infection with canine distemper virus are killed humanely to avoid unnecessary suffering. The test is not valid and must be repeated if one or more of the control animals do not either die of distemper or display typical signs of serious infection. The vaccine complies with the test if the vaccinated animals remain in good health.

Ph Eur

Canine Parainfluenza Virus Vaccine (Live)

(Ph Eur monograph 1955)

Ph Eur

DEFINITION

Canine parainfluenza virus vaccine (live) is a preparation of a suitable attenuated strain of canine parainfluenza virus for dogs. The vaccine is intended for the protection of dogs against respiratory signs of infection with parainfluenza virus of canine origin.

PRODUCTION

The virus is propagated in suitable cell cultures (*5.2.4*). The viral suspension is harvested, titrated and may be mixed with a suitable stabilising solution. The vaccine may be freeze-dried.

CHOICE OF VACCINE STRAIN

The vaccine is shown to be satisfactory with respect to safety, absence of increase in virulence and immunogenicity. The following tests may be used during demonstration of safety (*5.2.6*), absence of increase in virulence and immunogenicity (*5.2.7*).

Safety   The test is carried out for each route of administration stated on the label. Use not fewer than 5 susceptible puppies of the recommended minimum age for vaccination and that do not have antibodies against parainfluenza virus of canine origin. Administer to each puppy by a recommended route a quantity of virus corresponding to not less than 10 times the maximum titre that may be expected in a dose of vaccine. Observe the puppies for 21 days. The puppies remain in good health and there is no abnormal local or systemic reaction.

If the vaccine is intended for use in pregnant bitches, administer the virus to not fewer than 5 bitches at the recommended stage or stages of pregnancy and according to the recommended schedule. Prolong the observation period until 1 day after whelping. The dogs remain in good health and there is no abnormal local or systemic reaction. No adverse effects on the pregnancy or the offspring are noted.

Increase in virulence   Administer intranasally and by a recommended route to each of 2 puppies, 5 to 7 weeks old and which do not have antibodies against parainfluenza virus of canine origin, a quantity of virus that will allow recovery of virus for the passages described below. Use vaccine virus at the least attenuated passage level that will be present in a batch of the vaccine. Collect nasal swabs from each dog daily from 3 to 10 days after inoculation. Inoculate the suspension from the swabs into suitable cell cultures to verify the presence of virus. Use the suspension from the swabs that contain the maximum amount of virus and administer intranasally 1 ml of the suspension into each of 2 other puppies of the same age and susceptibility. This operation is then repeated at least 5 times. If the virus is not recovered at a given passage level, a second series of passages is carried out. Inoculate virus from the highest recovered passage level to not fewer than 5 puppies, observe for 21 days and compare any reactions that occur with those seen in the test for safety described above. There is no indication of an increase in virulence as compared with the non-passaged virus.

Immunogenicity   The test described under Potency is suitable to demonstrate the immunogenicity of the strain.

BATCH TESTING

If the test for potency has been carried out with satisfactory results on a representative batch of vaccine, this test may be omitted as a routine control on other batches of vaccine prepared from the same seed lot.

IDENTIFICATION

Carry out an immunofluorescence test in suitable cell cultures, using a monospecific antiserum.

TESTS
Safety
Use 2 puppies not older than the minimum age recommended for vaccination and which do not have antibodies against parainfluenza virus of canine origin. Administer a volume containing 10 doses of the vaccine into each puppy by a recommended route. Observe for 14 days. The puppies remain in good health and no abnormal local or systemic reaction occurs.

Extraneous viruses
Neutralise the vaccine virus using a monospecific antiserum and inoculate into cell cultures known for their susceptibility to viruses pathogenic for the dog. Carry out a passage after 6 to 8 days and maintain the cultures for a total of 14 days. No cytopathic effect develops and the cells show no evidence of the presence of haemadsorbing agents.

Bacterial and fungal contamination
The vaccine, reconstituted if necessary, complies with the test for sterility prescribed in the monograph on *Vaccines for veterinary use (0062)*.

Mycoplasmas (2.6.7)
The vaccine, reconstituted if necessary, complies with the test for mycoplasmas.

Virus titre
Reconstitute the vaccine, if necessary, and titrate in suitable cell cultures. 1 dose of the vaccine contains not less than the quantity of virus equivalent to the minimum virus titre stated on the label.

POTENCY
Use not fewer than 15 susceptible puppies of the minimum age recommended for vaccination and which do not have antibodies against parainfluenza virus of canine origin. Vaccinate not fewer than 10 of the puppies according to the instructions for use. Keep not fewer than 5 other puppies as controls. Observe all the animals for not less than 21 days after the last vaccination. Administer by the intratracheal or intranasal route to each animal a quantity of a virulent strain of parainfluenza virus of canine origin sufficient to establish infection with the virus in a susceptible dog. Observe the animals for a further 14 days. Collect nasal swabs or washings from each dog daily from day 2 to 10 after challenge and test these samples for the presence of excreted virus. Use a scoring system to record the incidence of coughing in each dog. The test is not valid if more than 1 of the control animals shows neither coughing nor the excretion of the challenge virus. The vaccine complies with the test if the scores for coughing or virus excretion for the vaccinated animals are significantly lower than in the controls.

Ph Eur

Canine Parvovirus Vaccine, Inactivated

(Canine Parvovirosis Vaccine (Inactivated), Ph Eur monograph 0795)

Ph Eur

DEFINITION
Inactivated canine parvovirosis vaccine is a liquid or freeze-dried preparation of canine parvovirus inactivated by a suitable method.

PRODUCTION
The virus is propagated in suitable cell cultures (5.2.4). The virus may be purified and concentrated.

A test for residual live virus is carried out on the bulk harvest of each batch to confirm inactivation of the canine parvovirus. The quantity of inactivated virus used in the test is equivalent to not less than 100 doses of the vaccine. The vaccine is inoculated into suitable non-confluent cells; after incubation for 8 days, a subculture is made using trypsinised cells. After incubation for a further 8 days, the cultures are examined for residual live parvovirus by an immunofluorescence test. The immunofluorescence test may be supplemented by a haemagglutination test or other suitable tests on the supernatant of the cell cultures. No live virus is detected.

The vaccine may contain an adjuvant or adjuvants.

CHOICE OF VACCINE COMPOSITION
The vaccine is shown to be satisfactory with respect to safety and immunogenicity in dogs. The following test may be used in the demonstration of efficacy (5.2.7).

Immunogenicity 7 susceptible dogs of the minimum age recommended for vaccination are used. A blood sample is drawn from each dog and tested individually for antibodies against canine parvovirus to determine susceptibility. 5 dogs are vaccinated according to the recommended schedule. 2 dogs are kept as controls. 20 to 22 days after the last vaccination each of the dogs receives by the oronasal route a suspension of pathogenic canine parvovirus. The dogs are observed for 14 days. Haemagglutination tests are carried out to detect virus in the faeces. The test is not valid unless the 2 control dogs show typical signs of the disease or leucopenia and excretion of the virus. The vaccine complies with the test if the 5 vaccinated dogs remain in excellent health and show no sign of the disease nor leucopenia and if the maximum titre of virus excreted in the faeces is less than 1/100 of the geometric mean of the maximum titres found in the controls.

IDENTIFICATION
When injected into dogs, the vaccine stimulates the production of antibodies against canine parvovirus.

TESTS
Safety
Use dogs of the minimum age recommended for vaccination and preferably having no canine parvovirus antibodies or, where justified, use dogs with a low level of such antibodies as long as they have not been vaccinated against canine parvovirus and administration of the vaccine does not cause an anamnestic response. Administer a double dose of vaccine by a recommended route to each of 2 dogs. Observe the animals for 14 days. No abnormal local or systemic reaction occurs.

Sterility
The vaccine complies with the test for sterility prescribed in the monograph on *Vaccines for veterinary use (0062)*.

POTENCY
Carry out test A or test B.

A. Inject subcutaneously into each of 5 guinea-pigs, free from specific antibodies, half of the dose stated on the label. After 14 days, inject again half of the dose stated on the label. 14 days later, collect blood samples and separate the serum. Inactivate each serum by heating at 56 °C for 30 min. To 1 volume of each serum add 9 volumes of a 200 g/l suspension of *light kaolin R* in *phosphate buffered saline pH 7.4 R*. Shake each mixture for 20 min. Centrifuge, collect the supernatant liquid and mix with 1 volume of a concentrated suspension of pig erythrocytes. Allow to stand at 4 °C for 60 min and centrifuge. The dilution of the serum obtained is 1:10. Using each serum, prepare a series of twofold dilutions. To 0.025 ml of each of the latter dilutions add 0.025 ml of a suspension of canine parvovirus antigen containing 4 haemagglutinating units. Allow to stand at 37 °C for 30 min and add 0.05 ml of a suspension of pig erythrocytes containing 30×10^6 cells per millilitre. Allow to stand at 4 °C for 90 min and note the last dilution of serum that still completely inhibits haemagglutination. The vaccine complies with the test if the median antibody titre of the sera collected after the second vaccination is not less than 1/80.

B. Vaccinate, according to the schedule stated on the label, 2 healthy susceptible dogs, 8 to 12 weeks old and having antibody titres less than $4 \, ND_{50}$ (50 per cent neutralising dose) per 0.1 ml of serum measured by the method described below. 14 days after vaccination, examine the serum of each animal as follows. Heat the serum at 56 °C for 30 min and prepare serial dilutions using a medium suitable for canine cells. Add to each dilution an equal volume of a virus suspension containing an amount of virus such that when the volume of serum-virus mixture appropriate for the assay system is inoculated into cell cultures, each culture receives approximately $10^4 \, CCID_{50}$. Incubate the mixtures at 37 °C for 1 h and inoculate 4 canine cell cultures with a suitable volume of each mixture. Incubate the cell cultures at 37 °C for 7 days, passage and incubate for a further 7 days. Examine the cultures for evidence of specific cytopathic effects and calculate the antibody titre. The vaccine complies with the test if the mean titre is not less than $32 \, ND_{50}$ per 0.1 ml of serum. If one dog fails to respond, repeat the test using 2 more dogs and calculate the result as the mean of the titres obtained from all of the 3 dogs that have responded.

Ph Eur

Canine Parvovirus Vaccine, Living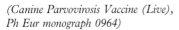

(Canine Parvovirosis Vaccine (Live),
Ph Eur monograph 0964)

Ph Eur _____

DEFINITION
Canine parvovirosis vaccine (live) is a preparation of a strain of canine parvovirus that is attenuated for the dog.

PRODUCTION
The attenuated virus is grown in suitable cell cultures (5.2.4).

The viral suspension is harvested, titrated and mixed with a suitable stabilising solution. The vaccine may be freeze-dried.

CHOICE OF VACCINE STRAIN
Only a virus strain shown to be satisfactory with respect to safety, irreversibility of attenuation, and immunogenicity may be used in the preparation of the vaccine. The following tests are used in the demonstration of safety (5.2.6) and efficacy (5.2.7).

Safety   Each test is carried out for each recommended route of administration.

5 susceptible puppies of the minimum age recommended for vaccination and having no haemagglutination-inhibiting antibodies against canine parvovirus are used for the test. A count of white blood cells in circulating blood is made on days 4, 2 and 0 before injection of the vaccine strain. Each puppy receives by a recommended route a quantity of

virus corresponding to not less than 10 times the maximum virus titre that may be expected in a batch of vaccine and at the lowest passage level. The puppies are observed for 21 days. A count of white blood cells in circulating blood is made on days 3, 5, 7 and 10 after the injection. The puppies remain in good health and there is no abnormal local or systemic reaction. Any diminution in the number of circulating white blood cells is not greater than 50 per cent of the initial number determined as the average of the 3 values found before injection of the vaccine strain.

A quantity of virus corresponding to not less than 10 times the maximum titre that may be expected in a batch of vaccine and at the lowest passage level is administered by one of the recommended routes to each of 5 susceptible puppies. Five puppies are kept as controls. 2 puppies from each group are killed at 14 days and the 3 remaining puppies from each group at 21 days and histological examination of the thymus of each animal is carried out. Slight hypoplasia of the thymus may be evident after 14 days. The strain is not acceptable if damage is evident after 21 days.

Irreversibility of attenuation   Use 2 susceptible puppies of the minimum age recommended for vaccination and which do not have haemagglutination-inhibiting antibodies against canine parvovirus. Administer to each puppy, by a recommended route, a quantity of virus corresponding to 10 times the maximum titre that may be expected in a batch of vaccine. From the second to the tenth day after administration of the virus, the faeces are collected from each puppy and checked for the presence of the virus; faeces containing virus are pooled. 1 ml of the suspension of pooled faeces is administered by the oronasal route to each of 2 other puppies of the same age and susceptibility; this operation is carried out 4 times. The presence of virus is verified at each passage. If the virus is not found, a second identification of passages is carried out; if the virus is not found in one of the second identification of passages, the vaccine strain complies with the test. No puppy dies or shows signs attributable to the vaccine. No indication of increase of virulence compared to the original vaccinal virus is observed; account is taken, notably, of the count of white blood cells, of results of histological examination of the thymus and of the titre of excreted virus.

Immunogenicity   The test described under Potency is suitable to demonstrate immunogenicity of the strain.

BATCH TESTING
If the test for potency has been carried out with satisfactory results on a representative batch of vaccine, this test may be omitted as a routine control on other batches of vaccine prepared from the same seed lot, subject to agreement by the competent authority.

IDENTIFICATION
The vaccine is grown in a susceptible cell line in a substrate suitable for presenting for fluorescent antibody or immunoperoxidase tests. Suitable controls are included. A proportion of the cells is tested with a monoclonal antibody specific for canine parvovirus and a proportion of the cells tested with a monoclonal antibody specific for feline parvovirus. Canine parvovirus antigen is detected but no feline parvovirus is detected in the cells inoculated with the vaccine.

TESTS
Safety
Use 2 dogs of the minimum age recommended for vaccination and having no haemagglutination-inhibiting antibodies against canine parvovirus. Administer 10 doses of

the vaccine to each dog by a recommended route. Observe for 14 days. No abnormal local or systemic reaction occurs.

Extraneous viruses

Mix the vaccine with a suitable antiserum against canine parvovirus and inoculate into cell cultures known for their susceptibility to viruses pathogenic for the dog. No cytopathic effect develops. There is no sign of haemagglutinating or haemadsorbing agents and no other sign of the presence of extraneous viruses.

Bacterial and fungal contamination

The vaccine, reconstituted if necessary, complies with the test for sterility prescribed in the monograph on *Vaccines for veterinary use (0062)*.

Mycoplasmas (2.6.7)

The vaccine, reconstituted if necessary, complies with the test for mycoplasmas.

Virus titre

Reconstitute the vaccine, if necessary, as stated on the label and titrate in suitable cell cultures. One dose of the vaccine contains not less than the quantity of virus equivalent to the minimum virus titre stated on the label.

POTENCY

Use 7 susceptible puppies of the minimum age recommended for vaccination and which do not have haemagglutination-inhibiting antibodies against canine parvovirus. Keep 2 of the puppies as controls and to each of the others inject by a recommended route the quantity of virus equivalent to the minimum titre stated on the label. Observe all the puppies for 20 to 22 days and then inoculate to each of them by the oronasal route a suspension of virulent canine parvovirus. Observe all the animals for 14 days. Carry out a haemagglutination test for the virus in the faeces. The test is not valid unless the 2 control puppies show typical signs of the disease and/or leucopenia and excretion of the virus. The vaccine complies with the test if the 5 vaccinated puppies remain in excellent health and show no sign of the disease nor leucopenia and if the maximum titre of virus excreted in the faeces is less than 1/100 of the geometric mean of the maximum titres found in the controls.

Ph Eur

Clostridium Botulinum Vaccine

Botulinum Vaccine

(*Clostridium Botulinum Vaccine for Veterinary Use, Ph Eur monograph 0360*)

When Clostridium Botulinum Vaccine or Botulinum Vaccine is prescribed or demanded and the types to be present are not stated, Clostridium Botulinum Vaccine prepared from types C and D shall be dispensed or supplied.

Ph Eur

DEFINITION

Clostridium botulinum vaccine for veterinary use is prepared from a culture in liquid medium of *Clostridium botulinum* type C or type D or a mixture of these types. The whole culture or its filtrate or a mixture of the two is inactivated in such a manner that toxicity is eliminated and immunogenic activity is retained.

The preparation may be adsorbed, precipitated or concentrated. It may be treated with a suitable adjuvant and may be freeze-dried.

The identification, the tests and the determination of potency apply to the liquid preparation and to the freeze-dried preparation reconstituted as stated on the label.

IDENTIFICATION

When injected into a healthy susceptible animal, the vaccine provokes the formation of specific antibodies against the type or types of *C. botulinum* from which the vaccine was prepared.

TESTS

Safety

Use 2 animals of one of the species for which the vaccine is intended and that have not been vaccinated against *C. botulinum*. Administer to each animal, by a recommended route, twice the maximum dose stated on the label. Observe the animals for 7 days. No abnormal local or systemic reaction occurs.

Residual toxicity

Inject 0.5 ml of the vaccine subcutaneously into each of 5 mice, each weighing 17 g to 22 g. Observe the animals for 7 days. No abnormal local or systemic reaction occurs.

Sterility

It complies with the test for sterility prescribed in the monograph on *Vaccines for veterinary use (0062)*.

POTENCY

Use healthy white mice from a uniform stock, each weighing 18 g to 20 g. Use as challenge dose a quantity of a toxin of *C. botulinum* of the same type as that used in the preparation of the vaccine corresponding to 25 times the paralytic dose 50 per cent, a paralytic dose 50 per cent being the quantity of toxin which, when injected intraperitoneally into mice, causes paralysis in 50 per cent of the animals within an observation period of 7 days. If 2 types of *C. botulinum* have been used in the preparation of the vaccine, carry out the potency determination for each. Dilute the vaccine to be examined 1 in 8 using a 9 g/l solution of *sodium chloride R*. Inject 0.2 ml of the dilution subcutaneously into each of 20 mice. After 21 days, inject the challenge dose intraperitoneally into each of the vaccinated mice and into each of 10 control mice. Observe the mice for 7 days and record the number of animals which show signs of botulism. All the control mice show signs of botulism during the observation period. The vaccine passes the test if not fewer than 80 per cent of the vaccinated mice are protected.

LABELLING

The label states:
— the type or types of *C. botulinum* from which the vaccine has been prepared,
— whether the preparation is a toxoid or a vaccine prepared from a whole inactivated culture or a mixture of the two,
— that the preparation be shaken before use.

Ph Eur

Clostridium Chauvoei Vaccine

Blackleg Vaccine

(*Clostridium Chauvoei Vaccine for Veterinary Use, Ph Eur monograph 0361*)

Ph Eur

DEFINITION

Clostridium chauvoei vaccine for veterinary use is prepared from a culture in liquid medium of one or more suitable strains of *Clostridium chauvoei*. The whole culture is inactivated in such a manner that toxicity is eliminated and immunogenic activity is retained. Inactivated cultures may be treated with a suitable adjuvant.

IDENTIFICATION
The vaccine protects susceptible animals against infection with *C. chauvoei*.

TESTS
Safety
Use 2 animals of one of the species for which the vaccine is intended and that have not been vaccinated against *C. chauvoei*. Administer to each animal at a single site, by a recommended route, twice the maximum dose stated on the label. Observe the animals for 7 days. No abnormal local or systemic reaction occurs.

Sterility
It complies with the test for sterility prescribed in the monograph on *Vaccines for veterinary use (0062)*.

POTENCY
Inject subcutaneously into not fewer than 10 healthy guinea-pigs, each weighing 350 g to 450 g, a quantity of the vaccine not exceeding the minimum dose stated on the label as the first dose. After 28 days, inject into the same animals a quantity of the vaccine not exceeding the minimum dose stated on the label as the second dose. 14 days after the second vaccination, inoculate intramuscularly into each of the vaccinated guinea-pigs and into each of 5 control animals a suitable quantity of a virulent culture, or of a spore suspension, of *C. chauvoei*, activated if necessary with an activating agent such as calcium chloride. The vaccine complies with the test if not more than 10 per cent of the vaccinated guinea-pigs die from *C. chauvoei* infection within 5 days and all the control animals die from *C. chauvoei* infection within 48 h of challenge or within 72 h if a spore suspension was used for the challenge. If more than 10 per cent but not more than 20 per cent of the vaccinated animals die, repeat the test. The vaccine complies with the test if not more than 10 per cent of the second group of vaccinated animals die within 5 days and all of the second group of control animals die within 48 h of challenge or within 72 h if a spore suspension was used for the challenge. To avoid unnecessary suffering following virulent challenge, moribund animals are killed and are then considered to have died from *C. chauvoei* infection.

LABELLING
The label states that the preparation is to be shaken before use.

Ph Eur

Clostridium Novyi Type B Vaccine

Black Disease Vaccine

(Clostridium Novyi (Type B) Vaccine for Veterinary Use, Ph Eur monograph 0362)

Ph Eur

DEFINITION
Clostridium novyi (type B) vaccine for veterinary use is prepared from a liquid culture of a suitable strain of *Clostridium novyi* (type B).

PRODUCTION
The whole culture or its filtrate or a mixture of the two is inactivated in such a manner that toxicity is eliminated and immunogenic activity is retained. Toxoids and/or inactivated cultures may be treated with a suitable adjuvant, after concentration if necessary.

CHOICE OF VACCINE COMPOSITION
The vaccine is shown to be satisfactory with respect to safety (5.2.6) and efficacy (5.2.7). For the latter, it shall be demonstrated that for each target species the vaccine, when administered according to the recommended schedule, stimulates an immune response (for example, induction of antibodies) consistent with the claims made for the product.

BATCH TESTING
Residual toxicity
The test for residual toxicity may be omitted by the manufacturer, since a test for detoxification is carried out immediately after the detoxification process and, when there is risk of reversion, a second test is carried out at as late a stage as possible during the production process.

Batch potency test
The test described under Potency is not necessarily carried out for routine testing of batches of vaccine. It is carried out for a given vaccine on one or more occasions as decided by or with the agreement of the competent authority. Where the test is not carried out, a suitable validated alternative test is carried out, the criteria for acceptance being set with reference to a batch of vaccine that has given satisfactory results in the test described under Potency and that has been shown to be satisfactory with respect to immunogenicity in the target species. The following test may be used after a satisfactory correlation with the test described under Potency has been established.

Vaccinate rabbits as described under Potency and prepare sera. Determine the level of antibodies against the alpha toxin of *C. novyi* in the individual sera by a suitable method such as an immunochemical method (2.7.1) or neutralisation in cell cultures. Use a homologous reference serum calibrated in International Units of *C. novyi* alpha antitoxin. *Clostridia (multicomponent) rabbit antiserum BRP* is suitable for use as a reference serum. The vaccine complies with the test if the level of antibodies is not less than that found for a batch of vaccine that has given satisfactory results in the test described under Potency and that has been shown to be satisfactory with respect to immunogenicity in the target species.

IDENTIFICATION
The vaccine stimulates the formation of novyi alpha antitoxin when injected into animals that do not have this antitoxin.

TESTS
Safety
Administer by a recommended route, to each of 2 sheep that have not been vaccinated against *C. novyi* (type B) twice the maximum dose of the vaccine stated on the label. Observe the animals for not less than 14 days. No abnormal local or systemic reaction occurs.

Residual toxicity
Inject 0.5 ml of the vaccine subcutaneously into each of 5 mice, each weighing 17 g to 22 g. Observe the animals for 7 days. No abnormal local or systemic reaction occurs.

Sterility
It complies with the test for sterility prescribed in the monograph on *Vaccines for veterinary use (0062)*.

POTENCY

Inject subcutaneously into each of not fewer than 10 healthy rabbits, 3 to 6 months old, a quantity of vaccine not exceeding the minimum dose stated on the label as the first dose. After 21 to 28 days, inject into the same animals a quantity of the vaccine not exceeding the minimum dose stated on the label as the second dose. 10 to 14 days after the second injection, bleed the rabbits and pool the sera.

The potency of the pooled sera is not less than 3.5 IU/ml.

The International Unit is the specific neutralising activity for *C. novyi* alpha toxin contained in a stated amount of the International Standard, which consists of a quantity of dried immune horse serum. The equivalence in International Units of the International Standard is stated by the World Health Organisation.

The potency of the pooled sera obtained from the rabbits is determined by comparing the quantity necessary to protect mice or other suitable animals against the toxic effects of a fixed dose of *C. novyi* alpha toxin with the quantity of a reference preparation of Clostridium novyi alpha antitoxin, calibrated in International Units, necessary to give the same protection. For this comparison, a suitable preparation of *C. novyi* alpha toxin for use as a test toxin is required. The dose of the test toxin is determined in relation to the reference preparation; the potency of the serum to be examined is determined in relation to the reference preparation using the test toxin.

Clostridia (multicomponent) rabbit antiserum BRP is suitable for use as a reference serum.

Preparation of test toxin

Prepare the test toxin from a sterile filtrate of an approximately 5-day culture in liquid medium of *C. novyi* type B and dry by a suitable method. Select the test toxin by determining for mice the L+/10 dose and the LD_{50}, the observation period being 72 h.

A suitable alpha toxin contains not less than one L+/10 dose in 0.05 mg and not less than 10 LD_{50} in each L+/10 dose.

Determination of test dose of toxin

Prepare a solution of the reference preparation in a suitable liquid so that it contains 1 IU/ml. Prepare a solution of the test toxin in a suitable liquid so that 1 ml contains a precisely known amount such as 1 mg. Prepare mixtures of the solution of the reference preparation and the solution of the test toxin such that each mixture contains 1.0 ml of the solution of the reference preparation (1 IU), one of a series of graded volumes of the solution of the test toxin and sufficient of a suitable liquid to bring the total volume to 2.0 ml. Allow the mixtures to stand at room temperature for 60 min. Using not fewer than 2 mice, each weighing 17 g to 22 g, for each mixture, inject a dose of 0.2 ml intramuscularly or subcutaneously into each mouse. Observe the mice for 72 h. If all the mice die, the amount of toxin present in 0.2 ml of the mixture is in excess of the test dose. If none of the mice die, the amount of toxin present in 0.2 ml of the mixture is less than the test dose. Prepare fresh mixtures such that 2.0 ml of each mixture contains 1.0 ml of the solution of the reference preparation (1 IU) and one of a series of graded volumes of the solution of the test toxin separated from each other by steps of not more than 20 per cent and covering the expected end-point. Allow the mixtures to stand at room temperature for 60 min. Using not fewer than two mice for each mixture, inject a dose of 0.2 ml intramuscularly or subcutaneously into each mouse. Observe the mice for 72 h. Repeat the determination at least once and combine the results of the separate tests that have been made with

mixtures of the same composition so that a series of totals is obtained, each total representing the mortality due to a mixture of a given composition.

The test dose of toxin is the amount present in 0.2 ml of that mixture which causes the death of one half of the total number of mice injected with it.

Determination of the potency of the serum obtained from rabbits

Preliminary test Dissolve a quantity of the test toxin in a suitable liquid so that 1 ml contains 10 times the test dose (solution of the test toxin). Prepare a series of mixtures of the solution of the test toxin and of the serum to be examined such that each mixture contains 1.0 ml of the solution of the test toxin, one of a series of graded volumes of the serum to be examined and sufficient of a suitable liquid to bring the final volume to 2.0 ml. Allow the mixtures to stand at room temperature for 60 min. Using not fewer than 2 mice for each mixture, inject a dose of 0.2 ml intramuscularly or subcutaneously into each mouse. Observe the mice for 72 h. If none of the mice dies, 0.2 ml of the mixture contains more than 0.1 IU. If all the mice die, 0.2 ml of the mixture contains less than 0.1 IU.

Final test Prepare a series of mixtures of the solution of the test toxin and of the serum to be examined such that 2.0 ml of each mixture contains 1.0 ml of the solution of the test toxin and one of a series of graded volumes of the serum to be examined, separated from each other by steps of not more than 20 per cent and covering the expected end-point as determined by the preliminary test. Prepare further mixtures of the solution of the test toxin and of the solution of the reference preparation such that 2.0 ml of each mixture contains 1.0 ml of the solution of the test toxin and one of a series of graded volumes of the solution of the reference preparation, in order to confirm the test dose of the toxin. Allow the mixtures to stand at room temperature for 60 min. Using not fewer than 2 mice for each mixture, proceed as described in the preliminary test. The test mixture which contains 0.1 IU in 0.2 ml is that mixture which kills the same or almost the same number of mice as the reference mixture containing 0.1 IU in 0.2 ml. Repeat the determination at least once and calculate the average of all valid estimates. The test is valid only if the reference preparation gives a result within 20 per cent of the expected value.

The confidence limits ($P = 0.95$) have been estimated to be:

— 85 per cent and 114 per cent when 2 animals per dose are used,
— 91.5 per cent and 109 per cent when 4 animals per dose are used,
— 93 per cent and 108 per cent when 6 animals per dose are used.

LABELLING

The label states:

— whether the product is a toxoid, a vaccine prepared from a whole inactivated culture or a mixture of the two,
— that the preparation is to be shaken before use,
— for each target species, the immunising effect produced (for example, antibody production, protection against signs of disease or infection).

Ph Eur

Clostridium Perfringens Vaccines

*(Clostridium Perfringens Vaccine for Veterinary Use,
Ph Eur monograph 0363)*

The following titles may be used for appropriate vaccines:

Clostridium Perfringens Type B Vaccine; Lamb Dysentery Vaccine;

Clostridium Perfringens Type C Vaccine; Struck Vaccine;

Clostridium Perfringens Type D Vaccine; Pulpy Kidney Vaccine

Ph Eur _____

DEFINITION

Clostridium perfringens vaccine for veterinary use is prepared from liquid cultures of suitable strains of *Clostridium perfringens* type B, *C. perfringens* type C or *C. perfringens* type D or a mixture of these types.

PRODUCTION

The whole cultures or their filtrates or a mixture of the two are inactivated in such a manner that toxicity is eliminated and immunogenic activity is retained. Toxoids and/or inactivated cultures may be treated with a suitable adjuvant.

CHOICE OF VACCINE COMPOSITION

The vaccine is shown to be satisfactory with respect to safety (5.2.6) and efficacy (5.2.7). For the latter, it shall be demonstrated that for each target species the vaccine, when administered according to the recommended schedule, stimulates an immune response (for example, induction of antibodies) consistent with the claims made for the product.

BATCH TESTING
Residual toxicity

The test for residual toxicity may be omitted by the manufacturer, since a test for detoxification is carried out immediately after the detoxification process and, when there is risk of reversion, a second test is carried out at as late a stage as possible during the production process.

Batch potency test

The test described under Potency is not necessarily carried out for routine testing of batches of vaccine. It is carried out for a given vaccine on one or more occasions as decided by or with the agreement of the competent authority. Where the test is not carried out, a suitable validated alternative test is carried out, the criteria for acceptance being set with reference to a batch of vaccine that has given satisfactory results in the test described under Potency and that has been shown to be satisfactory with respect to immunogenicity in the target species. The following test may be used after a satisfactory correlation with the test described under Potency has been established.

Vaccinate rabbits as described under Potency and prepare sera. Determine the level of antibodies against the beta and/or epsilon toxins of *C. perfringens* in the individual sera by a suitable method such as an immunochemical method (2.7.1) or neutralisation in cell cultures. Use a homologous reference serum calibrated in International Units of *C. perfringens* beta and/or epsilon antitoxin. *Clostridia (multicomponent) rabbit antiserum BRP* is suitable for use as a reference serum. The vaccine complies with the test if the level or levels of antibodies are not less than that found for a batch of vaccine that has given satisfactory results in the test described under Potency and that has been shown to be satisfactory with respect to immunogenicity in the target species.

IDENTIFICATION

Type B   The vaccine stimulates the formation of beta and epsilon antitoxins when injected into animals that do not have these antitoxins.

Type C   The vaccine stimulates the formation of beta antitoxin when injected into animals that do not have this antitoxin.

Type D   The vaccine stimulates the formation of epsilon antitoxin when injected into animals that do not have this antitoxin.

TESTS
Safety

Use 2 animals of one of the species for which the vaccine is intended and that have not been vaccinated against *C. perfringens*. Administer by a recommended route to each animal, twice the maximum dose stated on the label. Observe the animals for 14 days. No abnormal local or systemic reaction occurs.

Residual toxicity

Inject 0.5 ml of the vaccine subcutaneously into each of 5 mice, each weighing 17 g to 22 g. Observe the animals for 7 days. No abnormal local or systemic reaction occurs.

Sterility

It complies with the test for sterility prescribed in the monograph on *Vaccines for veterinary use (0062)*.

POTENCY

Inject subcutaneously into each of not fewer than 10 healthy rabbits, 3 to 6 months old, a quantity of vaccine not exceeding the minimum dose stated on the label as the first dose. After 21 to 28 days inject into the same animals a quantity of the vaccine not exceeding the minimum dose stated on the label as the second dose. 10 to 14 days after the second injection, bleed the rabbits and pool the sera.

Type B   The potency of the pooled sera is not less than 10 IU of beta antitoxin and not less than 5 IU of epsilon antitoxin per millilitre.

Type C   The potency of the pooled sera is not less than 10 IU of beta antitoxin per millilitre.

Type D   The potency of the pooled sera is not less than 5 IU of epsilon antitoxin per millilitre.

International standard for clostridium perfringens beta antitoxin

The International Unit is the specific neutralising activity for *C. perfringens* beta toxin contained in a stated amount of the International Standard which consists of a quantity of dried immune horse serum. The equivalence in International Units of the International Standard is stated by the World Health Organisation.

International standard for clostridium perfringens epsilon antitoxin

The International Unit is the specific neutralising activity for *C. perfringens* epsilon toxin contained in a stated amount of the International Standard which consists of a quantity of dried immune horse serum. The equivalence in International Units of the International Standard is stated by the World Health Organisation.

The potency of the pooled sera obtained from the rabbits is determined by comparing the quantity necessary to protect mice or other suitable animals against the toxic effects of a fixed dose of *C. perfringens* beta toxin or *C. perfringens* epsilon toxin with the quantity of a reference preparation of clostridium perfringens beta antitoxin or clostridium perfringens epsilon antitoxin, as appropriate, calibrated in

International Units, necessary to give the same protection. For this comparison, a suitable preparation of *C. perfringens* beta or epsilon toxin for use as a test toxin is required. The dose of the test toxin is determined in relation to the appropriate reference preparation; the potency of the serum to be examined is determined in relation to the appropriate reference preparation using the appropriate test toxin.

Clostridia (multicomponent) rabbit antiserum BRP is suitable for use as a reference serum.

Preparation of test toxin

Prepare the test toxin from a sterile filtrate of an early culture in liquid medium of *C. perfringens* type B, type C or type D as appropriate and dry by a suitable method. Use a beta or epsilon toxin as appropriate. Select the test toxin by determining for mice the L+ and the LD_{50} for the beta toxin and the L+/10 dose and the LD_{50} for the epsilon toxin, the observation period being 72 h.

A suitable beta toxin contains not less than one L+ in 0.2 mg and not less than 25 LD_{50} in one L+ dose. A suitable epsilon toxin contains not less than one L+/10 dose in 0.005 mg and not less than 20 LD_{50} in one L+/10 dose.

Determination of test dose of toxin

Prepare a solution of the reference preparation in a suitable liquid so that it contains 5 IU/ml for clostridium perfringens beta antitoxin and 0.5 IU/ml for clostridium perfringens epsilon antitoxin. Prepare a solution of the test toxin in a suitable liquid so that 1 ml contains a precisely known amount such as 10 mg for beta toxin and 1 mg for epsilon toxin. Prepare mixtures of the solution of the reference preparation and the solution of the test toxin such that each contains 2.0 ml of the solution of the reference preparation, one of a series of graded volumes of the solution of the test toxin and sufficient of a suitable liquid to bring the total volume to 5.0 ml. Allow the mixtures to stand at room temperature for 30 min. Using not fewer than 2 mice, each weighing 17 g to 22 g, for each mixture, inject a dose of 0.5 ml intravenously or intraperitoneally into each mouse. Observe the mice for 72 h. If all the mice die, the amount of toxin present in 0.5 ml of the mixture is in excess of the test dose. If none of the mice dies the amount of toxin present in 0.5 ml of the mixture is less than the test dose. Prepare fresh mixtures such that 5.0 ml of each mixture contains 2.0 ml of the solution of the reference preparation and one of a series of graded volumes of the solution of the test toxin separated from each other by steps of not more than 20 per cent and covering the expected end-point. Allow the mixtures to stand at room temperature for 30 min. Using not fewer than two mice for each mixture, inject a dose of 0.5 ml intravenously or intraperitoneally into each mouse. Observe the mice for 72 h. Repeat the determination at least once and add together the results of the separate tests that have been made with mixtures of the same composition so that a series of totals is obtained, each total representing the mortality due to a mixture of given composition.

The test dose of toxin is the amount present in 0.5 ml of that mixture which causes the death of one half of the total number of mice injected with it.

Determination of the potency of the serum obtained from rabbits

Preliminary test Dissolve a quantity of the test toxin in a suitable liquid so that 2.0 ml contains 10 times the test dose (solution of the test toxin). Prepare a series of mixtures of the solution of the test toxin and of the serum to be examined such that each contains 2.0 ml of the solution of the test toxin, one of a series of graded volumes of the serum to be

examined and sufficient of a suitable liquid to bring the final volume to 5.0 ml. Allow the mixtures to stand at room temperature for 30 min. Using not fewer than 2 mice for each mixture, inject a dose of 0.5 ml intravenously or intraperitoneally into each mouse. Observe the mice for 72 h. If none of the mice die, 0.5 ml of the mixture contains more than 1 IU of beta antitoxin or 0.1 IU of epsilon antitoxin. If all the mice die, 0.5 ml of the mixture contains less than 1 IU of beta antitoxin or 0.1 IU of epsilon antitoxin.

Final test Prepare a series of mixtures of the solution of the test toxin and the serum to be examined such that 5.0 ml of each mixture contains 2.0 ml of the solution of the test toxin and one of a series of graded volumes of the serum to be examined separated from each other by steps of not more than 20 per cent and covering the expected end-point as determined by the preliminary test. Prepare further mixtures of the solution of the test toxin and of the solution of the reference preparation such that 5.0 ml of each mixture contains 2.0 ml of the solution of the test toxin and one of a series of graded volumes of the solution of the reference preparation, in order to confirm the test dose of the toxin. Allow the mixtures to stand at room temperature for 30 min. Using not fewer than 2 mice for each mixture proceed as described in the preliminary test.

Beta antitoxin The test mixture which contains 1 IU in 0.5 ml is that mixture which kills the same or almost the same number of mice as the reference mixture containing 1 IU in 0.5 ml.

Epsilon antitoxin The test mixture which contains 0.1 IU in 0.5 ml is that mixture which kills the same or almost the same number of mice as the reference mixture containing 0.1 IU in 0.5 ml. Repeat the determination at least once and calculate the average of all valid estimates. The test is valid only if the reference preparation gives a result within 20 per cent of the expected value.

The confidence limits ($P = 0.95$) have been estimated to be:
— 85 per cent and 114 per cent when 2 animals per dose are used,
— 91.5 per cent and 109 per cent when 4 animals per dose are used,
— 93 per cent and 108 per cent when 6 animals per dose are used.

LABELLING
The label states:
— the type or types of *C. perfringens* from which the vaccine has been prepared,
— whether the preparation is a toxoid or a vaccine prepared from a whole inactivated culture or a mixture of the two,
— that the preparation is to be shaken before use,
— for each target species, the immunising effect produced (for example, antibody production, protection against signs of disease or infection).

_____ *Ph Eur*

Clostridium Septicum Vaccine

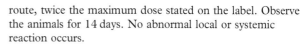

Braxy Vaccine

(*Clostridium Septicum Vaccine for Veterinary Use,*
Ph Eur monograph 0364)

Ph Eur _____

DEFINITION
Clostridium septicum vaccine for veterinary use is prepared
from a liquid culture of a suitable strain of *Clostridium*
septicum.

PRODUCTION
The whole culture or its filtrate or a mixture of the two is
inactivated in such a manner that toxicity is eliminated and
immunogenic activity is retained. Toxoid and/or inactivated
cultures may be treated with a suitable adjuvant.

CHOICE OF VACCINE COMPOSITION
The vaccine is shown to be satisfactory with respect to safety
(*5.2.6*) and efficacy (*5.2.7*). For the latter, it shall be
demonstrated that for each target species the vaccine, when
administered according to the recommended schedule,
stimulates an immune response (for example, induction of
antibodies) consistent with the claims made for the product.

BATCH TESTING
Residual toxicity
The test for residual toxicity may be omitted by the
manufacturer, since a test for detoxification is carried out
immediately after the detoxification process and, when there
is risk of reversion, a second test is carried out at as late a
stage as possible during the production process.

Batch potency test
The test described under Potency is not necessarily carried
out for routine testing of batches of vaccine. It is carried out
for a given vaccine on one or more occasions as decided by
or with the agreement of the competent authority. Where the
test is not carried out, a suitable validated alternative test is
carried out, the criteria for acceptance being set with
reference to a batch of vaccine that has given satisfactory
results in the test described under Potency and that has been
shown to be satisfactory with respect to immunogenicity in
the target species. The following test may be used after a
satisfactory correlation with the test described under Potency
has been established.

Vaccinate rabbits as described under Potency and prepare
sera. Determine the level of antibodies against the toxin of
C. septicum in the individual sera by a suitable method such
as an immunochemical method (*2.7.1*) or neutralisation in
cell cultures. Use a homologous reference serum calibrated
in International Units of *C. septicum* antitoxin.
Clostridia (multicomponent) rabbit antiserum BRP is suitable for
use as a reference serum. The vaccine complies with the test
if the level of antibodies is not less than that found for a
batch of vaccine that has given satisfactory results in the test
described under Potency and that has been shown to be
satisfactory with respect to immunogenicity in the target
species.

IDENTIFICATION
The vaccine stimulates the formation of *C. septicum* antitoxin
when injected into animals that do not have this antitoxin.

TESTS
Safety
Use 2 animals of one of the species for which the vaccine is
intended and that have not been vaccinated against
C. septicum. Administer to each animal, by a recommended

route, twice the maximum dose stated on the label. Observe
the animals for 14 days. No abnormal local or systemic
reaction occurs.

Residual toxicity
Inject 0.5 ml of the vaccine subcutaneously into each of
5 mice, each weighing 17 g to 22 g. Observe the animals for
7 days. No abnormal local or systemic reaction occurs.

Sterility
It complies with the test for sterility prescribed in the
monograph on *Vaccines for veterinary use (0062).*

POTENCY
Inject subcutaneously into each of not fewer than 10 healthy
rabbits, 3 to 6 months old, a quantity of vaccine not
exceeding the minimum dose stated on the label as the first
dose. After 21 to 28 days, inject into the same animals a
quantity of the vaccine not exceeding the minimum dose
stated on the label as the second dose. 10 to 14 days after
the second injection, bleed the rabbits and pool the sera.

The potency of the pooled sera is not less than 2.5 IU/ml.

The International Unit is the specific neutralising activity
for *C. septicum* toxin contained in a stated amount of the
International Standard which consists of a quantity of dried
immune horse serum. The equivalence in International Units
of the International Standard is stated by the World Health
Organisation.

The potency of the pooled sera obtained from the rabbits is
determined by comparing the quantity necessary to protect
mice or other suitable animals against the toxic effects of a
dose of *C. septicum* toxin with the quantity of a reference
preparation of clostridium septicum antitoxin, calibrated in
International Units, necessary to give the same protection.
For this comparison, a suitable preparation of *C. septicum*
toxin for use as a test toxin is required. The dose of the test
toxin is determined in relation to the reference preparation;
the potency of the serum to be examined is determined in
relation to the reference preparation using the test toxin.
Clostridia (multicomponent) rabbit antiserum BRP is suitable
for use as a reference serum.

Preparation of test toxin
Prepare the test toxin from a sterile filtrate of a 1- to 3-day
culture of *C. septicum* in liquid medium and dry by a suitable
method. Select the test toxin by determining for mice the
$L+/5$ dose and the LD_{50} the observation period being 72 h.

A suitable toxin contains not less than one $L+/5$ dose in
1.0 mg and not less than 10 LD_{50} in each $L+/5$ dose.

Determination of test dose of toxin
Prepare a solution of the reference preparation in a suitable
liquid so that it contains 1.0 IU/ml. Prepare a solution of the
test toxin in a suitable liquid so that 1 ml contains a precisely
known amount, such as 4 mg. Prepare mixtures of the
solution of the reference preparation and the solution of
the test toxin such that each mixture contains 2.0 ml of the
solution of the reference preparation (2 IU), one of a series of
graded volumes of the solution of the test toxin and sufficient
of a suitable liquid to bring the total volume to 5.0 ml. Allow
the mixtures to stand at room temperature for 60 min.
Using not fewer than 2 mice, each weighing 17 g to 22 g, for
each mixture, inject a dose of 0.5 ml intravenously or
intraperitoneally into each mouse. Observe the mice for 72 h.
If all the mice die, the amount of toxin present in 0.5 ml of
the mixture is in excess of the test dose. If none of the mice
die, the amount of toxin present in 0.5 ml of the mixture is
less than the test dose. Prepare fresh mixtures such that
5.0 ml of each mixture contains 2.0 ml of the reference

preparation (2 IU) and one of a series of graded volumes of the solution of the test toxin separated from each other by steps of not more than 20 per cent and covering the expected end-point. Allow the mixtures to stand at room temperature for 60 min. Using not fewer than 2 mice for each mixture, inject a dose of 0.5 ml intravenously or intraperitoneally into each mouse. Observe the mice for 72 h. Repeat the determination at least once and add together the results of the separate tests that have been made with mixtures of the same composition so that a series of totals is obtained, each total representing the mortality due to a mixture of a given composition.

The test dose of toxin is the amount present in 0.5 ml of that mixture which causes the death of one half of the total number of mice injected with it.

Determination of the potency of the serum obtained from rabbits

Preliminary test Dissolve a quantity of the test toxin in a suitable liquid so that 2.0 ml contains ten times the test dose (solution of the test toxin). Prepare a series of mixtures of the solution of the test toxin and of the serum to be examined such that each contains 2.0 ml of the solution of the test toxin, one of a series of graded volumes of the serum to be examined and sufficient of a suitable liquid to bring the final volume to 5.0 ml. Allow the mixtures to stand at room temperature for 60 min. Using not fewer than 2 mice for each mixture, inject a dose of 0.5 ml intravenously or intraperitoneally into each mouse. Observe the mice for 72 h. If none of the mice dies, 0.5 ml of the mixture contains more than 0.2 IU. If all the mice die, 0.5 ml of the mixture contains less than 0.2 IU.

Final test Prepare a series of mixtures of the solution of the test toxin and of the serum to be examined such that 5.0 ml of each mixture contains 2.0 ml of the solution of the test toxin and one of a series of graded volumes of the serum to be examined, separated from each other by steps of not more than 20 per cent and covering the expected end-point as determined by the preliminary test. Prepare further mixtures of the solution of the test toxin and of the solution of the reference preparation such that 5.0 ml of each mixture contains 2.0 ml of the solution of the test toxin and one of a series of graded volumes of the solution of the reference preparation to confirm the test dose of the toxin. Allow the mixtures to stand at room temperature for 60 min. Using not fewer than 2 mice for each mixture proceed as described in the preliminary test. The test mixture which contains 0.2 IU in 0.5 ml is that mixture which kills the same or almost the same number of mice as the reference mixture containing 0.2 IU in 0.5 ml. Repeat the determination at least once and calculate the average of all valid estimates. The test is valid only if the reference preparation gives a result within 20 per cent of the expected value.

The confidence limits ($P = 0.95$) have been estimated to be:
— 85 per cent and 114 per cent when 2 animals per dose are used,
— 91.5 per cent and 109 per cent when 4 animals per dose are used,
— 93 per cent and 108 per cent when 6 animals per dose are used.

LABELLING

The label states:
— whether the preparation is a toxoid or a vaccine prepared from a whole inactivated culture, or a mixture of the two,
— that the preparation is to be shaken before use,

— for each target species, the immunising effect produced (for example, antibody production, protection against signs of disease or infection).

Ph Eur

Clostridium Tetani Vaccines

Tetanus Toxoids (Veterinary)

(*Tetanus Vaccine for Veterinary Use, Ph Eur monograph 0697*)

The name Clostridium Tetani Vaccine for Equidae (Tetanus Toxoid for Equidae) may be used for vaccines with an appropriate potency.

When Tetanus Toxoid is demanded for veterinary use, Clostridium Tetani Vaccine shall be supplied.

Ph Eur

DEFINITION

Tetanus vaccine for veterinary use is a preparation of the neurotoxin of *Clostridium tetani* treated in a manner that eliminates toxicity while maintaining adequate immunogenic properties.

PRODUCTION

The *C. tetani* strain used for production is cultured in a suitable medium. The toxin is purified and then detoxified or it may be detoxified before purification. The antigenic purity is determined in Lf units of tetanus toxoid per milligram of protein and shown to be not less than the value approved for the particular product.

CHOICE OF VACCINE COMPOSITION

The *C. tetani* strain used in the preparation of the vaccine is shown to be satisfactory with respect to the production of the neurotoxin. The vaccine is shown to be satisfactory with respect to safety and immunogenicity for each species of animal for which it is intended. As part of the studies to demonstrate these characteristics, the tests described below may be used.

Production of antigens The production of the neurotoxin of *C. tetani* is verified by a suitable immunochemical method (*2.7.1*) carried out on the neurotoxin obtained from the vaccine strain under the conditions used for the production of the vaccine.

Safety Carry out the test for each recommended route of administration and species of animal for which the vaccine is intended; use animals of the minimum age recommended for vaccination and of the most sensitive category for the species.

Use not fewer than 15 animals, free from antitoxic antibodies for each test. Administer a double dose of vaccine to each animal. Administer a single dose of vaccine to each animal after the interval stated on the label. Observe the animals until 14 days after the last administration. If the vaccine is intended for use in pregnant animals, vaccinate the animals at the stage of pregnancy and according to the scheme stated on the label and prolong the observation period until 1 day after parturition. The vaccine complies with the test if no animal shows abnormal local or systemic signs of disease or dies from causes attributable to the vaccine. If the vaccine is intended for use in pregnant animals, in addition no significant effects on the gestation and the offspring are demonstrated.

Immunogenicity The test described under Potency may be used to demonstrate immunogenicity. It shall also be demonstrated for each target species that the vaccine, administered by the recommended route, stimulates an immune response consistent with the claims for the product (for example, induction of antitoxic antibodies or induction of protective levels of antitoxic antibodies).

DETOXIFIED HARVEST

Absence of toxin and irreversibility of toxoid   Carry out a test for reversion to toxicity on the detoxified harvest using 2 groups of 5 guinea-pigs, each weighing 350-450 g; if the vaccine is adsorbed, carry out the test with the shortest practical time interval before adsorption. Prepare a dilution of the detoxified harvest so that the guinea-pigs each receive 10 times the amount of toxoid (measured in Lf units) that will be present in a dose of vaccine. Divide the dilution into 2 equal parts. Keep one part at 5 ± 3 °C and the other at 37 °C for 6 weeks. Attribute each dilution to a separate group of guinea-pigs and inject into each guinea-pig the dilution attributed to its group. Observe the animals for 21 days. The toxoid complies with the test if no guinea-pig shows clinical signs of disease or dies from causes attributable to the neurotoxin of *C. tetani*.

BATCH POTENCY TEST

Where the test described under Potency is used as the batch potency test, the vaccine complies with the test if the antibody titre in International Units is not less than that found for a batch of vaccine shown to be satisfactory with respect to immunogenicity in the target species.

IDENTIFICATION

If the nature of the adjuvant allows it, carry out test A. Otherwise carry out test B.

A. Dissolve in the vaccine sufficient *sodium citrate R* to give a 100 g/l solution. Maintain the solution at 37 °C for about 16 h and centrifuge until a clear supernatant liquid is obtained. The supernatant reacts with a suitable tetanus antitoxin, giving a precipitate.

B. When injected into susceptible animals, the vaccine provokes the formation of antibodies against the neurotoxin of *C. tetani*.

TESTS
Safety

Inject 5 ml of the vaccine subcutaneously as 2 equal divided doses, at separate sites into each of 5 healthy guinea-pigs, each weighing 350-450 g, that have not previously been treated with any material that will interfere with the test. No abnormal local or systemic reaction occurs. If within 21 days of the injection any of the animals shows signs of or dies from tetanus, the vaccine does not comply with the test. If more than one animal dies from non-specific causes, repeat the test. If any animal dies in the second test, the vaccine does not comply with the test.

Sterility

The vaccine complies with the test for sterility prescribed in the monograph on *Vaccines for veterinary use (0062)*.

POTENCY

Administer 1 dose of vaccine subcutaneously to each of at least 5 susceptible guinea-pigs or rabbits. After 28 days, administer again 1 dose subcutaneously to each animal. 14 days after the second dose, collect blood from each animal and prepare serum samples. Determine for each serum the titre of antibodies against the neurotoxin of *C. tetani* using a suitable immunochemical method *(2.7.1)* such as a toxin-binding-inhibition test (ToBI test) and a homologous reference serum. Determine the average antibody titre of the serum samples.

Clostridia (multicomponent) rabbit antiserum BRP, Clostridium tetani guinea-pig antiserum for vaccines for veterinary use BRP and *Clostridium tetani rabbit antiserum BRP* are suitable as reference sera.

Tetanus vaccine intended for use in animals other than horses complies with the test if the average antibody titre in guinea-pigs is not less than 7.5 IU/ml.

Tetanus vaccine intended for use in horses complies with the test if the average antibody titre in guinea-pigs is not less than 30 IU/ml.

For tetanus vaccine presented as a combined vaccine for use in animals other than horses, the above test may be carried out in susceptible rabbits instead of guinea-pigs. The vaccine complies with the test if the average antibody titre in rabbits is not less than 2.5 IU/ml.

_____ *Ph Eur*

Contagious Pustular Dermatitis Vaccine, Living

Orf Vaccine

DEFINITION

Contagious Pustular Dermatitis Vaccine, Living is a preparation of a suitable strain of orf virus (contagious pustular dermatitis virus) for administration to sheep, by skin scarification.

PRODUCTION

The vaccinal organisms are obtained from the vesiculo-pustular lesions produced on the skin of lambs inoculated with the seed virus or prepared in suitable cell cultures (Appendix XV J(Vet) 1). If lambs are used for production, they are obtained from a flock known to be free from the natural disease, are healthy and have not been exposed previously to orf virus. Both the flock and the lambs are monitored for freedom from infectious diseases, the range of diseases in each case being agreed with the competent authority.

The harvested material may be freeze-dried. The finished preparation administered to the animals may contain glycerol and may contain an approved dye.

CHOICE OF VACCINE STRAIN

The vaccine strain is shown to be satisfactory with respect to safety and immunogenicity for the animals for which the vaccine is intended. The following tests may be used during the demonstration of safety, Appendix XV K(Vet) 1, reversion to virulence and immunogenicity, Appendix XV K(Vet) 2.

Safety   Carry out a test in each category of animal for which the vaccine is to be recommended. Vaccinate at least five animals that do not have antibodies to orf virus. Administer to each, by skin scarification of one site or a small number of contiguous sites, a quantity of virus containing not less than ten times the maximum virus titre likely to be contained in a dose of the vaccine. Observe the animals for 4 weeks. No systemic or local reactions occur except for mild localised lesions of orf which resolve in less than three weeks after vaccination to leave no more than a small area of scar tissue. If the vaccine is for use or may be used in pregnant animals, for the test in this category, administer the vaccine at the relevant stage or stages of pregnancy, prolong the observation period up to the time of parturition and note any effects on gestation or the offspring.

Reversion to virulence Administer by skin scarification a quantity of virus containing not less than one dose of the vaccine to each of two lambs of the minimum age to be recommended for vaccination and that do not have antibodies to orf virus. Six to eight days later, anaesthetise the lambs and remove, pool and homogenise the orf lesions in buffer containing suitable antibiotics and inoculate into two more lambs. Repeat this passage operation four more times. If the virus disappears (no lesions develop) a second series of passages is carried out. Observe the lambs given the last passage material for four weeks. The vaccine complies with the test if the virus from the last passage produces no systemic reactions and the local reactions observed are no more severe than those seen in the lambs given the unpassaged material.

Immunogenicity Carry out a test in each category of animal for which the vaccine is to be recommended. Vaccinate, by skin scarification, at least five animals that do not have antibodies to orf virus, with a quantity of virus containing the minimum virus titre likely to be contained in a dose of vaccine. Maintain separately at least two animals of the same age and from the same source as unvaccinated controls. Eighteen to twenty four days later, challenge all the animals by skin scarification with a sufficient quantity of virulent strain of orf virus to cause disease in the controls. Observe the animals for 21 days and monitor and score the skin lesions. The test is not valid unless there are marked lesions of orf in both the control animals after challenge.

The vaccine complies with the test if, after challenge, there are no more than mild transient lesions of orf in the vaccinates.

BATCH TESTING

Extraneous bacteria and fungi:

A. Vaccines produced in lambs For each batch, the number of non-pathogenic organisms per dose shall be within the limits set for the product and shown to be safe.

B. Vaccines produced in cell cultures Each batch complies with the test described under Veterinary Vaccines.

Virus titre Where the nature of the vaccine strain allows a satisfactory test to be conducted *in vitro*, the test for Potency may be omitted as a routine control on each batch of vaccine. Where the Potency test is not carried out, an alternative validated *in vitro* test is conducted on each batch to measure the virus content. The batch complies with the tests if the titre of the batch is not less than the minimum titre stated on the label.

The vaccine complies with the requirements stated under Veterinary Vaccines with the following modifications.

IDENTIFICATION

Produces the characteristic lesions of contagious pustular dermatitis when applied to a scarified area of the skin of lambs.

TESTS

Extraneous bacteria and fungi

The vaccine is shown by appropriate methods to be free from pathogenic organisms.

Mycoplasmas

Complies with the test for absence of mycoplasmas, Appendix XVI B(Vet) 3.

Safety

Administer by skin scarification of one site or a small number of contiguous sites, ten doses of the vaccine to each of two lambs of the minimum age to be recommended for vaccination and that are free from antibodies to orf virus.

Observe the lambs for two weeks. No systemic or local reactions occur except for mild local lesions of orf.

Extraneous viruses

Neutralise the vaccine if necessary. Inoculate the vaccine onto suitable cell cultures that are susceptible to ovine viruses, make at least one passage and maintain the cultures for at least 14 days. No cytopathic effect develops. Conduct a test for freedom from haemadsorbing agents. The cell cultures show no signs of viral contamination.

POTENCY

Vaccinate each of no fewer than two healthy susceptible sheep, 6 to 12 months old, with serial dilutions of the vaccine applied to the scarified skin. Characteristic lesions of contagious pustular dermatitis appearing on the fourth to eighth day after inoculation are recorded. The vaccine contains not less than 100 MID in the dose stated on the label.

STORAGE

When stored in the prescribed conditions the vaccine may be expected to retain its potency for at least a year.

Duck Plague Vaccine (Live)

(*Ph Eur monograph 1938*)

Ph Eur

1 DEFINITION

Duck plague vaccine (live) is a preparation of a suitable strain of duck plague virus (anatid herpesvirus 1). This monograph applies to vaccines intended for the active immunisation of ducks.

2 PRODUCTION

2-1 Preparation of the vaccine

The vaccine virus is grown in embryonated hens' eggs or in cell cultures. The vaccine may be freeze-dried.

2-2 Substrate for virus propagation

2-2-1 Embryonated hens' eggs

If the vaccine virus is grown in embryonated hens' eggs, they are obtained from flocks free from specified pathogens (SPF) (*5.2.2*).

2-2-2 Cell cultures

If the vaccine virus is grown in cell cultures, they comply with the requirements for cell cultures for production of veterinary vaccines (*5.2.4*).

2-3 Seed lots

2-3-1 Extraneous agents

The master seed lot complies with the test for extraneous agents in seed lots (*2.6.24*). In these tests on the master seed lot, the organisms used are not more than 5 passages from the master seed lot at the start of the tests.

2-4 Choice of vaccine virus

The vaccine virus shall be shown to be satisfactory with respect to safety (*5.2.6*) and efficacy (*5.2.7*) for the ducks for which the vaccine is intended.

The following tests for safety (section 2-4-1), increase in virulence (section 2-4-2) and immunogenicity (section 2-4-3) may be used during demonstration of safety and immunogenicity.

2-4-1 Safety

Carry out the test for each route and method of administration to be recommended for vaccination, using in each case ducks from a species considered to be the most susceptible among the species to be recommended for vaccination and not older than the youngest age to be recommended for vaccination. Use vaccine virus at the least attenuated passage level that will be present in a batch of vaccine. For each test, use not fewer than 20 susceptible ducks that do not have antibodies against duck plague virus. Administer to each duck a quantity of vaccine virus equivalent to not less than 10 times the maximum virus titre likely to be contained in 1 dose of the vaccine. Observe the ducks at least daily for 21 days. The test is not valid if more than 10 per cent of the ducks die from causes not attributable to the vaccine virus. The vaccine virus complies with the test if no duck shows notable signs of duck plague or dies from causes attributable to the vaccine virus.

2-4-2 Increase in virulence

The test for increase in virulence consists of the administration of the vaccine virus, at the least attenuated passage level that will be present between the master seed lot and a batch of vaccine, to a group of 5 domestic ducks that do not have antibodies against duck plague virus and of an age suitable for the multiplication of the virus then its sequential passage, 5 times where possible, to further similar groups of ducks of an age suitable for the multiplication of the virus and testing of the final recovered virus for increase in virulence. If the properties of the vaccine virus allow sequential passage to 5 groups via natural spreading, this method may be used, otherwise passage as described below is carried out and the maximally passaged virus that has been recovered is tested for increase in virulence. Care must be taken to avoid contamination by virus from previous passages. Administer by a recommended route a quantity of the vaccine virus that will allow recovery of virus for the passages described below. 2 to 4 days later, take samples of liver and spleen from each duck and pool all samples. Administer 0.1 ml of the pooled suspension by the oro-nasal or a parenteral route to each of 5 other domestic ducks of the same age that do not have antibodies against duck plague virus. Carry out this passage operation not fewer than 5 times; verify the presence of the virus at each passage. If the virus is not found at a passage level, carry out a second series of passages. Carry out the test for safety (section 2-4-1) using the unpassaged vaccine virus and the maximally passaged vaccine virus that has been recovered. The vaccine virus complies with the test if no indication of increase in virulence of the maximally passaged virus compared with the unpassaged virus is observed. If virus is not recovered at any passage level in the first and second series of passages, the vaccine virus also complies with the test.

2-4-3 Immunogenicity

A test is carried out for each route and method of administration to be recommended for vaccination, using in each case domestic ducks not older than the youngest age to be recommended for vaccination. The quantity of the vaccine virus administered to each duck is not greater than the minimum virus titre to be stated on the label and the virus is at the most attenuated passage level that will be present in a batch of the vaccine. For each test, use not fewer than 30 ducks of the same origin and that do not have antibodies against duck plague virus. Vaccinate by a recommended route not fewer than 20 ducks. Maintain not fewer than 10 ducks as controls. After 5 days, challenge each duck by a suitable route with a sufficient quantity of virulent duck plague virus. Observe the ducks at least daily for 14 days after challenge. Record the deaths and the number of surviving ducks that show clinical signs of disease. The test

is not valid if during the observation period after challenge fewer than 80 per cent of the control ducks die or show typical signs of duck plague and/or if during the period between the vaccination and challenge more than 10 per cent of control or vaccinated ducks show abnormal clinical signs of disease or die from causes not attributable to the vaccine. The vaccine virus complies with the test if during the observation period after challenge not fewer than 80 per cent of the vaccinated ducks survive and show no notable clinical signs of duck plague.

3 BATCH TESTS

3-1 Identification
The vaccine, diluted if necessary and mixed with a monospecific duck plague virus antiserum, no longer infects embryonated hens' eggs from an SPF flock (5.2.2) or susceptible cell cultures (5.2.4) into which it is inoculated.

3-2 Bacteria and fungi
The vaccine and, where applicable, the liquid supplied with it comply with the requirement for sterility prescribed in the monograph *Vaccines for veterinary use (0062)*.

3-3 Mycoplasmas
The vaccine complies with the test for mycoplasmas (2.6.7).

3-4 Extraneous agents
The vaccine complies with the tests for extraneous agents in batches of finished product (2.6.25).

3-5 Safety
Use not fewer than 10 domestic ducks that do not have antibodies against duck plague virus and not older than the minimum age recommended for vaccination. Administer by a recommended route and method to each duck 10 doses of the vaccine in a volume suitable for the test. Observe the ducks at least daily for 21 days. The test is not valid if more than 20 per cent of the ducks show abnormal clinical signs of disease or die from causes not attributable to the vaccine. The vaccine complies with the test if no duck shows notable clinical signs of disease or dies from causes attributable to the vaccine.

3-6 Virus titre
Titrate the vaccine virus by inoculation into embryonated hens' eggs from an SPF flock (5.2.2) or into suitable cell cultures (5.2.4). The vaccine complies with the test if 1 dose contains not less than the minimum virus titre stated on the label.

3-7 Potency
The vaccine complies with the test prescribed under immunogenicity (section 2-4-3), when administered by a recommended route and method. It is not necessary to carry out the potency test for each batch of the vaccine if it has been carried out on a representative batch using a vaccinating dose containing not more than the minimum virus titre stated on the label.

Ph Eur

Duck Viral Hepatitis Type I Vaccine (Live)

(Ph Eur monograph 1315)

Ph Eur

1. DEFINITION

Duck viral hepatitis type I vaccine (live) is a preparation of a suitable strain of duck hepatitis virus type I. This monograph applies to vaccines intended for the active immunisation of breeder ducks in order to protect passively their progeny and/or for the active immunisation of ducklings.

2. PRODUCTION

2-1. PREPARATION OF THE VACCINE

The vaccine virus is grown in embryonated hens' eggs or in cell cultures.

2-2. SUBSTRATE FOR VIRUS PROPAGATION

2-2-1. Embryonated hens' eggs

If the vaccine virus is grown in embryonated hens' eggs, they are obtained from flocks free from specified pathogens (SPF) (5.2.2).

2-2-2. Cell cultures

If the vaccine virus is grown in cell cultures, they comply with the requirements for cell cultures for production of veterinary vaccines (5.2.4).

2-3. SEED LOTS

2-3-1. Extraneous agents

The master seed lot complies with the tests for extraneous agents in seed lots (2.6.24). In these tests on the master seed lot, the organisms used are not more than 5 passages from the master seed lot at the start of the tests.

2-4. CHOICE OF VACCINE VIRUS

The vaccine virus shall be shown to be satisfactory with respect to safety (5.2.6) and efficacy (5.2.7) for the ducks for which it is intended.

The following tests for safety (section 2-4-1), increase in virulence (section 2-4-2) and immunogenicity (section 2-4-3) may be used during demonstration of safety and immunogenicity.

2-4-1. Safety

Carry out the test for each route and method of administration to be recommended for vaccination using in each case ducks not older than the youngest age to be recommended for vaccination. Use vaccine virus at the least attenuated passage level that will be present between the master seed lot and a batch of the vaccine. For each test, use not fewer than 20 susceptible domestic ducklings (*Anas platyrhynchos*) that do not have antibodies against duck hepatitis virus type I. Administer to each duckling a quantity of vaccine virus equivalent to not less than 10 times the maximum virus titre likely to be contained in 1 dose of vaccine. Observe the ducklings at least daily for 21 days. The test is not valid if more than 10 per cent of the ducklings die from causes not attributable to the vaccine virus. The vaccine virus complies with the test if no duckling shows notable signs of duck viral hepatitis or dies from causes attributable to the vaccine virus.

2-4-2. Increase in virulence

The test for increase in virulence consists of the administration of the vaccine virus at the least attenuated passage level that will be present between the master seed lot and a batch of vaccine to a group of five 1-day-old domestic ducklings that do not have antibodies against duck hepatitis virus type I, sequential passages, 5 times where possible, to further similar groups of 1-day-old ducklings and testing of the final recovered virus for increase in virulence. If the properties of the vaccine virus allow sequential passage to 5 groups via natural spreading, this method may be used, otherwise passage as described below is carried out and the maximally passaged virus that has been recovered is tested for increase in virulence. Care must be taken to avoid contamination by virus from previous passages. Administer by the oro-nasal route a quantity of vaccine virus that will

allow recovery of virus for the passages described below. 2 to 4 days later, take samples of liver from each duckling and pool the samples. Administer 1 ml of the pooled liver suspension by the oro-nasal route to each of five 1-day-old seronegative domestic ducklings. Carry out this operation 5 times. Verify the presence of the virus at each passage. If the virus is not found at a passage level, carry out a second series of passages. Observe the ducklings given the last passage at least daily for 21 days. Compare the results obtained with unpassaged virus in the safety studies and those obtained with maximally passaged virus to assess the degree of increase in virulence. If the virus is not recovered at any passage level in the first and second series of passages, it is considered not to show increase in virulence.

2-4-3. Immunogenicity

A test is carried out for each route and method of administration to be recommended, using in each case domestic ducks not older than the youngest age to be recommended for vaccination. The quantity of the vaccine virus administered to each bird is not greater than the minimum virus titre to be stated on the label and the virus is at the most attenuated passage level that will be present in a batch of the vaccine.

2-4-3-1. Vaccines for passive immunisation of ducklings Use for the test not fewer than 15 laying ducks or ducks intended for laying, as appropriate, of the same origin and that do not have antibodies against duck hepatitis virus type I. Vaccinate by a recommended route not fewer than 10 ducks using the schedule to be recommended. Maintain not fewer than 5 ducks as controls. Starting from 4 weeks after onset of lay, collect embryonated eggs from vaccinated and control ducks and incubate them. Challenge not fewer than twenty 1-week-old ducklings representative of the vaccinated group and not fewer than 10 from the control group by the oro-nasal route with a sufficient quantity of virulent duck hepatitis virus type I. Observe the ducklings at least daily for 14 days after challenge. Record the deaths and the number of surviving ducklings that show clinical signs of disease.

The test is not valid if:
— during the observation period after challenge fewer than 70 per cent of the challenged ducklings from the control ducks die or show typical signs of the disease,
— and/or during the period between vaccination and collection of the eggs more than 10 per cent of the control or vaccinated ducks show abnormal clinical signs or die from causes not attributable to the vaccine.

The vaccine virus complies with the test if during the observation period after challenge the percentage relative protection calculated using the following expression is not less than 80 per cent:

$$\frac{V - C}{100 - C} \times 100$$

V = percentage of challenged ducklings from vaccinated ducks that survive to the end of the observation period without clinical signs of the disease.
C = percentage of challenged ducklings from unvaccinated control ducks that survive to the end of the observation period without clinical signs of the disease.

2-4-3-2. Vaccines for active immunisation of ducklings Use for the test not fewer than 30 ducklings of the same origin and that do not have antibodies against duck hepatitis virus type I. Vaccinate by a recommended route not fewer than 20 ducklings. Maintain not fewer than 10 ducklings as controls. Challenge each duckling after at least 5 days by the oro-nasal route with a sufficient quantity of virulent duck hepatitis virus type I. Observe the ducklings at least daily for 14 days after challenge. Record the deaths and the number of surviving ducklings that show clinical signs of disease.

The test is not valid if:
— during the observation period after challenge fewer than 70 per cent of the control ducklings die or show typical signs of the disease,
— and/or during the period between vaccination and challenge more than 10 per cent of the control or vaccinated ducklings show abnormal clinical signs or die from causes not attributable to the vaccine.

The vaccine virus complies with the test if during the observation period after challenge the percentage relative protection calculated using the following expression is not less than 80 per cent:

$$\frac{V - C}{100 - C} \times 100$$

V = percentage of challenged vaccinated ducklings that survive to the end of the observation period without clinical signs of the disease.

C = percentage of challenged unvaccinated control ducklings that survive to the end of the observation period without clinical signs of the disease.

3. BATCH TESTS

3-1. Identification
The vaccine, diluted if necessary and mixed with a monospecific duck hepatitis virus type I antiserum, no longer infects embryonated hens' eggs from an SPF flock (5.2.2) or susceptible cell cultures (5.2.4) into which it is inoculated.

3-2. Bacteria and fungi
Vaccines intended for administration by injection comply with the test for sterility prescribed in the monograph *Vaccines for veterinary use (0062)*.

Vaccines not intended for administration by injection either comply with the test for sterility prescribed in the monograph *Vaccines for veterinary use (0062)* or with the following test: carry out a quantitative test for bacterial and fungal contamination; carry out identification tests for micro-organisms detected in the vaccine; the vaccine does not contain pathogenic micro-organisms and contains not more than 1 non-pathogenic micro-organism per dose.

Any liquid supplied with the vaccine complies with the test for sterility prescribed in the monograph *Vaccines for veterinary use (0062)*.

3-3. Mycoplasmas
The vaccine complies with the test for mycoplasmas (2.6.7).

3-4. Extraneous agents
The vaccine complies with the tests for extraneous agents in batches of finished product (2.6.25).

3-5. Safety
Use not fewer than 10 domestic ducks that do not have antibodies against duck hepatitis virus type I and of the youngest age recommended for vaccination. For vaccines recommended for use in ducks older than 2 weeks, ducks 2 weeks old may be used. Administer by a recommended route and method to each duck 10 doses of the vaccine. Observe the ducks at least daily for 21 days. The test is not valid if more than 20 per cent of ducks show abnormal clinical signs or die from causes not attributable to the vaccine. The vaccine complies with the test if no duck

shows notable clinical signs of disease or dies from causes attributable to the vaccine.

3-6. Virus titre
Titrate the vaccine virus by inoculation into embryonated hens' eggs from an SPF flock (5.2.2) or into suitable cell cultures (5.2.4). The vaccine complies with the test if 1 dose contains not less than the minimum virus titre stated on the label.

3-7. Potency
Depending on the indications, the vaccine complies with 1 or both of the tests prescribed under Immunogenicity (section 2-4-3), when administered by a recommended route and method. It is not necessary to carry out the potency test for each batch of the vaccine if it has been carried out on a representative batch using a vaccinating dose containing not more than the minimum virus titre stated on the label.

4. LABELLING
If it has been found that the vaccine may show reversion to virulence, the label indicates the precautions necessary to avoid transmission of virulent virus to unvaccinated ducklings.

Ph Eur

Egg Drop Syndrome 76 (Adenovirus) Vaccine

(Egg Drop Syndrome '76 Vaccine (Inactivated), Ph Eur monograph 1202)

CAUTION *Accidental injection of oily vaccine can cause serious local reactions in man. Expert medical advice should be sought immediately and the doctor should be informed that the vaccine is an oil emulsion.*

Ph Eur

DEFINITION
Egg drop syndrome '76 vaccine (inactivated) consists of an emulsion or a suspension of a suitable strain of egg drop syndrome '76 virus (haemagglutinating avian adenovirus) which has been inactivated in such a manner that immunogenic activity is retained.

PRODUCTION
The vaccine strain is propagated in fertilised hen or duck eggs from healthy flocks or in suitable cell cultures (5.2.4).

The test for inactivation is carried out in fertilised duck eggs from a flock free from egg drop syndrome '76 virus infection or hen eggs from a flock free from specified pathogens (5.2.2), or in suitable cell cultures, whichever is the most sensitive for the vaccine strain; the quantity of virus used in the test is equivalent to not less than ten doses of the vaccine. No live virus is detected.

The vaccine may contain adjuvants.

CHOICE OF VACCINE COMPOSITION
The vaccine is shown to be satisfactory with respect to safety and immunogenicity. The following test may be used during demonstration of efficacy (5.2.7).

Immunogenicity The test described under Potency is suitable to demonstrate immunogenicity.

BATCH TESTING
The test described under Potency is not necessarily carried out for routine testing of batches of vaccine. It is carried out, for a given vaccine, on one or more occasions, as decided by or with the agreement of the competent authority; where the

test is not carried out, an alternative validated method is used, the criteria for acceptance being set with reference to a batch of vaccine that has given satisfactory results in the test described under Potency. The following test may be used after a satisfactory correlation with the test described under Potency has been established.

Batch potency test
Vaccinate not fewer than ten 14- to 28-day-old chickens from a flock free from specified pathogens (5.2.2) with one dose of vaccine by one of the recommended routes. Four weeks later, collect serum samples from each bird and from five unvaccinated control birds of the same age and from the same source. Measure the antibody response in a haemagglutination (HA) inhibition test on each serum using four HA units of antigen and chicken erythrocytes. The test is not valid if there are specific antibodies in the sera of the unvaccinated birds. The vaccine complies with the test if the mean titre of the vaccinated group is not less than that found previously for a batch of vaccine that has given satisfactory results in the test described under Potency.

IDENTIFICATION

In chickens with no antibodies to egg drop syndrome '76 virus, the vaccine stimulates the production of specific antibodies.

TESTS

Safety
Inject a double dose by a recommended route into each of 10 chickens, 14 to 28 days old, from a flock free from specified pathogens (5.2.2). Observe the birds for 21 days. No abnormal local or systemic reaction occurs.

Inactivation
A. For a vaccine prepared in eggs, carry out the test in fertilised duck eggs from a flock free from egg drop syndrome '76 virus infection or, if it is known to provide a more sensitive test system, in hen eggs from a flock free from specified pathogens (5.2.2).

Inject two-fifths of a dose into the allantoic cavity of each of ten 10- to 14-day-old fertilised eggs that are free from parental antibodies to egg drop syndrome '76 virus. Incubate the eggs and observe for 8 days. Pool separately the allantoic fluid from eggs containing live embryos, and that from eggs containing dead embryos, excluding those that die from non-specific causes within 24 h of the injection.

Inject into the allantoic cavity of each of ten 10- to 14-day-old fertilised eggs that are free from parental antibodies to egg drop syndrome '76 virus, 0.2 ml of the pooled allantoic fluid from the live embryos and into each of ten similar eggs, 0.2 ml of the pooled allantoic fluid from the dead embryos and incubate for 8 days. Examine the allantoic fluid from each egg for the presence of haemagglutinating activity using chicken erythrocytes.

If more than 20 per cent of the embryos die at either stage, repeat that stage. The vaccine complies with the test if there is no evidence of haemagglutinating activity and if, in any repeat test, not more than 20 per cent of the embryos die from non-specific causes.

Antibiotics may be used in the test to control extraneous bacterial infection.

B. For a vaccine adapted to growth in cell cultures, inoculate ten doses into suitable cell cultures. If the vaccine contains an oily adjuvant, eliminate it by suitable means. Incubate the cultures at $38 \pm 1\ °C$ for 7 days. Make a passage on another set of cell cultures and incubate at $38 \pm 1\ °C$ for 7 days. Examine the cultures regularly and at the end of the incubation period examine the supernatant liquid for the presence of haemagglutinating activity. The vaccine complies with the test if the cell cultures show no sign of infection and if the there is no haemagglutinating activity in the supernatant liquid.

Extraneous agents
Use the chickens from the test for safety. 21 days after injection of the double dose of vaccine, inject one dose by the same route into each chicken. Collect serum samples from each chicken 2 weeks later and carry out tests for antibodies to the following agents by the methods prescribed for chicken flocks free from specified pathogens (5.2.2):
avian encephalomyelitis virus, avian leucosis viruses, infectious bronchitis virus, infectious bursal disease virus, infectious laryngotracheitis virus, influenza A virus, Marek's disease virus, Newcastle disease virus and, for vaccine produced in duck eggs, *Chlamydia* (by a complement-fixation test or agar gel precipitation test), duck hepatitis virus type I (by a fluorescent-antibody test or serum-neutralisation test) and Derzsy's disease virus (by a serum-neutralisation test). The vaccine does not stimulate the formation of antibodies against these agents.

Sterility
The vaccine complies with the test for sterility prescribed in the monograph on *Vaccines for veterinary use (0062)*.

POTENCY

Vaccinate each of 2 groups of 30 hens from a flock free from specified pathogens (5.2.2) and of the age at which vaccination is recommended. Maintain two control groups one of 10 hens and the other of 30 hens, of the same age and from the same source as the vaccinates. Keep individual egg production records from point of lay until 4 weeks after challenge.

At 30 weeks of age, 1 group of 30 vaccinates and the group of 10 control birds are challenged with a dose of egg drop syndrome '76 virus sufficient to cause a well marked drop in egg production and/or quality. The vaccine complies with the test if the vaccinated birds show no marked drop in egg production and/or quality. The test is not valid unless there is a well marked drop in egg production and/or quality in the control birds.

When the second group of vaccinated birds and the group of 30 control birds are nearing the end of lay, challenge these birds, as before. The vaccine complies with the test if the vaccinated birds show no marked drop in egg production and/or quality. The test is not valid unless there is a well marked drop in egg production and/or quality in the control birds.

Carry out serological tests on serum samples obtained at the time of vaccination, 4 weeks later and just prior to challenge. The test is not valid if antibodies to egg drop syndrome '76 virus are detected in any sample from control birds.

LABELLING

The label states whether the strain in the vaccine is duck- or hen-embryo-adapted or cell-culture-adapted.

Ph Eur

Equine Herpesvirus Vaccine, Inactivated

(Equine Herpesvirus Vaccine (Inactivated), Ph Eur monograph 1613)

Ph Eur _____

DEFINITION

Equine herpesvirus vaccine (inactivated) is a preparation of one or more suitable strains of equid herpesvirus 1 and/or equid herpesvirus 4 inactivated without impairing their immunogenic activity or a suspension of an inactivated fraction of the virus.

PRODUCTION

Each strain of virus is propagated separately in suitable cell cultures (5.2.4). The viral suspensions may be purified and concentrated and are inactivated; they may be treated to fragment the virus and the viral fragments may be purified and concentrated.

The test for residual infectious equid herpesvirus is carried out using 2 passages in the same type of cell culture as that used in the production or in cell cultures shown to be at least as sensitive. The quantity of inactivated virus used in the test is equivalent to not less than 25 doses of the vaccine. No live virus is detected.

The vaccine may contain a suitable adjuvant.

CHOICE OF VACCINE COMPOSITION

The vaccine is shown to be satisfactory with respect to safety (5.2.6) and immunogenicity (5.2.7) in horses. Where a particular breed of horse is known to be especially sensitive to the vaccine, horses from that breed are included in the test for safety. The following tests may be used during demonstration of safety and immunogenicity.

Safety A test is carried out in each category of animals for which the vaccine is intended and by each recommended route. 2 doses of vaccine are administered to each of not fewer than 10 animals which have not been previously vaccinated with an equine herpesvirus vaccine, which have at most a low antibody titre not indicative of recent infection and which do not excrete equid herpesvirus. After 14 days, 1 dose of vaccine is injected into each of the animals. The animals are observed for a further 14 days. During the 28 days of the test, no abnormal or systemic reaction occurs. If the vaccine is intended for use in pregnant horses, for the test in this category of animal, mares are vaccinated during the relevant trimester or trimesters of pregnancy and the observation period is prolonged up to foaling; any effects on gestation or the offspring are noted.

Immunogenicity The claims of the product reflect the type of immunogenicity demonstrated (protection against the disease of the respiratory tract and/or protection against abortion). The tests described under Potency are suitable to demonstrate the immunogenicity of the strains present in the vaccine.

BATCH TESTING

The test described under Potency is not carried out for routine testing of batches of vaccine. It is carried out, for a given vaccine on one or more occasions; where the test is not carried out, an alternative validated method is used, the criteria for acceptance being set with reference to a batch of vaccine that has given satisfactory results in the tests described under Potency. The following test may be used.

Batch potency test

Vaccinate not fewer than 5 rabbits, guinea-pigs or mice with a single injection of a suitable dose. Where the schedule stated on the label requires a second injection to be given, the recommended schedule may be used in laboratory animals provided it has been demonstrated that this will still provide a suitably sensitive test system. At a given interval within the range of 14 to 21 days after the last injection, collect blood from each animal and prepare serum samples. Use a suitable validated test such as an enzyme-linked immunosorbent assay to measure the response to each of the antigens stated on the label. The antibody levels are not significantly less than those obtained with a batch that has given satisfactory results in the test described under Potency.

IDENTIFICATION

In animals having no antibodies against equid herpesvirus 1 and equid herpesvirus 4 or a fraction of the viruses, the vaccine stimulates the production of specific antibodies against the virus type or types included in the product. The method used must distinguish between antibodies against equid herpesviruses 1 and 4.

TESTS

Safety

Use for the test horses that have not been vaccinated against equid herpesviruses 1 and 4. Administer by a recommended route twice the vaccinating dose into each of not fewer than 2 horses. After 2 weeks, administer a single dose to each of the animals. Observe the animals for a further 10 days. The animals remain in good health and no abnormal local or systemic reaction occurs.

Inactivation

Carry out a test for residual infectious equid herpesvirus using not less than 25 doses of vaccine by inoculating cell cultures sensitive to equid herpesviruses 1 and 4; make a passage after 5 to 7 days and maintain the cultures for 14 days. No live virus is detected. If the vaccine contains an adjuvant, separate the adjuvant from the liquid phase, by a method that does not inactivate or otherwise interfere with the detection of live virus, or carry out a test for inactivation on the mixture of bulk antigens before addition of the adjuvant.

Sterility

The vaccine complies with the test for sterility prescribed in the monograph on *Vaccines for veterinary use (0062)*.

POTENCY

The type of potency test depends on the claims for the product. For vaccines intended to protect against the disease of the respiratory tract carry out test A, using equid herpesvirus 1 and/or equid herpesvirus 4 depending on the claims for protection. For vaccines intended to protect against abortion carry out test B.

Use horses which have not been vaccinated with an equine herpesvirus vaccine, which have at most a low antibody titre not indicative of recent infection, and which do not excrete equid herpesvirus. To demonstrate that no recent infection occurs, immediately before vaccination: draw a blood sample from each animal and test individually for antibodies against equid herpesviruses 1 and 4; collect 10 ml of heparinised blood and test the washed leucocytes for equid herpesviruses 1 and 4; collect a nasopharyngeal swab and test for equid herpesviruses 1 and 4. There is no indication of an active infection. Immediately before challenge collect a nasopharyngeal swab and test for equid herpesviruses 1 and 4. If there is an indication of virus excretion remove the animal from the test. Keep the horses in strict isolation.

A. Use not fewer than 10 horses, not less than 6 months old. Vaccinate not fewer than 6 horses using the recommended schedule. Keep not fewer than 4 unvaccinated horses as controls. At least 2 weeks after the last vaccination, administer by nasal instillation to all horses a quantity of equid herpesvirus 1 or 4, sufficient to produce in a susceptible horse characteristic signs of the disease such as pyrexia and virus excretion (and possibly nasal discharge and coughing). Observe the horses for 14 days. Collect nasopharyngeal swabs daily from each individual animal to isolate the virus. The vaccinated horses show no more than slight signs; the signs in vaccinates are less severe than in controls. The average number of days on which virus is excreted, and the respective virus titres are significantly lower in vaccinated horses than in controls.

B. Use not fewer than 10 pregnant mares. In addition to the testing described above, 6, 4, 3, 2 and 1 month before the first vaccination draw a blood sample from each horse and test individually for antibodies against equid herpesvirus 1 and equid herpesvirus 4. There is no evidence of recent infection or virus excretion. Vaccinate not fewer than 6 mares using the recommended schedule. Keep not fewer than 4 horses as unvaccinated controls. Between day 260 and 290 of pregnancy but not earlier than 3 weeks after the last vaccination administer by nasal instillation to all horses a quantity of equid herpesvirus 1 sufficient to produce abortion in susceptible mares. Observe the mares up to foaling or abortion. Collect samples of fetal lung and liver tissues from aborted fetuses and carry out tests for virus in cell cultures. The test is invalid if more than one control horse gives birth to a healthy foal and if the challenge virus is not isolated from the aborted fetuses. The vaccine complies with the test if not more than one vaccinated mare aborts.

LABELLING

The label states:
— the strains of virus included in the vaccine,
— the claims of protection.

Ph Eur

Equine Influenza Vaccine, Inactivated

(*Equine Influenza Vaccine (Inactivated)*, *Ph Eur monograph 0249*)

Ph Eur

DEFINITION

Equine influenza vaccine (inactivated) is a preparation of one or more suitable strains of equine influenza virus, inactivated in such a manner that immunogenic activity is maintained. Suitable strains contain both haemagglutinin and neuraminidase.

PRODUCTION

Each strain of virus is propagated separately in fertilised hen eggs from healthy flocks or in suitable cell cultures (5.2.4). The viral suspensions may be purified and concentrated. The antigen content of the vaccine is based on the haemagglutinin content of the viral suspensions determined as described under In-process Tests; the amount of haemagglutinin for each strain is not less than that in the vaccine shown to be satisfactory in the test for potency.

The test for residual infectious influenza virus is carried out using method A or method B whichever is the more sensitive.

The quantity of inactivated virus used is equivalent to not less than 10 doses of vaccine.

A. The vaccine is inoculated into suitable cells; after incubation for 8 days, a subculture is made. It is incubated for a further 6 to 8 days. Harvest about 0.1 ml of the supernatant and examine for live virus by a haemagglutination test. If haemagglutination is found, carry out a further passage in cell culture and test for haemagglutination; no haemagglutination occurs.

B. Inoculate 0.2 ml into the allantoic cavity of each of 10 fertilised eggs and incubate at 33 °C to 37 °C for 3 to 4 days. The test is not valid unless not fewer than 8 of the 10 embryos survive. Harvest 0.5 ml of the allantoic fluid from each surviving embryo and pool the fluids. Inoculate 0.2 ml of the pooled fluid into a further 10 fertilised eggs and incubate at 33 °C to 37 °C for 3 to 4 days. The test is not valid unless at least 8 of the 10 embryos survive. Harvest about 0.1 ml of the allantoic fluid from each surviving embryo and examine each individual harvest for live virus by a haemagglutination test. If haemagglutination is found for any of the fluids, carry out a further passage of that fluid in eggs and test for haemagglutination; no haemagglutination occurs.

The vaccine may contain suitable adjuvants.

CHOICE OF VACCINE COMPOSITION

The choice of strains used in the vaccine is based on epidemiological data. The Office international des épizooties reviews the epidemiological data periodically and if necessary recommends new strains corresponding to prevailing epidemiological evidence. Such strains are used in accordance with the regulations in force in the signatory States of the Convention on the Elaboration of a European Pharmacopoeia.

The vaccine is shown to be satisfactory with respect to safety and immunogenicity in horses. Where a particular breed of horse is known to be especially sensitive to the vaccine, horses from that breed are included in the tests for safety. The following tests may be used during demonstration of safety (5.2.6) and efficacy (5.2.7).

Safety

A test is carried out in each category of animals for which the vaccine is intended and by each recommended route. Use animals that preferably have no equine influenza antibodies or, where justified, use animals with a low level of such antibodies as long as they have not been vaccinated against equine influenza and administration of the vaccine does not cause an anamnestic response. 2 doses of vaccine are injected by the intended route into each of not fewer than 10 animals. After 14 days, 1 dose of vaccine is injected into each of the animals. The animals are observed for a further 14 days. During the 28 days of the test, no abnormal local or systemic reaction occurs. If the vaccine is intended for use in pregnant horses, for the test in this category of animal, horses are vaccinated during the relevant trimester or trimesters of pregnancy and the observation period is prolonged up to foaling; any effects on gestation or the offspring are noted.

Immunogenicity

The test described under Potency is suitable to demonstrate the immunogenicity of the strains present in the vaccine.

A test with virulent challenge is carried out for at least one vaccine strain. For other strains in the vaccine, demonstration of immunogenicity may, where justified, be based on the serological response induced in horses by the vaccine; justification for protection against these strains may be based on published data on the correlation of the antibody titre with protection against antigenically related strains.

Where serology is used, the test is carried out as described under Potency but instead of virulent challenge, a blood sample is drawn 2 weeks after the last vaccination and the antibody titre of each serum is determined by a suitable immunochemical method (2.7.1), such as the single radial haemolysis test or the haemagglutination-inhibition test shown below; a reference serum is used to validate the test. The acceptance criteria depend on the strain and are based on available data; for A/equine-2 virus, vaccines have usually been found satisfactory if the antibody titre of each serum is not less than 85 mm^2 where the single radial haemolysistest is used, or not less than 1:64 (before mixture with the suspension of antigen and erythrocytes) where the haemagglutination-inhibition test is used.

Equine influenza subtype I horse antiserum BRP, equine influenza subtype 2 American-like horse antiserum BRP and *equine influenza subtype 2 European-like horse antiserum BRP* are suitable for use as reference sera for the single radial haemolysis test.

The claims for the product reflect the type of immunogenicity demonstrated (protection against challenge or antibody production).

Single radial haemolysis

Heat each serum at 56 °C for 30 min. Perform tests on each serum using respectively the antigen or antigens prepared from the strain(s) used in the production of the vaccine. Mix 1 ml of sheep erythrocyte suspension in barbital buffer solution (1 volume of erythrocytes in 10 volumes of final suspension) with 1 ml of a suitable dilution of the influenza virus strain in barbital buffer solution and incubate the mixture at 4 °C for 30 min. To 2 ml of the virus/erythrocyte mixture, add 1 ml of a 3 g/l solution of *chromium(III) chloride hexahydrate R*, mix and allow to stand for 10 min. Heat the sensitised erythrocytes to 47 °C in a water-bath. Mix 15 ml of a 10 g/l solution of *agarose for electrophoresis R* in barbital buffer solution, 0.7 ml of sensitised erythrocyte suspension and the appropriate amount of diluted guinea-pig complement in barbital buffer solution at 47 °C. Pour the mixture into Petri dishes and allow the agar to set. Punch holes in the agar layer and place in each hole, 5 µl of the undiluted serum to be tested or control serum. Incubate the Petri dishes at 37 °C for 18 h. Measure the diameter of the haemolysis zone and calculate its area, which expresses the antibody titre, in square millimetres.

Equine influenza subtype I horse antiserum BRP, equine influenza subtype 2 American-like horse antiserum BRP and *equine influenza subtype 2 European-like horse antiserum BRP* are suitable for use as reference sera for the single radial haemolysis test.

Haemagglutination-inhibition test

Inactivate each serum by heating at 56 °C for 30 min. To one volume of each serum add three volumes of *phosphate-buffered saline pH 7.4 R* and four volumes of a 250 g/l suspension of *light kaolin R* in the same buffer solution. Shake each mixture for 10 min. Centrifuge, collect the supernatant liquid and mix with a concentrated suspension of chicken erythrocytes. Allow to stand at 37 °C for 60 min and centrifuge. The dilution of the serum obtained is 1:8. Perform tests on each serum using each antigen prepared from the strains used in the production of the vaccine. Using each diluted serum, prepare a series of twofold dilutions. To 0.025 ml of each of the latter dilutions add 0.025 ml of a suspension of antigen treated with *ether R*

and containing four haemagglutinating units. Allow the mixture to stand for 30 min and add 0.05 ml of a suspension of chicken erythrocytes containing 2×10^7 erythrocytes/ml. Allow to stand for 1 h and note the last dilution of serum that still completely inhibits haemagglutination.

IN-PROCESS TESTS

The content of haemagglutinin in the inactivated virus suspension, after purification and concentration where applicable, is determined by a suitable immunochemical method (2.7.1), such as single radial immunodiffusion, using a suitable haemagglutinin reference preparation; the content is shown to be within the limits shown to allow preparation of a satisfactory vaccine. For vaccines produced in eggs, the content of bacterial endotoxins is determined on the virus harvest to monitor production.

BATCH TESTING

The test described under Potency is not carried out for routine testing of batches of vaccine. It is carried out, for a given vaccine, on one or more occasions, as decided by or with the agreement of the competent authority; where the test is not carried out, an alternative validated method is used, the criteria for acceptance being set with reference to a batch of vaccine that has given satisfactory results in the test described under Potency. The following test may be used.

Batch potency test

Inject one dose of vaccine subcutaneously into each of 5 guinea-pigs free from specified antibodies. 21 days later, collect blood samples and separate the serum. Carry out tests on the serum for specific antibodies by a suitable immunochemical method (2.7.1) such as single radial haemolysis or haemagglutinin inhibition, using reference sera to validate the test. The antibody titres are not significantly lower than those obtained in guinea-pigs with a reference batch of vaccine shown to have satisfactory potency in horses.

IDENTIFICATION

In susceptible animals, the vaccine stimulates the production of specific antibodies.

TESTS
Safety

Use horses that preferably have no equine influenza virus antibodies or, where justified, use horses with a low level of such antibodies as long as they have not been vaccinated against equine influenza and administration of the vaccine does not cause an anamnestic response. Administer by a recommended route a double dose of vaccine to each of not fewer than 2 horses. After 2 weeks, administer a single dose to each horse. Observe the animals for a further 10 days. No abnormal local or systemic reaction occurs.

Inactivation

Inoculate 0.2 ml of the vaccine into the allantoic cavity of each of 10 fertilised eggs and incubate at 33 °C to 37 °C for 3 to 4 days. The test is not valid unless at least 8 of the 10 embryos survive. Harvest 0.5 ml of the allantoic fluid from each surviving embryo and pool the fluids. Inoculate 0.2 ml of the pooled fluid into a further 10 fertilised eggs and incubate at 33 °C to 37 °C for 3 to 4 days. The test is not valid unless not fewer than 8 of the 10 embryos survive. Harvest about 0.1 ml of the allantoic fluid from each surviving embryo and examine each individual harvest for live virus by a haemagglutination test. If haemagglutination is found for any of the fluids, carry out for that fluid a further passage in eggs and test for haemagglutination; no haemagglutination occurs.

Sterility

The vaccine complies with the test for sterility prescribed in the monograph on *Vaccines for veterinary use (0062)*.

POTENCY

Carry out the potency test using a challenge strain against which the vaccine is stated to provide protection. Use where possible a recent isolate.

Use 10 horses, at least 6 months old, that do not have specific antibodies against equine influenza virus. Draw a blood sample from each animal and test individually for antibodies against equine influenza virus to determine seronegativity. Vaccinate 6 animals using the recommended schedule. Draw a second blood sample from each animal 7 days after the first vaccination and test individually for antibodies against equine influenza virus, to detect an anamnestic sero-response. Animals showing sero-conversion at this stage are excluded from the test. At least 2 weeks after the last vaccination, administer by aerosol to the 10 animals a quantity of equine influenza virus sufficient to produce characteristic signs of disease such as fever, nasal discharge and coughing in a susceptible animal. Observe the animals for 14 days. Collect nasal swabs daily from each individual animal to isolate the virus. The vaccinated animals show no more than slight signs; the controls show characteristic signs. The average number of days on which virus is excreted, and the respective virus titres are significantly lower in vaccinated animals than in control animals.

LABELLING

The label states:
— the age at which animals should be vaccinated,
— the period of time that should elapse between the first and second injections,
— any booster injections required,
— the strains of virus included in the vaccine.

————————————————————— Ph Eur

Feline Calicivirus Vaccine, Inactivated

(Feline Calicivirosis Vaccine (Inactivated) Ph Eur monograph 1101)

Ph Eur —————————————————————————————

DEFINITION

Inactivated feline calicivirosis vaccine is a suspension of one or more suitable strains of feline calicivirus which have been inactivated while maintaining adequate immunogenic properties or of fractions of one or more strains of feline calicivirus with adequate immunogenic properties.

PRODUCTION

The virus is grown in suitable cell lines (*5.2.4*). The viral suspension is harvested and inactivated.

The test for residual infectious calicivirus is carried out using 2 passages in cell cultures of the same type as those used for preparation of the vaccine or in cell cultures shown to be at least as sensitive; the quantity of inactivated virus used in the test is equivalent to not less than 25 doses of vaccine. No live virus is detected.

The vaccine may contain one or more suitable adjuvants.

CHOICE OF VACCINE COMPOSITION

The vaccine is shown to be satisfactory with respect to safety and immunogenicity in cats. The following test may be used during demonstration of efficacy (*5.2.7*).

Immunogenicity The test described under Potency is suitable to demonstrate immunogenicity of the vaccine.

BATCH TESTING

Batch potency test

The test described under Potency is not carried out for routine testing of batches of vaccine. It is carried out, for a given vaccine, on one or more occasions, as decided by or with the agreement of the competent authority; where the test is not carried out, a suitable validated alternative test is carried out, the criteria for acceptance being set with reference to a batch of vaccine that has given satisfactory results in the test described under Potency. The following test may be used after a satisfactory correlation with the test described under Potency has been established.

Use groups of 15 seronegative mice. Administer half a dose of the vaccine to each mouse and 7 days later repeat the administration. 21 days after the first injection, take blood samples and determine the level of antibodies against feline calicivirus by an immunofluorescence technique using pools of serum from groups of 3 mice. The antibody levels are not significantly lower than those obtained with a batch of vaccine that has given satisfactory results in the test described under Potency.

IDENTIFICATION

When injected into susceptible animals, the vaccine stimulates the formation of specific antibodies against feline calicivirus.

TESTS

Safety

Use cats 8 to 12 weeks old and preferably having no feline calicivirus antibodies or, where justified, use cats with a low level of such antibodies as long as they have not been vaccinated against feline calicivirosis and administration of the vaccine does not cause an anamnestic response. Administer a double dose of vaccine by a recommended route to each of 2 cats. Observe the cats for 14 days. No abnormal local or systemic reaction occurs.

Inactivation

Carry out a test for residual infectious calicivirus using 10 doses of vaccine and 2 passages in cell cultures of the same type as those used for preparation of the vaccine or in cell cultures shown to be at least as sensitive. No live virus is detected. If the vaccine contains an adjuvant that would interfere with the test, where possible separate the adjuvant from the liquid phase by a method that does not inactivate or otherwise interfere with detection of live virus.

Sterility

The reconstituted vaccine complies with the test for sterility prescribed in *Vaccines for veterinary use (0062)*.

POTENCY

Carry out a potency test for each strain of feline calicivirus in the vaccine.

Use cats 8 to 12 weeks old and that do not have antibodies against feline calicivirus. Vaccinate 10 cats by a recommended route and according to the recommended schedule. Keep 10 cats as controls. 4 weeks after the last injection, administer intranasally to each vaccinated and control cat a quantity of a virulent strain of calicivirus of the same type as the vaccine strain sufficient to produce typical signs of the disease (hyperthermia, buccal ulcers, respiratory signs) in at least 8 of the control cats. Observe the cats for

14 days after challenge; collect nasal washings daily on days 2 to 14 to test for virus excretion. Note daily the body temperature and signs of disease using the scoring system shown below. The vaccine complies with the test if the score for the vaccinated cats is significantly lower than that for the controls.

Observed signs	Score
Death	10
Depressed state	2
Temperature $\geq 39.5\,^{\circ}\mathrm{C}$	1
Temperature $\leq 37\,^{\circ}\mathrm{C}$	2
Ulcer (nasal or oral)	
– small and few in number	1
– large and numerous	3
Nasal discharge	
– slight	1
– copious	2
Ocular discharge	1
Weight loss	2
Virus excretion (total number of days):	
≤ 4 days	1
5-7 days	2
> 7 days	3

Ph Eur

Feline Calicivirus Vaccine, Living

(Feline Calicivirosis Vaccine (Live), Freeze-Dried, Ph Eur monograph 1102)

Ph Eur

DEFINITION
Freeze-dried feline calicivirosis vaccine (live) is a preparation of one or more suitable strains of feline calicivirus.

PRODUCTION
The virus is grown in suitable cell lines (5.2.4). The viral suspension is harvested and mixed with a suitable stabilising solution. The mixture is subsequently freeze-dried.

CHOICE OF VACCINE STRAIN
The vaccine strain shall have been shown to be satisfactory with respect to safety (including safety for pregnant queens if such use is not contra-indicated), absence of reversion to virulence, and immunogenicity. The following tests may be used during demonstration of safety (5.2.6) and efficacy (5.2.7).

Safety To 10 cats of the minimum age stated for vaccination and which do not have antibodies against feline calicivirus, administer by a recommended route, a quantity of virus equivalent to 10 times the maximum titre that may be expected in a batch of vaccine. Observe the cats for 21 days. No abnormal local or systemic reaction occurs.

Reversion to virulence To 2 cats which do not have antibodies against feline calicivirus administer by a recommended route a quantity of virus (for example, approximately 10 doses) that will allow maximum recovery of virus for the passages described below. 5 days later, kill the cats, remove the nasal mucus, tonsils and the trachea, mix, homogenise in 10 ml of buffered saline and decant; inoculate the supernatant intranasally into 2 other cats; carry out this operation five times. Verify the presence of virus at each passage. If the virus is not recovered, carry out a second series of passages. Observe the cats given the last passage for 21 days and compare the reactions observed with those seen

in the cats in the safety test described above. The strain complies with the test if no evidence of an increase in virulence is seen compared to the original virus.

Immunogenicity The test described under Potency is suitable to demonstrate immunogenicity.

BATCH TESTING
If the test for potency has been carried out with satisfactory results on a representative batch of vaccine, this test may be omitted as a routine control on other batches of vaccine prepared from the same seed lot, subject to agreement by the competent authority.

IDENTIFICATION
When neutralised by one or more monospecific antisera, the reconstituted vaccine no longer infects susceptible cell cultures into which it is inoculated.

TESTS
Safety
Administer 10 doses of vaccine, by a recommended route to 2 cats, 8 to 12 weeks old and having no antibodies against feline calicivirus. Observe the cats for 14 days. No abnormal local or systemic reaction occurs.

Bacterial and fungal contamination
The reconstituted vaccine complies with the test for sterility prescribed in *Vaccines for veterinary use (0062)*.

Mycoplasmas (2.6.7)
The reconstituted vaccine complies wtith the test for mycoplasmas.

Extraneous viruses
Neutralise the vaccine using one or more monospecific antisera and inoculate into suitable cell cultures; make at least one passage and maintain the cultures for 14 days. Examine the cultures for cytopathic effects and carry out tests for haemadsorbing agents. No signs of viral contamination occur in the cell cultures.

Virus titre
Titrate the reconstituted vaccine in susceptible cell cultures at a temperature favourable to replication of the virus. One dose of the vaccine contains not less than the quantity of virus equivalent to the minimum titre stated on the label.

POTENCY
Carry out a potency test for each strain of feline calicivirus in the vaccine.

Use cats 8 to 12 weeks old that do not have antibodies against feline calicivirus. Vaccinate 10 cats by one of the recommended routes and according to the recommended schedule. Keep 10 cats as controls. 4 weeks after the last injection, administer intranasally to each vaccinated and control cat a quantity of a virulent strain of calicivirus of the same type as the vaccine strain sufficient to produce typical signs of the disease (hyperthermia, buccal ulcers, respiratory signs) in not fewer than 8 of the control cats. Observe the cats for 14 days after challenge; collect nasal washings daily on days 2 to 14 to test for virus excretion. Note daily the body temperature and signs of disease using the scoring system shown below. The vaccine complies with the test if the score for the vaccinated cats is significantly lower than that for the controls.

Observed signs	Score
Death	10
Depressed state	2
Temperature $\geq 39.5\,^{\circ}\mathrm{C}$	1
Temperature $\leq 37\,^{\circ}\mathrm{C}$	2
Ulcer (nasal or oral)	

– small and few in number	1
– large and numerous	3
Nasal discharge	
– slight	1
– copious	2
Ocular discharge	1
Weight loss	2
Virus excretion (total number of days):	
$\leqslant$ 4 days	1
5-7 days	2
> 7 days	3

Ph Eur

Feline Chlamydiosis Vaccine (Inactivated)

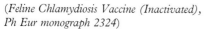

(*Feline Chlamydiosis Vaccine (Inactivated)*,
Ph Eur monograph 2324)

Ph Eur

1. DEFINITION

Feline chlamydiosis vaccine (inactivated) is a preparation of one or more suitable strains of *Chlamydophila felis*, which have been inactivated by a suitable method. This monograph applies to vaccines intended for administration to cats for active immunisation.

2. PRODUCTION

2-1. PREPARATION OF THE VACCINE

The seed material is cultured in embryonated hens' eggs from a healthy flock or in suitable cell cultures (*5.2.4*). If the vaccine contains more than one strain of bacterium, the different strains are grown and harvested separately.
The bacterial harvests are inactivated using suitable and validated methods. The suspensions may be treated to fragment the micro-organisms and the fragments may be purified and concentrated. The vaccine may contain adjuvants.

2-2. CHOICE OF VACCINE COMPOSITION

The vaccine is shown to be satisfactory with respect to safety (*5.2.6*) and efficacy (*5.2.7*) in cats for which it is intended.

The following test for immunogenicity (section 2-2-1) may be used during the demonstration of efficacy.

2-2-1. Immunogenicity

Carry out the test for each route and method of administration to be recommended for vaccination, using in each case cats not older than the minimum age recommended for vaccination and which do not have antibodies against *C. felis*. Vaccinate 10 cats according to the instructions for use and keep 10 cats as controls. Not later than 4 weeks after the last administration of vaccine, administer by a suitable route to each cat a quantity of a virulent strain of *C. felis* sufficient to produce in susceptible cats typical signs of disease such as conjunctivitis and nasal discharge. Observe the cats for 28 days. Where reduction of chlamydophila excretion is to be claimed, collect nasal washings and/or conjunctival swabs on days 7, 14, 17, 21, 24 and 28 after challenge to test for chlamydophila excretion. The duration of excretion for the vaccinated animals is significantly lower than for the controls. Note daily the body temperature and signs of disease using a suitable scoring system. The vaccine complies with the test if the score for the vaccinated cats is significantly lower than that for the controls.

2-3. MANUFACTURER'S TESTS

2-3-1. Batch potency test

It is not necessary to carry out the potency test (section 3-5) for each batch of the vaccine if it has been carried out using a batch of vaccine with a minimum potency. Where the test is not carried out on a batch, an alternative validated method is used, the criteria for acceptance being set with reference to a batch of vaccine that has given satisfactory results in the potency test (section 3-5). The following test may be used.

Inject a suitable dose by a suitable route into each of 5 seronegative cats or another suitable species. Where the schedule stated on the label requires a booster injection to be given, a booster vaccination may also be given in this test provided it has been demonstrated that this will still provide a suitably sensitive test system. Before the vaccination and at a given interval usually within the range of 14-21 days after the last injection, collect blood from each animal and prepare serum samples. Determine individually for each serum the titre of antibodies against each strain stated on the label, using a suitable test such as enzyme-linked immunosorbent assay (*2.7.1*). The vaccine complies with the test if the antibody levels are not significantly lower than those obtained for a batch that has given satisfactory results in the potency test (section 3-5).

2-3-2. Bacterial endotoxins

A test for bacterial endotoxins (*2.6.14*) is carried out on the final lot or, where the nature of the adjuvant prevents performance of a satisfactory test, on the bulk antigen or the mixture of bulk antigens immediately before addition of the adjuvant. The maximum acceptable amount of bacterial endotoxins is that found for a batch of vaccine that has been shown to be satisfactory in the safety test (section 3-4). The method chosen for determining the maximum acceptable amount of bacterial endotoxins is subsequently used for the testing of each batch.

3. BATCH TESTS

3-1. Identification

When injected into seronegative animals, the vaccine stimulates the production of antibodies against each of the strains of *C. felis* present in the vaccine.

3-2. Residual live chlamydophila

The vaccine complies with a suitable test for residual live chlamydophila.

3-3. Bacteria and fungi

The vaccine complies with the test for sterility prescribed in the monograph *Vaccines for veterinary use (0062)*.

3-4. Safety

Use 2 cats not older than the minimum age recommended for vaccination and free from antibodies against *C. felis*. Administer to each cat by a recommended route a double dose of the vaccine. Observe the cats at least daily for 2 weeks. The vaccine complies with the test if the cats remain in good health and no abnormal local or systemic reactions occur.

3-5. Potency

The vaccine complies with the test for immunogenicity (section 2-2-1).

Ph Eur

Feline Infectious Enteritis Vaccine, Inactivated

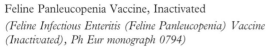

Feline Panleucopenia Vaccine, Inactivated

(Feline Infectious Enteritis (Feline Panleucopenia) Vaccine (Inactivated), Ph Eur monograph 0794)

Ph Eur

DEFINITION

Feline infectious enteritis (feline panleucopenia) vaccine (inactivated) is a liquid or freeze-dried preparation of feline panleucopenia virus or canine parvovirus inactivated by a suitable method.

PRODUCTION

The virus is propagated in suitable cell cultures (5.2.4). The virus is harvested and may be purified and concentrated.

The test for inactivation is carried out using a quantity of inactivated virus equivalent to not less than 100 doses of the vaccine by a validated method such as the following: inoculate into suitable non-confluent cells and after incubation for 8 days, make a subculture using trypsinised cells. After incubation for a further 8 days, examine the cultures for residual live parvovirus by an immunofluorescence test. The immunofluorescence test may be supplemented by a haemagglutination test or other suitable tests on the supernatant of the cell cultures. No live virus is detected.

The vaccine may contain an adjuvant and may be freeze-dried.

CHOICE OF VACCINE COMPOSITION

The vaccine is shown to be satisfactory with respect to safety (5.2.6) and efficacy (5.2.7) in cats. The following test may be used during demonstration of immunogenicity.

Immunogenicity Use 10 susceptible cats, 8 to 12 weeks old. Draw a blood sample from each cat and test individually for antibodies against feline panleucopenia virus and canine parvovirus to determine susceptibility. Vaccinate 5 cats by the recommended schedule. Carry out leucocyte counts 8 days and 4 days before challenge and calculate the mean of the 2 counts to serve as the initial value. 20 to 22 days after the last vaccination, challenge each cat by the intraperitoneal injection of a suspension of pathogenic feline panleucopenia virus. Observe the cats for 14 days. Carry out leucocyte counts on the fourth, sixth, eighth and tenth days after challenge. The test is not valid unless the 5 control cats all show on not fewer than one occasion a diminution in the number of leucocytes of at least 75 per cent of the initial value; these animals may die from panleucopenia. The vaccine complies with the test if the 5 vaccinated cats remain in excellent health and show no sign of leucopenia; that is to say, the diminution in the number of leucocytes does not exceed, in any of the four counts, 50 per cent of the initial value.

BATCH TESTING

Batch potency test

For routine testing of batches of vaccine a test based on production of haemagglutination-inhibiting antibodies in guinea-pigs may be used instead of test A or B described under Potency if a satisfactory correlation with the test for immunogenicity has been established.

IDENTIFICATION

When injected into animals, the vaccine stimulates the production of antibodies against the parvovirus present in the vaccine.

TESTS

Safety

Use cats of the minimum age recommended for vaccination and preferably having no antibodies against feline panleucopenia virus or against canine parvovirus or, where justified, use cats with a low level of such antibodies as long as they have not been vaccinated against feline panleucopenia virus or against canine parvovirus, and administration of the vaccine does not cause an anamnestic response. Administer by a recommended route a double dose of vaccine to each of 2 cats. Observe the animals for 14 days. No abnormal local or systemic reaction occurs.

Sterility

The vaccine complies with the test for sterility prescribed in the monograph on *Vaccines for veterinary use (0062)*.

POTENCY

Carry out test A or test B.

A. Use 4 cats, 8 to 12 weeks old. Draw a blood sample from each cat and test individually for antibodies against feline panleucopenia virus and canine parvovirus to determine susceptibility. Inject by a recommended route one dose of vaccine into each of 2 cats. After 21 days, draw a blood sample from each cat and separate the serum from each sample. Inactivate each serum by heating at 56 °C for 30 min. To 1 volume of each serum add 9 volumes of a 200 g/l suspension of *light kaolin R* in *phosphate buffered saline pH 7.4 R*. Shake each mixture for 20 min. Centrifuge, collect the supernatant liquid and mix with 1 volume of a concentrated suspension of pig erythrocytes. Allow to stand at 4 °C for 60 min and centrifuge. The dilution of the serum obtained is 1:10. Using each serum, prepare a series of twofold dilutions. To 0.025 ml of each of the latter dilutions add 0.025 ml of a suspension of canine parvovirus or feline panleucopenia virus antigen containing 4 haemagglutinating units. Allow to stand at 37 °C for 30 min and add 0.05 ml of a suspension of pig erythrocytes containing 30×10^6 cells per millilitre. Allow to stand at 4 °C for 90 min and note the last dilution of serum that still completely inhibits haemagglutination. The vaccine complies with the test if both vaccinated cats have developed titres of at least 1:20. The test is not valid if either control cat develops antibodies against canine parvovirus or feline panleucopenia virus.

B. Vaccinate according to the recommended schedule, 2 cats, 8 to 12 weeks old and having antibody titres less than 4 ND_{50} (neutralising dose 50 per cent) per 0.1 ml of serum measured by the method described below. 14 days after vaccination, examine the serum of each animal as follows. Heat the serum at 56 °C for 30 min and prepare serial dilutions using a medium suitable for feline cells. Add to each dilution an equal volume of a virus suspension containing an amount of virus such that when the volume of serum-virus mixture appropriate for the assay system is inoculated into cell cultures, each culture receives approximately 10^4 $CCID_{50}$. Incubate the mixtures at 37 °C for 1 h and inoculate four feline cell cultures with a suitable volume of each mixture. Incubate the cell cultures at 37 °C for 7 days, passage and incubate for a further 7 days. Examine the cultures for evidence of specific cytopathic effects and calculate the antibody titre. The vaccine complies with the test if the mean titre is not less than 32 ND_{50} per 0.1 ml of serum. If one cat fails to respond, repeat the test using 2 more cats and calculate the result as the mean of the titres obtained from all of the 3 cats that have responded.

Ph Eur

Feline Infectious Enteritis Vaccine, Living

Feline Panleucopenia Vaccine, Living

(*Feline Infectious Enteritis (Feline Panleucopenia) Vaccine (Live), Ph Eur monograph 0251*)

Ph Eur

DEFINITION

Feline infectious enteritis (feline panleucopenia) vaccine (live) is a preparation of a suitable strain of feline panleucopenia virus.

PRODUCTION

The virus is propagated in suitable cell cultures (*5.2.4*). The virus suspension is harvested and may be purified and concentrated. It is mixed with a suitable stabilising solution. The vaccine may be freeze-dried.

CHOICE OF VACCINE STRAIN

The vaccine strain shall have been shown to be satisfactory with respect to safety (including safety for pregnant queens if such use is not contra-indicated or if the virus is excreted in the faeces), absence of increase in virulence and immunogenicity.

The following tests may be used during demonstration of safety (*5.2.6*) and efficacy (*5.2.7*).

Safety   Each test is carried out for each recommended route of administration. Use 5 cats, of the minimum age recommended for vaccination and free from specific haemagglutination-inhibiting antibodies against feline panleucopenia virus and canine parvovirus. Make counts of leucocytes in circulating blood on days 8 and 4 before injection of the vaccine strain and calculate the mean of the 2 counts to serve as the initial value. Administer to each cat by a recommended route a quantity of virus corresponding to at least 10 times the maximum virus titre that may be expected in a batch of vaccine and at the lowest level of attenuation. Observe the animals for 21 days. Make leucocyte counts on the fourth, sixth, eighth and tenth days after inoculation. The strain complies with the test if: the cats remain in good health and there is no abnormal local or systemic reaction; for each animal and for each blood count, the number of leucocytes is not less than 50 per cent of the initial value.

Increase in virulence   Use 2 cats of the minimum age recommended for vaccination and which do not have haemagglutination-inhibiting antibodies against feline panleucopenia virus and canine parvovirus. Administer to each cat, by a recommended route, a quantity of virus suitable to allow maximum recovery of the virus for subsequent passages. From the second to the tenth day after administration of the virus, collect the faeces from each cat and check for the presence of the virus; pool faeces containing virus. Administer 1 ml of the suspension of pooled faeces by the oronasal route to each of 2 other cats of the same age and susceptibility; repeat this operation a further 4 times. Verify the presence of virus at each passage. If the virus is not found, carry out a second series of passages; if the virus is not found in one of the second series of passages, the vaccine strain complies with the test.

The vaccine strain complies with the test if: no cat dies or shows signs attributable to the vaccine; no indication of increase of virulence compared to the original vaccinal virus is observed; account is taken, notably, of the count of white blood cells, of results of histological examination of the thymus and of the titre of excreted virus.

Immunogenicity   The test described under Potency is suitable to demonstrate immunogenicity of the strain.

BATCH TESTING

If the test for potency has been carried out with satisfactory results on a representative batch of vaccine, this test may be omitted as a routine control on other batches of vaccine prepared from the same seed lot, subject to agreement by the competent authority.

IDENTIFICATION

Carry out replication of the vaccine virus in a susceptible cell line in a substrate suitable for a fluorescent antibody test or peroxidase test. Prepare suitable controls. Test a proportion of the cells with monoclonal antibodies specific for feline panleucopenia virus and a proportion with monoclonal antibodies specific for canine parvovirus.
Feline panleucopenia virus is detected but no canine parvovirus is detected in the cells inoculated with the vaccine.

TESTS

Safety

Use 2 cats of the minimum age recommended for vaccination and having no antibodies against feline panleucopenia virus or against canine parvovirus. Administer 10 doses of the vaccine to each cat, by a recommended route. Observe the animals for 14 days. No abnormal local or systemic reaction occurs.

Extraneous viruses

Neutralise the vaccine using a suitable monospecific antiserum against feline panleucopenia virus and inoculate into suitable cell cultures; make at least one passage and maintain the cultures for 14 days. Examine the cultures for cytopathic effects and carry out tests for haemadsorbing agents. No signs of viral contamination occur in the cell cultures.

Bacterial and fungal contamination

The vaccine, reconstituted if necessary, complies with the test for sterility prescribed in the monograph on *Vaccines for veterinary use (0062)*.

Mycoplasmas (*2.6.7*)

The vaccine complies with the test for mycoplasmas.

Virus titre

Reconstitute the vaccine, if necessary, and titrate in suitable cell cultures. One dose of vaccine contains not less than the quantity of virus equivalent to the minimum titre stated on the label.

POTENCY

Use 10 susceptible cats, 8 to 12 weeks old. Draw a blood sample from each cat and test individually for antibodies against feline panleucopenia virus and canine parvovirus to determine susceptibility. Vaccinate 5 cats by the recommended schedule. Carry out leucocyte counts 8 days and 4 days before challenge and calculate the mean of the 2 counts to serve as the initial value. 20 to 22 days after the last vaccination, challenge each cat by the intraperitoneal injection of a suspension of pathogenic feline panleucopenia virus. Observe the cats for 14 days. Carry out leucocyte counts on the fourth, sixth, eighth and tenth days after challenge. The test is not valid unless the 5 control cats all show on not fewer than one occasion a diminution in the number of leucocytes of at least 75 per cent of the initial value; these animals may die from panleucopenia.
The vaccine complies with the test if the 5 vaccinated cats remain in excellent health and show no sign of leucopenia; that is to say, the diminution in the number of leucocytes

does not exceed, in any of the four counts, 50 per cent of the initial value.

LABELLING

The label states that the vaccine should not be used in pregnant queens (unless it has been shown to be safe in such conditions).

Ph Eur

Feline Leukaemia Vaccine, Inactivated

(Feline Leukaemia Vaccine (Inactivated), Ph Eur monograph 1321)

Ph Eur

DEFINITION

Feline leukaemia vaccine (inactivated) is a preparation of immunogens from a suitable strain of feline leukaemia virus.

PRODUCTION

The immunogens consist either of a suitable strain of feline leukaemia virus inactivated in such a manner that adequate immunogenicity is maintained or of a fraction of the virus with adequate immunogenic properties; the immunogenic fraction may be produced by recombinant DNA technology.

Where applicable, the test for inactivation is carried out using a quantity of inactivated virus equivalent to not less than 25 doses of vaccine and two passages in the same type of cell cultures as used for the production of the vaccine or in cell cultures shown to be at least as sensitive; no live virus is detected.

The vaccine may contain an adjuvant.

CHOICE OF VACCINE COMPOSITION

The choice of the feline leukaemia virus strains and/or of the antigens included in the vaccine composition is made in such a manner as to ensure the safety (5.2.6) (including safety for pregnant queens if the vaccine may be used in such animals) and immunogenicity (5.2.7) of the vaccine. The following tests may be used during demonstration of safety and immunogenicity.

Safety Carry out the test for each intended route of administration. Use animals that do not have antibodies against gp 70 antigen of feline leukaemia virus nor display viraemia or antigenaemia at the time of the test; absence of antibodies and antigen is demonstrated by enzyme-linked immunosorbent assay (2.7.1).

A. Vaccinate, according to the intended schedule, not fewer than ten cats of the minimum age recommended for vaccination. Keep five cats as controls. Record the rectal temperature of each cat on the day before each vaccination, at the time of vaccination, 4 h and 8 h later, and once per day during the four following days. Observe the animals for at least 4 weeks after the last vaccination. No abnormal local or systemic reaction occurs during the test. 1, 2 and 4 weeks after the last vaccination, submit the animals to suitable tests for evidence of an immunosuppressive effect. The vaccine complies with the test if no significant difference is observed in vaccinated animals compared with controls.

B. Inject two doses of vaccine by one of the intended routes to not fewer than ten cats of the minimum age recommended for vaccination. At the end of the period of time stated in the instructions for use, inject one dose of vaccine to each animal. Where the instructions for use recommend it, administer a third injection after the period indicated. Observe the animals for 14 days after the last administration. The vaccine complies with the test if no abnormal local or systemic reaction occurs during the test.

C. If the vaccine is not contra-indicated for use in pregnant queens, inject two doses of vaccine into each of not fewer than ten cats at different stages of pregnancy. Observe the cats until parturition and note any effects on gestation and the offspring. The vaccine complies with the test if no abnormal local or systemic reaction occurs during the test.

Immunogenicity The test described under Potency is suitable to demonstrate immunogenicity of the vaccine.

IN-PROCESS CONTROL TESTS

During production, suitable immunochemical tests are carried out for the evaluation of the quality and purity of the viral antigens included in the vaccine composition. The values found are within the limits approved for the particular vaccine.

BATCH TESTING
Potency

The test described under Potency is not carried out for routine testing of batches of vaccine. It is carried out, for a given vaccine, on one or more occasions, as decided by or with the agreement of the competent authority; where the test is not carried out, a suitable validated alternative method is used, the criteria for acceptance being set with reference to a batch of vaccine that has given satisfactory results in the test described under Potency.

Bacterial endotoxins

For vaccines produced by recombinant DNA technology with a bacterial host cell such as *Escherichia coli*, a test for bacterial endotoxins (2.6.14) is carried out on each final lot or, where the nature of the adjuvant prevents performance of a satisfactory test, on the antigen immediately before addition of the adjuvant. The value found is within the limit approved for the particular vaccine and which has been shown to be safe for cats.

IDENTIFICATION

When injected into healthy, seronegative cats, the vaccine stimulates the production of specific antibodies against the antigen or antigens stated on the label.

TESTS
Safety

Use two cats of the minimum age recommended for vaccination and that do not have antibodies against feline leukaemia virus. Inject by a recommended route a double dose of vaccine into each animal. Observe the animals for 14 days. The vaccine complies with the test if no abnormal local or systemic reaction is produced.

Inactivation

If the vaccine contains inactivated virus, carry out a test for residual live feline leukaemia virus by making two passages on susceptible cell cultures. No virus is detected. If the vaccine contains an adjuvant, if possible separate the adjuvant from the liquid phase by a method that does not inactivate the virus nor interfere in any other way with the detection of virus.

Sterility

The vaccine complies with the test for sterility prescribed in *Vaccines for veterinary use (0062)*.

POTENCY

Use not fewer than twenty-five susceptible cats of the minimum age recommended for vaccination, free from antibodies against the antigens of feline leukaemia virus and against the feline oncogene membrane antigen (anti-FOCMA antibodies), and showing no viraemia or antigenaemia at the time of the test. Vaccinate not fewer than fifteen cats by a recommended route in accordance with the instructions for use. Keep not fewer than ten cats as controls. Observe the animals for at least 14 days after the last administration of vaccine. Inject by the peritoneal or oronasal route, on one or several occasions, a quantity of a virulent strain of feline leukaemia virus sufficient to induce persistent viraemia or antigenaemia in not fewer than 80 per cent of susceptible animals; use for the challenge an epidemiologically relevant strain consisting predominantly of type A virus. Observe the animals for 15 weeks and, from the third week onwards, test each week for viraemia or antigenaemia (p27 protein) by suitable methods such as immunofluorescence on circulating leucocytes or enzyme-linked immunosorbent assay. A cat is considered persistently infected if it shows positive viraemia or antigenaemia for three consecutive weeks or on five occasions, consecutively or not, between the third and the fifteenth week. The test is not valid if fewer than 80 per cent of the control cats are persistently infected. The vaccine complies with the test if not fewer than 80 per cent of the vaccinated cats show no persistent infection.

LABELLING

The label states the antigen or antigens contained in the vaccine.

Ph Eur

Feline Viral Rhinotracheitis Vaccine, Inactivated

(*Feline Viral Rhinotracheitis Vaccine (Inactivated), Ph Eur monograph 1207*)

Ph Eur

1 DEFINITION

Feline viral rhinotracheitis vaccine (inactivated) is a preparation of a suitable strain of feline rhinotracheitis virus (feline herpesvirus 1), inactivated while maintaining adequate immunogenic properties, or of an inactivated fraction of the virus having adequate immunogenic properties. This monograph applies to vaccines intended for the active immunisation of cats against feline viral rhinotracheitis.

2 PRODUCTION

2-1 PREPARATION OF THE VACCINE

The vaccine virus is grown in cell cultures. The virus harvest is inactivated; the virus may be fragmented and the fragments purified and concentrated. The vaccine may be adjuvanted.

2-2 SUBSTRATE FOR VIRUS PROPAGATION
2-2-1 Cell cultures

The cell cultures comply with the requirements for cell cultures for production of veterinary vaccines (*5.2.4*).

2-3 CHOICE OF VACCINE COMPOSITION

The vaccine is shown to be satisfactory with respect to safety (*5.2.6*) and efficacy (*5.2.7*) for the cats for which it is intended.

The following test for immunogenicity (2-3-1) may be used during the demonstration of efficacy.

2-3-1 Immunogenicity

A test is carried out for each route and method of administration to be recommended for vaccination, using in each case cats 8-12 weeks old. The vaccine administered to each cat is of minimum antigen content and/or potency.

Use for the test not fewer than 20 cats that do not have antibodies against feline herpesvirus 1 or against a fraction of the virus. Vaccinate not fewer than 10 cats, according to the schedule to be recommended. Maintain not fewer than 10 cats as controls. Challenge each cat after 4 weeks by the intranasal route with a sufficient quantity of a suspension of virulent feline herpesvirus 1. Observe the cats at least daily for 14 days after challenge. Collect nasal washings daily on days 2 to 14 after challenge to test for virus excretion. Note daily the body temperature and signs of disease using the scoring system shown below. The vaccine complies with the test if the score for the vaccinated cats is significantly lower than that for the controls.

Sign	Score
Death	10
Depressed state	2
Temperature:	
39.5 °C - 40.0 °C	1
$\geqslant$ 40.0 °C	2
$\leqslant$ 37.0 °C	3
Glossitis	3
Nasal discharge, slight	1
Nasal discharge, copious	2
Cough	2
Sneezing	1
Sneezing, paroxysmal	2
Ocular discharge, slight	1
Ocular discharge, serious	2
Conjunctivitis	2
Weight loss $\geqslant$ 5.0 per cent	5
Virus excretion (total number of days):	
$\leqslant$ 4 days	1
5-7 days	2
> 7 days	3

2-4 MANUFACTURER'S TESTS
2-4-1 Residual live virus

The test for residual live virus is carried out using 2 passages in cell cultures of the same type as those used for preparation of the vaccine or in cell cultures shown to be at least as sensitive; the quantity of inactivated virus harvest used in the test is equivalent to not less than 25 doses of vaccine.

The vaccine complies with the test if no live virus is detected.

2-4-2 Batch potency test

It is not necessary to carry out the Potency test (section 3-5) for each batch of the vaccine if it has been carried out using a batch of vaccine with a minimum potency. Where the test is not carried out, an alternative validated method is used, the criteria for acceptance being set with reference to a batch of vaccine that has given satisfactory results in the test described under Potency. The following test may be used.

Use for the test a group of 15 seronegative mice. Administer to each mouse half a dose of the vaccine to be recommended and, 7 days later, repeat the administration. 21 days after the first injection, take blood samples and determine the level of antibodies against feline herpesvirus 1 by a suitable immunochemical method (*2.7.1*), such as an immunofluorescence technique using pools of serum from groups of 3 mice. The vaccine complies with the test if the antibody levels are not significantly lower than those obtained with a batch of vaccine that has given satisfactory results in the test described under Potency.

3 BATCH TESTS

3-1 Identification

When administered to susceptible animals, the vaccine stimulates the production of specific serum antibodies against feline herpesvirus 1 or against the fraction of the virus used to produce the vaccine.

3-2 Bacteria and fungi

The vaccine and, where applicable, the liquid supplied with it comply with the test for sterility prescribed in the monograph *Vaccines for veterinary use (0062).*

3-3 Safety

Use 2 cats, 8-12 weeks old and preferably that do not have antibodies against feline herpesvirus 1 or against a fraction of the virus or, where justified, use cats that have a low level of such antibodies as long as they have not been vaccinated against feline rhinotracheitis and administration of the vaccine does not cause an anamnestic response. Administer to each cat by a recommended route a double dose of the vaccine. Observe the cats at least daily for 14 days.

The vaccine complies with the test if no cat shows notable signs of disease or dies from causes attributable to the vaccine.

3-4 Residual live virus

Carry out a test for residual live feline herpesvirus 1 using 10 doses of vaccine and 2 passages in cell cultures of the same type as those used for preparation of the vaccine, or in other suitably sensitive cell cultures. The vaccine complies with the test if no live virus is detected. If the vaccine contains an adjuvant that interferes with the test, where possible separate the adjuvant from the liquid phase by a method that does not inactivate or otherwise interfere with detection of live virus.

3-5 Potency

The vaccine complies with the requirements of the test prescribed under Immunogenicity (section 2-3-1) when administered by a recommended route and method. It is not necessary to carry out the potency test for each batch of the vaccine if it has been carried out on a representative batch with minimum potency.

_____ *Ph Eur*

Feline Viral Rhinotracheitis Vaccine, Living

(Feline Viral Rhinotracheitis Vaccine (Live), Freeze-dried, Ph Eur monograph 1206)

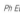 *Ph Eur* _____

1 DEFINITION

Feline viral rhinotracheitis vaccine (live) is a preparation of a suitable strain of feline rhinotracheitis virus (feline herpesvirus 1). This monograph applies to vaccines intended for the active immunisation of cats against feline viral rhinotracheitis.

2 PRODUCTION

2-1 PREPARATION OF THE VACCINE

The vaccine virus is grown in cell cultures.

2-2 SUBSTRATE FOR VIRUS PROPAGATION

2-2-1 Cell cultures

The cell cultures comply with the requirements for cell cultures for production of veterinary vaccines (5.2.4).

2-3 CHOICE OF VACCINE VIRUS

The vaccine virus is shown to be satisfactory with respect to safety (5.2.6) and efficacy (5.2.7) for the cats for which it is intended (including safety for pregnant queens if such use is not contra-indicated).

The following tests for safety (section 2-3-1), increase in virulence (section 2-3-2) and immunogenicity (2-3-3) may be used during the demonstration of safety and efficacy.

2-3-1 Safety

Carry out the test for each route and method of administration to be recommended for vaccination, using in each case cats of the minimum age to be recommended. Use vaccine virus at the least attenuated passage level that will be present between the master seed lot and a batch of the vaccine.

For each test, use not fewer than 10 cats that do not have antibodies against feline herpesvirus 1. Administer to each cat a quantity of the vaccine virus equivalent to not less than 10 times the maximum virus titre likely to be contained in one dose of the vaccine. Observe the cats at least daily for 21 days.

The vaccine virus complies with the test if no cat shows notable signs of disease or dies from causes attributable to the vaccine virus.

2-3-2 Increase in virulence

The test for increase in virulence consists of the administration of the vaccine virus at the least attenuated passage level that will be present between the master seed lot and a batch of the vaccine to 2 cats that do not have antibodies against feline herpesvirus 1, sequential passages, 5 times where possible, to further similar groups and testing of the final recovered virus for increase in virulence. If the properties of the vaccine virus allow sequential passage to 5 groups via natural spreading, this method may be used, otherwise passage as described below is carried out and the maximally passaged virus that has been recovered is tested for increase in virulence. Care must be taken to avoid contamination by virus from previous passages.

Administer to each cat by a route to be recommended a quantity of the vaccine virus that will allow recovery of virus for the passages described below. After 2-4 days, prepare a suspension from the nasal mucus, tonsils and local lymphatic ganglia and the trachea of each cat and pool the samples. Mix, homogenise in 10 ml of buffered saline and decant. Administer 1 ml of the supernatant by the intranasal route to each of 2 other cats. Carry out this passage operation not fewer than 5 times; verify the presence of the virus at each passage. If the virus is not found at a passage level, carry out a second series of passages.

Carry out the test for safety (section 2-3-1) using unpassaged vaccine virus and the maximally passaged virus that has been recovered. Administer the virus by the route to be recommended for vaccination most likely to lead to reversion of virulence.

The vaccine virus complies with the test if no indication of increased virulence of the maximally passaged virus compared with the unpassaged virus is observed. If virus is not recovered at any passage level in the first and second series of passages, the vaccine virus also complies with the test.

2-3-3 Immunogenicity

A test is carried out for each route and method of administration to be recommended for vaccination, using in each case cats 8-12 weeks old. The quantity of vaccine virus to be administered to each cat is not greater than the minimum virus titre to be stated on the label and the virus is at the most attenuated passage level that will be present in a batch of vaccine.

Use for the test not fewer than 20 cats that do not have antibodies against feline herpesvirus 1. Vaccinate not fewer than 10 cats, according to the schedule to be recommended. Maintain not fewer than 10 cats as controls. Challenge each cat after 4 weeks by the intranasal route with a sufficient quantity of a suspension of virulent feline herpesvirus 1. Observe the cats at least daily for 14 days after challenge. Collect nasal washings daily on days 2 to 14 after challenge to test for virus excretion. Note daily the body temperature and signs of disease using the scoring system shown below. The vaccine virus complies with the test if, during the observation period after challenge, the score for the vaccinated cats is significantly lower than that for the controls.

Sign	Score
Death	10
Depressed state	2
Temperature:	
39.5 °C - 40.0 °C	1
⩾ 40.0 °C	2
⩽ 37.0 °C	3
Glossitis	3
Nasal discharge, slight	1
Nasal discharge, copious	2
Cough	2
Sneezing	1
Sneezing, paroxysmal	2
Ocular discharge, slight	1
Ocular discharge, serious	2
Conjunctivitis	2
Weight loss ⩾ 5.0 per cent	5
Virus excretion (total number of days):	
⩽ 4 days	1
5-7 days	2
> 7 days	3

3 BATCH TESTS
3-1 Identification
When mixed with a monospecific antiserum, the vaccine no longer infects susceptible cell cultures into which it is inoculated.

3-2 Bacteria and fungi
The vaccine and, where applicable, the liquid supplied with it comply with the test for sterility prescribed in the monograph *Vaccines for veterinary use (0062)*.

3-3 Mycoplasmas (2.6.7)
The vaccine complies with the test for mycoplasmas.

3-4 Extraneous agents
Neutralise the vaccine virus with a suitable monospecific antiserum against feline herpesvirus 1 and inoculate into cell cultures known for their susceptibility to viruses pathogenic for the cat. Carry out at least one passage and maintain the cultures for 14 days. The vaccine complies with the test if no cytopathic effect develops and there is no sign of the presence of haemadsorbing agents.

3-5 Safety
Use 2 cats, 8-12 weeks old, that do not have antibodies against feline herpesvirus 1. Administer to each cat by a recommended route 10 doses of the vaccine. Observe the cats at least daily for 14 days.

The vaccine complies with the test if no cat shows notable signs of disease or dies from causes attributable to the vaccine.

3-6 Virus titre
Titrate the vaccine virus in suitable cell cultures and at a temperature favourable to replication of the virus. The vaccine complies with the test if one dose contains not less than the minimum virus titre stated on the label.

3-7 Potency
The vaccine complies with the requirements of the test prescribed under Immunogenicity when administered by a recommended route and method. It is not necessary to carry out the potency test for each batch of the vaccine if it has been carried out on a representative batch using a vaccinating dose containing not more than the minimum virus titre stated on the label.

Ph Eur

Ferret and Mink Distemper Vaccine, Living

(Distemper Vaccine (Live) for Mustelids, Freeze-dried, Ph Eur monograph 0449)

Ph Eur

DEFINITION
Freeze-dried distemper vaccine (live) for mustelids is a preparation of a strain of distemper virus that is attenuated for ferrets.

PRODUCTION
The attenuated strain is grown in suitable cell cultures (5.2.4) or in fertilised hen eggs, obtained from healthy flocks.

CHOICE OF VACCINE STRAIN
Only a virus strain shown to be satisfactory with respect to attenuation and immunogenicity may be used in the preparation of the vaccine. The following tests may be used during demonstration of safety (5.2.6) and immunogenicity (5.2.7).

Attenuation When a volume of a viral suspension equivalent to five doses of the vaccine is injected intramuscularly into each of two susceptible ferrets, it does not provoke pathogenic effects within 21 days.

Immunogenicity The test described under Potency is suitable to demonstrate the immunogenicity of the strain.

BATCH TESTING
If the test for potency has been carried out with satisfactory results on a representative batch of vaccine, this test may be omitted as a routine control on other batches of vaccine prepared from the same seed lot, subject to agreement by the competent authority.

IDENTIFICATION
The vaccine reconstituted as stated on the label and mixed with a specific distemper antiserum no longer provokes cytopathic effects in susceptible cell cultures or lesions on the chorio-allantoic membranes of fertilised hen eggs 9 to 11 days old.

TESTS
Safety
Inject by the route stated on the label twice the dose of the reconstituted vaccine into each of two susceptible ferrets free from distemper-virus-neutralising antibodies. Observe the

animals for 21 days. They remain in normal health and no abnormal local or systemic reaction occurs.

Extraneous viruses

Mix the reconstituted vaccine with a monospecific antiserum. It no longer provokes cytopathic effects in susceptible cell cultures. It shows no evidence of haemagglutinating or haemadsorbing agents.

Bacterial and fungal contamination

The reconstituted vaccine complies with the test for sterility prescribed in the monograph on *Vaccines for veterinary use (0062)*.

Mycoplasmas (*2.6.7*)

The reconstituted vaccine complies with the test for mycoplasmas.

Virus titre

Titrate the reconstituted vaccine in suitable cell cultures or fertilised hen eggs 9 to 11 days old. One dose of the vaccine contains not less than the quantity of virus equivalent to the minimum titre stated on the label.

POTENCY

Use seven susceptible ferrets free from distemper-virus-neutralising antibodies. Vaccinate five of the ferrets according to the instructions for use. Keep the two other animals as controls. Observe all the animals for 21 days. Inject intramuscularly into each animal a quantity of distemper virus sufficient to cause the death of a susceptible ferret. Observe the animals for a further 21 days. The test is invalid if one or both of the control ferrets do not die of distemper. The vaccine complies with the test if the vaccinated ferrets remain in normal health.

Ph Eur

Foot and Mouth Disease (Ruminants) Vaccine

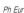

(Foot-and-Mouth Disease (Ruminants) Vaccine (Inactivated), Ph Eur monograph 0063)

Ph Eur

DEFINITION

Foot-and-mouth disease (ruminants) vaccine (inactivated) is a liquid preparation containing one or more serotypes of foot-and-mouth disease virus inactivated without impairing their immunogenic activity. This monograph applies to vaccines intended for protection of ruminants against foot-and-mouth disease.

PRODUCTION

PREPARATION OF THE VACCINE

The virus is grown in suitable cell cultures (*5.2.4*) and then separated from cellular material by filtration or other suitable procedures. The harvested virus is inactivated in suitable conditions and may be concentrated and purified. It is used for the preparation of vaccine immediately or after storage at a temperature shown to be consistent with antigen stability. The vaccine is prepared from inactivated virus by blending with one or more adjuvants. For a given antigen, the quantity of 146S antigen blended in each batch of vaccine is not lower than that of a batch of vaccine that has been found satisfactory with respect to Immunogenicity or in the test described under Potency.

Substrate for virus propagation

The substrate complies with the requirements for cell cultures for production of veterinary vaccines (*5.2.4*).

Validation of the inactivation procedure

During inactivation, the virus titre is monitored by a sensitive and reproducible technique. The inactivation procedure is not satisfactory unless the decrease in virus titre, plotted logarithmically, is linear and extrapolation indicates that there is less than 1 infectious virus unit per 10^4 litres of liquid preparation at the end of inactivation.

CHOICE OF VACCINE COMPOSITION

The vaccine shall be shown to be satisfactory with respect to safety (*5.2.6*) and efficacy (*5.2.7*) in each species for which the vaccine is intended.

Safety

Carry out a safety test for each recommended route and for each species for which the vaccine is intended. Use animals of the minimum age recommended for vaccination and that are free from antibodies against foot-and-mouth disease virus. Inject a double dose of vaccine into not fewer than 10 animals. Observe the animals at least daily for 14 days after the injection. No abnormal local or systemic reaction occurs. If the vaccine is intended for use or may be used in pregnant animals, carry out the test in these animals at the beginning of each trimester for which the use is not contra-indicated and extend the observation period to parturition. No undesirable effect on gestation or the offspring occurs.

Immunogenicity

The test for potency carried out for each recommended route is suitable to demonstrate immunogenicity of the vaccine for cattle.

BULK INACTIVATED ANTIGEN

Identification

The bulk inactivated antigen is identified by a suitable immunochemical method (*2.7.1*).

Residual live virus

The limit of detection of the cell cultures to be used with respect to the virus to be tested is established by determining the number of $CCID_{50}$ and the 146S antigen content of a sample of live virus. The cells are not suitable if an amount of virus corresponding to 1 µg of 146S antigen has less than 10^6 $CCID_{50}$. A proportion of each batch of bulk inactivated antigen representing at least 200 doses is tested for freedom from infectious virus by inoculation into suitable cell cultures. A passage is made during culture of the cells. For this purpose, the sample of the inactivated antigen may be concentrated to allow testing of such large samples in cell cultures. It must be shown that the selected concentration and assay systems are not detrimental to detection of infectious virus within the test sample and that the concentrated inactivated antigen does not interfere with virus replication or cause toxic changes. A positive control is included in each test.

Antigen content

The 146S antigen content of each batch of bulk inactivated antigen is determined by an *in vitro* method (for example, by sucrose density gradient centrifugation and ultraviolet spectrophotometry at 259 nm).

BATCH TESTING

Batch potency test

The test described under Potency is not necessarily carried out for routine testing of batches of vaccine. It is carried out on one or more occasions as decided by or with the agreement of the competent authority. Where the test is not carried out, a suitable validated alternative test is carried out, the criteria for acceptance being set with reference to a batch of vaccine that has given satisfactory results in the test described under Potency and has been shown to be satisfactory with respect to immunogenicity in the target species. The following test may be used after a satisfactory pass level for a given antigen has been established. Once a pass level has been established for a given antigen, the same level may be used when this antigen is formulated in combination with any other provided that the formulation of the vaccine differs only in the antigens included.

Vaccines for use in cattle   Use cattle of the minimum age recommended for vaccination obtained from areas free from foot-and-mouth disease, which have never been vaccinated against foot-and-mouth disease and are free from antibodies neutralising the different serotypes of foot-and-mouth disease virus. Vaccinate not fewer than 5 cattle by the route stated on the label. Use a suitable dose of the vaccine for each animal. After a defined period, not greater than 28 days following vaccination, draw a blood sample and determine individually in each serum the level of antibodies against each serotype used in the preparation of the vaccine by a validated technique (e.g. sero-neutralisation test, ELISA). Titres at least equal to the pass level shall be measured in at least 50 per cent of the animals.

Vaccines for use in other ruminants   The potency of each batch shall be demonstrated in a suitable, validated test. A test in cattle, following the procedures outlined above for vaccines for use in cattle, may be suitable.

Emergency use
In situations of extreme urgency and subject to agreement by the competent authority, a batch of vaccine may be released before completion of the tests and the determination of potency if a test for sterility has been carried out on the bulk inactivated antigen and all other components of the vaccine and if the test for safety and the determination of potency have been carried out on a representative batch of vaccine prepared from the same bulk inactivated antigen. In this context, a batch is not considered to be representative unless it has been prepared with not more than the amount of antigen or antigens and with the same formulation as the batch to be released.

IDENTIFICATION
The serum of a susceptible animal that has been immunised with the vaccine neutralises the serotypes of the virus used to prepare the vaccine, when tested by a suitably sensitive method.

TESTS
Safety
Use 2 non-vaccinated animals of one of the species for which the vaccine is intended, not less than 6 months old, having serum free from foot-and-mouth disease antibodies and coming from regions free from foot-and-mouth disease. Administer a double dose of vaccine to each animal by a recommended route. Observe the animals for 14 days. No abnormal local or systemic reaction occurs.

Sterility
It complies with the test for sterility prescribed in the monograph on *Vaccines for veterinary use (0062)*.

POTENCY
The potency of the vaccine is expressed as the number of 50 per cent cattle protective doses (PD_{50}) contained in the dose stated on the label. The PD_{50} is determined in animals given primary vaccination and challenged by the inoculation of 10 000 ID_{50} of virulent bovine virus of the same serotype as that used in the preparation of the vaccine in the

conditions described below. The vaccine strain may be used for challenge.

The potency is not less than that stated on the label; the minimum potency stated on the label is not less than 3 PD_{50} per dose for cattle.

Carry out a potency test for each serotype of foot-and-mouth disease virus that may be included in the vaccine. The Potency test carried out for a particular serotype will be valid for other vaccines provided that they have the same basic composition and that they have a batch potency with regard to that particular serotype that is not lower than that of the vaccine that has given satisfactory results in the Potency test.

Use cattle not less than 6 months old, obtained from areas free from foot-and-mouth disease, which have never been vaccinated against foot-and-mouth disease and are free from antibodies neutralising the different serotypes of foot-and-mouth disease virus. Vaccinate not fewer than 3 groups of not fewer than 5 cattle per group by the route stated on the label. Use a different dose of the vaccine for each group. Administer the different doses by injecting different volumes of the vaccine and not by dilution of the vaccine. For example, if the label states that the injection of 2 ml corresponds to the administration of 1 dose of vaccine, a 1/4 dose of vaccine would be obtained by injecting 0.5 ml, and a 1/10 dose would be obtained by injecting 0.2 ml. 3 weeks after the vaccination, challenge the vaccinated animals and a control group of 2 animals with a suspension of virus that has been obtained from cattle and that is fully virulent and of the same serotype as that used in the preparation of the vaccine, by inoculating a dose equivalent to approximately 10 000 ID_{50} intradermally into 2 sites on the upper surface of the tongue (0.1 ml per site). Observe the animals for 8 days and then slaughter. Unprotected animals show lesions at sites other than the tongue. Protected animals may display lingual lesions. The test is not valid unless each control animal shows lesions on at least 3 feet. From the number of protected animals in each group, calculate the PD_{50} content of the vaccine.

LABELLING
The label states:
— the serotypes of virus used to prepare the vaccine,
— the minimum potency (PD_{50} per dose) for each serotype of virus used to prepare the vaccine.

Ph Eur

Fowl Cholera Vaccine (Inactivated)

(Ph Eur monograph 1945)

Ph Eur

1 DEFINITION
Fowl cholera vaccine (inactivated) is a preparation of 1 or more suitable strains of 1 or more serovars of *Pasteurella multocida*. This monograph applies to vaccines intended for the active immunisation of chickens, turkeys, ducks and geese against acute fowl cholera.

2 PRODUCTION
2-1 PREPARATION OF THE VACCINE
The seed material is cultured in a suitable medium. If the vaccine contains more than 1 strain of bacterium, the different strains are grown and harvested separately. The bacterial harvests are inactivated. The vaccine may contain an adjuvant.

2-2 CHOICE OF VACCINE COMPOSITION

The vaccine is shown to be satisfactory with respect to safety (5.2.6) and efficacy (5.2.7) for the species for which it is intended. The following tests for safety (section 2-2-1) and immunogenicity (section 2-2-2) may be used during the demonstration of safety and efficacy.

2-2-1 Safety

The test is carried out for each route of administration to be recommended for vaccination and for each avian species for which the vaccine is intended. For each test, use not fewer than 20 birds not older than the minimum age to be recommended for vaccination. In the case of chickens, use chickens from a flock free from specified pathogens (SPF) (5.2.2) and in the case of turkeys, ducks or geese, use birds that have not been vaccinated and that are free from antibodies against *P. multocida*. Administer by a recommended route and method to each bird a double dose of vaccine. If the recommended schedule requires a second dose, administer 1 dose after the recommended interval. Observe the birds at least daily until 21 days after the last administration of the vaccine. The test is not valid if more than 10 per cent of the birds show abnormal clinical signs of disease or die from causes not attributable to the vaccine.
The vaccine complies with the test if no bird shows abnormal clinical signs of disease or dies from causes attributable to the vaccine.

2-2-2 Immunogenicity

The test is carried out for each route of administration to be recommended for vaccination, for each avian species for which the vaccine is intended and for each serovar of *P. multocida* against which protection is claimed. Use for each test not fewer than 30 birds not older than the youngest age to be recommended for vaccination. Use birds that have not been vaccinated and that are free from antibodies against *P. multocida*. For each test, administer to each of not fewer than 20 birds a quantity of the vaccine not greater than 1 dose. If re-vaccination is recommended, repeat this operation after the recommended interval. Maintain not fewer than 10 birds as controls. Challenge each of the birds of both groups 21 days after the last administration by the intramuscular route with a sufficient quantity of virulent *P. multocida*. Observe the birds at least daily for 14 days after challenge. The test is not valid if during the observation period after challenge, fewer than 70 per cent of the control birds die or show signs of infection (such as either clinical signs or bacterial re-isolation in organs) or if during the period before challenge, more than 10 per cent of the birds from the control group or from the vaccinated group show abnormal clinical signs of disease or die from causes not attributable to the vaccine. The vaccine complies with the test if, at the end of the observation period after challenge, not fewer than 70 per cent of the birds from the vaccinated group survive and show no clinical signs of disease. Mild signs that do not persist beyond the observation period may be tolerated.

2-3 Batch potency

It is not necessary to carry out the Potency test (section 3-4) for each batch of the vaccine if it has been carried out using a batch of vaccine with minimum potency. Where the test is not carried out, an alternative validated method is used, the criteria for acceptance being set with reference to a batch of vaccine that has given satisfactory results in the test described under Immunogenicity (section 2-2-2). The following test may be used.

Use not fewer than 15 SPF chickens (5.2.2), 3 to 4 weeks old. Collect serum samples from each vaccinated and control chicken just before vaccination and check the absence of antibodies against each serovar of *P. multocida* in the vaccine. Administer to each of 10 chickens 1 dose of the vaccine by the subcutaneous route. Maintain 5 chickens as controls. Collect serum samples 5 weeks after vaccination from each vaccinated and control chicken. Measure the titres of serum antibodies against each serovar of *P. multocida* stated on the label using a suitable validated serological method. Calculate the mean titres for the group of vaccinates. The test is not valid if specific *P. multocida* antibodies are found: before vaccination in 1 or more sera from chickens to be vaccinated or from controls; in 1 or more sera from control chickens 5 weeks after the time of administration of the vaccine. The vaccine complies with the test if the mean antibody titres of the group of vaccinates are equal to or greater than the titres obtained with a batch that has given satisfactory results in the test described under Immunogenicity (section 2-2-2).

2-4 Bacterial endotoxins

A test for bacterial endotoxins (2.6.14) is carried out on the final lot or, where the nature of the adjuvant prevents performance of a satisfactory test, on the bulk antigen or the mixture of bulk antigens immediately before addition of the adjuvant. The maximum acceptable amount of bacterial endotoxins is that found for a batch of vaccine that has been shown satisfactory in safety test (section 2-2-1). The method chosen for determining the maximum acceptable amount of bacterial endotoxins is used subsequently for testing each batch.

3 BATCH TESTS

3-1 IDENTIFICATION

The vaccine injected into SPF chickens (5.2.2) stimulates the production of antibodies against each of the serovars of *P. multocida* in the vaccine.

3-2 BACTERIA AND FUNGI

The vaccine complies with the test for sterility prescribed in the monograph *Vaccines for veterinary use (0062)*.

3-3 SAFETY

For vaccines recommended for use in chickens, use not fewer than 10 chickens from an SPF flock (5.2.2) and of the minimum age recommended for vaccination. For vaccines recommended for use only in turkeys, ducks or geese, use not fewer than 10 birds of the species likely to be most sensitive to fowl cholera, that do not have antibodies against *P. multocida* and of the minimum age recommended for vaccination. Administer to each bird by a recommended route a double dose of the vaccine. Observe the birds at least daily for 21 days. The test is not valid if more than 20 per cent of the birds show abnormal clinical signs or die from causes not attributable to the vaccine. The vaccine complies with the test if no bird shows notable clinical signs of disease or dies from causes attributable to the vaccine.

3-4 POTENCY

The vaccine complies with the requirements of the test mentioned under Immunogenicity (section 2-2-2) using 1 dose of the vaccine administered by a recommended route.

LABELLING

The label states:
— the serovar(s) used to prepare the vaccine,
— the serovar(s) against which protection is claimed.

Fowl Pox Vaccine, Living

(Fowl-pox Vaccine (Live), Ph Eur monograph 0649)

Ph Eur ___

1. DEFINITION

Fowl-pox vaccine (live) is a preparation of a suitable strain of avian pox virus. This monograph applies to vaccines intended for administration to chickens for active immunisation.

2. PRODUCTION

2-1. PREPARATION OF THE VACCINE

The vaccine virus is grown in embryonated hens' eggs or in cell cultures.

2-2. SUBSTRATE FOR VIRUS PROPAGATION

2-2-1. Embryonated hens' eggs

If the vaccine virus is grown in embryonated hens' eggs, they are obtained from flocks free from specified pathogens (SPF) (5.2.2).

2-2-2. Cell cultures

If the vaccine virus is grown in cell cultures, they comply with the requirements for cell cultures for production of veterinary vaccines (5.2.4).

2-3. SEED LOTS

2-3-1. Extraneous agents

The master seed lot complies with the tests for extraneous agents in seed lots (2.6.24). In these tests on the master seed lot, the organisms used are not more than 5 passages from the master seed lot at the start of the tests.

2-4. CHOICE OF VACCINE VIRUS

The vaccine virus shall be shown to be satisfactory with respect to safety (5.2.6) and efficacy (5.2.7) for the chickens for which it is intended.

The following tests for safety (section 2-4-1), increase in virulence (section 2-4-2) and immunogenicity (section 2-4-3) may be used during demonstration of safety and immunogenicity.

2-4-1. Safety

Carry out the test for each route and method of administration to be recommended for vaccination using in each case chickens not older than the youngest age to be recommended for vaccination. Use vaccine virus at the least attenuated passage level that will be present between the master seed lot and a batch of the vaccine. For each test use not fewer than 20 chickens, from an SPF flock (5.2.2). Administer to each chicken a quantity of the vaccine virus equivalent to not less than 10 times the maximum virus titre likely to be contained in a dose of the vaccine. Observe the chickens at least daily for 21 days. The test is not valid if more than 10 per cent of the chickens die from causes not attributable to the vaccine virus. The vaccine virus complies with the test if no chicken shows notable clinical signs of fowl pox or dies from causes attributable to the vaccine virus.

2-4-2. Increase in virulence

Administer by a suitable route a quantity of the vaccine virus that will allow recovery of virus for the passages described below to each of 5 chickens not older than the minimum age to be recommended for vaccination and from an SPF flock (5.2.2). Use the vaccine virus at the least attenuated passage level that will be present between the master seed lot and a batch of the vaccine. Prepare 4 to 7 days after administration a suspension from the induced skin lesions of each chicken and pool these samples. Administer 0.2 ml of the pooled samples by cutaneous scarification of the comb or other unfeathered part of the body, or by another suitable method to each of 5 other chickens not older than the minimum age

to be recommended for vaccination and from an SPF flock (5.2.2). Carry out this passage operation not fewer than 5 times; verify the presence of the virus at each passage. Care must be taken to avoid contamination by virus from previous passages. If the virus is not found at a passage level, carry out a second series of passages. Carry out the test for safety (section 2-4-1) using the unpassaged vaccine virus and the maximally passaged virus that has been recovered. Administer the virus by the route recommended for vaccination likely to be the least safe. The vaccine virus complies with the test if no indication of increase in virulence of the maximally passaged virus compared with the unpassaged virus is observed. If virus is not recovered at any passage level in the first and second series of passages, the vaccine virus also complies with the test.

2-4-3. Immunogenicity

A test is carried out for each route and method of administration to be recommended using in each case chickens not older than the youngest age to be recommended for vaccination. The quantity of the vaccine virus administered to each chicken is not greater than the minimum virus titre to be stated on the label and the virus is at the most attenuated passage level that will be present in a batch of the vaccine. Use for the test not fewer than 30 chickens of the same origin and from an SPF flock (5.2.2). Vaccinate by a recommended route not fewer than 20 chickens. Maintain not fewer than 10 chickens as controls. Challenge each chicken after 21 days by the feather-follicle route with a sufficient quantity of virulent fowl-pox virus. Observe the chickens at least daily for 21 days after challenge. Record the deaths and the number of surviving chickens that show clinical signs of disease. Examine each surviving chicken for macroscopic lesions: cutaneous lesions of the comb, wattle and other unfeathered areas of the skin and diphtherical lesions of the mucous membranes of the oro-pharyngeal area.

The test is not valid if:
— during the observation period after challenge fewer than 90 per cent of the control chickens die or show severe clinical signs of fowl pox, including notable macroscopical lesions of the skin or mucous membranes of the oro-pharyngeal area,
— and/or during the period between vaccination and challenge, more than 10 per cent of the control or vaccinated chickens show abnormal clinical signs or die from causes not attributable to the vaccine.

The vaccine virus complies with the test if during the observation period after challenge not less than 90 per cent of the vaccinated chickens survive and show no notable clinical signs of disease, including macroscopical lesions of the skin and mucous membranes of the oro-pharyngeal area.

3. BATCH TESTS

3-1. Identification

Carry out an immunostaining test in cell cultures to demonstrate the presence of the vaccine virus. For egg adapted strains, inoculate the vaccine into eggs and notice the characteristic lesions.

3-2. Bacteria and fungi

Vaccines intended for administration by injection, scarification or piercing of the wing web comply with the test for sterility prescribed in the monograph *Vaccines for veterinary use (0062)*.

Vaccines not intended for administration by injection, scarification or piercing of the wing web either comply with the test for sterility prescribed in the monograph *Vaccines for veterinary use (0062)* or with the following test: carry out a quantitative test for bacterial and fungal contamination; carry out identification tests for microorganisms detected in the vaccine; the vaccine does not contain pathogenic microorganisms and contains not more than 1 non-pathogenic microorganism per dose.

Any liquid supplied with the vaccine complies with the test for sterility prescribed in the monograph *Vaccines for veterinary use (0062)*.

3-3. Mycoplasmas

The vaccine complies with the test for mycoplasmas *(2.6.7)*.

3-4. Extraneous agents

The vaccine complies with the tests for extraneous agents in batches of finished product *(2.6.25)*.

3-5. Safety

Use not fewer than 10 chickens from an SPF flock *(5.2.2)* of the youngest age recommended for vaccination. For vaccines recommended for use in chickens older than 6 weeks, chickens 6 weeks old may be used. Administer 10 doses of the vaccine to each chicken by a recommended route. Observe the chickens at least daily for 21 days. The test is not valid if more than 20 per cent of the chickens show abnormal clinical signs or die from causes not attributable to the vaccine.

The vaccine complies with the test if no chicken shows notable clinical signs of disease or dies from causes attributable to the vaccine.

3-6. Virus titre

Titrate the vaccine virus by inoculation into embryonated hens' eggs from an SPF flock *(5.2.2)* or into suitable cell cultures *(5.2.4)*. The vaccine complies with the test if 1 dose contains not less than the minimum virus titre stated on the label.

3-7. Potency

The vaccine complies with the requirements of the test prescribed under Immunogenicity (section 2-4-3) when administered according to the recommended schedule by a recommended route and method. It is not necessary to carry out the potency test for each batch of the vaccine if it has been carried out on a representative batch using a vaccinating dose containing not more than the minimum virus titre stated on the label.

Ph Eur

Furunculosis Vaccine for Salmonids, Inactivated

(Furunculosis Vaccine (Inactivated, Oil-Adjuvanted, Injectable) for Salmonids, Ph Eur monograph 1521)

Ph Eur

DEFINITION

Furunculosis vaccine (inactivated, oil-adjuvanted, injectable) for salmonids is prepared from cultures of one or more suitable strains of *Aeromonas salmonicida* subsp. *salmonicida*.

PRODUCTION

The strains of *A. salmonicida* are cultured and harvested separately. The harvests are inactivated by a suitable method. They may be purified and concentrated. Whole or disrupted cells may be used and the vaccine may contain extracellular products of the bacterium released into the growth medium. The vaccine contains an oily adjuvant.

CHOICE OF VACCINE COMPOSITION

The strains included in the vaccine are shown to be suitable with respect to production of antigens of assumed immunological importance. The vaccine is shown to be satisfactory with respect to safety *(5.2.6)* and efficacy *(5.2.7)* in the species of fish for which it is intended. The following tests may be used during demonstration of safety and immunogenicity.

Safety A. During development of the vaccine, safety is tested on 3 different batches. A test is carried out in each species of fish for which the vaccine is intended. The fish used are from a population that does not have specific antibodies against *A. salmonicida* subsp. *salmonicida* and has not been vaccinated against or exposed to furunculosis. The test is carried out in the conditions recommended for the use of the vaccine with a water temperature not less than 10 °C. An amount of vaccine corresponding to twice the recommended dose per mass unit is administered intraperitoneally into each of not fewer than 50 fish of the minimum body mass recommended for vaccination. The fish are observed for 21 days. No abnormal local or systemic reaction occurs. The test is invalid if more than 6 per cent of the fish die from causes not attributable to the vaccine.

B. Safety is also demonstrated in field trials by administering the intended dose to a sufficient number of fish in not fewer than 2 sets of premises. Samples of 30 fish are taken on 3 occasions (after vaccination, at the middle of the rearing period and at slaughter) and examined for local reactions in the body cavity. Moderate lesions involving localised adhesions between viscera or between viscera and the abdominal wall and slight opaqueness and/or sparse pigmentation of the peritoneum are acceptable. Extensive lesions including adhesions between greater parts of the abdominal organs, massive pigmentation and/or obvious thickening and opaqueness of greater areas of the peritoneum are unacceptable if they occur in more than 10 per cent of the fish in any sample. Such lesions include adhesions that give the viscera a "one-unit" appearance and/or lead to manifest laceration of the peritoneum following evisceration.

Immunogenicity The test described under Potency is suitable to demonstrate the immunogenicity of the vaccine.

BATCH TESTING

Batch potency test

For routine testing of batches of vaccine, the test described under Potency may be carried out using not fewer than 30 fish per group; alternatively, a suitable validated test based on antibody response may be carried out, the criteria being set with reference to a batch of vaccine that has given satisfactory results in the test described under Potency. The following test may be used after a satisfactory correlation with the test described under Potency has been established.

Use fish from a population that does not have specific antibodies against *A. salmonicida* subsp. *salmonicida* and that are within defined limits for body mass. Carry out the test at a defined temperature. Inject intraperitoneally into each of not fewer than 25 fish one dose of vaccine, according to the instructions for use. Perform mock vaccination on a control group of not fewer than 10 fish. Collect blood samples at a defined time after vaccination. Determine for each sample the level of specific antibodies against *A. salmonicida* subsp. *salmonicida* by a suitable immunochemical method *(2.7.1)*. The vaccine complies with the test if the mean level of antibodies is not significantly lower than that found for a batch that gave satisfactory results in the test described under Potency. The test is not valid if the control group shows antibodies against *A. salmonicida* subsp. *salmonicida*.

IDENTIFICATION

When injected into fish that do not have specific antibodies against *A. salmonicida*, the vaccine stimulates the production of such antibodies.

TESTS

Safety

Use not fewer than 10 fish of one of the species for which the vaccine is intended, having, where possible, the minimum body mass recommended for vaccination; if fish of the minimum body mass are not available, use fish not greater than twice this mass. Use fish from a population that preferably does not have specific antibodies against *A. salmonicida* subsp. *salmonicida* or, where justified, use fish from a population with a low level of such antibodies as long as they have not been vaccinated against or exposed to furunculosis and administration of the vaccine does not cause an anamnestic response. Carry out the test in the conditions recommended for use of the vaccine with a water temperature not less than 10 °C. Administer intraperitoneally to each fish an amount of vaccine corresponding to twice the recommended dose per mass unit. Observe the animals for 21 days. No abnormal local or systemic reaction attributable to the vaccine occurs. The test is invalid if more than 10 per cent of the fish die from causes not attributable to the vaccine.

Sterility

The vaccine complies with the test for sterility prescribed in the monograph on *Vaccines for veterinary use (0062)*.

POTENCY

Carry out the test according to a protocol defining limits of body mass for the fish, water source, water flow and temperature limits, and preparation of a standardised challenge. Vaccinate not fewer than 100 fish by a recommended route, according to the instructions for use. Perform mock vaccination on a control group of not fewer than 100 fish; mark vaccinated and control fish for identification. Keep all the fish in the same tank or mix equal numbers of controls and vaccinates in each tank if more than one tank is used. Carry out challenge by injection at a fixed time interval after vaccination, defined according to the statement regarding development of immunity. Use for challenge a culture of *A. salmonicida* subsp. *salmonicida* whose virulence has been verified. Observe the fish daily until at least 60 per cent specific mortality is reached in the control group. Plot for both vaccinates and controls a curve of specific mortality against time from challenge and determine by interpolation the time corresponding to 60 per cent specific mortality in controls. The test is invalid if the specific mortality is less than 60 per cent in the control group 21 days after the first death in the fish. Read from the curve for vaccinates the mortality (*M*) at the time corresponding to 60 per cent mortality in controls. Calculate the relative percentage survival (RPS) from the expression:

$$\left(1 - \frac{M}{60}\right) \times 100$$

The vaccine complies with the test if the RPS is not less than 80 per cent.

LABELLING

The label states information on the time needed for development of immunity after vaccination under the range of conditions corresponding to the recommended use.

Infectious Avian Encephalomyelitis Vaccine, Living

Epidemic Tremor Vaccine, Living

(Avian Infectious Encephalomyelitis Vaccine (Live), Ph Eur monograph 0588)

Ph Eur ___

1. DEFINITION

Avian infectious encephalomyelitis vaccine (live) is a preparation of a suitable strain of avian encephalomyelitis virus. This monograph applies to vaccines intended for administration to non-laying breeder chickens to protect passively their future progeny and/or to prevent vertical transmission of virus via the egg.

2. PRODUCTION

2-1. PREPARATION OF THE VACCINE

The vaccine virus is grown in embryonated hens' eggs or in cell cultures.

2-2. SUBSTRATE FOR VIRUS PROPAGATION

2-2-1. Embryonated hens' eggs

If the vaccine virus is grown in embryonated hens' eggs, they are obtained from flocks free from specified pathogens (SPF) (*5.2.2*).

2-2-2. Cell cultures

If the vaccine virus is grown in cell cultures, they comply with the requirements for cell cultures for production of veterinary vaccines (*5.2.4*).

2-3. SEED LOTS

2-3-1. Extraneous agents

The master seed lot complies with the tests for extraneous agents in seed lots (*2.6.24*). In these tests on the master seed lot, the organisms used are not more than 5 passages from the master seed lot at the start of the tests.

2-4. CHOICE OF VACCINE VIRUS

The vaccine virus shall be shown to be satisfactory with respect to safety (*5.2.6*) and efficacy (*5.2.7*) for the chickens for which it is intended.

The following tests for safety (section 2-4-1), increase in virulence (section 2-4-2) and immunogenicity (section 2-4-3) may be used during the demonstration of safety and immunogenicity.

2-4-1. Safety

Carry out the test for each route and method of administration to be recommended for vaccination using in each case non-laying breeder chickens not older than the youngest age to be recommended for vaccination. Use vaccine virus at the least attenuated passage level that will be present between the master seed lot and a batch of the vaccine. For each test, use not fewer than 20 chickens from an SPF flock (*5.2.2*). Administer to each chicken a quantity of the vaccine virus equivalent to not less than 10 times the maximum virus titre likely to be contained in 1 dose of the vaccine. Observe the chickens at least daily for 21 days. The test is not valid if more than 10 per cent of the chickens show abnormal clinical signs or die from causes not attributable to the vaccine virus. The vaccine virus complies with the test if no chicken shows notable clinical signs of avian infectious encephalomyelitis or dies from causes attributable to the vaccine virus.

2-4-2. Increase in virulence

The test for increase in virulence consists of the administration of the vaccine virus at the least attenuated passage level that will be present between the master seed lot and a batch of vaccine to a group of five 1-day-old chickens from an SPF flock (5.2.2), sequential passages, 5 times where possible, to further similar groups of 1-day-old chickens, and testing of the final recovered virus for increase in virulence. If the properties of the vaccine virus allow sequential passage to 5 groups via natural spreading, this method may be used, otherwise passage as described below is carried out and the maximally passaged virus that has been recovered is tested for increase in virulence. Care must be taken to avoid contamination by virus from previous passages. Administer by a recommended route and method, a quantity of the vaccine virus that will allow recovery of virus for the passages described below. 5 to 7 days later, prepare a suspension from the brain of each chick and pool these samples. Administer a suitable volume of the pooled samples by the oral route to each of 5 other chickens of the same age and origin. Carry out this passage operation not fewer than 5 times; verify the presence of the virus at each passage. If the virus is not found at a passage level, carry out a second series of passages. Carry out the test for safety (section 2-4-1) using the unpassaged vaccine virus and the maximally passaged vaccine virus that has been recovered. The vaccine virus complies with the test if no indication of increase in virulence of the maximally passaged virus compared with the unpassaged virus is observed. If virus is not recovered at any passage level in the first and second series of passages, the vaccine virus also complies with the test.

2-4-3. Immunogenicity

If the vaccine is recommended for passive protection of future progeny carry out test 2-4-3-1. If the vaccine is recommended for prevention of vertical transmission of virus via the egg, carry out test 2-4-3-2. A test is carried out for each route and method of administration to be recommended, using in each case chickens from an SPF flock (5.2.2) not older than the youngest age to be recommended for vaccination. The quantity of the vaccine virus administered to each chicken is not greater than the minimum titre to be stated on the label and the virus is at the most attenuated passage level that will be present in a batch of the vaccine.

2-4-3-1. Passive immunity in chickens Vaccinate not fewer than 20 breeder chickens from an SPF flock (5.2.2). Maintain separately not fewer than 10 breeder chickens of the same age and origin as controls. At the peak of lay, hatch not fewer than 25 chickens from eggs from vaccinated breeder chickens and 10 chickens from non-vaccinated breeder chickens. At 2 weeks of age, challenge each chicken by the intracerebral route with a sufficient quantity of virulent avian encephalomyelitis virus. Observe the chickens at least daily for 21 days after challenge. Record the deaths and the number of surviving chickens that show clinical signs of disease. The test is not valid if:

— during the observation period after challenge fewer than 80 per cent of the control chickens die or show severe clinical signs of avian infectious encephalomyelitis,

— and/or during the period between the vaccination and challenge more than 15 per cent of control or vaccinated chickens show abnormal clinical signs or die from causes not attributable to the vaccine.

The vaccine virus complies with the test if during the observation period after challenge not fewer than 80 per cent of the progeny of vaccinated chickens survive and show no notable clinical signs of disease.

2-4-3-2. Passive immunity in embryos Vaccinate not fewer than 20 breeder chickens from an SPF flock (5.2.2). Maintain separately not fewer than 10 breeder chickens of the same age and origin as controls. At the peak of lay, incubate not fewer than 36 eggs from the 2 groups, vaccinated and controls, and carry out an embryo sensitivity test. On the sixth day of incubation inoculate $100\,EID_{50}$ of the Van Roekel strain of avian encephalomyelitis virus into the yolk sacs of the eggs. 12 days after inoculation examine the embryos for specific lesions of avian encephalomyelitis (muscular atrophy). Deaths during the first 24 h are considered to be non-specific. The test is not valid if fewer than 80 per cent of the control embryos show lesions of avian encephalomyelitis. The test is not valid if fewer than 80 per cent of the embryos can be given an assessment. The vaccine virus complies with the test if not fewer than 80 per cent of the embryos in the vaccinated group show no lesions of avian encephalomyelitis.

3. BATCH TESTS

3-1. Identification

The vaccine, diluted if necessary and mixed with a monospecific avian encephalomyelitis virus antiserum, no longer infects embryonated hens' eggs from an SPF flock (5.2.2) or susceptible cell cultures (5.2.4) into which it is inoculated.

3-2. Bacteria and fungi

Vaccines intended for administration by injection comply with the test for sterility prescribed in the monograph *Vaccines for veterinary use (0062)*.

Vaccines not intended for administration by injection either comply with the test for sterility prescribed in the monograph *Vaccines for veterinary use (0062)* or with the following test: carry out a quantitative test for bacterial and fungal contamination; carry out identification tests for microorganisms detected in the vaccine; the vaccine does not contain pathogenic microorganisms and contains not more than 1 non-pathogenic microorganism per dose.

Any liquid supplied with the vaccine complies with the test for sterility prescribed in the monograph *Vaccines for veterinary use (0062)*.

3-3. Mycoplasmas

The vaccine complies with the test for mycoplasmas (2.6.7).

3-4. Extraneous agents

The vaccine complies with the tests for extraneous agents in batches of finished product (2.6.25).

3-5. Safety

Use not fewer than 10 chickens not older than the minimum age recommended for vaccination and from an SPF flock (5.2.2). Administer by a recommended route and method to each chicken 10 doses of the vaccine. Observe the chickens at least daily for 21 days. The test is not valid if more than 20 per cent of the chickens show abnormal clinical signs or die from causes not attributable to the vaccine. The vaccine complies with the test if no chicken shows notable clinical signs of disease or dies from causes attributable to the vaccine.

3-6. Virus titre

Titrate the vaccine virus by inoculation into embryonated hens' eggs from an SPF flock (5.2.2) or into suitable cell cultures (5.2.4). The vaccine complies with the test if 1 dose contains not less than the minimum virus titre stated on the label.

3-7. Potency

Depending on the indications, the vaccine complies with the requirements of 1 or both of the tests prescribed under Immunogenicity (section 2-4-3-1, 2-4-3-2), when administered by a recommended route and method. It is not necessary to carry out the potency test for each batch of the vaccine if it has been carried out on a representative batch using a vaccinating dose containing not more than the minimum virus titre stated on the label.

Ph Eur

Infectious Bovine Rhinotracheitis Vaccine, Living

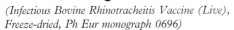

(Infectious Bovine Rhinotracheitis Vaccine (Live), Freeze-dried, Ph Eur monograph 0696)

Ph Eur

DEFINITION

Freeze-dried infectious bovine rhinotracheitis vaccine (live) is a preparation of one or more attenuated strains of infectious bovine rhinotracheitis virus (bovine herpesvirus 1).

PRODUCTION

The virus is grown in suitable cell cultures (*5.2.4*). The viral suspension is collected and mixed with a suitable stabilising solution. The mixture is subsequently freeze-dried.

CHOICE OF VACCINE STRAIN

Only a virus strain shown to be satisfactory with respect to the following characteristics may be used in the preparation of the vaccine: safety (including absence of abortigenicity and passage through the placenta); reversion to virulence and immunogenicity. The strain may have markers.

The following tests may be used during demonstration of safety (*5.2.6*) and efficacy (*5.2.7*)

Safety   Use 5 calves 3 months old, or of the minimum age to be recommended for vaccination if this is less than 3 months, and that do not have antibodies against infectious bovine rhinotracheitis virus. Administer to each calf, by the intended route, a quantity of virus corresponding to 10 doses of vaccine. The calves are observed for 21 days. No abnormal local or systemic reaction occurs.

Abortigenicity and passage through the placenta   24 pregnant cows that do not have antibodies against infectious bovine rhinotracheitis virus are used for the test: 8 of the cows are in the fourth month of pregnancy, 8 in the fifth month and 8 in the sixth or seventh month. A quantity of virus equivalent to ten doses of vaccine is administered by the intended route to each cow. The cows are observed until the end of pregnancy. If abortion occurs, tests for infectious bovine rhinotracheitis virus are carried out; neither the virus nor viral antigens are present in the foetus or placenta. A test for antibodies against infectious bovine rhinotracheitis virus is carried out on calves born at term before ingestion of colostrum; no such antibodies are found.

Reversion to virulence   Suitable samples are taken from the 5 calves used for the test for safety at a time when the vaccinal virus can be easily detected. The presence and titre of virus in the samples are verified. The samples are then mixed and administered intranasally to 2 other calves of the same age having no antibodies against bovine rhinotracheitis virus. 5 further serial passages are carried out. The presence of the virus is verified at each passage. No abnormal local or systemic reaction occurs.

Immunogenicity   The test described under Potency is suitable to demonstrate immunogenicity.

BATCH TESTING

If the test for potency has been carried out with satisfactory results on a representative batch of vaccine, this test may be omitted as a routine control on other batches of vaccine prepared from the same seed lot, subject to agreement by the competent authority.

IDENTIFICATION

A. Reconstitute the vaccine as stated on the label. When mixed with a suitable quantity of a monospecific antiserum, the reconstituted vaccine is no longer able to infect susceptible cell cultures into which it is inoculated.

B. Any markers of the strain are verified.

TESTS

Safety

Use 2 calves 3 months old or of the minimum age recommended for vaccination if this is less than 3 months, having no antibodies against bovine rhinotracheitis virus. Administer 10 doses of the reconstituted vaccine to each calf by a recommended route. Observe the calves for 21 days. No abnormal local or systemic reaction occurs.

Bacterial and fungal contamination

The reconstituted vaccine complies with the test for sterility prescribed in the monograph on *Vaccines for veterinary use (0062)*.

Mycoplasmas (*2.6.7*)

The reconstituted vaccine complies with the test for mycoplasmas.

Extraneous viruses

Neutralise the vaccine using a monospecific antiserum and inoculate into suitable cell cultures. Maintain the cultures for 14 days and make a passage at 7 days. The cell cultures show no signs of viral contamination.

Virus titre

Titrate the reconstituted vaccine in susceptible cell cultures at a temperature favourable to replication of the virus. One dose of the vaccine contains not less than the quantity of virus equivalent to the minimum virus titre stated on the label.

POTENCY

Use susceptible calves, 2 to 3 months old and free from antibodies neutralising infectious bovine rhinotracheitis virus. Administer to five calves, by the route stated on the label a volume of the reconstituted vaccine containing a quantity of virus equivalent to the minimum virus titre stated on the label. Keep 2 calves as controls. After 21 days, administer intranasally to the seven calves a quantity of infectious bovine rhinotracheitis virus sufficient to produce typical signs of disease such as fever, ocular and nasal discharge and ulceration of the nasal mucosa in a susceptible calf. Observe the animals for 21 days. The vaccinated calves show no more than mild signs; the controls show typical signs. In not fewer than 4 of the 5 vaccinated calves, the maximum virus titre found in the nasal mucus is at least 100 times lower than the average of the maximum titres found in the control calves; the average number of days on which virus is excreted is at least 3 days less in vaccinated calves than in the control calves.

Ph Eur

Infectious Bursal Disease Vaccine, Inactivated

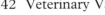

Gumboro Disease Vaccine, Inactivated

(Avian Infectious Bursal Disease Vaccine (Inactivated),
Ph Eur monograph 0960)

CAUTION *Accidental Injection of oily vaccine can cause serious local reactions in man. Expert medical advice should be sought immediately and the doctor should be informed that the vaccine is an oil emulsion.*

Ph Eur _____

DEFINITION

Inactivated infectious avian bursal disease vaccine consists of an emulsion or a suspension of a suitable strain of infectious avian bursal disease virus type 1 which has been inactivated in such a manner that immunogenic activity is retained. The vaccine is for use in breeding domestic fowl to protect their progeny from infectious avian bursal disease.

PRODUCTION

The virus is propagated in fertilised eggs from healthy flocks, in suitable cell cultures (5.2.4) or in chickens from a flock free from specified pathogens (5.2.2).

An amplification test for residual live infectious avian bursal disease virus is carried out on each batch of antigen immediately after inactivation and on the final bulk vaccine or, if the vaccine contains an adjuvant, on the bulk antigen or the mixture of bulk antigens immediately before the addition of any adjuvant, to confirm inactivation; the test is carried out in fertilised hen eggs or in suitable cell cultures or, where chickens have been used for production of the vaccine, in chickens from a flock free from specified pathogens (5.2.2); the quantity of inactivated virus used in the test is equivalent to not less than ten doses of the vaccine. No live virus is detected.

The vaccine may contain one or more suitable adjuvants.

CHOICE OF VACCINE COMPOSITION

The vaccine is shown to be satisfactory with respect to safety (5.2.6) and immunogenicity (5.2.7). The following test may be used during demonstration of efficacy.

Immunogenicity Each of at least twenty chickens from a flock free from specified pathogens (5.2.2), and of the recommended age for vaccination (close to the point of lay), is injected with the minimum recommended dose of vaccine by one of the recommended routes. 4 to 6 weeks later serum samples are collected from each bird and the antibody response is measured in a serum-neutralisation (SN) test. A suitable standard, calibrated in Ph. Eur. Units against *infectious avian bursal disease serum BRP*, is included in the test. The vaccine complies with the test if the mean antibody level in the sera from the vaccinated birds is at least 10 000 Ph. Eur. Units per millilitre.

Eggs are collected for hatching 5 to 7 weeks after vaccination and the test described below is carried out with 3-week-old chickens from that egg collection. Eggs are collected again towards the end of the period of lay and the test is repeated with chickens from that egg collection which are at least 15 days old.

Twenty-five chickens from vaccinated hens and ten control chickens of the same breed and age from unvaccinated hens are challenged with an eye-drop application of a quantity of a virulent strain of infectious avian bursal disease virus sufficient to produce severe signs of disease, including lesions of the bursa of Fabricius, in all unvaccinated chickens. 3 to 4 days after challenge, the bursa of Fabricius is removed from each chicken. The bursae are examined for evidence of infection by histological examination or by testing for the presence of infectious avian bursal disease antigen in an agar-gel precipitation test. The vaccine complies with the test if three or fewer of the chickens from vaccinated hens show evidence of infectious avian bursal disease infection. The test is not valid unless all the chickens from unvaccinated hens are affected.

Where there is more than one recommended route of administration, the test described under Potency is carried out in parallel with the above immunogenicity test, using different groups of birds for each recommended route. The serological response of the birds inoculated by routes other than that used in the immunogenicity test is not significantly less than that of the group vaccinated by that route.

IDENTIFICATION

In chickens with no antibodies to infectious avian bursal disease virus type 1, the vaccine stimulates the production of specific antibodies.

TESTS
Safety

Inject twice the vaccinating dose by one of the recommended routes into each of ten chickens, 14 to 28 days old, from flocks free from specified pathogens (5.2.2). Observe the birds for 21 days. No abnormal local or systemic reaction occurs. *Note: this test may be omitted if inactivation test C is carried out.*

Inactivation

A. For vaccine prepared with embryo-adapted strains of virus, inject two-fifths of a dose into the allantoic cavity or onto the chorio-allantoic membrane of ten 9- to 11-day-old fertilised hen eggs from a flock free from specified pathogens (SPF eggs) (5.2.2). Incubate the eggs and observe for 6 days. Pool separately the allantoic liquid or membranes from eggs containing live embryos, and that from eggs containing dead embryos, excluding those that die from non-specific causes within 24 h of the injection.

Inject into the allantoic cavity or onto the chorio-allantoic membrane of each of ten 9- to 11-day-old SPF eggs 0.2 ml of the pooled allantoic liquid or crushed chorio-allantoic membranes from the live embryos and, into each of ten similar eggs, 0.2 ml of the pooled liquid or membranes from the dead embryos and incubate for 6 days. Examine each embryo for lesions of infectious avian bursal disease.

If more than 20 per cent of the embryos die at either stage repeat that stage. The vaccine complies with the test if there is no evidence of lesions of infectious avian bursal disease and if, in any repeat test, not more than 20 per cent of the embryos die from non-specific causes.

Antibiotics may be used in the test to control extraneous bacterial infection.

B. For vaccine prepared with cell-culture-adapted strains of virus, inoculate ten doses of the vaccine into suitable cell cultures. If the vaccine contains an oil adjuvant, eliminate it by suitable means. Incubate at 38 ± 1 °C for 7 days. Make a passage on another set of cell cultures and incubate at 38 ± 1 °C for 7 days. The cultures show no signs of infection.

C. For vaccine prepared with strains of virus not adapted to embryos or cell cultures, inject two doses intramuscularly into each of twenty 14- to 28-day-old chickens from flocks free from specified pathogens (5.2.2). 4 days later, kill ten of the chickens and remove the bursa of Fabricius from each chicken. Pool the bursae and homogenise in an equal volume of a suitable liquid. Inject 1 ml of the bursal homogenate into each of a further ten chickens of the same age and from the same source. Examine microscopically the bursa of Fabricius of each remaining chicken from the first group and of each chicken from the second group 21 days after the injection; there is no evidence of infectious avian bursal disease infection. In addition there are no signs of any disease attributable to the vaccine and no abnormal local reaction develops. The chickens of the second group do not have antibodies against infectious avian bursal disease virus when examined 21 days after the injection.

Extraneous agents

Collect serum samples from each of the birds used in the safety test or inactivation test C, three weeks after vaccination. Carry out tests for antibodies to the following agents by the methods prescribed for *chicken flocks free from specified pathogens for the production and quality control of vaccines (5.2.2)*: avian encephalomyelitis virus, avian leucosis viruses, haemagglutinating avian adenovirus, infectious bronchitis virus, infectious laryngotracheitis virus, influenza A virus, Marek's disease virus, Newcastle disease virus. The vaccine does not stimulate the formation of antibodies against these agents.

Sterility

The vaccine complies with the test for sterility prescribed in the monograph on *Vaccines for veterinary use (0062)*.

POTENCY

Vaccinate each of not fewer than ten chickens, 4 weeks of age and from a flock free from specified pathogens (5.2.2), with one dose of vaccine by one of the recommended routes. 4 to 6 weeks later, collect serum samples from each bird and ten unvaccinated control birds of the same age and from the same source. Measure the antibody response in a serum-neutralisation test. Include in the test a suitable standard, calibrated in Ph.Eur. Units against *infectious avian bursal disease serum BRP*. The mean antibody level in the sera from the vaccinated birds is not less than 10 000 Ph. Eur. Units per millilitre. There are no antibodies in the sera of the unvaccinated birds.

LABELLING

The label states whether the strain in the vaccine is embryo-adapted or cell-culture-adapted.

_____ *Ph Eur*

Infectious Bursal Disease Vaccine, Living

Gumboro Disease Vaccine, Living

(*Avian Infectious Bursal Disease Vaccine (Live)*, Ph Eur monograph 0587)

Ph Eur _____

1. DEFINITION

Avian infectious bursal disease vaccine (live) [Gumboro disease vaccine (live)] is a preparation of a suitable strain of infectious bursal disease virus type 1. This monograph applies to vaccines intended for administration to chickens for active immunisation; it applies to vaccines containing strains of low virulence but not to those containing strains of higher virulence that may be needed for disease control in certain epidemiological situations.

2. PRODUCTION

2-1. PREPARATION OF THE VACCINE

The vaccine virus is grown in embryonated hens' eggs or in cell cultures.

2-2. SUBSTRATE FOR VIRUS PROPAGATION

2-2-1. Embryonated hens' eggs

If the vaccine virus is grown in embryonated hens' eggs, they are obtained from flocks free from specified pathogens (SPF) (5.2.2).

2-2-2. Cell cultures

If the vaccine virus is grown in cell cultures, they comply with the requirements for cell cultures for production of veterinary vaccines (5.2.4).

2-3. SEED LOTS

2-3-1. Extraneous agents

The master seed lot complies with the tests for extraneous agents in seed lots (2.6.24). In these tests on the master seed lot, the organisms used are not more than 5 passages from the master seed lot at the start of the tests.

2-4. CHOICE OF VACCINE VIRUS

The vaccine virus shall be shown to be satisfactory with respect to safety (5.2.6) and efficacy (5.2.7) for the chickens for which it is intended.

The following tests for safety (section 2-4-1), damage to the bursa of Fabricius (section 2-4-2), immunosuppression (section 2-4-3), increase in virulence (section 2-4-4) and immunogenicity (section 2-4-5) may be used during the demonstration of safety and immunogenicity.

2-4-1. Safety

Carry out the test for each route and method of administration to be recommended for vaccination using in each case chickens not older than the youngest age to be recommended for vaccination. Use vaccine virus at the least attenuated passage level that will be present between the master seed lot and a batch of the vaccine. For each test, use not fewer than 20 chickens from an SPF flock (5.2.2). Administer to each chicken a quantity of the vaccine virus equivalent to not less than 10 times the maximum virus titre likely to be contained in 1 dose of the vaccine. Observe the chickens at least daily for 21 days. The test is not valid if more than 10 per cent of the chickens die from causes not attributable to the vaccine virus. The vaccine virus complies with the test if no chicken shows notable clinical signs of avian infectious bursal disease or dies from causes attributable to the vaccine virus.

2-4-2. Damage to the bursa of Fabricius

Carry out the test for the route to be recommended for vaccination likely to be the least safe using chickens not older than the youngest age to be recommended for vaccination. Use virus at the least attenuated passage level that will be present between the master seed lot and a batch of the vaccine. Use not fewer than 20 chickens from an SPF flock (5.2.2). Administer to each chicken a quantity of the vaccine virus equivalent to 10 times the maximum titre likely to be contained in a dose of the vaccine. On each of days 7, 14, 21 and 28 after administration of the vaccine virus, kill not fewer than 5 chickens and prepare a section from the site with the greatest diameters of the bursa of Fabricius of each chicken. Carry out histological examination of the section and score the degree of bursal damage using the following scale.

0   No lesion, normal bursa.

1   1 per cent to 25 per cent of the follicles show lymphoid depletion (i.e. less than 50 per cent depletion in 1 affected follicle) influx of heterophils in lesions.

2   26 per cent to 50 per cent of the follicles show nearly complete lymphoid depletion (i.e. more than 75 per cent depletion in 1 affected follicle), affected follicles show necrosis and severe influx of heterophils may be detected.

3   51 per cent to 75 per cent of the follicles show lymphoid depletion; affected follicles show necrosis and severe influx of heterophils is detected.

4   76 per cent to 100 per cent of the follicles show nearly complete lymphoid depletion, hyperplasia and cyst structures are detected; affected follicles show necrosis and severe influx of heterophils is detected.

5   100 per cent of the follicles show nearly complete lymphoid depletion; complete loss of follicular structure, thickened and folded epithelium, fibrosis of bursal tissue.

Calculate the average score for each group of chickens. The vaccine virus complies with the test if:
— no chicken shows notable clinical signs of disease or dies from causes attributable to the vaccine virus,
— the average score for bursal damage 21 days after administration of the vaccine virus is less than or equal to 2.0 and 28 days after administration is less than or equal to 0.6,
— during the 21 days after administration a notable repopulation of the bursae by lymphocytes has taken place.

2-4-3. Immunosuppression

Carry out the tests for the route recommended for vaccination likely to be the least safe using chickens not older than the youngest age recommended for vaccination. Use vaccine virus at the least attenuated passage level that will be present between the master seed lot and a batch of the vaccine. Use not fewer than 30 chickens from an SPF flock (5.2.2). Divide them randomly into 3 groups each of not fewer than 10 and maintain the groups separately. Administer by eye-drop to each chicken of 1 group a quantity of the vaccine virus equivalent to not less than the maximum titre likely to be contained in 1 dose of the vaccine. At the time after administration when maximal bursal damage is likely to be present, as judged from the results obtained in the test for damage to the bursa of Fabricius (section 2-4-2), administer to each vaccinated chicken and to each chicken of another group 1 dose of Hitchner B1 strain Newcastle disease vaccine (live). Determine the seroresponse of each chicken of the 2 groups to the Newcastle disease virus 14 days after administration. Challenge each chicken of the 3 groups by the intramuscular route with not less than 10^5 EID_{50} of virulent Newcastle disease virus and note the degree of protection in the 2 groups vaccinated with Hitchner B1 strain Newcastle vaccine compared with the non-vaccinated group. The test is not valid if 1 or more of the non-vaccinated chickens does not die within 7 days of challenge. The degree of immunosuppression is estimated from the comparative seroresponses and protection rates of the 2 Hitchner B1 vaccinated groups. The vaccine complies with the test if there is no significant difference between the 2 groups.

2-4-4. Increase in virulence

The test for increase in virulence consists of the administration of the vaccine virus at the least attenuated passage level that will be present between the master seed lot and a batch of the vaccine to a group of 5 chickens from an SPF flock (5.2.2) and not older than the youngest age to be recommended for vaccination, sequential passages, 5 times where possible, to further similar groups and testing of the final recovered virus for increase in virulence. If the

properties of the vaccine virus allow sequential passage to 5 groups via natural spreading, this method may be used, otherwise passage as described below is carried out and the maximally passaged virus that has been recovered is tested for increase in virulence. Care must be taken to avoid contamination by virus from previous passages. Administer by eye-drop a quantity of the vaccine virus that will allow recovery of virus for the passages described below. Prepare 3 to 4 days after administration a suspension from the bursa of Fabricius of each chicken and pool these samples. Administer 0.05 ml of the pooled samples by eye-drop to each of 5 other chickens of the same age and origin. Carry out this passage operation not fewer than 5 times; verify the presence of the virus at each passage. If the virus is not found at a passage level, carry out a second series of passages. Carry out the test for damage to the bursa of Fabricius (section 2-4-2) using the unpassaged vaccine virus and the maximally passaged virus that has been recovered. Administer the virus by the route recommended for vaccination likely to be the least safe. The vaccine virus complies with the test if no indication of increasing virulence of the maximally passaged virus compared with the unpassaged virus is observed. If virus is not recovered at any passage level in the first and second series of passages, the vaccine virus also complies with the test.

2-4-5. Immunogenicity

A test is carried out for each route and method of administration to be recommended using in each case chickens not older than the youngest age to be recommended for vaccination. The quantity of vaccine virus administered to each chicken is not greater than the minimum virus titre to be stated on the label and the virus is at the most attenuated passage level that will be present in a batch of the vaccine. Use not fewer than 30 chickens of the same origin and from an SPF flock (5.2.2). Vaccinate by a recommended route not fewer than 20 chickens. Maintain not fewer than 10 chickens as controls. Challenge each chicken after 14 days by eye-drop with a sufficient quantity of virulent avian infectious bursal disease virus. Observe the chickens at least daily for 10 days after challenge. Record the deaths due to infectious bursal disease and the surviving chickens that show clinical signs of disease. At the end of the observation period, kill all the surviving chickens and carry out histological examination for lesions of the bursa of Fabricius. The test is not valid if one or more of the following applies:
— during the observation period following challenge, fewer than 50 per cent of the control chickens show characteristic signs of avian infectious bursal disease,
— 1 or more of the surviving control chickens does not show degree 3 lesions of the bursa of Fabricius,
— during the period between the vaccination and challenge more than 10 per cent of the vaccinated or control chickens show abnormal clinical signs or die from causes not attributable to the vaccine.

The vaccine virus complies with the test if during the observation period after challenge not fewer than 90 per cent of the vaccinated chickens survive and show no notable clinical signs of disease nor degree 3 lesions of the bursa of Fabricius.

3. BATCH TESTS

3-1. Identification

The vaccine, diluted if necessary and mixed with a monospecific infectious bursal disease virus type 1 antiserum, no longer infects embryonated hens' eggs from an SPF flock

(*5.2.2*) or susceptible cell cultures (*5.2.4*) into which it is inoculated.

3-2. Bacteria and fungi

Vaccines intended for administration by injection comply with the test for sterility prescribed in the monograph *Vaccines for veterinary use (0062)*.

Vaccines not intended for administration by injection either comply with the test for sterility prescribed in the monograph *Vaccines for veterinary use (0062)* or with the following test: carry out a quantitative test for bacterial and fungal contamination; carry out identification tests for microorganisms detected in the vaccine; the vaccine does not contain pathogenic microorganisms and contains not more than 1 non-pathogenic microorganism per dose.

Any liquid supplied with the vaccine complies with the test for sterility prescribed in the monograph *Vaccines for veterinary use (0062)*.

3-3. Mycoplasmas

The vaccine complies with the test for mycoplasmas (*2.6.7*).

3-4. Extraneous agents

The vaccine complies with the tests for extraneous agents in batches of finished product (*2.6.25*).

3-5. Safety

Use not fewer than 10 chickens from an SPF flock (*5.2.2*) and of the youngest age recommended for vaccination. Administer by a recommended route and method to each chicken 10 doses of the vaccine. Observe the chickens at least daily for 21 days. The test is not valid if more than 20 per cent of the chickens show abnormal clinical signs or die from causes not attributable to the vaccine. The vaccine complies with the test if no chicken shows notable clinical signs of disease or dies from causes attributable to the vaccine.

3-6. Virus titre

Titrate the vaccine virus by inoculation into embryonated hens' eggs from an SPF flock (*5.2.2*) or into suitable cell cultures (*5.2.4*). The vaccine complies with the test if 1 dose contains not less than the minimum virus titre stated on the label.

3-7. Potency

The vaccine complies with the requirements of the test prescribed under Immunogenicity (section 2-4-5) when administered by a recommended route and method. It is not necessary to carry out the potency test for each batch of the vaccine if it has been carried out on a representative batch using a vaccinating dose containing not more than the minimum virus titre stated on the label.

Ph Eur

Infectious Chicken Anaemia Vaccine (Live)

(*Ph Eur monograph 2038*)

Ph Eur

1. DEFINITION

Infectious chicken anaemia vaccine (live) is a preparation of a suitable strain of chicken anaemia virus. This monograph applies to vaccines intended for administration to breeder chickens for active immunisation, to prevent excretion of the virus, to prevent or reduce egg transmission and to protect passively their future progeny.

2. PRODUCTION

2-1. PREPARATION OF THE VACCINE

The vaccine virus is grown in embryonated hens' eggs or in cell cultures.

2-2. SUBSTRATE FOR VIRUS PROPAGATION

2-2-1. Embryonated hens' eggs

If the vaccine virus is grown in embryonated hens' eggs, they are obtained from flocks free from specified pathogens (SPF) (*5.2.2*).

2-2-2. Cell cultures

If the vaccine virus is grown in cell cultures, they comply with the requirements for cell cultures for production of veterinary vaccines (*5.2.4*).

2-3. SEED LOTS

2-3-1. Extraneous agents

The master seed lot complies with the tests for extraneous agents in seed lots (*2.6.24*). In these tests on the master seed lot, the organisms used are not more than 5 passages from the master seed lot at the start of the tests.

2-4. CHOICE OF VACCINE VIRUS

The vaccine virus shall be shown to be satisfactory with respect to safety (*5.2.6*) and efficacy (*5.2.7*) for the chickens for which it is intended.

The following tests for safety (section 2-4-1), increase in virulence (section 2-4-2) and immunogenicity (section 2-4-3) may be used during the demonstration of safety and immunogenicity.

2-4-1. Safety

2-4-1-1. General test Carry out the test for each route and method of administration to be recommended for vaccination in chickens not older than the youngest age to be recommended for vaccination and from an SPF flock (*5.2.2*). Use vaccine virus at the least attenuated passage level that will be present between the master seed lot and a batch of the vaccine. For each test use not fewer than 20 chickens. Administer to each chicken a quantity of the vaccine virus not less than 10 times the maximum virus titre likely to be contained in 1 dose of the vaccine. 14 days after vaccination, collect blood samples from half of the chickens and determine the haematocrit value. Kill these chickens and carry out post-mortem examination. Note any pathological changes attributable to chicken anaemia virus, such as thymic atrophy and specific bone-marrow lesions. Observe the remaining chickens at least daily for 21 days. The vaccine virus complies with the test if during the observation period no chicken shows notable clinical signs of chicken anaemia or dies from causes attributable to the vaccine virus.

2-4-1-2. Safety for young chicks Use not fewer than twenty 1-day-old chicks from an SPF flock (*5.2.2*). Administer to each chick by the oculonasal route a quantity of the vaccine virus equivalent to not less than the maximum titre likely to be contained in 1 dose of the vaccine. Observe the chicks at least daily. Record the incidence of any clinical signs attributable to the vaccine virus, such as depression, and any deaths. 14 days after vaccination, collect blood samples from half of the chicks and determine the haematocrit value. Kill these chicks and carry out post-mortem examination. Note any pathological changes attributable to chicken anaemia virus, such as thymic atrophy and specific bone marrow lesions. Observe the remaining chicks at least daily for 21 days. Assess the extent to which the vaccine strain is pathogenic for 1-day-old susceptible chicks from the results of the clinical observations and mortality rates and the proportion of chicks examined at 14 days that show anaemia (haematocrit value less than 27 per cent) and signs of infectious chicken anaemia on post-mortem examination. The results are used to formulate the label statement on safety for young chicks.

2-4-2. Increase in virulence
The test for increase in virulence consists of the administration of the vaccine virus at the least attenuated passage level that will be present between the master seed lot and a batch of the vaccine to a group of five 1-day-old chicks from an SPF flock (5.2.2), sequential passages, 5 times where possible, to further similar groups of 1-day-old chicks and testing of the final recovered virus for increase in virulence. If the properties of the vaccine virus allow sequential passage to 5 groups via natural spreading, this method may be used, otherwise passage as described below is carried out and the maximally passaged virus that has been recovered is tested for increase in virulence. Care must be taken to avoid contamination by virus from previous passages. Administer by the intramuscular route a quantity of the vaccine virus that will allow recovery of virus for the passages described below. Prepare 7 to 9 days after administration a suspension from the liver of each chick and pool these samples. Depending on the tropism of the virus, other tissues such as spleen or bone marrow may be used. Administer 0.1 ml of the pooled samples by the intramuscular route to each of 5 other chicks of the same age and origin. Carry out this passage operation at least 5 times; verify the presence of the virus at each passage. If the virus is not found at a passage level, carry out a second series of passages. Carry out the tests for safety (section 2-4-1) using the unpassaged vaccine virus and the maximally passaged vaccine virus that has been recovered. The vaccine virus complies with the test if no indication of increase in virulence of the maximally passaged virus compared with the unpassaged virus is observed.
If virus is not recovered at any passage level in the first and second series of passages, the vaccine virus also complies with the test.

2-4-3. Immunogenicity
A test is carried out for each route and method of administration to be recommended using chickens from an SPF flock (5.2.2) not older than the youngest age to be recommended for vaccination. The test for prevention of virus excretion is intended to demonstrate absence of egg transmission. The quantity of the vaccine virus administered to each chicken is not greater than the minimum titre to be stated on the label and the virus is at the most attenuated passage level that will be present in a batch of the vaccine.

2-4-3-1. Passive immunisation of chickens Vaccinate according to the recommended schedule not fewer than 10 breeder chickens not older than the minimum age recommended for vaccination and from an SPF flock (5.2.2); keep not fewer than 10 unvaccinated breeder chickens of the same origin and from an SPF flock (5.2.2). At a suitable time after excretion of vaccine virus has ceased, collect fertilised eggs from each vaccinated and control breeder chicken and incubate them. Challenge at least 3 randomly chosen 1-day-old chickens from each vaccinated and control breeder chicken by intramuscular administration of a sufficient quantity of virulent chicken anaemia virus. Observe the chickens at least daily for 14 days after challenge. Record the deaths and the surviving chickens that show clinical signs of disease. At the end of the observation period determine the haematocrit value of each surviving chicken. Kill these chickens and carry out post-mortem examination. Note any pathological signs attributable to chicken anaemia virus, such as thymic atrophy and specific bone-marrow lesions. The test is not valid if:

— during the observation period after challenge fewer than 90 per cent of the chickens of the control breeder chickens die or show severe clinical signs of infectious chicken anaemia, including haematocrit value under 27 per cent, and/or notable macroscopic lesions of the bone marrow and thymus,
— and/or during the period between vaccination and egg collection more than 10 per cent of vaccinated or control breeder chickens show notable clinical signs of disease or die from causes not attributable to the vaccine.

The vaccine complies with the test if during the observation period after challenge not fewer than 90 per cent of the chickens of the vaccinated breeder chickens survive and show no notable clinical signs of disease and/or macroscopic lesions of the bone marrow and thymus.

2-4-3-2. Prevention of virus excretion Vaccinate according to the recommended schedule not fewer than 10 chickens not older than the minimum age recommended for vaccination and from an SPF flock (5.2.2). Maintain separately not fewer than 10 chickens of the same age and origin as controls. At a suitable time after excretion of vaccine virus has ceased, challenge all the chickens by intramuscular administration of a sufficient quantity of virulent chicken anaemia virus. Collect blood and faecal samples from the chickens on days 3, 5 and 7 after challenge and carry out a test for virus isolation to determine whether or not the chickens are viraemic and are excreting the virus. The test is not valid if:
— fewer than 70 per cent of the control chickens are viraemic and excrete the virus at one or more times of sampling,
— and/or during the period between vaccination and challenge more than 10 per cent of control or vaccinated chickens show abnormal clinical signs or die from causes not attributable to the vaccine.

The vaccine complies with the test if not fewer than 90 per cent of the vaccinated chickens do not develop viraemia or excrete the virus.

3. BATCH TESTING
3-1. Identification
The vaccine, diluted if necessary and mixed with a monospecific chicken anaemia virus antiserum, no longer infects susceptible cell cultures or eggs from an SPF flock (5.2.2) into which it is inoculated.

3-2. Bacteria and fungi
Vaccines intended for administration by injection comply with the test for sterility prescribed in the monograph *Vaccines for veterinary use (0062)*.

Vaccines not intended for administration by injection either comply with the test for sterility prescribed in the monograph *Vaccines for veterinary use (0062)* or with the following test: carry out a quantitative test for bacterial and fungal contamination; carry out identification tests for microorganisms detected in the vaccine; the vaccine does not contain pathogenic microorganisms and contains not more than 1 non-pathogenic microorganism per dose.

Any liquid supplied with the vaccine complies with the test for sterility prescribed in the monograph *Vaccines for veterinary use (0062)*.

3-3. Mycoplasmas
The vaccine complies with the test for mycoplasmas (2.6.7).

3-4. Extraneous agents
The vaccine complies with the tests for extraneous agents in batches of finished product (2.6.25).

3-5. Safety

Use not fewer than 10 chickens not older than the minimum age recommended for vaccination and from an SPF flock (5.2.2). Administer by a recommended route to each chicken 10 doses of the vaccine. Observe the chickens at least daily for 21 days. The test is not valid if more than 20 per cent of the chickens show abnormal clinical signs or die from causes not attributable to the vaccine. The vaccine complies with the test if no chicken shows notable clinical signs of disease or dies from causes attributable to the vaccine.

3-6. Virus titre

Titrate the vaccine virus by inoculation into suitable cell cultures (5.2.4) or eggs from an SPF flock (5.2.2). The vaccine complies with the test if 1 dose contains not less than the minimum virus titre stated on the label.

3-7. Potency

The vaccine complies with the requirements of the tests prescribed under Immunogenicity (sections 2-4-3-1 and 2-4-3-2) when administered by a recommended route and method. It is not necessary to carry out the potency test for each batch of the vaccine if it has been carried out on a representative batch using a vaccinating dose containing not more than the minimum virus titre stated on the label.

4. LABELLING

The label states to which extent the vaccine virus causes disease if it spreads to susceptible young chicks.

Ph Eur

Laryngotracheitis Vaccine, Living

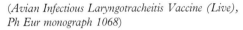

(*Avian Infectious Laryngotracheitis Vaccine (Live)*, *Ph Eur monograph 1068*)

Ph Eur

1. DEFINITION

Avian infectious laryngotracheitis vaccine (live) is a preparation of a suitable strain of avian infectious laryngotracheitis virus (gallid herpesvirus 1). This monograph applies to vaccines intended for administration to chickens for active immunisation.

2. PRODUCTION

2-1. PREPARATION OF THE VACCINE

The vaccine virus is grown in embryonated hens' eggs or in cell cultures.

2-2. SUBSTRATE FOR VIRUS PROPAGATION

2-2-1. Embryonated hens' eggs

If the vaccine virus is grown in embryonated hens' eggs, they are obtained from flocks free from specified pathogens (SPF) (5.2.2).

2-2-2. Cell cultures

If the vaccine virus is grown in cell cultures, they comply with the requirements for cell cultures for production of veterinary vaccines (5.2.4).

2-3. SEED LOTS

2-3-1. Extraneous agents

The master seed lot complies with the tests for extraneous agents in seed lots (2.6.24). In these tests on the master seed lot, the organisms used are not more than 5 passages from the master seed lot at the start of the tests.

2-4. CHOICE OF VACCINE VIRUS

The vaccine virus shall be shown to be satisfactory with respect to safety (5.2.6) and efficacy (5.2.7) for the chickens for which it is intended.

The following tests for index of respiratory virulence (section 2-4-1), safety (section 2-4-2), increase in virulence (section 2-4-3) and immunogenicity (section 2-4-4) may be used during the demonstration of safety and immunogenicity.

2-4-1. Index of respiratory virulence

Use for the test not fewer than sixty 10-day-old chickens from an SPF flock (5.2.2). Divide them randomly into 3 groups, maintained separately. Prepare 2 tenfold serial dilutions starting from a suspension of the vaccine virus having a titre of 10^5 EID$_{50}$ or 10^5 CCID$_{50}$ per 0.2 ml or, if not possible, having the maximum attainable titre. Use vaccine virus at the least attenuated passage level that will be present in a batch of the vaccine. Allocate the undiluted virus suspension and the 2 virus dilutions each to a different group of chickens. Administer by the intratracheal route to each chicken 0.2 ml of the virus suspension attributed to its group. Observe the chickens for 10 days after administration and record the number of deaths. The index of respiratory virulence is the total number of deaths in the 3 groups divided by the total number of chickens. The vaccine virus complies with the test if its index of respiratory virulence is not greater than 0.33.

2-4-2. Safety

Carry out the test for each route and method of administration to be recommended for vaccination, using in each case chickens not older than the youngest age to be recommended for vaccination. Use vaccine virus at the least attenuated passage level that will be present between the master seed lot and a batch of the vaccine. For each test use not fewer than 20 chickens, from an SPF flock (5.2.2). Administer to each chicken a quantity of the vaccine virus equivalent to not less than 10 times the maximum virus titre likely to be contained in 1 dose of the vaccine. Observe the chickens at least daily for 21 days. The test is not valid if more than 10 per cent of the chickens die from causes not attributable to the vaccine virus. The vaccine virus complies with the test if no chicken shows notable clinical signs of avian infectious laryngotracheitis or dies from causes attributable to the vaccine virus.

2-4-3. Increase in virulence

The test for increase in virulence consists of the administration of the vaccine virus at the least attenuated passage level that will be present between the master seed lot and a batch of the vaccine to a group of 5 chickens not more than 2 weeks old, from an SPF flock (5.2.2), sequential passages, 5 times where possible, to further similar groups and testing of the final recovered virus for increase in virulence. If the properties of the vaccine virus allow sequential passage to 5 groups via natural spreading, this method may be used, otherwise passage as described below is carried out and the maximally passaged virus that has been recovered is tested for increase in virulence. Care must be taken to avoid contamination by virus from previous passages. Administer by eye-drop a quantity of the vaccine virus that will allow recovery of virus for the passages described below. After the period shown to correspond to maximum replication of the virus, prepare a suspension from the mucosae of suitable parts of the respiratory tract of each chicken and pool these samples. Administer 0.05 ml of the pooled samples by eye-drop to each of 5 other chickens that are 2 weeks old and from an SPF flock (5.2.2). Carry out this passage operation not fewer than 5 times; verify the presence of the virus at each passage. If the virus is not found at a passage level, carry out a second series of passages. Determine the index of respiratory virulence (section 2-4-1) using the unpassaged vaccine virus and the maximally passaged virus that has been recovered; if the titre of the maximally passaged virus is less than 10^5 EID$_{50}$ or 10^5 CCID$_{50}$, prepare the tenfold, serial dilutions using the highest titre available. The vaccine virus complies with the test if no indication of increase in virulence of the maximally passaged virus compared with the unpassaged virus is observed. If virus is not recovered at any passage level in the first and second series of passages, the vaccine virus also complies with the test.

2-4-4. Immunogenicity

A test is carried out for each route and method of administration to be recommended using in each case chickens not older than the youngest age to be recommended for vaccination. The quantity of the vaccine virus administered to each chicken is not greater than the minimum virus titre to be stated on the label and the virus is at the most attenuated passage level that will be present in a batch of the vaccine. Use for the test not fewer than 30 chickens of the same origin and from an SPF flock (5.2.2). Vaccinate by a recommended route not fewer than 20 chickens. Maintain not fewer than 10 chickens as controls. Challenge each chicken after 21 days by the intratracheal route with a sufficient quantity of virulent infectious laryngotracheitis virus. Observe the chickens at least daily for 7 days after challenge. Record the deaths and the number of surviving chickens that show clinical signs of disease. At the end of the observation period kill all the surviving chickens and carry out examination for macroscopic lesions: mucoid, haemorrhagic and pseudomembraneous inflammation of the trachea and orbital sinuses. The test is not valid if:

— during the observation period after challenge fewer than 90 per cent of the control chickens die or show severe clinical signs of avian infectious laryngotracheitis or notable macroscopic lesions of the trachea and orbital sinuses,

— or if during the period between the vaccination and challenge more than 10 per cent of the vaccinated or control chickens show notable clinical signs of disease or die from causes not attributable to the vaccine.

The vaccine virus complies with the test if during the observation period after challenge not fewer than 90 per cent of the vaccinated chickens survive and show no notable clinical signs of disease and/or macroscopical lesions of the trachea and orbital sinuses.

3. BATCH TESTS

3-1. Identification

The vaccine, diluted if necessary and mixed with a monospecific infectious laryngotracheitis virus antiserum, no longer infects embryonated hens' eggs from an SPF flock (5.2.2) or susceptible cell cultures (5.2.4) into which it is inoculated.

3-2. Bacteria and fungi

Vaccines intended for administration by injection comply with the test for sterility prescribed in the monograph *Vaccines for veterinary use (0062)*.

Vaccines not intended for administration by injection either comply with the test for sterility prescribed in the monograph *Vaccines for veterinary use (0062)* or with the following test: carry out a quantitative test for bacterial and fungal contamination; carry out identification tests for micro-

organisms detected in the vaccine; the vaccine does not contain pathogenic micro-organisms and contains not more than 1 non-pathogenic micro-organism per dose.

Any liquid supplied with the vaccine complies with test for sterility in the monograph *Vaccines for veterinary use (0062)*.

3-3. Mycoplasmas

The vaccine complies with the test for mycoplasmas (2.6.7).

3-4. Extraneous agents

The vaccine complies with the tests for extraneous agents in batches of finished product (2.6.25).

3-5. Safety

Use not fewer than 10 chickens from an SPF flock (5.2.2) and of the youngest age recommended for vaccination. Administer by eye-drop to each chicken 10 doses of the vaccine. Observe the chickens at least daily for 21 days. The test is not valid if more than 20 per cent of the chickens show abnormal clinical signs or die from causes not attributable to the vaccine. The vaccine complies with the test if no chicken shows notable clinical signs of disease or dies from causes attributable to the vaccine.

3-6. Virus titre

Titrate the vaccine virus by inoculation into embryonated hens' eggs from an SPF flock (5.2.2) or into suitable cell cultures (5.2.4). The vaccine complies with the test if 1 dose contains not less than the minimum titre stated on the label.

3-7. Potency

The vaccine complies with the requirements of the test prescribed under Immunogenicity (section 2-4-4) when administered according to the recommended schedule by a recommended route and method. It is not necessary to carry out the potency test for each batch of the vaccine if it has been carried out on a representative batch using a vaccinating dose containing not more than the minimum virus titre stated on the label.

Ph Eur

Bovine Leptospirosis Vaccine (Inactivated)

(Ph Eur monograph 1939)

Ph Eur

DEFINITION

Bovine leptospirosis vaccine (inactivated) is a suspension of inactivated whole organisms and/or antigenic extract(s) of one or more suitable strains of one or more of *Leptospira borgpetersenii* serovar hardjo, *Leptospira interrogans* serovar hardjo or other *L. interrogans* serovars, inactivated and prepared in such a way that adequate immunogenicity is maintained. This monograph applies to vaccines intended for active immunisation of cattle against leptospirosis.

PRODUCTION

The seed material is cultured in a suitable medium; each strain is cultivated separately. During production, various parameters such as growth rate are monitored by suitable methods; the values are within the limits approved for the particular product. Purity and identity are verified on the harvest using suitable methods. After cultivation, the bacterial harvest is inactivated by a suitable method. The antigen may be concentrated. The vaccine may contain an adjuvant.

CHOICE OF VACCINE COMPOSITION

The vaccine is shown to be satisfactory with respect to safety (*5.2.6*) and efficacy (*5.2.7*) in cattle. As part of the studies to demonstrate the suitability of the vaccine with respect to these characteristics the following tests may be carried out.

Safety

A. The test is carried out for each route of administration to be stated on the label and in animals of each category (for example, young calves, pregnant cattle) for which the vaccine is intended. For each test, use not fewer than 10 animals that do not have antibodies against *L. borgpetersenii* serovar hardjo and the principal serovars of *L. interrogans* (icterohaemorrhagiae, canicola, grippotyphosa, sejroe, hardjo, hebdomonadis, pomona, australis and autumnalis). Use a batch of vaccine containing not less than the maximum potency that may be expected in a batch of vaccine. Administer to each animal a double dose of vaccine. If the recommended schedule requires a second dose, administer 1 dose after the recommended interval. Observe the animals for at least 14 days after the last administration. Record body temperatures the day before each vaccination, at vaccination, 4 h later and daily for 4 days. If the vaccine is intended for use or may be used in pregnant cattle, vaccinate the animals at the relevant stages of pregnancy and prolong the observation period until 1 day after calving. The vaccine complies with the test if no animal shows an abnormal local or systemic reaction or clinical signs of disease or dies from a cause attributable to the vaccine. In addition, if the vaccine is for use in pregnant animals, no adverse effects on the pregnancy and offspring are noted.

B. The animals used for the field trials are also used to evaluate safety. Use not fewer than 3 groups of 20 animals with corresponding groups of not fewer than 10 controls in 3 different locations. Examine the injection sites for local reactions after vaccination. Record body temperatures the day before vaccination, at vaccination and on the 2 days following vaccination. The vaccine complies with the test if no animal shows an abnormal local or systemic reaction or clinical signs of disease or dies from a cause attributable to the vaccine. In addition, if the vaccine is for use in pregnant animals, no adverse effects on the pregnancy and offspring are noted.

Immunogenicity

As part of the studies to demonstrate the suitability of the vaccine with respect to immunogenicity and in support of the claims for a beneficial effect on the rates of infection and urinary excretion, the test described under Potency may be carried out for each proposed route of administration, using vaccine of minimum potency. Urine samples are collected from each animal on days 0, 14, 21, 28 and 35 post-challenge. For leptospiral species other than *L. borgpetersenii* serovar hardjo, appropriate days are determined by the characteristics of the challenge model. In the case of other serovars for which there is published evidence that the serovar has a lower tropism for the urinary tract, a lower rate of infection may be justified. Depending on their tissue tropism, for some leptospira serovars, samples from other tissues/body fluids can be used to establish whether the animals are infected or not by the challenge organism. If claims are to be made for protection against reproductive or production losses, further specific studies will be required.

BATCH POTENCY TEST

The test described under Potency is not carried out for routine testing of batches of vaccine. It is carried out, for a given vaccine, on one or more occasions, as decided by or with the agreement of the competent authority; where the test is not carried out, a suitable validated test is carried out, the criteria for acceptance being set with reference to a batch of vaccine that has given satisfactory results in the test described under Potency. The following test may be used after a suitable correlation with the test described under Potency has been established.

For each of the serovars for which protection is claimed, the antibody response from vaccinated animals is measured. Use guinea pigs weighing 250-350 g which do not have antibodies to *L. borgpetersenii* serovar hardjo and the principal serovars of *L. interrogans* (icterohaemorrhagiae, canicola, grippotyphosa, sejroe, hardjo, hebdomonadis, pomona, australis and autumnalis) and which have been obtained from a regularly tested and certified leptospira-free source. The dose to be administered to the animals is that fraction of a cattle dose which has been shown in the validation studies to provide a suitably sensitive test. Vaccinate each of 10 animals with the suitable dose. Maintain not fewer than 2 guinea-pigs as unvaccinated controls. At a given interval within the range of 19 to 23 days after the injection, collect blood from each animal and prepare serum samples. Use a suitable validated method such as a micro-agglutination test to measure the antibody responses in each sample. The antibody levels are equal to or greater than those obtained with a batch that has given satisfactory results in the test described under Potency and there is no significant increase in antibody titre in the controls.

IDENTIFICATION

When injected into healthy seronegative animals, the vaccine stimulates the production of specific antibodies to the leptospira serovar(s) present in the vaccine.

TESTS

Safety

For vaccines recommended for use in cattle older than 6 months of age, use cattle not older than the minimum age recommended for vaccination and not younger than 6 months of age. For vaccines recommended for use in cattle less than 6 months of age, use cattle of the minimum age recommended for vaccination. Inject 2 doses of the vaccine into each of 2 cattle, free from specific antibodies to the leptospira serovar(s) present in the vaccine, by a recommended route. Observe the animals for 14 days. The animals remain in good health and no abnormal local or systemic reaction occurs.

Inactivation

Carry out a test for live leptospirae by inoculation of a specific medium. Inoculate 1 ml of the vaccine into 100 ml of the medium. Incubate at 30 °C for 14 days, subculture into a further quantity of the medium and incubate both media at 30 °C for 14 days: no growth occurs in either medium. At the same time, carry out a control test by inoculating a further quantity of the medium with the vaccine together with a quantity of a culture containing approximately 100 leptospirae and incubating at 30 °C: growth of leptospirae occurs within 14 days.

Sterility

The vaccine complies with the test for sterility prescribed in the monograph *Vaccines for veterinary use (0062)*.

POTENCY

Carry out a separate test for each of the serovars for which a claim is made for a beneficial effect on the rates of infection and urinary excretion.

Use not fewer than 15 cattle of the minimum age recommended for vaccination and free from specific antibodies against *L. borgpetersenii* serovar hardjo and the principal serovars of *L. interrogans* (icterohaemorrhagiae, canicola, grippotyphosa, sejroe, hardjo, hebdomonadis, pomona, australis and autumnalis). Vaccinate not fewer than 10 animals by a recommended route and according to the recommended schedule. Keep not fewer than 5 animals as controls. 21 days after the last vaccination, infect all the animals by a suitable mucosal route with a suitable quantity of a virulent strain of the relevant serovar. Observe the animals for a further 35 days. Collect urine samples from each animal on days 0, 14, 21, 28 and 35 post-challenge. Kill surviving animals at the end of the observation period. Carry out post-mortem examination on any animal that dies and on those killed at the end of the observation period.

In particular, examine the kidneys for macroscopic and microscopic signs of leptospira infection. A sample of each kidney is collected and each urine and kidney sample is tested for the presence of the challenge organisms by re-isolation or by another suitable method.

For the test conducted with *L. borgpetersenii* serovar hardjo, control animals are regarded as infected if the challenge organisms are re-isolated from at least 2 samples. The test is invalid if infection has been established in fewer than 80 per cent of the control animals.

The vaccine complies with the requirements of the test if the challenge organisms are re-isolated from any urine or kidney sample from not more than 20 per cent of the vaccinated animals.

LABELLING
The label states:
— the serovar(s) used to prepare the vaccine,
— the serovar(s) against which protection is claimed.

Ph Eur

Canine Leptospirosis Vaccine (Inactivated)

(*Ph Eur monograph 0447*)

Ph Eur

DEFINITION
Canine leptospirosis vaccine (inactivated) is a suspension of inactivated whole organisms and/or antigenic extract(s) of one or more suitable strains of one or more of *Leptospira interrogans* serovar canicola, serovar icterohaemorrhagiae or any other epidemiologically appropriate serovar, inactivated and prepared in such a way that adequate immunogenicity is maintained. This monograph applies to vaccines intended for active immunisation of dogs against leptospirosis.

PRODUCTION
The seed material is cultured in a suitable medium; each strain is cultivated separately. During production, various parameters such as growth rate are monitored by suitable methods; the values are within the limits approved for the particular product. Purity and identity are verified on the harvest using suitable methods. After cultivation, the bacterial harvests are collected separately and inactivated by a suitable method. The antigen may be concentrated. The vaccine may contain an adjuvant.

CHOICE OF VACCINE COMPOSITION
The vaccine is shown to be satisfactory with respect to safety (*5.2.6*) and efficacy (*5.2.7*) in dogs. As part of the studies to demonstrate the suitability of the vaccine with respect to these characteristics the following tests may be carried out.

Safety
The test is carried out for each route of administration to be stated on the label and in animals of each category for which the vaccine is intended. For each test, use not fewer than 10 dogs that do not have antibodies against the principal *L. interrogans* serovars (icterohaemorrhagiae, canicola, grippotyphosa, sejroe, hardjo, hebdomonadis, pomona, australis and autumnalis). Use a batch of vaccine containing not less than the maximum antigen content and/or potency that may be expected in a batch of vaccine. Administer to each animal a double dose of vaccine. If the recommended schedule requires a second dose, administer 1 dose after the recommended interval. Observe the animals for at least 14 days after the last administration. Record body temperatures the day before each vaccination, at vaccination, 4 h later and daily for 4 days. If the vaccine is intended for use or may be used in pregnant bitches, vaccinate the animals at the recommended stage of pregnancy or at a range of stages of pregnancy and prolong the observation period until 1 day after whelping. The vaccine complies with the test if no animal shows an abnormal local or systemic reaction or clinical signs of disease or dies from a cause attributable to the vaccine. In addition, if the vaccine is for use in pregnant animals, no adverse effects on the pregnancy and offspring are noted.

Immunogenicity
As part of the studies to demonstrate the suitability of the vaccine with respect to immunogenicity and compliance with the claims to be stated on the label, the test described under Potency may be carried out for each proposed route of administration and using vaccine of minimum antigen content and/or potency.

BATCH POTENCY TEST
The test described under Potency is not carried out for routine testing of batches of vaccine. It is carried out, for a given vaccine, on one or more occasions, as decided by or with the agreement of the competent authority. Where the test is not carried out, one of the following tests may be used.

A. For vaccines with or without adjuvants

If leptospira from more than 1 serovar (for example *L. interrogans* serovar canicola and serovar icterohaemorrhagiae) has been used to prepare the vaccine, carry out a batch potency test for each serovar against which protective immunity is claimed on the label. Inject 1/40 of the dose for dogs stated on the label subcutaneously into each of 5 healthy hamsters not more than 3 months old, which do not have antibodies to the principal serovars of *L. interrogans* (icterohaemorrhagiae, canicola, grippotyphosa, sejroe, hardjo, hebdomonadis, pomona, australis and autumnalis) and which have been obtained from a regularly tested and certified leptospira-free source. After 15-20 days, inoculate intraperitoneally into each of the vaccinated animals and into an equal number of non-vaccinated controls derived from the same certified leptospira-free source, a suitable quantity of a virulent culture of leptospirae of the serovar against which protective immunity is claimed on the label. The vaccine complies with the test if not fewer than 4 of the 5 control animals die showing typical signs of leptospira infection within 14 days of receiving the challenge suspension and if not fewer than 4 of the 5 vaccinated animals remain in good health for 14 days after the death of 4 control animals.

B. For vaccines with or without adjuvants

A suitable validated sero-response test may be carried out. Vaccinate each animal in a group of experimental animals with a suitable dose. Collect blood samples after a suitable, fixed time after vaccination. For each of the serovars present in the vaccine, an *in vitro* test is carried out on individual blood samples to determine the antibody response to one or more antigenic components which are indicators of protection and which are specific for that serovar. The criteria for acceptance are set with reference to a batch of vaccine that has given satisfactory results in the test described under Potency.

C. For vaccines without adjuvants

For each of the serovars present in the vaccine, a suitable validated *in vitro* test may be carried out to determine the content of one or more antigenic components which are indicators of protection and which are specific for that serovar. The criteria for acceptance are set with reference to a batch of vaccine that has given satisfactory results in the test described under Potency.

IDENTIFICATION
When injected into healthy seronegative animals, the vaccine stimulates the production of specific antibodies to the leptospira serovar(s) present in the vaccine. If test C is used for batch potency test, it also serves to identify the vaccine.

TESTS
Safety
Use 2 dogs of the minimum age recommended for vaccination and which do not have antibodies to the leptospira serovar(s) present in the vaccine. Administer 2 doses of the vaccine to each dog by a recommended route. Observe the animals for 14 days. The animals remain in good health and no abnormal local or systemic reaction occurs.

Inactivation
Carry out a test for live leptospirae by inoculation of a specific medium. Inoculate 1 ml of the vaccine into 100 ml of the medium. Incubate at 30 °C for 14 days, subculture into a further quantity of the medium and incubate both media at 30 °C for 14 days: no growth occurs in either medium. At the same time, carry out a control test by inoculating a further quantity of the medium with the vaccine together with a quantity of a culture containing approximately 100 leptospirae and incubating at 30 °C: growth of leptospirae occurs within 14 days.

Sterility
The vaccine complies with the test for sterility prescribed in the monograph *Vaccines for veterinary use (0062)*.

POTENCY
For each type of the serovars against which protective immunity is claimed on the label, carry out a separate test with a challenge strain representative of that serovar.

Use not fewer than 12 dogs of the minimum age recommended for vaccination and free from specific antibodies against the principal serovars of *L. interrogans* (icterohaemorrhagiae, canicola, grippotyphosa, sejroe, hardjo, hebdomadis, pomona, australis and autumnalis). Vaccinate half of the animals by a recommended route and according to the recommended schedule. Keep the remaining animals as controls. 25-28 days after the last vaccination, infect all the animals by the conjunctival and/or intraperitoneal route with a suitable quantity of a virulent strain of the relevant

L. interrogans serovar. Observe the animals for a further 28 days. Examine the dogs daily and record and score clinical signs observed post-challenge and any deaths that occur. If an animal shows marked signs of disease, it is killed. Monitor body temperatures each day for the first week after challenge. Collect blood samples from each animal on days 0, 2, 3, 4, 5, 8 and 11 post challenge. Collect urine samples from each animal on days 0, 3, 5, 8, 11, 14, 21 and 28 post challenge. Kill surviving animals at the end of the observation period. Carry out post-mortem examination on any animal that dies during the observation period and on the remainder when killed at the end of the observation period. In particular, examine the liver and kidneys for macroscopic and microscopic signs of leptospira infection. A sample of each kidney is collected and each blood, urine and kidney sample is tested for the presence of challenge organisms by re-isolation or by another suitable method. The blood samples are also analysed to detect biochemical and haematological changes indicative of infection and these are also scored.

The test is invalid if: samples give positive results on day 0; *L. interrogans* serovar challenge strain is re-isolated from or demonstrated by another suitable method to be present in fewer than 2 samples on fewer than 2 different days, to show infection has been established in fewer than 80 per cent of the control animals.

The vaccine complies with the test if: at least 80 per cent of the vaccinates show no more than mild signs of disease (for example, transient hyperthermia) and, depending on the *L interrogans* serovar used for the challenge, one or more of the following is also shown:
— where the vaccine is intended to have a beneficial effect against clinical signs, the clinical scores and haematological and biochemical scores are statistically lower for the vaccinates than for the controls,
— where the vaccine is intended to have a beneficial effect against infection, the number of days that the organisms are detected in the blood is statistically lower for the vaccinates than for the controls,
— where the vaccine is intended to have a beneficial effect against urinary tract infection and excretion, the number of days that the organisms are detected in the urine and the number of kidney samples in which the organisms are detected is statistically lower for the vaccinates than for the controls.

LABELLING
The label states:
— the serovar(s) used to prepare the vaccine,
— the serovar(s) against which the protection is claimed.

_____ *Ph Eur*

Louping-ill Vaccine
DEFINITION
Louping-ill Vaccine is a preparation of a suitable strain of louping-ill virus which has been inactivated in such a manner that immunogenic activity is retained.

PRODUCTION
The virus strain is grown in suitable cell cultures, Appendix XV J(Vet)1. The viral suspension is harvested and inactivated. A test for residual infectious louping-ill virus is carried out on each batch of antigen immediately after inactivation. A mouse inoculation test may provide a suitably

sensitive test if there is no suitably sensitive *in vitro* test for the strain.

The vaccine contains an adjuvant.

CHOICE OF VACCINE COMPOSITION

This vaccine is shown to be satisfactory with respect to safety and immunogenicity for the animals for which the vaccine is intended. The following tests may be used during the demonstration of safety, Appendix XV J(Vet) 1 and immunogenicity, Appendix XV J(Vet) 2.

Safety

Carry out a test in each category of each species of animal for which the vaccine is to be recommended and by each recommended route of administration. Vaccinate at least five animals that do not have antibodies to louping-ill virus. Use for the test a batch of vaccine with the maximum potency likely to be included in a dose of the vaccine. Administer a double dose of vaccine to each animal and observe them for two weeks. No abnormal local or systemic reactions occur. If the vaccine is for use or may be used in pregnant animals, for the test in this category, administer the vaccine at the relevant stage or stages of pregnancy, prolong the observation period up to the time of parturition and note any effects on gestation or on the offspring.

Immunogenicity

The tests to demonstrate immunogenicity are carried out in each category of each species of animal for which the vaccine is to be recommended and by each recommended route of administration and using a batch or batches with the minimum potency likely to be included in a dose of the vaccine. The efficacy claims made on the label (e.g. protection from clinical signs of the disease) reflect the type of data generated.

BATCH TESTING

Inactivation

Carry out a suitable validated test for residual louping-ill virus on the bulk antigen blend immediately before the addition of the adjuvant. No live virus is detected.

The vaccine complies with the requirements stated under Veterinary Vaccines with the following modifications.

IDENTIFICATION

When injected into healthy seronegative animals, the vaccine stimulates the production of specific haemagglutinating antibodies against louping-ill virus.

TESTS

Extraneous bacteria and fungi

The vaccine complies with the test for sterility described under Veterinary Vaccines.

Safety

Use two lambs of the minimum age recommended for vaccination and that do not have antibodies to louping-ill virus. Administer a double dose of vaccine to each of the lambs by a route recommended on the label and observe the animals for two weeks. No abnormal local or systemic reactions occur.

POTENCY

Inject subcutaneously each of no fewer than six healthy sheep, free from louping-ill haemagglutination-inhibiting (HI) antibodies, with the dose stated on the label. Between 14 and 28 days after injection the serum of at least five of the sheep contains HI antibodies at dilutions of 1 in 20 or greater against 4 to 8 haemagglutinating units.

STORAGE

When stored under the prescribed conditions the vaccine may be expected to retain its potency for at least 1 year.

Lungworm (Dictyocaulus Viviparus) Oral Vaccine, Living

DEFINITION

Lungworm (Dictyocaulus Viviparus) Oral Vaccine, Living is an aqueous preparation containing approximately 1000 modified *Dictyocaulus viviparus* larvae per dose.

PRODUCTION

The vaccinal organisms are produced in calves. The calves used for production are obtained from a known, defined source that is monitored for freedom from certain diseases, as agreed with the competent authority. The calves are healthy, have not been exposed previously to *Dictyocaulus viviparus* and have been shown to be free from a range of infectious diseases, as agreed with the competent authority.

The third stage larvae are harvested from the faeces, purified, partially inactivated by ionising radiation, then diluted as necessary.

CHOICE OF VACCINE STRAIN

The suspension of irradiated vaccinal organisms is shown to be satisfactory with respect to safety and immunogenicity for the animals for which the vaccine is intended. The following tests may be used during the demonstration of safety, Appendix XV K(Vet) 1 and immunogenicity, Appendix XV K(Vet) 2.

Safety

Carry out a test in at least five calves of the minimum age to be recommended for vaccination that do not have antibodies to *Dictyocaulus viviparus*. Administer orally, to each calf, a quantity of irradiated vaccinal organisms corresponding to twice the maximum number of organisms likely to be included in a dose of the vaccine. Observe the calves for 6 weeks. They remain in good health and show no more than transient respiratory signs approximately one week after vaccination. Collect faecal samples from each calf 4, 5 and 6 weeks after vaccination and examine separately for the presence of *D. viviparus* larvae. No larvae are detected.

Immunogenicity

The test described under Potency is suitable to demonstrate immunogenicity when carried out using the minimum number of organisms likely to be included in a dose of the vaccine.

BATCH TESTING

If Identification test B and the test for Potency have been carried out with satisfactory results on a representative batch of vaccine, these tests may be omitted as a routine control on other batches of vaccine subject to the agreement of the competent authority.

Subject to the agreement of the competent authority, Test A described below under Safety, may be conducted on representative batches, selected at defined periods during the production season, rather than as a routine test on every batch.

Extraneous bacteria

For each batch, the number of non-pathogenic organisms per dose is shown to be within the limits set for the product and shown to be safe.

The vaccine complies with the requirements stated under Veterinary Vaccines with the following modifications.

IDENTIFICATION

A. Produces petechial haemorrhages in the lungs of guinea-pigs within 48 hours of oral administration. Adult worms do not develop.

B. Protects calves against *D. viviparus* infection and does not cause parasitic bronchitis.

TESTS

Extraneous bacteria and fungi

The vaccine is shown by appropriate methods to be free from pathogenic organisms including *Brucella*, *Mycobacteria* and *Salmonella* species.

Extraneous viruses

Inoculate the vaccine onto suitable cell cultures susceptible to bovine viruses, make at least one passage and maintain the cultures for at least 14 days. No cytopathic effect develops.

Carry out a specific test for freedom from bovine viral diarrhoea. No evidence of bovine viral diarrhoea is found.

Carry out a test for freedom from haemadsorbing agents. The cell cultures show no signs of viral contamination.

Safety

A. Administer orally to each of two healthy susceptible calves of the minimum age for vaccination and free from antibodies to *D. viviparus*, twice the dose stated on the label and repeat four weeks later. The animals remain free from clinical signs during 60 days after the second dose and show no post-mortem signs of parasitic bronchitis when subsequently killed.

B. Administer orally to each of four healthy susceptible guinea-pigs the larval contents of 5 calf doses of vaccine. Kill two guinea-pigs on day 2 and the other two on day 10 after dosing. Examine the lungs. The vaccine complies with the test if at day 2 there are petechial haemorrhages in the lungs and at day 10 there are no more than a very small number of fifth-stage larvae.

Viable larvae

The number of viable larvae is not less than 1000 per dose determined by microscopic examination.

POTENCY

Use calves of the minimum age for vaccination recommended on the label and that do not have antibodies to *D. viviparus*. Vaccinate at least ten calves as recommended on the label. Maintain at least five calves as unvaccinated controls. Observe the calves for 40 days and monitor and score the calves for signs of respiratory disease (e.g. increased respiratory rate, coughing). Carry out post-mortem examination of the lungs of any animal that dies during the observation period. At the end of the observation period, kill the surviving calves and examine the lungs. The test is not valid unless the control calves show typical signs of respiratory disease due to lungworm infection and, at post-mortem examination, there are noticeable, typical lesions in the lungs (e.g. areas of consolidation) and in calves submitted to post-mortem examination in the later stages, adult worms are present.

The vaccine complies with the test if the vaccinated calves show no more than very mild respiratory signs after challenge and, at post-mortem examination, there are no or only very limited lesions in the lungs (e.g. areas of consolidation) and no or very few adult worms are present.

STORAGE

When stored under the prescribed conditions the parasites may be expected to survive for 45 days.

Mannheimia Vaccine (Inactivated) for Cattle

(Ph Eur monograph 1944)

Ph Eur

DEFINITION

Mannheimia vaccine (inactivated) for cattle is a preparation from cultures of one or more suitable strains of *Mannheimia haemolytica* (formerly *Pasteurella haemolytica*). This monograph applies to vaccines intended for administration to cattle of different ages for protection against respiratory diseases caused by *M. haemolytica*.

PRODUCTION

Production of the vaccine is based on a seed-lot system. The seed material is cultured in a suitable medium; each strain is cultivated separately and identity is verified using a suitable method. During production, various parameters such as growth rate are monitored by suitable methods; the values are within the limits approved for the particular product. Purity and identity of the harvest are verified using suitable methods. After cultivation, the bacterial suspensions are collected separately and inactivated by a suitable method. The vaccine may contain an adjuvant and may be freeze-dried.

CHOICE OF VACCINE COMPOSITION

The choice of composition and the strains to be included in the vaccine is based on epidemiological data on the prevalence of the different serovars of *M. haemolytica* and on the claims being made. The vaccine is shown to be satisfactory with respect to safety (*5.2.6*) and efficacy (*5.2.7*) in cattle. As part of the studies to demonstrate the suitability of the vaccine with respect to these characteristics the following tests may be carried out.

Safety

A. The test is carried out for each route of administration to be stated on the label and in animals of each category for which the vaccine is intended.

For each test, use not fewer than 10 animals that preferably do not have antibodies against the serovars of *M. haemolytica* or against the leucotoxin present in the vaccine. Where justified, animals with a known history of no previous mannheimia vaccination and with low antibody titres (measured in a sensitive test system such as an ELISA) may be used.

Administer to each animal a double dose of vaccine containing not less than the maximum potency that may be expected in a batch of vaccine. Administer a single dose of vaccine to each animal after the recommended interval. Observe the animals for at least 14 days after the last administration. Record body temperature the day before vaccination, at vaccination, 2 h, 4 h and 6 h later and then daily for 4 days; note the maximum temperature increase for each animal. No abnormal local or systemic reaction occurs; the average body temperature increase for all animals does not exceed 1.5 °C and no animal shows a rise greater than 2 °C. If the vaccine is intended for use or may be used in pregnant cows, vaccinate the cows at the relevant stages of pregnancy and prolong the observation period until 1 day after parturition.

The vaccine complies with the test if no animal shows abnormal local or systemic reactions or clinical signs of disease or dies from causes attributable to the vaccine. In addition, if the vaccine is intended for use in pregnant cows, no significant effects on the pregnancy and offspring are demonstrated.

B. The animals used for the field trials are also used to evaluate safety. Carry out a test in each category of animals for which the vaccine is intended. Use not fewer than 3 groups of 20 animals with corresponding groups of not fewer than 10 controls in 3 different locations. Examine the injection sites for local reactions after vaccination. Record body temperatures the day before vaccination, at vaccination and on the 2 days following vaccination. The vaccine complies with the test if no animal shows abnormal local or systemic reactions or clinical signs of disease or dies from causes attributable to the vaccine. The average body temperature increase for all animals does not exceed 1.5 °C and no animal shows a rise greater than 2 °C. In addition, if the vaccine is intended for use in pregnant cows, no significant effects on the pregnancy and offspring are demonstrated.

Immunogenicity   As part of the studies to demonstrate the suitability of the vaccine with respect to immunogenicity, the test described under Potency may be carried out for each proposed route of administration and using vaccine of minimum potency.

BATCH TESTING
Batch potency test
The test described under Potency is not carried out for routine testing of batches of vaccine. It is carried out, for a given vaccine, on one or more occasions, as decided by or with the agreement of the competent authority. Where the test is not carried out, a suitable validated test is carried out, the criteria for acceptance being set with reference to the results obtained with a batch of vaccine that has given satisfactory results in the test described under Potency.

Bacterial endotoxins
A test for bacterial endotoxins (*2.6.14*) is carried out on the final lot or, where the nature of the adjuvant prevents performance of a satisfactory test, on the bulk antigen or the mixture of bulk antigens immediately before addition of the adjuvant. The maximum acceptable amount of bacterial endotoxins is that found for a batch of vaccine that has been shown satisfactory in safety test A given under Choice of vaccine composition or in the safety test described under Tests, carried out using 10 animals. Where the latter test is used, note the maximum temperature increase for each animal; the average body temperature increase for all animals does not exceed 1.5 °C. The method chosen for determining the amount of bacterial endotoxin present in the vaccine batch used in the safety test for determining the maximum acceptable level of endotoxin is used subsequently for testing of each batch.

IDENTIFICATION
When injected into healthy seronegative animals, the vaccine stimulates the production of specific antibodies against the serovars of *M. haemolytica* and/or against the leucotoxin present in the vaccine.

TESTS
Safety
Use 2 cattle of the minimum age recommended for vaccination that have not been vaccinated against mannheimiosis. Administer a double dose of vaccine to each animal by a recommended route. Observe the animals for 14 days. Record body temperature the day before vaccination, at vaccination, 2 h, 4 h and 6 h later and then daily for 2 days. The animals remain in good health and no abnormal local or systemic reaction occurs; a transient temperature increase not exceeding 2 °C may occur.

Sterility
It complies with the test for sterility prescribed in the monograph on *Vaccines for veterinary use (0062)*.

POTENCY
Carry out a test for each serovar for which protection is claimed on the label.

Use not fewer than 16 animals of the minimum age recommended for vaccination, free from antibodies against *M. haemolytica* and against the leucotoxin of *M. haemolytica*. Vaccinate not fewer than 8 of the animals by a recommended route and according to the recommended schedule. Keep 8 animals as controls. 21 days after the last vaccination, challenge all the animals by the intratracheal route or by another appropriate route, with a suitable quantity of a low-passage, virulent strain of a serovar of *M. haemolytica*. Observe the animals for a further 7 days; to avoid unnecessary suffering, severely ill animals are killed and are then considered to have died from the disease. During the observation period, the animals are examined for signs of disease for example, increased body temperature, dullness, abnormal breathing and the mortality is recorded. Kill surviving animals at the end of the observation period. Post-mortem examination is carried out on any animal that dies and those killed at the end of the observation period.

The lungs are examined and the extent of lung lesions due to mannheimiosis is evaluated. Samples of lung tissue are collected for re-isolation of the challenge organisms.

The clinical observations and lung lesions are scored and the results obtained for these parameters and the bacterial re-isolation results compared for the 2 groups.

The test is invalid if signs of *M. haemolytica* infection occur in less than 70 per cent of the control animals.

The vaccine complies with the requirements of the test if there is a significant difference between the scores obtained for the clinical and post-mortem observations in the vaccinates compared to the controls. For vaccines with a claim for a beneficial effect on the extent of infection against the serovar, the results for the infection rates are also significantly better for the vaccinates compared to the controls.

LABELLING
The label states:
— the serovar(s) of *M. haemolytica* against which protection is claimed,
— the serovar(s) of *M. haemolytica* and/or the leucotoxin present in the vaccine.

Ph Eur

Mannheimia Vaccine (Inactivated) for Sheep

(Ph Eur monograph 1946)

Ph Eur _____

DEFINITION

Mannheimia vaccine (inactivated) for sheep is a preparation of one or more suitable strains of *Mannheimia haemolytica* (formerly *Pasteurella haemolytica*). This monograph applies to vaccines intended for administration to sheep for active immunisation and to protect passively their future progeny against disease caused by *M. haemolytica*.

PRODUCTION

Production of the vaccine is based on a seed lot system. The seed material is cultured in a suitable medium; each strain is cultivated separately and identity is verified using a suitable method. During production, various parameters such as growth rate are monitored by suitable methods; the values are within the limits approved for the particular product. Purity and identity of the harvest are verified using suitable methods. After cultivation, the bacterial suspensions are collected separately and inactivated by a suitable method. The vaccine may contain an adjuvant and may be freeze-dried.

CHOICE OF VACCINE COMPOSITION

The choice of composition and the strains to be included in the vaccine is based on epidemiological data on the prevalence of the different serovars of *M. haemolytica* and on the claims being made for the product, for example active and/or passive protection. The vaccine is shown to be satisfactory with respect to safety (5.2.6) and efficacy (5.2.7) in sheep. As part of the studies to demonstrate the suitability of the vaccine with respect to these characteristics the following tests may be carried out.

Safety

A. The test is carried out for each of the routes of administration to be stated on the label and in animals of each category (for example, young sheep, pregnant ewes) for which the vaccine is intended.

For each test, use not fewer than 10 animals that preferably do not have antibodies against the serovars of *M. haemolytica* or against the leucotoxin present in the vaccine. Where justified, animals with a known history of no previous mannheimia vaccination and with low antibody titres (measured in a sensitive test system such as an ELISA) may be used.

Administer to each animal a double dose of vaccine containing not less than the maximum potency that may be expected in a batch of vaccine. Administer a single dose of vaccine to each animal after the recommended interval. Observe the animals for at least 14 days after the last administration. Record body temperature the day before vaccination, at vaccination, 2 h, 4 h and 6 h later and then daily for 4 days; note the maximum temperature increase for each animal. No abnormal local or systemic reaction occurs; the average body temperature increase for all animals does not exceed 1.5 °C and no animal shows a rise greater than 2 °C. If the vaccine is intended for use or may be used in pregnant ewes, vaccinate the ewes at the relevant stages of pregnancy and prolong the observation period until 1 day after lambing.

The vaccine complies with the test if no animal shows abnormal local reactions or clinical signs of disease or dies from causes attributable to the vaccine. In addition, if the vaccine is intended for use in pregnant ewes, no significant effects on the pregnancy and offspring are demonstrated.

B. The animals used for the field trials are also used to evaluate safety. Carry out a test in each category of animals for which the vaccine is intended. Use not fewer than 3 groups of 20 animals with corresponding groups of not fewer than 10 controls in 3 different locations. Examine the injection sites for local reactions after vaccination. Record body temperatures the day before vaccination, at vaccination and on the 2 days following vaccination. The vaccine complies with the test if no animal shows abnormal local or systemic reactions or clinical signs of disease or dies from causes attributable to the vaccine. The average body temperature increase for all animals does not exceed 1.5 °C and no animal shows a rise greater than 2 °C. In addition, if the vaccine is intended for use in pregnant ewes, no significant effects on the pregnancy and offspring are demonstrated.

Immunogenicity As part of the studies to demonstrate the suitability of the vaccine with respect to immunogenicity, the tests described under Potency may be carried out for each proposed route of administration and using vaccine of minimum potency.

BATCH TESTING

Batch potency test

The relevant test or tests described under Potency are not carried out for routine testing of batches of vaccine. They are carried out, for a given vaccine, on one or more occasions, as decided by or with the agreement of the competent authority. Where the relevant test or tests are not carried out, a suitable validated batch potency test is carried out, the criteria for acceptance being set with reference to the results obtained with a batch of vaccine that has given satisfactory results in the test(s) described under Potency.

Bacterial endotoxins

A test for bacterial endotoxins (2.6.14) is carried out on the final lot or, where the nature of the adjuvant prevents performance of a satisfactory test, on the bulk antigen or the mixture of bulk antigens immediately before addition of the adjuvant. The maximum acceptable amount of bacterial endotoxins is that found for a batch of vaccine that has been shown satisfactory in safety test A given under Choice of vaccine composition or in the safety test described under Tests, carried out using 10 animals. Where the latter test is used, note the maximum temperature increase for each animal; the average body temperature increase for all animals does not exceed 1.5 °C. The method chosen for determining the amount of bacterial endotoxin present in the vaccine batch used in the safety test for determining the maximum acceptable level of endotoxin is used subsequently for testing of each batch.

IDENTIFICATION

When injected into healthy seronegative animals, the vaccine stimulates the production of specific antibodies against the serovars of *M. haemolytica* and/or against the leucotoxin present in the vaccine.

TESTS

Safety

Use 2 sheep of the minimum age recommended for vaccination or, if not available, of an age as close as possible to the minimum recommended age, and that have not been vaccinated against mannheimiosis. Administer a double dose of vaccine to each animal by a recommended route. Observe the animals for 14 days. Record body temperature the day before vaccination, at vaccination, 2 h, 4 h and 6 h later and then daily for 2 days. The animals remain in good health and no abnormal local or systemic reaction occurs; a transient temperature increase not exceeding 2 °C may occur.

Sterility
It complies with the test for sterility prescribed in the monograph on *Vaccines for veterinary use (0062)*.

POTENCY
Active immunisation
For vaccines with claims for active immunisation due to *M. haemolytica*, carry out a test for each serovar of *M. haemolytica* for which protection is claimed on the label.

Use not fewer than 20 lambs of the minimum age recommended for vaccination, free from antibodies against *M. haemolytica* and against the leucotoxin of *M. haemolytica*. Vaccinate not fewer than 10 of the animals by a recommended route and according to the recommended schedule. Keep 10 animals as controls. 21 days after the last vaccination, challenge all the lambs by the intratracheal route or by another appropriate route, with a suitable quantity of a low-passage, virulent strain of a serovar of *M. haemolytica*. Where necessary for a given serovar, prechallenge with parainfluenza type 3 (PI3) virus or another appropriate respiratory pathogen may be used. Observe the animals for a further 7 days; to avoid unnecessary suffering, severely ill animals are killed and are then considered to have died from the disease. During the observation period, the animals are examined for signs of disease (for example, increased body temperature, dullness, abnormal respiration) and the mortality is recorded. Kill surviving animals at the end of the observation period. Post-mortem examination is carried out on any animal that dies and those killed at the end of the observation period. The lungs are examined and the extent of lung lesions due to mannheimiosis is evaluated. Samples of lung tissue are collected for re-isolation of the challenge organisms. The clinical observations and lung lesions are scored and the results obtained for these parameters and the bacterial re-isolation results compared for the 2 groups.

The test is invalid if signs of *M. haemolytica* infection occur in less than 70 per cent of the control lambs.

The vaccine complies with the requirements of the test if there is a significant difference between the scores obtained for the clinical and post-mortem observations in the vaccinates compared to the controls. For vaccines with a claim for a beneficial effect on the extent of infection against the serovar, the results for the infection rates are also significantly better for the vaccinates compared to the controls.

Passive protection
For vaccines with claims for passive protection against mannheimiosis carry out a test for each serovar of *M. haemolytica* for which protection is claimed on the label.

Use at least 6 ewes that preferably do not have antibodies against the serovars of *M. haemolytica* or against the leucotoxin present in the vaccine. Where justified, animals with a known history of no previous mannheimia vaccination, from a source with a low incidence of respiratory disease and with low antibody titres (measured in a sensitive test system such as an ELISA) may be used. Vaccinate the animals by 1 of the recommended routes, at the recommended stages of pregnancy and according to the recommended schedule. A challenge study is conducted with 20 newborn, colostrum-deprived lambs. 10 of these lambs are given colostrum from the vaccinated ewes and 10 control lambs are given colostrum or colostrum substitute without detectable antibodies to *M. haemolytica*. When the lambs are at the age claimed for the duration of the passive protection, challenge by the intratracheal route with a suitable quantity of a low-passage, virulent strain of a serovar of *M. haemolytica*. Observe the animals for a further 7 days; to avoid unnecessary suffering, severely ill animals are killed and are then considered to have died from the disease. Observe the animals and assess the effect of the challenge on the offspring of the vaccinates and the controls as described in the test for active immunisation.

The test is invalid if clinical signs or lesions of *M. haemolytica* infection occur in less than 70 per cent of the control lambs.

The vaccine complies with the requirements of the test if there is a significant difference between the scores obtained for the clinical and post-mortem observations in the lambs from the vaccinates compared to those from the controls. For vaccines with a claim for a beneficial effect on the extent of infection against the serovar, the results for the infection rates are also significantly better for the lambs from the vaccinates compared to those from the controls.

LABELLING
The label states:
— the serovar(s) of *M. haemolytica* against which protection is claimed,
— the serovar(s) of *M. haemolytica* and/or the leucotoxin present in the vaccine,
— for vaccines for passive protection, the length of time for which the passive protection is claimed.

Ph Eur

Marek's Disease Vaccine, Living

Marek's Disease Vaccine (Turkey Herpes Virus)
Marek's Disease Vaccine, Living (HVT)
(*Marek's Disease Vaccine (Live)*, Ph Eur monograph 0589)

Ph Eur

1. DEFINITION
Marek's disease vaccine (live) is a preparation of a suitable strain or strains of Marek's disease virus (gallid herpesvirus 2 or 3) and/or turkey herpesvirus (meleagrid herpesvirus 1). This monograph applies to vaccines intended for administration to chickens and/or chicken embryos for active immunisation.

2. PRODUCTION
2-1. PREPARATION OF THE VACCINE
The vaccine virus is grown in cell cultures. If the vaccine contains more than one type of virus, the different types are grown separately. The vaccine may be freeze-dried or stored in liquid nitrogen.

2-2. SUBSTRATE FOR VIRUS PROPAGATION
2-2-1. Cell cultures
The cell cultures comply with the requirements for cell cultures for production of veterinary vaccines (*5.2.4*).

2-3. SEED LOTS
2-3-1. Extraneous agents
The master seed lot complies with the tests for extraneous agents in seed lots (*2.6.24*). In these tests on the master seed lot, the organisms used are not more than 5 passages from the master seed lot at the start of the tests.

2-4. CHOICE OF VACCINE VIRUS

The vaccine virus shall be shown to be satisfactory with respect to safety (5.2.6) and efficacy (5.2.7) for the chickens and/or chicken embryos for which it is intended.

The tests shown below for residual pathogenicity of the strain (section 2-4-1), increase in virulence (section 2-4-2) and immunogenicity (section 2-4-3) may be used during the demonstration of safety and immunogenicity. Additional testing may be needed to demonstrate safety in breeds of chickens known to be particularly susceptible to Marek's disease virus, unless the vaccine is to be contra-indicated.

2-4-1. Residual pathogenicity of the strain

Carry out the test for the route to be recommended for vaccination that is likely to be the least safe and in the category of chickens for which the vaccine is intended that is likely to be the most susceptible for Marek's disease. Carry out the test in chickens if the vaccine is intended for chickens; carry out the test in chicken embryos if the vaccine is intended for chicken embryos; carry out the test in chickens and in chicken embryos if the vaccine is intended for both. Use vaccine virus at the least attenuated passage level that will be present between the master seed lot and a batch of the vaccine.

Vaccines intended for use in chickens   Use not fewer than 80 one-day-old chickens from a flock free from specified pathogens (SPF) (5.2.2). Divide them randomly into 2 groups of not fewer than 40 chickens and maintain the groups separately. Administer by a suitable route to each chicken of one group (I) a quantity of the vaccine virus equivalent to not less than 10 times the maximum virus titre likely to be contained in 1 dose of the vaccine. Administer by a suitable route to each chicken of the other group (II) a quantity of virulent Marek's disease virus that will cause mortality and/or severe macroscopic lesions of Marek's disease in not fewer than 70 per cent of the effective number of chickens within 70 days (initial number reduced by the number that die within the first 7 days of the test).

Vaccines intended for use in chicken embryos   Use not fewer than 150 embryonated eggs from an SPF flock (5.2.2). Divide them randomly into 3 groups of not fewer than 50 embryonated eggs and maintain the groups separately but under identical incubation conditions. Not later than the recommended day of vaccination, administer by the recommended method to each embryonated egg of one group (I) a quantity of the vaccine virus equivalent to not less than 10 times the maximum virus titre likely to be contained in 1 dose of the vaccine. Administer by a suitable route to each embryonated egg of another group (II) a quantity of virulent Marek's disease virus that will cause mortality and/or severe macroscopic lesions of Marek's disease in not fewer than 70 per cent of the effective number of hatched chickens within 70 days (initial number reduced by the number that die within the first 7 days after hatching). Keep the last group (III) non-inoculated. The test is invalid if there is a significant difference in hatchability between groups I and III and the hatchability in any of the 3 groups is less than 80 per cent.

Provided that the chickens and chicken embryos are derived from the same flock, a common control group for *in ovo* and parenteral administration can be used.

Irrespective of whether the vaccine was administered to chickens or chicken embryos, observe the chickens of group II at least daily for 70 days and those of group I at least daily for 120 days. The test is invalid if one or more of the following apply:

— more than 10 per cent of the chickens in any of the 3 groups die within the first 7 days;
— fewer than 70 per cent of the effective number of chickens in group II show macroscopic lesions of Marek's disease.

The vaccine virus complies with the test if:
— no chicken of group I shows notable clinical signs or macroscopic lesions of Marek's disease or dies from causes attributable to the vaccine virus;
— at 120 days the number of surviving chickens of group I is not fewer than 80 per cent of the effective number.

2-4-2. Increase in virulence

The test for increase in virulence is required for Marek's disease virus vaccine strains but not for turkey herpesvirus vaccine strains, which are naturally apathogenic. Use vaccine virus at the least attenuated passage level that will be present between the master seed lot and a batch of the vaccine.

Vaccines intended for use in chickens   Administer by the intramuscular route a quantity of the vaccine virus that will allow recovery of virus for the passages described below to each of 5 one-day-old chickens from an SPF flock (5.2.2).

Vaccines intended for use only in chicken embryos or intended for use in chickens and in chicken embryos   Administer by the *in ovo* route, using the recommended method, a quantity of the vaccine virus that will allow recovery of virus for the passages described below to each of 5 embryonated eggs not later than the recommended day for vaccination.

5-7 days after administering the vaccine to chickens or 5-7 days after hatching when the vaccine has been administered *in ovo*, prepare a suspension of white blood cells from each chicken and pool these samples. Administer a suitable volume of the pooled samples by the intraperitoneal route to each of 5 other chickens that are 1 dayold and from an SPF flock (5.2.2). Carry out this passage operation not fewer than 5 times; verify the presence of the virus at each passage. Care must be taken to avoid contamination by virus from previous passages. If the virus is not found at a passage level, carry out a second series of passages. Carry out the test for residual pathogenicity (section 2-4-1) using the unpassaged vaccine virus and the maximally passaged virus that has been recovered. Administer the virus by the route to be recommended for vaccination that is likely to be the least safe for use in these chickens or chicken embryos.

The vaccine virus complies with the test if no indication of increase in virulence of the maximally passaged virus compared with the unpassaged virus is observed. If virus is not recovered at any passage level in the first and second series of passages, the vaccine virus also complies with the test.

2-4-3. Immunogenicity

A test is carried out for each route and method of administration to be recommended, using in each case chickens of the youngest age to be recommended for vaccination or chicken embryos. The quantity of the vaccine virus administered to each chicken or chicken embryo is not greater than the minimum virus titre to be stated on the label and the virus is at the most attenuated passage level that will be present in a batch of the vaccine.

Vaccines intended for use in chickens   Use not fewer than 60 chickens of the same origin and from an SPF flock (5.2.2). Vaccinate by a recommended route not fewer than 30 chickens. Maintain not fewer than 30 chickens as controls.

Vaccines intended for use in chicken embryos   Use embryonated chickens of the same origin and from an SPF flock (5.2.2). Vaccinate by the *in ovo* route using the method to be

---

recommended, 50 per cent of the embryonated eggs. Maintain 50 per cent of the embryonated eggs as controls. The test is invalid if any group consists of fewer than 30 hatched chicks.

Irrespective of whether the vaccine was administered to chickens or chicken embryos, challenge each chicken not later than 9 days after vaccination by a suitable route with a sufficient quantity of virulent Marek's disease virus. Observe the chickens at least daily for 70 days after challenge. Record the deaths and the number of surviving chickens that show clinical signs of disease. At the end of the observation period, euthanise all the surviving chickens and carry out an examination for macroscopic lesions of Marek's disease. The test is not valid if:

— during the observation period after challenge, fewer than 70 per cent of the control chickens die or show severe clinical signs or macroscopic lesions of Marek's disease;
— and/or, during the period between the vaccination and challenge, more than 10 per cent of the control or vaccinated chickens show abnormal clinical signs or die from causes not attributable to the vaccine.

The vaccine virus complies with the test if the relative protection percentage, calculated using the following expression, is not less than 80 per cent:

$$\frac{V - C}{100 - C} \times 100$$

V = percentage of challenged vaccinated chickens that survive to the end of the observation period without notable clinical signs or macroscopic lesions of Marek's disease;

C = percentage of challenged control chickens that survive to the end of the observation period without notable clinical signs or macroscopic lesions of Marek's disease.

3. BATCH TESTS
3-1. Identification
Carry out an immunostaining test in cell cultures using monoclonal antibodies to demonstrate the presence of each type of virus stated on the label.

3-2. Bacteria and fungi
The vaccine and, where applicable, the liquid supplied with it comply with the test for sterility prescribed in the monograph *Vaccines for veterinary use (0062)*.

3-3. Mycoplasmas
The vaccine complies with the test for mycoplasmas (*2.6.7*).

3-4. Extraneous agents
The vaccine complies with the tests for extraneous agents in batches of finished product (*2.6.25*).

3-5. Safety
Administer by a recommended route and method to each chicken or chicken embryo 10 doses of the vaccine.

Vaccines intended for use in chickens Use not fewer than 10 chickens from an SPF flock (*5.2.2*) and not older than the youngest age recommended for vaccination.

Vaccines intended for use only in chicken embryos or intended for use in chickens and in chicken embryos Use embryonated eggs from an SPF flock (*5.2.2*) at not later than the recommended day of vaccination of embryos. The test is invalid if the group consists of fewer than 10 hatched chicks and hatchability is less than 80 per cent.

Irrespective of whether the vaccine was administered to chickens or embryos, observe the chickens at least daily for 21 days after vaccination or hatching, as appropriate. The test is not valid if more than 20 per cent of the chickens show abnormal clinical signs or die from causes not attributable to the vaccine. The vaccine complies with the test if no chicken shows notable clinical signs of disease or dies from causes attributable to the vaccine.

3-6. Virus titre
3-6-1. *Vaccines containing one type of virus* Titrate the vaccine virus by inoculation into suitable cell cultures (*5.2.4*). If the virus titre is determined in plaque-forming units (PFU), only primary plaques are taken into consideration. The vaccine complies with the test if one dose contains not less than the minimum virus titre stated on the label.

3-6-2. *Vaccines containing more than one type of virus* For vaccines containing more than one type of virus, titrate each virus by inoculation into suitable cell cultures (*5.2.4*), reading the results by immunostaining using antibodies. The vaccine complies with the test if one dose contains for each vaccine virus not less than the minimum virus titre stated on the label.

3-7. Potency
The vaccine complies with the test for immunogenicity (section 2-4-3) when administered according to the recommended schedule by a recommended route and method. It is not necessary to carry out the potency test for each batch of the vaccine if it has been carried out on a representative batch using a vaccinating dose containing not more than the minimum virus titre stated on the label.

Ph Eur

Mycoplasma Gallisepticum Vaccine (Inactivated)

(*Mycoplasma Gallisepticum Vaccine (Inactivated),* Ph Eur monograph 1942)

Ph Eur

1. DEFINITION
Mycoplasma gallisepticum vaccine (inactivated) is a preparation of one or more suitable strains of *Mycoplasma gallisepticum* that have been inactivated while maintaining adequate immunogenic properties. This monograph applies to vaccines intended for the active immunisation of chickens and/or turkeys.

2. PRODUCTION
2-1. PREPARATION OF THE VACCINE
Production of the vaccine is based on a seed-lot system. The seed material is cultured in a suitable solid and/or liquid medium to ensure optimal growth under the chosen incubation conditions. Each strain is cultivated separately and identity is verified using a suitable method. During production, various parameters such as growth rate are monitored by suitable methods; the values are within the limits approved for the particular vaccine. Purity and identity of the harvest are verified using suitable methods. After cultivation, the mycoplasma suspensions are collected separately and inactivated by a suitable method.

The mycoplasma suspensions may be treated to fragment the mycoplasmas and the fragments may be purified and concentrated. The vaccine may contain an adjuvant.

2-2. CHOICE OF VACCINE COMPOSITION
The vaccine is shown to be satisfactory with respect to safety (*5.2.6*) and efficacy (*5.2.7*) in the target animals.

The following test for immunogenicity (section 2-2-1) may be used during the demonstration of efficacy. If the indications for the vaccine include protection against a drop in laying performance or protection against infectious sinusitis in turkeys, further suitable immunogenicity testing is necessary.

2-2-1. Immunogenicity

The test is carried out for each recommended route of administration and for each avian species for which the vaccine is intended. Use for each test not fewer than 40 birds not older than the youngest age to be recommended for vaccination. Use chickens from a flock free from specified pathogens (SPF) (5.2.2) or turkeys that have not been vaccinated and are free from antibodies against *M. gallisepticum*. For each test, administer to each of not fewer than 20 birds a quantity of the vaccine not greater than a single dose. If re-vaccination is recommended, repeat this operation after the recommended interval. Maintain not fewer than 20 birds as controls. Challenge each bird from both groups not more than 28 days after the last administration by a suitable route with a sufficient quantity of virulent *M. gallisepticum* (R-strain). Observe the birds at least daily for 14 days after challenge. Evaluation is carried out 14 days after challenge, at which point the birds are euthanised. Record the deaths and the number of surviving birds that show clinical signs of disease (e.g. respiratory distress, nasal discharge), and record air sac lesions.

The test is invalid if:
— during the observation period after challenge, fewer than 70 per cent of the controls die or show lesions or clinical signs of disease;
— and/or during the period between vaccination and challenge, more than 10 per cent of the birds from the control group or from the vaccinated group show abnormal clinical signs of disease or die from causes not attributable to the vaccine.

Thoracic and abdominal air sacs are evaluated individually on each side of the animal. The scoring system presented below may be used. The vaccine complies with the test if the score for the vaccinated birds is significantly lower than that for the controls and if the reduction is not less than 30 per cent.

0 no air sac lesions
1 in a limited area of 1 or 2 air sacs: cloudiness with slight thickening of the air sac membrane or flecks of yellowish exudate
2 in 1 air sac or portions of 2 air sacs: greyish or yellow, sometimes foamy exudate, with thickening of the air sac membrane
3 in 3 air sacs: extensive exudate, with clear thickening of most air sacs
4 severe air-sacculitis with considerable exudate and thickening of most air sacs.

2-3. MANUFACTURER'S TESTS
2-3-1. Batch potency test

It is not necessary to carry out the potency test (section 3-5) for each batch of the vaccine if it has been carried out using a batch of vaccine with a minimum potency. Where the test is not carried out on a batch, an alternative validated method is used, the criteria for acceptance being set with reference to a batch of vaccine that has given satisfactory results in the potency test (section 3-5). The following test may be used.

Use not fewer than 15 chickens, 3-4 weeks old, from an SPF flock (5.2.2) or not fewer than 15 turkeys, 3-4 weeks old, that have not been vaccinated against *M. gallisepticum*, do not

have antibodies against *M. gallisepticum*, and are obtained from a healthy flock. Collect serum samples from each vaccinate and control bird just before vaccination and check for the absence of antibodies against *M. gallisepticum*. Administer to each of not fewer than 10 birds 1 dose of the vaccine by a recommended route. Maintain not fewer than 5 birds as controls. Collect serum samples 5 weeks after vaccination from each vaccinated and control bird. Measure the titres of serum antibodies against *M. gallisepticum* using a suitable method. Calculate the mean titres for the group of vaccinates. The test is invalid if specific *M. gallisepticum* antibodies are found in any serum samples from the control birds 5 weeks after the time of administration of the vaccine. The vaccine complies with the test if the mean antibody titres of the group of vaccinates are equal to or greater than the titres obtained with a batch that has given satisfactory results in the potency test (section 3-5).

3. BATCH TESTS
3-1. Identification

When injected into chickens from an SPF flock (5.2.2) or turkeys from healthy flocks, the vaccine stimulates the production of antibodies against one or more strains of *M. gallisepticum*.

3-2. Bacteria and fungi

The vaccine complies with the test for sterility prescribed in the monograph *Vaccines for veterinary use (0062)*.

3-3. Residual live mycoplasmas

The vaccine complies with a validated test for residual live *M. gallisepticum* carried out by a culture method (see for example *2.6.7*, using media shown to be suitable for *M. gallisepticum*).

3-4. Safety

Use not fewer than 10 chickens from an SPF flock (5.2.2) or, if the vaccine is intended only for turkeys, not fewer than 10 turkeys of the minimum age recommended for vaccination from an unvaccinated flock that is free from antibodies against *M. gallisepticum*. Administer to each bird by a recommended route a double dose of the vaccine. Observe the birds at least daily for 21 days. The vaccine complies with the test if all the birds remain in good health and no abnormal local or systemic reaction occurs.

3-5. Potency

The vaccine complies with the test for immunogenicity (section 2-2-1).

_____ Ph Eur

Myxomatosis Vaccine (Live) for Rabbits

(*Ph Eur monograph 1943*)

Ph Eur _____

DEFINITION

Myxomatosis vaccine (live) for rabbits is a preparation of a suitable strain of either myxoma virus that is attenuated for rabbits or Shope fibroma virus. The vaccine is intended for the active immunisation of rabbits against myxomatosis.

PRODUCTION

The virus is propagated in suitable cell cultures (5.2.4). The viral suspension is harvested, titrated and may be mixed with a suitable stabilising solution. The vaccine may be freeze-dried.

CHOICE OF VACCINE STRAIN

The vaccine is shown to be satisfactory with respect to safety, absence of increase in virulence and immunogenicity.

The following tests may be used during demonstration of safety, absence of increase in virulence (5.2.6) and efficacy (5.2.7).

Safety   The test is carried out for each route of administration to be stated on the label. Use at least 10 rabbits of the minimum age to be recommended for vaccination and that do not have antibodies against myxoma virus. Administer to each rabbit by a recommended route a quantity of virus corresponding to not less than 10 times the maximum titre that may be expected in a dose of vaccine. Observe the rabbits for 28 days. Record the body temperature the day before vaccination, at vaccination, 4 h after vaccination and then daily for 4 days; note the maximum temperature increase for each animal.

No abnormal local or systemic reaction occurs; the average temperature increase does not exceed 1 °C and no animal shows a rise greater than 2 °C. A local reaction lasting less than 28 days may occur.

If the vaccine is intended for use in pregnant rabbits, administer the virus to not less than 10 pregnant rabbits according to the schedule to be recommended on the label. Prolong the observation period until 1 day after parturition. The rabbits remain in good health and there is no abnormal local or systemic reaction. No adverse effects on the pregnancy or the offspring are noted.

Increase in virulence   (*This test is performed only for vaccines based on attenuated strains of myxoma virus*). Administer by a recommended route to each of 2 rabbits, 5 to 7 weeks old and which do not have antibodies against myxoma virus, a quantity of virus that will allow recovery of virus for the passages described below. Use vaccine virus at the least attenuated passage level that will be present between the master seed lot and a batch of the vaccine. Kill the rabbits 5 to 10 days after inoculation and remove from each rabbit organs, or tissues with sufficient virus to allow passage; homogenise the organs and tissues in a suitable buffer solution, centrifuge the suspension and use the supernatant for further passages. Inoculate the supernatant into suitable cell cultures to verify the presence of virus. Administer by an appropriate route, at a suitable rate, a suitable volume of the supernatant to each of 2 other rabbits of the same age and the same susceptibility. This operation is then repeated at least 5 times. If the virus has disappeared, a second series of passages is carried out. Inoculate virus from the highest recovered passage level to rabbits, observe for 28 days and compare any reactions that occur with those seen in the test for safety described above. There is no indication of an increase in virulence as compared with the non-passaged virus. If virus is not recovered in either of 2 series of passages, the vaccine virus also complies with the test.

Immunogenicity   The test described under Potency may be used to demonstrate the immunogenicity of the strain.

BATCH POTENCY TEST

If the test for potency has been carried out with satisfactory results on a representative batch of vaccine, using a vaccinating dose containing not more than the minimum virus titre stated on the label, this test may be omitted as a routine control on other batches of vaccine prepared from the same seed lot.

IDENTIFICATION

Carry out an immunofluorescence test in suitable cell cultures, using a monospecific antiserum.

TESTS
Safety

Use not fewer than 2 rabbits, not older than the minimum age recommended for vaccination, that do not have antibodies against myxoma virus and rabbit haemorrhagic disease virus and that have been reared in suitable isolation conditions to avoid contact with myxoma virus. Administer by a recommended route to each rabbit 10 doses of vaccine. Observe the rabbits at least daily for 14 days. No abnormal local or systemic reaction occurs.

Extraneous agents

At the end of the 14 day observation period of the safety test, administer by a recommended route to each rabbit, a further 10 doses of vaccine. After 14 days take a blood sample from each rabbit and carry out a test for antibodies against rabbit haemorrhagic disease virus. No antibodies are found.

Bacterial and fungal contamination

The vaccine, reconstituted if necessary, complies with the test for sterility prescribed in the monograph on *Vaccines for Veterinary Use (0062)*.

Mycoplasmas (2.6.7)

The vaccine, reconstituted if necessary, complies with the test for mycoplasmas.

Virus titre

Reconstitute the vaccine, if necessary, and titrate in suitable cell cultures. 1 dose of the vaccine contains not less than the quantity of virus equivalent to the minimum virus titre stated on the label.

POTENCY

Use not fewer than 15 susceptible rabbits of the minimum age to be recommended for vaccination, free from antibodies against myxoma virus and reared in suitable isolation conditions to ensure absence of contact with myxoma virus. Administer 1 dose of vaccine to each of not fewer than 10 of the rabbits according to the instructions for use. Keep not less than 5 other rabbits as controls. Not less than 21 days after the last vaccination, administer by a suitable route to each rabbit a quantity of a virulent strain of myxoma virus sufficient to cause typical signs of myxomatosis in a susceptible rabbit. Observe the rabbits for a further 21 days. The test is not valid if fewer than 90 per cent of the control rabbits display typical signs of myxomatosis. A vaccine containing myxoma virus complies with the test if not fewer than 90 per cent of vaccinated rabbits show no signs of myxomatosis. A vaccine containing Shope fibroma virus complies with the test if not fewer than 75 per cent of vaccinated rabbits show no signs of myxomatosis.

LABELLING

The label states, where applicable, that a local reaction may occur.

Ph Eur

Newcastle Disease and Avian Infectious Bronchitis Vaccine, Living

The use of Newcastle Disease and Avian Infectious Bronchitis Vaccine Living is restricted in the United Kingdom by the Agricultural Departments.

DEFINITION

Newcastle Disease and Avian Infectious Bronchitis Vaccine, Living is a mixed preparation derived from separate groups of eggs infected with suitable strains of Newcastle disease virus and of avian infectious bronchitis virus. The Newcastle disease virus seed is either a modified strain, such as Hitchner B1 or La Sota, or a naturally occurring strain of low pathogenicity. The avian infectious bronchitis virus seed is a strain of the Massachusetts type[1] and it may be used at various levels of attenuation. The vaccine is prepared immediately before use by reconstitution from the dried vaccine with a suitable liquid.

PRODUCTION

For vaccine production the virus is propagated in embryonated eggs derived from chicken flocks free from specified pathogens. The final product is freeze dried.

Provided that the test for potency described below has been performed with satisfactory results on a representative batch of vaccine it may be omitted by the manufacturer as a routine control on other batches of vaccine prepared from the same seed lot, subject to the agreement of the competent authority.

CAUTION *The vaccine is not dangerous to man, but it is advisable to avoid undue exposure to the Newcastle disease virus and to infected birds, as the Newcastle disease virus may cause a type of conjuctivitis or, more rarely, may cause symptoms similar to those characteristic of influenza.*

The vaccine, reconstituted with a suitable liquid to provide a concentration appropriate to the particular test, complies with the requirements stated under Veterinary Vaccines with the following modifications.

IDENTIFICATION

When mixed with a mixture of monospecific Newcastle disease virus antiserum and avian infectious bronchitis virus antiserum, the vaccine no longer infects susceptible 10- to 11-day-old embryonated eggs.

TESTS

Mycoplasmas

Complies with the *test for absence of mycoplasmas*, Appendix XVI B(Vet) 3.

Sterility

Carry out the test described under Veterinary Vaccines using solid media in place of liquid media. The vaccine contains no pathogenic organisms and not more than one organism of a non-pathogenic species per bird dose.

Absence of extraneous pathogens

The neutralised vaccine complies with the *test for Avian Live Virus Vaccines: Tests for Extraneous Agents in Batches of Finished Product*, Appendix XVI B(Vet) 5.

Safety

Inoculate each of 10 chicks of the minimum age for vaccination from a flock free from specified pathogens with 10 doses of the vaccine by intranasal instillation and observe for 14 days. No abnormal reaction develops.

Virus titre

For the Newcastle disease component Neutralise the vaccine with monospecific avian infectious bronchitis virus antiserum. Inoculate serial dilutions of neutralised vaccine into the allantoic cavity of 10- to 11-day-old embryonated eggs derived from chicken flocks free from specified pathogens. Incubate the eggs for 3 days at 37° and then examine the embryos for evidence of virus infection, which is shown by the presence of chick red cell haemagglutinins. The vaccine contains not less than $10^{6.0}$ EID$_{50}$ of virus per bird dose.

For the avian infectious bronchitis component Neutralise the vaccine with monospecific Newcastle disease virus antiserum. Inoculate serial dilutions of neutralised vaccine into the allantoic cavity of 10- to 11-day-old embryonated eggs derived from chicken flocks free from specified pathogens. Incubate the eggs at 37° for 7 days and then examine the embryos for lesions typical of avian infectious bronchitis. The vaccine contains not less than $10^{3.5}$ EID$_{50}$ of virus per bird dose.

POTENCY

For the Newcastle disease component

Vaccinate each of twenty-five 5- to 10-day-old chicks from flocks free from specified pathogens, by the nasal instillation of one dose of vaccine. Twenty-one days later challenge the vaccinated chicks as well as 10 control birds by the intramuscular inoculation of at least $10^{6.0}$ EID$_{50}$ of Herts (Weybridge 33/56) strain of Newcastle disease virus and observe for 10 days. All the control birds die within 6 days and no fewer than 23 of the vaccinated birds survive the observation period without showing signs of Newcastle disease.

For the avian infectious bronchitis component

Vaccinate each of 10 healthy 3- to 4-week-old chickens from flocks free from specified pathogens, by nasal or ocular instillation such that each chicken receives one dose of vaccine. Twenty-one to twenty-eight days later challenge the vaccinated chickens, as well as 10 control birds that are kept separate from the vaccinated birds, by nasal or ocular instillation of $10^{3.0}$ to $10^{3.5}$ EID$_{50}$ of the Massachusetts 41 strain of virulent infectious bronchitis virus.

Between the 4th and 7th day after challenge, take a tracheal swab from each bird. Place each swab in a test tube containing 3 ml of broth to which suitable antibiotics have been added to inhibit the growth of bacterial contaminants and test for the presence of infectious bronchitis virus by the inoculation of 0.2 ml of inoculum into the allantoic cavity of 9- to 11-day-old embryonated eggs using at least five eggs for each swab. A tracheal swab is positive if 20% or more of the embryos inoculated from it show lesions typical of infectious bronchitis virus. If more than one embryo but fewer than 20% of those inoculated from any one swab show lesions similar to those of infectious bronchitis, inoculate at least five additional embryonated eggs with allantoic fluid from each of the suspect embryos. The swab is positive if 20% or more of these additional embryos show lesions typical of infectious bronchitis virus.

Not less than 80% of the control birds give positive tracheal swabs, and no more than 20% of the vaccinated chickens give positive tracheal swabs.

STORAGE

When stored under the prescribed conditions the dried vaccine may be expected to retain its potency for not less than 12 months. The reconstituted vaccine should be used immediately.

LABELLING

The label states (1) the names of the strains of virus used in the vaccine; (2) that the reconstituted vaccine should be used immediately.

---

[1] Vaccine prepared using avian infectious bronchitis virus seed of the Connecticut type may be used in some countries but is not permitted in the United Kingdom.

Newcastle Disease Vaccine, Inactivated

(Newcastle Disease Vaccine (Inactivated),
Ph Eur monograph 0870)

Ph Eur _____

1. DEFINITION

Newcastle disease vaccine (inactivated) (also known as avian paramyxovirus 1 vaccine (inactivated) for vaccines intended for some species) consists of an emulsion or a suspension of a suitable strain of Newcastle disease virus (avian paramyxovirus 1) that has been inactivated in such a manner that immunogenic activity is retained.

2. PRODUCTION

2-1. PREPARATION OF THE VACCINE

The vaccine virus is grown in embryonated hens' eggs or in cell cultures. The virus harvest is inactivated. The vaccine may contain adjuvants.

2-2. SUBSTRATE FOR VIRUS PROPAGATION

2-2-1. Embryonated hens' eggs

If the vaccine virus is grown in embryonated hens' eggs, they are obtained from healthy flocks.

2-2-2. Cell cultures

If the vaccine virus is grown in cell cultures, they comply with the requirements for cell cultures for production of veterinary vaccines (*5.2.4*).

2-3. CHOICE OF VACCINE COMPOSITION

The vaccine is shown to be satisfactory with respect to safety (*5.2.6*) and efficacy (*5.2.7*) for each species and category of birds for which it is intended. The following tests for immunogenicity (section 2-3-1) may be used during the demonstration of efficacy.

2-3-1. Immunogenicity

For chickens, the test for vaccines for use in chickens (section 2-3-1-1) is suitable for demonstrating immunogenicity. For other species of birds (for example, pigeons or turkeys), the test for vaccines for use in species other than the chicken (section 2-3-1-2) is suitable for demonstrating immunogenicity.

2-3-1-1. *Vaccines for use in chickens*   Use not fewer than 70 chickens, 21-28 days old, of the same origin and from a flock free from specified pathogens (SPF) (*5.2.2*). For vaccination, use not fewer than 3 groups, each of not fewer than 20 chickens. Choose a number of different volumes of the vaccine corresponding to the number of groups: for example, volumes equivalent to 1/25, 1/50 and 1/100 of a dose. Allocate a different volume to each vaccination group. Vaccinate each chicken by the intramuscular route with the volume of vaccine allocated to its group. Maintain not fewer than 10 chickens as controls. Challenge each chicken after 17-21 days by the intramuscular route with 6 $\log_{10}$ embryo LD_{50} of the Herts (Weybridge 33/56) strain of avian paramyxovirus 1. Observe the chickens at least daily for 21 days after challenge. At the end of the observation period, calculate the PD_{50} by standard statistical methods from the number of chickens that survive in each vaccinated group without showing any signs of Newcastle disease during the 21 days. The vaccine complies with the test if the smallest dose stated on the label corresponds to not less than 50 PD_{50} and the lower confidence limit is not less than 35 PD_{50} per dose. If the lower confidence limit is less than 35 PD_{50} per dose, repeat the test; the vaccine must be shown to contain not less than 50 PD_{50} in the repeat test.

The test is not valid unless all the control birds die within 6 days of challenge.

2-3-1-2. *Vaccines for use in species other than the chicken*   Use not fewer than 30 birds of the target species, of the same origin and of the same age, that do not have antibodies against avian paramyxovirus 1. Vaccinate in accordance with the recommendations for use not fewer than 20 birds. Maintain not fewer than 10 birds as controls. Challenge each bird after 4 weeks by the intramuscular route with a sufficient quantity of virulent avian paramyxovirus 1. The test is invalid if serum samples obtained at the time of the first vaccination show the presence of antibodies against avian paramyxovirus 1 in either vaccinates or controls, or if tests carried out at the time of challenge show such antibodies in controls. The test is not valid if fewer than 70 per cent of the control birds die or show serious signs of Newcastle disease. The vaccine complies with the test if not fewer than 90 per cent of the vaccinated birds survive and show no serious signs of avian paramyxovirus 1 infection.

2-4. MANUFACTURER'S TESTS

2-4-1. Inactivation

The test for inactivation is carried out in embryonated eggs or suitable cell cultures and the quantity of inactivated virus used is equivalent to not less than 10 doses of vaccine. No live virus is detected.

2-4-2. Batch potency test

It is not necessary to carry out the potency test (section 3-6) for each batch of vaccine if it has been carried out using a batch of vaccine with a minimum potency. The following tests may be used. Wherever possible, carry out the test for antigen content (section 2-4-2-1) together with the test for adjuvant (section 2-4-2-2).

Vaccines for use in chickens   The test for antigen content (section 2-4-2-1) together with the test for adjuvant (section 2-4-2-2) may be carried out; if the nature of the product does not allow valid results to be obtained with these tests, or if the vaccine does not comply, the test for serological assay (section 2-4-2-3) may be carried out. If the vaccine does not comply with the latter test, the test for vaccines for use in chickens (section 2-3-1-1) may be carried out. A test using fewer than 20 birds per group and a shorter observation period after challenge may be used if this has been shown to give a valid potency test.

Vaccines for use in species other than the chicken   Carry out a suitable test for which a satisfactory correlation has been established with the test for vaccines for use in species other than the chicken (section 2-3-1-2), the criteria for acceptance being set with reference to a batch that has given satisfactory results in the latter test. A test in chickens from an SPF flock (*5.2.2*) consisting of a measure of the serological response to graded amounts of vaccine (for example, 1/25, 1/50 and 1/100 of a dose with serum sampling 17-21 days later) may be used. Alternatively, the test for antigen content (section 2-4-2-1) together with the test for adjuvant (section 2-4-2-2) may be conducted if shown to provide a valid potency test.

2-4-2-1. *Antigen content*   The relative antigen content is determined by comparing the content of haemagglutinin-neuraminidase antigen per dose of vaccine with a haemagglutinin-neuraminidase antigen reference preparation, by enzyme-linked immunosorbent assay (*2.7.1*). For this comparison, *Newcastle disease virus reference antigen BRP, Newcastle disease virus control antigen BRP, Newcastle disease virus coating antibody BRP* and *Newcastle disease virus conjugated detection antibody BRP* are suitable. Before estimation, the antigen may be extracted from the emulsion

using *isopropyl myristate R* or another suitable method.
The vaccine complies with the test if the estimated antigen content is not significantly lower than that of a batch that has been found to be satisfactory with respect to immunogenicity (section 2-3-1).

2-4-2-2. *Adjuvant* If the immunochemical assay (section 2-4-2-1) is performed and if the vaccine is adjuvanted, the adjuvant is tested by suitable physical and chemical methods. For oil-adjuvanted vaccines, the adjuvant is tested in accordance with the monograph *Vaccines for veterinary use (0062)*. If the adjuvant cannot be adequately characterised, the antigen content determination cannot be used as the batch potency test.

2-4-2-3. *Serological assay* Use not fewer than 15 chickens, 21-28 days old, of the same origin and from an SPF flock (5.2.2). Vaccinate by the intramuscular route not fewer than 10 chickens with a volume of the vaccine equivalent to 1/50 of a dose. Maintain not fewer than 5 chickens as controls. Collect serum samples from each chicken after 17-21 days. Measure the antibody levels in the sera by the haemagglutination-inhibition (HI) test using the technique described below or an equivalent technique with the same numbers of haemagglutinating units and red blood cells. The test system used must include negative and positive control sera, the latter having an HI titre of $5.0 \log_2$ to $6.0 \log_2$. The vaccine complies with the test if the mean HI titre of the vaccinated group is equal to or greater than $4.0 \log_2$ and that of the unvaccinated group is $2.0 \log_2$ or less. If the HI titres are not satisfactory, carry out the test for vaccines for use in chickens (section 2-3-1-1).

Haemagglutination inhibition
Inactivate the test sera by heating at 56 °C for 30 min. Add 25 µl of inactivated serum to the first row of wells in a microtitre plate. Add 25 µl of a buffered 9 g/l solution of *sodium chloride R* at pH 7.2-7.4 to the rest of the wells. Prepare twofold dilutions of the sera across the plate. To each well add 25 µl of a suspension containing 4 haemagglutinating units of inactivated Newcastle disease virus. Incubate the plate at 4 °C for 1 h. Add 25 µl of a 1 per cent *V/V* suspension of red blood cells collected from chickens that are 3-4 weeks old and free from antibodies against Newcastle disease virus. Incubate the plate at 4 °C for 1 h. The HI titre is equal to the highest dilution that produces complete inhibition.

3. BATCH TESTS
3-1. Identification
When injected into animals free from antibodies against Newcastle disease virus, the vaccine stimulates the production of such antibodies.

3-2. Bacteria and fungi
The vaccine and, where applicable, the liquid supplied with it comply with the test for sterility prescribed in the monograph *Vaccines for veterinary use (0062)*.

3-3. Extraneous agents
Use 10 chickens, 14-28 days old, from an SPF flock (5.2.2). Vaccinate each chicken by a recommended route with a double dose of the vaccine. After 3 weeks, inject 1 dose by the same route. Collect serum samples from each chicken 2 weeks later and carry out tests for antibodies to the following agents by the methods prescribed for SPF chicken flocks (5.2.2): avian encephalomyelitis virus, avian infectious bronchitis virus, avian leucosis viruses, egg-drop syndrome virus, avian bursal disease virus, avian infectious laryngotracheitis virus, influenza A virus, Marek's disease

virus. The vaccine does not stimulate the formation of antibodies against these agents.

3-4. Safety
If the vaccine is intended for use in chickens, use 10 chickens, 14-28 days old, from an SPF flock (5.2.2). If the vaccine is not for use in chickens, use 10 birds of one of the species for which the vaccine is intended that do not have antibodies against Newcastle disease virus. Administer to each bird by a recommended route a double dose of the vaccine. Observe the birds at least daily for 21 days. The vaccine complies with the test if no bird shows notable signs of disease or dies from causes attributable to the vaccine.

3-5. Inactivation
Inject 2/5 of a dose into the allantoic cavity of each of 10 embryonated hen eggs that are 9-11 days old and from SPF flocks (5.2.2) (SPF eggs), and incubate. Observe for 6 days and pool separately the allantoic fluid from eggs containing live embryos and that from eggs containing dead embryos, excluding those dying within 24 h of the injection. Examine embryos that die within 24 h of injection for the presence of Newcastle disease virus: the vaccine does not comply with the test if Newcastle disease virus is found.

Inject into the allantoic cavity of each of 10 SPF eggs, 9-11 days old, 0.2 ml of the pooled allantoic fluid from the live embryos and, into each of 10 similar eggs, 0.2 ml of the pooled fluid from the dead embryos and incubate for 5-6 days. Test the allantoic fluid from each egg for the presence of haemagglutinins using chicken erythrocytes.

The vaccine complies with the test if there is no evidence of haemagglutinating activity and if not more than 20 per cent of the embryos die at either stage. If more than 20 per cent of the embryos die at one of the stages, repeat that stage; the vaccine complies with the test if there is no evidence of haemagglutinating activity and not more than 20 per cent of the embryos die at that stage.

Antibiotics may be used in the test to control extraneous bacterial infection.

3-6. Potency
The vaccine complies with the test for immunogenicity (section 2-3-1).

Ph Eur

Newcastle Disease Vaccine, Living

(Newcastle Disease Vaccine (Live),
Ph Eur monograph 0450)

The use of Newcastle Disease Vaccine, Living is restricted in the United Kingdom by the Agricultural Departments.

Ph Eur

1. DEFINITION
Newcastle disease vaccine (live) is a preparation of a suitable strain of Newcastle disease virus (avian paramyxovirus 1). This monograph applies to vaccines intended for administration to chickens and/or other avian species for active immunisation.

2. PRODUCTION
2-1. PREPARATION OF THE VACCINE
The vaccine virus is grown in embryonated hens' eggs or in cell cultures.

2-2. SUBSTRATE FOR VIRUS PROPAGATION

2-2-1. Embryonated hens' eggs

If the vaccine virus is grown in embryonated hens' eggs, they are obtained from flocks free from specified pathogens (SPF) (5.2.2).

2-2-2. Cell cultures

If the vaccine virus is grown in cell cultures, they comply with the requirements for cell cultures for production of veterinary vaccines (5.2.4).

2-3. SEED LOTS

2-3-1. Extraneous agents

The master seed lot complies with the tests for extraneous agents in seed lots (2.6.24). In these tests on the master seed lot, the organisms used are not more than 5 passages from the master seed lot at the start of the tests.

2-4. CHOICE OF VACCINE VIRUS

The vaccine virus shall be shown to be satisfactory with respect to safety (5.2.6) and efficacy (5.2.7) for the birds for which it is intended.

The following tests for intracerebral pathogenicity index (section 2-4-1), amino-acid sequence (section 2-4-2), safety (section 2-4-3), increase in virulence (section 2-4-4) and immunogenicity (section 2-4-5) may be used during the demonstration of safety and immunogenicity.

2-4-1. Intracerebral pathogenicity index

Use vaccine virus at the least attenuated passage level that will be present in a batch of the vaccine. Inoculate the vaccine virus into the allantoic cavity of embryonated hens' eggs, 9- to 11- days-old, from an SPF flock (5.2.2). Incubate the inoculated eggs for a suitable period and harvest and pool the allantoic fluids. Use not fewer than ten 1-day-old chickens (i.e. more than 24 h but less than 40 h after hatching), from an SPF flock (5.2.2). Administer by the intracerebral route to each chick 0.05 ml of the pooled allantoic fluids containing not less than $10^{8.0}$ EID$_{50}$ or, if this virus quantity cannot be achieved, not less than $10^{7.0}$ EID$_{50}$. Observe the chickens at least daily for 8 days after administration and score them once every 24 h. A score of 0 is attributed to a chicken if it is clinically normal, 1 if it shows clinical signs of disease and 2 if it is dead. The intracerebral pathogenicity index is the mean of the scores per chicken per observation over the 8 day period.

If an inoculum of not less than $10^{8.0}$ EID$_{50}$ is used, the vaccine virus complies with the test if its intracerebral pathogenicity index is not greater than 0.5; if an inoculum of not less than $10^{7.0}$ EID$_{50}$ but less than $10^{8.0}$ EID$_{50}$ is used, the vaccine virus complies with the test if its intracerebral pathogenicity index is not greater than 0.4.

2-4-2. Amino-acid sequence

Determine the sequence of a fragment of RNA from the vaccine virus containing the region encoding for the F0 cleavage site by a suitable method. The encoded amino-acid sequence is shown to be one of the following:

		F2					Cleavage site	F1		
Site	111	112	113	114	115	116	∨	117	118	119
	Gly	Gly	Lys	Gln	Gly	Arg		Leu	Ile	Gly
or	Gly	Gly	Arg	Gln	Gly	Arg		Leu	Ile	Gly
or	Gly	Glu	Arg	Gln	Glu	Arg		Leu	Val	Gly

or equivalent with leucine at 117 and no basic amino acids at sites 111, 112, 114 and 115.

2-4-3. Safety

Carry out the test for each route and method of administration to be recommended for vaccination and in each avian species for which the vaccine is intended, using in each case birds not older than the youngest age to be recommended for vaccination. Use vaccine virus at the least attenuated passage level that will be present between the master seed lot and a batch of the vaccine. For tests in chickens, use not fewer than 20 chickens, from an SPF flock (5.2.2). For species other than the chicken, use not fewer than 20 birds that do not have antibodies against Newcastle disease virus. Administer to each bird a quantity of the vaccine virus equivalent to not less than 10 times the maximum virus titre likely to be contained in 1 dose of the vaccine. Observe the birds at least daily for 21 days. The test is not valid if more than 10 per cent of the birds show abnormal clinical signs or die from causes not attributable to the vaccine virus. The vaccine virus complies with the test if no bird shows notable clinical signs of Newcastle disease or dies from causes attributable to the vaccine virus.

2-4-4. Increase in virulence

The test for increase in virulence consists of the administration of the vaccine virus at the least attenuated passage level that will be present between the master seed lot and a batch of the vaccine to a group of 5 birds not more than 2 weeks old, sequential passages, 5 times where possible, to further similar groups and testing of the final recovered virus for increase in virulence. If the properties of the vaccine virus allow sequential passage to 5 groups via natural spreading, this method may be used, otherwise passage as described below is carried out and the maximally passaged virus that has been recovered is tested for increase in virulence. Care must be taken to avoid contamination by virus from previous passages. Carry out the test in a target species, using the chicken if it is one of the target species. For the test in chickens, use chickens from an SPF flock (5.2.2). For other species, carry out the test in birds that do not have antibodies against Newcastle disease virus. Administer by eye-drop a quantity of the vaccine virus that will allow recovery of virus for the passages described below. Observe the birds for the period shown to correspond to maximum replication of the vaccine virus, kill them and prepare a suspension from the brain of each bird and from a suitable organ depending on the tropism of the strain (for example, mucosa of the entire trachea, intestine, pancreas); pool the samples. Administer 0.05 ml of the pooled samples by eye-drop to each of 5 other birds of the same species, age and origin. Carry out this passage operation not fewer than 5 times; verify the presence of the virus at each passage. If the virus is not found at a passage level, carry out a second series of passages.

A. Carry out the test for intracerebral pathogenicity index (section 2-4-1) using unpassaged vaccine virus and the maximally passaged virus that has been recovered.

B. Carry out the test for amino-acid sequence (section 2-4-2) using unpassaged vaccine virus and the maximally passaged virus that has been recovered.

C. Carry out the test for safety (section 2-4-3) using unpassaged vaccine virus and the maximally passaged virus that has been recovered. Administer the virus by the route to be recommended for vaccination likely to be the least safe and to the avian species for which the vaccine is intended that is likely to be the most susceptible to Newcastle disease.

The vaccine virus complies with the test if, in the tests 2-4-4A, 2-4-4B and 2-4-4C, no indication of increase in virulence of the maximally passaged virus compared with the unpassaged virus is observed. If virus is not recovered at any passage level in the first and second series of passages, the vaccine virus also complies with the test.

2-4-5. Immunogenicity

For each avian species for which the vaccine is intended, a test is carried out for each route and method of administration to be recommended using in each case birds not older than the youngest age to be recommended for vaccination. The quantity of the vaccine virus administered to each bird is not greater than the minimum titre to be stated on the label and the virus is at the most attenuated passage level that will be present in a batch of the vaccine.

2-4-5-1. Vaccines for use in chickens Use not fewer than 30 chickens of the same origin and from an SPF flock (5.2.2). Vaccinate by a recommended route not fewer than 20 chickens. Maintain not fewer than 10 chickens as controls. Challenge each chicken after 21 days by the intramuscular route with not less than $10^{5.0}$ embryo LD_{50} of the Herts (Weybridge 33/56) strain of Newcastle disease virus. Observe the chickens at least daily for 14 days after challenge. Record the deaths and the number of surviving chickens that show clinical signs of disease. The test is not valid if 6 days after challenge fewer than 100 per cent of the control chickens have died or if during the period between vaccination and challenge more than 10 per cent of the vaccinated or control chickens show abnormal clinical signs or die from causes not attributable to the vaccine. The vaccine virus complies with the test if during the observation period after challenge not fewer than 90 per cent of the vaccinated chickens survive and show no notable clinical signs of Newcastle disease.

2-4-5-2. Vaccines for use in avian species other than the chicken Use not fewer than 30 birds of the species for which the vaccine is intended for Newcastle disease, of the same origin and that do not have antibodies against avian paramyxovirus 1. Vaccinate by a recommended route not fewer than 20 birds. Maintain not fewer than 10 birds as controls. Challenge each bird after 21 days by the intramuscular route with a sufficient quantity of virulent avian paramyxovirus 1. Observe the birds at least daily for 21 days after challenge. Record the deaths and the surviving birds that show clinical signs of disease. The test is not valid if:

— during the observation period after challenge fewer than 90 per cent of the control birds die or show severe clinical signs of Newcastle disease,

— or if during the period between the vaccination and challenge more than 10 per cent of the vaccinated or control birds show abnormal clinical signs or die from causes not attributable to the vaccine.

The vaccine virus complies with the test if during the observation period after challenge not fewer than 90 per cent of the vaccinated birds survive and show no notable clinical signs of Newcastle disease. For species where there is published evidence that it is not possible to achieve this level of protection, the vaccine complies with the test if there is a significant reduction in morbidity and mortality of the vaccinated birds compared with the control birds.

3. BATCH TESTS

3-1. Identification

3-1-1. Identification of the vaccine virus The vaccine, diluted if necessary and mixed with a monospecific Newcastle disease virus antiserum, no longer provokes haemagglutination of chicken red blood cells or infects

embryonated hens' eggs from an SPF flock (5.2.2) or susceptible cell cultures (5.2.4) into which it is inoculated.

3-1-2. Identification of the virus strain The strain of vaccine virus is identified by a suitable method, for example using monoclonal antibodies.

3-2. Bacteria and fungi

Vaccines intended for administration by injection comply with the test for sterility prescribed in the monograph *Vaccines for veterinary use (0062)*.

Vaccines not intended for administration by injection either comply with the test for sterility prescribed in the monograph *Vaccines for veterinary use (0062)* or with the following test: carry out a quantitative test for bacterial and fungal contamination; carry out identification tests for microorganisms detected in the vaccine; the vaccine does not contain pathogenic microorganisms and contains not more than 1 non-pathogenic microorganism per dose.

Any liquid supplied with the vaccine complies with test for sterility prescribed in the monograph *Vaccines for veterinary use (0062)*.

3-3. Mycoplasmas

The vaccine complies with the test for mycoplasmas (2.6.7).

3-4. Extraneous agents

The vaccine complies with the tests for extraneous agents in batches of finished product (2.6.25).

3-5. Safety

For vaccines recommended for use in chickens, use not fewer than 10 chickens from an SPF flock (5.2.2) and of the youngest age recommended for vaccination. For vaccines recommended for use only in avian species other than the chicken, use not fewer than 10 birds of the species likely to be most sensitive to Newcastle disease, that do not have antibodies against Newcastle disease virus and of the minimum age recommended for vaccination. Administer to each bird by eye-drop, or parenterally if only parenteral administration is recommended, 10 doses of the vaccine in a volume suitable for the test. Observe the birds at least daily for 21 days. The test is not valid if more than 20 per cent of the birds show abnormal clinical signs or die from causes not attributable to the vaccine. The vaccine complies with the test if no bird shows notable clinical signs of disease or dies from causes attributable to the vaccine.

3-6. Virus titre

Titrate the vaccine virus by inoculation into embryonated hens' eggs from an SPF flock (5.2.2) or into suitable cell cultures (5.2.4). The vaccine complies with the test if 1 dose contains not less than the minimum virus titre stated on the label.

3-7. Potency

Depending on the indications, the vaccine complies with 1 or both of the tests prescribed under Immunogenicity (section 2-4-5) when administered according to the recommended schedule by a recommended route and method. If the test in section 2-4-5-2 *Vaccine for use in avian species other than the chicken* is conducted and the vaccine is recommended for use in more than 1 avian species, the test is carried out with birds of that species for which the vaccine is recommended which is likely to be the most susceptible to avian paramyxovirus 1. It is not necessary to carry out the potency test for each batch of the vaccine if it has been carried out on a representative batch using a vaccinating dose containing not more than the minimum virus titre stated on the label.

Ovine Enzootic Abortion Vaccine, Inactivated

DEFINITION

Ovine Enzootic Abortion Vaccine, Inactivated is a suspension of one or more strains of the chlamydia organisms of ovine enzootic abortion which have been inactivated in such a manner that the immunogenic activity is retained.

PRODUCTION

The *Chlamydia psittaci* organisms are grown in either suitable cell cultures, Appendix XV J(Vet) 1, or in the yolk sacs of embryonated eggs derived from healthy chicken flocks. The organisms are harvested and inactivated. A validated, suitably sensitive test for residual chlamydia is carried out in tissue cultures, on each batch of antigen immediately after inactivation.

The vaccine contains an adjuvant.

CHOICE OF VACCINE COMPOSITION

The vaccine is shown to be satisfactory with respect to safety and immunogenicity for the animals for which the vaccine is intended. The following tests may be used during the demonstration of safety, Appendix XV K(Vet) 1, and immunogenicity, Appendix XV K(Vet) 2.

Safety

Carry out a test in each category of animal for which the vaccine is to be recommended and by each recommended route of administration. Vaccinate at least five animals that do not have antibodies to *Chlamydia psittaci*. Use for the test, a batch of vaccine with the maximum potency likely to be included in a dose of the vaccine. Administer a double dose of vaccine to each animal and observe them for two weeks. No abnormal local or systemic reactions occur. If the vaccine is for use or may be used in pregnant animals, for the test in this category, administer the vaccine at the relevant stage or stages of pregnancy, prolong the observation period up to the time of parturition and note any effects on gestation or on the offspring.

Immunogenicity

The tests to demonstrate Immunogenicity are carried out in each category of animal for which the vaccine is to be recommended and by each recommended route of administration and using a batch or batches with the minimum potency likely to be included in a dose of the vaccine. The efficacy claims made on the label (e.g. protection from abortion) reflect the type of data generated.

BATCH TESTING

Inactivation

Carry out a suitable validated test in tissue cultures for residual *Chlamydia psittaci* on the bulk antigen blend immediately before the addition of the adjuvant. No live organisms are detected.

CAUTION *Accidental injection of oil emulsion vaccines can cause serious local reactions in man. Expert medical advice should be sought immediately and the doctor should be informed that the vaccine is an oil emulsion.*

The vaccine complies with the requirements stated under Veterinary Vaccines with the following modifications.

IDENTIFICATION

When injected into healthy seronegative animals, the vaccine stimulates the production of specific antibodies against *Chlamydia psittaci*.

TESTS

Extraneous bacteria and fungi

The vaccine complies with the test for sterility described under Veterinary Vaccines.

Safety

Use two lambs of the minimum age recommended for vaccination and that do not have antibodies to *Chlamydia psittaci*. Administer by a route recommended on the label, a double dose of vaccine to each of the lambs and observe the animals for two weeks. No abnormal local or systemic reactions occur.

POTENCY

Inject each of five healthy susceptible sheep according to the recommendations stated on the label. Maintain two unvaccinated sheep from the same source as the unvaccinated controls. Bleed all of the animals before vaccination and again not less than 28 days later. Using an appropriate serological test (complement-fixation or immunofluorescence is suitable) the serum of each sheep before vaccination is negative at a 2-fold dilution and, not less than 28 days after vaccination, the serum of no fewer than four of the vaccinated sheep gives a positive reaction at an 8-fold or greater dilution. The test is not valid if there is an increase in antibody levels in the controls.

STORAGE

When stored under the prescribed conditions the vaccine may be expected to retain its potency for at least 1 year.

Pasteurella Vaccine (Inactivated) for Sheep

(Ph Eur monograph 2072)

Ph Eur _____

DEFINITION

Pasteurella vaccine (inactivated) for sheep is a preparation of one or more suitable strains of *Pasteurella trehalosi*. This monograph applies to vaccines intended for administration to sheep to protect against disease caused by *P. trehalosi*.

PRODUCTION

Production of the vaccine is based on a seed-lot system. The seed material is cultured in a suitable medium; each strain is cultivated separately and identity is verified using a suitable method. During production, various parameters such as growth rate are monitored by suitable methods; the values are within the limits approved for the particular product. Purity and identity of the harvest are verified using suitable methods. After cultivation, the bacterial suspensions are collected separately and inactivated by a suitable method. The vaccine may contain an adjuvant and may be freeze-dried.

CHOICE OF VACCINE COMPOSITION

The choice of composition and the strains to be included in the vaccine is based on epidemiological data on the prevalence of the different serovars of *P. trehalosi*.

The vaccine is shown to be satisfactory with respect to safety (5.2.6) and efficacy (5.2.7) in sheep. As part of the studies to demonstrate the suitability of the vaccine with respect to these characteristics the following tests may be carried out.

Safety

A. The test is carried out for each of the routes of administration to be stated on the label and in animals of each category (for example, young sheep, pregnant ewes) for which the vaccine is intended.

For each test, use not fewer than 10 animals that preferably do not have antibodies against the serovars of *P. trehalosi* or against leucotoxin present in the vaccine. Where justified, animals with a known history of no previous pasteurella vaccination and with low antibody titres (measured in a sensitive test system such as an ELISA) may be used.

Administer to each animal a double dose of vaccine containing not less than the maximum potency that may be expected in a batch of vaccine. Administer a single dose of vaccine to each animal after the recommended interval. Observe the animals for at least 14 days after the last administration. Record body temperature the day before vaccination, at vaccination, 2 h, 4 h and 6 h later and then daily for 4 days; note the maximum temperature increase for each animal. No abnormal local or systemic reaction occurs; the average body temperature increase for all animals does not exceed 1.5 °C and no animal shows a rise greater than 2 °C. If the vaccine is intended for use or may be used in pregnant ewes, vaccinate the ewes at the relevant stages of pregnancy and prolong the observation period until 1 day after lambing.

The vaccine complies with the test if no animal shows abnormal local reactions or clinical signs of disease or dies from causes attributable to the vaccine. In addition, if the vaccine is intended for use in pregnant ewes, no significant effects on the pregnancy and offspring are demonstrated.

B. The animals used for the field trials are also used to evaluate safety. Carry out a test in each category of animals for which the vaccine is intended. Use not fewer than 3 groups of 20 animals with corresponding groups of not fewer than 10 controls in 3 different locations. Examine the injection sites for local reactions after vaccination. Record body temperatures the day before vaccination, at vaccination and on the 2 days following vaccination. The vaccine complies with the test if no animal shows abnormal local or systemic reactions or clinical signs of disease or dies from causes attributable to the vaccine. The average body temperature increase for all animals does not exceed 1.5 °C and no animal shows a rise greater than 2 °C. In addition, if the vaccine is intended for use in pregnant ewes, no significant effects on the pregnancy and offspring are demonstrated.

Immunogenicity As part of the studies to demonstrate the suitability of the vaccine with respect to immunogenicity, the test described under Potency may be carried out for each proposed route of administration and using vaccine of minimum potency.

BATCH TESTING
Batch potency test
The test described under Potency is not carried out for routine testing of batches of vaccine. It is carried out, for a given vaccine, on one or more occasions, as decided by or with the agreement of the competent authority. Where the test is not carried out, a suitable validated batch potency test is carried out, the criteria for acceptance being set with reference to the results obtained with a batch of vaccine that has given satisfactory results in the test described under Potency.

Bacterial endotoxins
A test for bacterial endotoxins (*2.6.14*) is carried out on the final lot or, where the nature of the adjuvant prevents performance of a satisfactory test, on the bulk antigen or the mixture of bulk antigens immediately before addition of the adjuvant. The maximum acceptable amount of bacterial endotoxins is that found for a batch of vaccine that has been shown satisfactory in safety test A given under Choice of vaccine composition or in the safety test described under Tests, carried out using 10 animals. Where the latter test is used, note the maximum temperature increase for each animal; the average body temperature increase for all animals does not exceed 1.5 °C. The method chosen for determining the amount of bacterial endotoxin present in the vaccine batch used in the safety test for determining the maximum acceptable level of endotoxin is used subsequently for testing of each batch.

IDENTIFICATION
When injected into healthy seronegative animals, the vaccine stimulates the production of specific antibodies against the serovars of *P. trehalosi* and/or against the leucotoxin present in the vaccine.

TESTS
Safety
Use 2 sheep of the minimum age recommended for vaccination or, if not available, of an age as close as possible to the minimum recommended age, and that have not been vaccinated against Pasteurella. Administer a double dose of vaccine to each animal by a recommended route. Observe the animals for 14 days. Record body temperature the day before vaccination, at vaccination, 2 h, 4 h and 6 h later and then daily for 2 days. The animals remain in good health and no abnormal local or systemic reaction occurs; a transient temperature increase not exceeding 2 °C may occur.

Sterility
It complies with the test for sterility prescribed in the monograph on *Vaccines for veterinary use (0062)*.

POTENCY
Carry out a test for each serovar of *P trehalosi* for which protection is claimed on the label.

Use not fewer than 20 lambs of the minimum age recommended for vaccination, free from antibodies against *P. trehalosi* and against the leucotoxin of *P. trehalosi*. Vaccinate not fewer than 10 of the animals by a recommended route and according to the recommended schedule. Keep 10 animals as controls. 21 days after the last vaccination, infect all the lambs by injection, using the subcutaneous or other suitable route, with a suitable quantity of a low-passage, virulent strain of a serovar of *P. trehalosi*. Observe the animals for a further 7 days; to avoid unnecessary suffering, severely ill animals are killed and are then considered to have died from the disease. During the observation period, the animals are examined for any signs of disease (for example, severe dullness, excess salivation) and the mortality is recorded. Kill surviving animals at the end of the observation period. Post-mortem examination is carried out on any animal that dies and those killed at the end of the observation period. The lungs, pleura, liver and spleen are examined for haemorrhages and the extent of lung consolidation due to pasteurellosis is evaluated. Samples of lung, liver and spleen tissue are collected for re-isolation of the challenge organisms. The mortality, clinical observations and the post-mortem lesions are scored and the results obtained for these parameters and the bacterial re-isolation results compared for the 2 groups.

The test is invalid if clinical signs or lesions of *P. trehalosi* infection occur in less than 70 per cent of the control lambs.

The vaccine complies with the requirements of the test if there is a significant difference between the scores obtained for the clinical and post-mortem observations in the vaccinates compared to the controls. For vaccines with a claim for a beneficial effect on the extent of infection against the serovar, the results for the infection rates are also significantly better for the vaccinates compared to the controls.

LABELLING
The label states:
— the serovar(s) of *P. trehalosi* against which protection is claimed,
— the serovar(s) of *P. trehalosi* and/or the leucotoxin present in the vaccine.

_____ Ph Eur

Porcine Actinobacillosis Vaccine, Inactivated

(Porcine Actinobacillosis Vaccine (Inactivated), Ph Eur monograph 1360)

Ph Eur _____

DEFINITION
Porcine actinobacillosis vaccine (inactivated) is a liquid preparation which has one or more of the following components: inactivated *Actinobacillus pleuropneumoniae* of a suitable strain or strains; toxins, proteins or polysaccharides derived from suitable strains of *A. pleuropneumoniae*, and treated to render them harmless; fractions of toxins derived from suitable strains of *A. pleuropneumoniae* and treated if necessary to render them harmless. This monograph applies to vaccines intended for protection of pigs against actinobacillosis.

PRODUCTION
The seed material is cultured in a suitable medium; each strain is cultivated separately. During production, various parameters such as growth rate, protein content and quantity of relevant antigens are monitored by suitable methods; the values are within the limits approved for the particular product. Purity and identity are verified on the harvest using suitable methods. After cultivation, the bacterial suspensions are collected separately and inactivated by a suitable method. They may be detoxified, purified and concentrated.
The vaccine may contain an adjuvant.

CHOICE OF VACCINE COMPOSITION
The choice of strains is based on epidemiological data. The vaccine is shown to be satisfactory with respect to safety (*5.2.6*) and efficacy (*5.2.7*) in pigs. The following tests may be used during demonstration of safety and immunogenicity.
Safety
A. Carry out a test in each category of animals for which the vaccine is intended and by each of the recommended routes of administration. Use animals that do not have antibodies against the serotypes of *A. pleuropneumoniae* or its toxins present in the vaccine. Administer a double dose of vaccine by a recommended route to each of not fewer than 10 animals. Administer a single dose of vaccine to each of the animals after the interval recommended in the instructions for use. Observe the animals for 14 days after vaccination. Record body temperature the day before vaccination, at vaccination, 2 h, 4 h and 6 h later and then daily for 4 days; note the maximum temperature increase for each animal. No abnormal local or systemic reaction occurs; the average temperature increase for all animals does not exceed 1.5 °C and no animal shows a rise greater than 2 °C. If the vaccine

is intended for use in pregnant sows, for the test in this category of animals, prolong the observation period up to farrowing and note any effects on gestation or the offspring.
B. The animals used for field trials are also used to evaluate safety. Carry out a test in each category of animals for which the vaccine is intended. Use not fewer than 3 groups each of not fewer than 20 animals with corresponding groups of not fewer than 10 controls. Examine the injection site for local reactions after vaccination. Record body temperature the day before vaccination, at vaccination, at the time interval after which a rise in temperature, if any, was seen in test A, and daily during the 2 days following vaccination; note the maximum temperature increase for each animal.
No abnormal local or systemic reaction occurs; the average temperature increase for all animals does not exceed 1.5 °C and no animal shows a rise greater than 2 °C.
Immunogenicity The test described under Potency may be used to demonstrate the immunogenicity of the vaccine.

BATCH TESTING
Batch potency test
The test described under Potency is not carried out for routine testing of batches of vaccine. It is carried out, for a given vaccine, on one or more occasions, as decided by or with the agreement of the competent authority; where the test is not carried out, a suitable validated test is carried out, the criteria for acceptance being set with reference to a batch of vaccine that has given satisfactory results in the test described under Potency. The following test may be used after a satisfactory correlation with the test described under Potency has been established.

Inject a suitable dose subcutaneously into each of 5 seronegative mice, weighing 18-20 g. Where the schedule stated on the label requires a booster injection to be given, a booster vaccination may also be given in this test provided it has been demonstrated that this will still provide a suitably sensitive test system. Before the vaccination and at a given interval within the range of 14-21 days after the last injection, collect blood from each animal and prepare serum samples. Determine individually for each serum the titre of specific antibodies against each antigenic component stated on the label, using a suitable validated test such as enzyme-linked immunosorbent assay (*2.7.1*). The vaccine complies with the test if the antibody levels are not significantly lower than those obtained for a batch that has given satisfactory results in the test described under Potency.

Bacterial endotoxins
A test for bacterial endotoxins (*2.6.14*) is carried out on the final bulk or, where the nature of the adjuvant prevents performance of a satisfactory test, on the bulk antigen or mixture of bulk antigens immediately before addition of the adjuvant. The maximum acceptable amount of bacterial endotoxins is that found for a batch of vaccine that has been shown satisfactory in safety test A described under Choice of vaccine composition or the safety test described under Tests, carried out using 10 pigs. Where the latter test is used, note the maximum temperature increase for each animal; the average temperature increase for all animals does not exceed 1.5 °C. The method chosen for determining the amount of bacterial endotoxin present in the vaccine batch used in the safety test for determining the maximum acceptable level of endotoxin is used subsequently for batch testing.

IDENTIFICATION
When injected into healthy seronegative animals, the vaccine stimulates the production of specific antibodies against the

antigenic components of *A. pleuropneumoniae* stated on the label.

TESTS

Safety

Use 2 pigs of the minimum age stated for vaccination and which do not have antibodies against the serotypes of *A. pleuropneumoniae* or its toxins present in the vaccine. Administer to each pig a double dose of vaccine by a recommended route. Observe the animals for 14 days. Record body temperature the day before vaccination, at vaccination, 2 h, 4 h and 6 h later and then daily for 2 days. No abnormal local or systemic reaction occurs; a transient temperature increase not exceeding 2 °C may occur.

Sterility

The vaccine complies with the test for sterility prescribed in the monograph on *Vaccines for veterinary use (0062)*.

POTENCY

The challenge strain for the potency test is chosen to ensure challenge with each Ap toxin[1] produced by the serotypes stated on the label; it may be necessary to carry out more than one test using a different challenge strain for each test.

Vaccinate according to the recommended schedule not fewer than 7 pigs, of the minimum age recommended for vaccination, which do not have antibodies against *A. pleuropneumoniae* and Ap toxins. Keep not fewer than 7 unvaccinated pigs of the same age as controls. 3 weeks after the last vaccination, challenge all the pigs intranasally or intratracheally or by aerosol with a suitable quantity of a serotype of *A. pleuropneumoniae*. Observe the animals for 7 days; to avoid unnecessary suffering, severely ill control animals are killed and are then considered to have died from the disease. Kill all surviving animals at the end of the observation period. Carry out a post-mortem examination on all animals. Examine the lungs, the tracheobronchial lymph nodes and the tonsils for the presence of *A. pleuropneumoniae*. Evaluate the extent of lung lesions at post-mortem examination. Each of the 7 lobes of the lungs is allotted a maximum possible lesion score[2] of 5. The area showing pneumonia and/or pleuritis of each lobe is assessed and expressed on a scale of 0 to 5 to give the pneumonic score per lobe (the maximum total score possible for each complete lung is 35). Calculate separately for the vaccinated and the control animals the total score (the maximum score per group is 245, if 7 pigs are used per group).

The vaccine complies with the test if the vaccinated animals, when compared with controls, show lower incidence of: mortality; typical clinical signs (dyspnoea, coughing and vomiting); typical lung lesions; re-isolation of *A. pleuropneumoniae* from the lungs, the tracheobronchial lymph nodes and the tonsils. Where possible, the incidence is analysed statistically and shown to be significantly lower for vaccinates.

LABELLING

The label states:
— the antigens present in the vaccine,
— the serotypes of *A. pleuropneumoniae* for which the vaccine affords protection.

---

[1] The nomenclature of the toxins of *A. pleuropneumoniae* is described by J. Frey *et al.*, *Journal of General Microbiology*, 1993, 139, 1723-1728.
[2] The system of lung scores is described in detail by P.C.T. Hannan, B.S. Bhogal, J.P. Fish, *Research in Veterinary Science*, 1982, 33, 76-88.

Porcine E. Coli Vaccine, Inactivated

Porcine Escherichia Coli Vaccine, Inactivated

(Neonatal Piglet Colibacillosis Vaccine (Inactivated), Ph Eur monograph 0962)

Ph Eur

DEFINITION

Neonatal piglet colibacillosis vaccine (inactivated) is prepared from cultures of one or more suitable strains of *Escherichia coli*, carrying one or more adhesins or enterotoxins. This monograph applies to vaccines administered by injection to sows and gilts for protection of newborn piglets against enteric forms of colibacillosis.

PRODUCTION

The *E. coli* strains used for production are cultured separately in a suitable medium. The cells or toxins are processed to render them safe and are blended.

The vaccine may contain one or more suitable adjuvants.

CHOICE OF VACCINE COMPOSITION

The *E. coli* strains used in the production of the vaccine are shown to be satisfactory with respect to expression of antigens and the vaccine is shown to be satisfactory with respect to safety and immunogenicity. The following tests may be used during demonstration of safety (*5.2.6*) and efficacy (*5.2.7*).

Expression of antigens The expression of antigens that stimulate a protective immune response is verified by a suitable immunochemical method (*2.7.1*) carried out on the antigen obtained from each of the vaccine strains under the conditions used for the production of the vaccine.

Safety

A. Administer a double dose of vaccine by a recommended route to each of not fewer than 10 pregnant sows that have not been vaccinated against colibacillosis. Administer 1 dose of vaccine to each of the animals after the recommended interval. Observe the animals until farrowing. Record body temperature the day before vaccination, at vaccination, 2 h, 4 h and 6 h later and then daily for 4 days; note the maximum temperature increase for each animal. Note any effects on gestation or the offspring. No abnormal local or systemic reaction occurs: the average temperature increase for all animals does not exceed 1.5 °C and no animal shows a rise greater than 2 °C.

B. The animals used for field trials are also used to evaluate safety. Use not fewer than 3 groups each of not fewer than 20 animals with corresponding groups of not fewer than 10 controls. Examine the injection site for local reactions after vaccination. Record body temperature the day before vaccination, at vaccination, at the time interval after which a rise in temperature, if any, was seen in test A, and daily during the 2 days following vaccination; note the maximum temperature increase for each animal. No abnormal local or systemic reaction occurs: the average temperature increase for all animals does not exceed 1.5 °C and no animal shows a rise greater than 2 °C.

Immunogenicity The suitability of the vaccine with respect to immunogenicity may be demonstrated by the test described under Potency.

BATCH TESTING

Batch potency test

The test described under Potency is not carried out for routine testing of batches of vaccine. It is carried out, for a given vaccine,

*on one or more occasions, as decided by or with the agreement
of the competent authority; where the test is not carried out, a
suitable validated test is carried out, the criteria for acceptance
being set with reference to a batch of vaccine that has given
satisfactory results in the test described under Potency.
The following test may be used after a suitable correlation with the
test described under Potency has been established by a statistical
evaluation.*

Use pigs not less than 3 weeks old and free from specific
antibodies against the antigens stated on the label: vaccinate
each of 5 pigs by the route and according to the schedule
stated on the label. Maintain 2 pigs as unvaccinated controls.
Alternatively, if the nature of the antigens allows reproducible
results to be obtained, a test in laboratory animals (for
example, guinea-pigs, mice, rabbits or rats) may be carried
out. To obtain a valid assay, it may be necessary to carry out
a test using several groups of animals, each receiving a
different dose. For each dose, carry out the test as follows.
Vaccinate not fewer than 5 animals with a single injection of
a suitable dose. Maintain not fewer than 2 animals as
unvaccinated controls. Where the schedule stated on the
label requires a booster injection to be given, a booster
vaccination may also be given in this test provided it has
been demonstrated that this will still provide a suitably
sensitive test system. At a given interval within the range of
14 to 21 days after the last injection, collect blood from each
animal and prepare serum samples. Use a suitable validated
test such as an enzyme-linked immunosorbent assay (*2.7.1*)
to measure the antibody response to each of the antigens
stated on the label. The antibody levels are not significantly
less than those obtained with a batch that has given
satisfactory results in the test described under Potency and
there is no significant increase in antibody titre in the
controls.

Where seronegative animals are not available, seropositive
animals may be used in the above test. During the
development of a test with seropositive animals, particular
care will be required during the validation of the test system
to establish that the test is suitably sensitive and to specify
acceptable pass, fail and retest criteria. It will be necessary to
take into account the range of possible prevaccination titres
and establish the acceptable minimum titre rise after
vaccination in relation to these.

Bacterial endotoxins

A test for bacterial endotoxins (*2.6.14*) is carried out on the
final lot or, where the nature of the adjuvant prevents
performance of a satisfactory test, on the bulk antigen or the
mixture of bulk antigens immediately before addition of the
adjuvant. The maximum acceptable amount of bacterial
endotoxins is that found for a batch of vaccine that has been
shown satisfactory in safety test A given under Choice of
vaccine composition or in the safety test described under
Tests, carried out using 10 piglets. Where the latter test is
used, note the maximum temperature increase for each
animal; the average temperature increase for all animals does
not exceed 1.5 °C. The method chosen for determining the
amount of bacterial endotoxin present in the vaccine batch
used in the safety test for determining the maximum
acceptable level of endotoxin is used subsequently for testing
of each batch.

IDENTIFICATION

In animals free from specific antibodies against the antigens
stated on the label, the vaccine stimulates the production of
antibodies against these antigens.

TESTS
Safety
Use pigs preferably having no specific antibodies against the
antigens stated on the label or, where justified, pigs with a
low level of such antibodies as long as they have not been
vaccinated against colibacillosis and administration of the
vaccine does not cause an anamnestic response. Administer
to each of 2 pigs a double dose of vaccine by a recommended
route. Observe the animals for 14 days. Record body
temperature before vaccination, at vaccination, 2 h, 4 h and
6 h later and then daily for 2 days. No abnormal local or
systemic reaction occurs; a transient temperature increase
not exceeding 2 °C may occur.

Sterility
The vaccine complies with the test for sterility prescribed
in the monograph on *Vaccines for veterinary use (0062)*.

POTENCY
Carry out the test with a challenge strain representing each
type of antigen against which the vaccine is intended to
protect: if a single strain with all the necessary antigens is not
available, repeat the test using different challenge strains.

Use not fewer than 8 susceptible gilts free from specific
antibodies against the antigens stated on the label. Take not
fewer than 4 at random and vaccinate these at the stage of
pregnancy and according to the recommended vaccination
scheme. Within 12 h of their giving birth, take not fewer than
15 healthy piglets from the vaccinated animals and 15 healthy
piglets from the unvaccinated controls, taking at least 3 from
each litter. Challenge all the piglets orally with a pathogenic
strain of *E. coli* before or after colostrum feeding and using
the same conditions for vaccinated animals and controls.
The strain used must not be one used in the manufacture of
the vaccine. Return the piglets to their dam and observe for
8 days.

On each day, note clinical signs in each piglet and score
using the following scale:

0	no signs
1	slight diarrhoea
2	marked diarrhoea (watery faeces)
3	dead

Total scores for each piglet over 8 days are calculated.
The test is not valid unless at least 40 per cent of the piglets
from the control animals die and not more than 15 per cent
of the piglets from the control animals show no signs of
illness. The vaccine complies with the test if there is a
significant reduction in score in the group of piglets from
the vaccinated gilts compared with the group from the
unvaccinated controls.

For some adhesins (for example, F5 and F41), there is
published evidence that high mortality cannot be achieved
under experimental conditions. If challenge has to be carried
out with a strain having such adhesins: the test is not valid if
fewer than 70 per cent of the control piglets show clinical
signs expected with the challenge strain; the vaccine complies
with the test if there is a significant reduction in score in the
group of piglets from the vaccinated gilts compared with the
group from the unvaccinated controls.

LABELLING
The label states the antigen or antigens contained in the
vaccine that stimulate a protective immune response.

Ph Eur

Porcine Parvovirus Vaccine, Inactivated

(Porcine Parvovirus Vaccine (Inactivated),
Ph Eur monograph 0965)

Ph Eur ___

DEFINITION
Inactivated porcine parvovirosis vaccine consists of a suspension of inactivated porcine parvovirus or of a noninfectious fraction of the virus.

PRODUCTION
The virus is grown in suitable cell cultures (5.2.4). The viral suspension is harvested; the virus is inactivated by a method that avoids destruction of the immunogenicity and may be fragmented (inactivation may be by fragmentation); the virus or viral fragments may be purified and concentrated at a suitable stage of the process.

A test for residual infectious porcine parvovirus is carried out on each batch of antigen immediately after inactivation and on the final bulk or, if the vaccine contains an adjuvant, on the bulk antigen or the mixture of bulk antigens immediately before the addition of adjuvant. The quantity used in the test is equivalent to not less than 100 doses of the vaccine. The bulk harvest is inoculated into suitable non-confluent cells; after incubation for 7 days, a subculture is made using trypsinised cells. After incubation for a further 7 days, the cultures are examined for residual live parvovirus by an immunfluorescence test. No live virus is detected.

The vaccine may contain one or more suitable adjuvants.

CHOICE OF VACCINE COMPOSITION
The vaccine is shown to be satisfactory with respect to safety (including absence of adverse effects on fertility, gestation, farrowing or offspring) and immunogenicity in pigs.
The following tests may be used during demonstration of safety (5.2.6) and efficacy (5.2.7).

Safety

A. A test is carried out in each category of animals for which the vaccine is intended and by each of the recommended routes. The animals used do not have antibodies against porcine parvovirus or against a fraction of the virus.
Two doses of vaccine are injected by the intended route into each of not fewer than ten animals. After 14 days, one dose of vaccine is injected into each of the animals. The animals are observed for a further 14 days. During the 28 days of the test, no abnormal local or systemic reaction occurs. If the vaccine is intended for use in pregnant sows, for the test in this category of animal, the observation period is prolonged up to farrowing and any effects on gestation or the offspring are noted.

B. The animals used in the test for immunogenicity are also used to evaluate safety. The rectal temperature of each vaccinated animal is measured at the time of vaccination and 24 h and 48 h later. No abnormal effect on body temperature is noted nor other systemic reactions (for example, anorexia). The injection site is examined for local reactions after vaccination and at slaughter. No abnormal local reaction occurs.

C. The animals used for field trials are also used to evaluate safety. A test is carried out in each category of animals for which the vaccine is intended (sows, gilts). Not fewer than three groups each of not fewer than twenty animals are used with corresponding groups of not fewer than ten controls. The rectal temperature of each animal is measured at the time of vaccination and 24 h and 48 h later. No abnormal

effect on body temperature is noted. The injection site is examined for local reactions after vaccination and at slaughter. No abnormal local reaction occurs.

Immunogenicity The test described under Potency may be used to demonstrate the immunogenicity of the vaccine.

BATCH POTENCY TEST
The test described below is not carried out for routine testing of batches of vaccine. It is carried out, for a given vaccine, on one or more occasions, as decided by or with the agreement of the competent authority; where the test is not carried out, a suitable validated test is carried out, the criteria for acceptance being set with reference to a batch of vaccine that has given satisfactory results in the test described underPotency. The following test may be used after a satisfactory correlation with the test described under Potency has been established by a statistical evaluation.

Vaccinate subcutaneously not fewer than five guinea-pigs, 5 to 7 weeks old, according to the vaccination scheme stated on the label using one-fourth of the prescribed dose volume. Take blood samples after the period corresponding to maximum antibody production and carry out tests on the serum for specific antibodies by a haemagglutination-inhibition test or other suitable test. The antibody titres are not less than those obtained with a batch of vaccine shown to be satisfactory in the test in pigs (see Potency).

IDENTIFICATION
The vaccine stimulates the formation of specific antibodies against porcine parvovirus or the fraction of the virus used in the production of the vaccine when injected into susceptible animals on one or, if necessary, more than one occasion.

TESTS
Safety
Use two pigs 6 weeks to 6 months old and having no antibodies against porcine parvovirus virus or against a fraction of the virus. Inject into each animal by one of the routes stated on the label a double dose of vaccine. Observe the animals for 14 days and then inject a single dose of vaccine into each pig. Observe the animals for a further 14 days. No abnormal local or systemic reaction occurs during the 28 days of the test.

Inactivation
This test may be omitted by the manufacturer if a test for inactivation has been carried out on the bulk vaccine, immediately before the addition of the adjuvant, where applicable. Use a quantity of vaccine equivalent to ten doses. If the vaccine contains an oily adjuvant, break the emulsion and separate the phases. If the vaccine contains a mineral adjuvant, carry out an elution to liberate the virus. Concentrate the viral suspension 100 times by ultrafiltration or ultracentrifugation. None of the above procedures must be such as to inactivate or otherwise interfere with detection of live virus. Carry out a test for residual live virus in suitable non-confluent cells; after incubation for 7 days, make a subculture using trypsinised cells. After incubation for a further 7 days, examine the cultures for residual live parvovirus by an immunfluorescence test. No live virus is detected.

Extraneous viruses
On the pigs used for the safety test carry out tests for antibodies. The vaccine does not stimulate the formation of antibodies - other than those against porcine parvovirus - against viruses pathogenic for pigs or against viruses which could interfere with the diagnosis of infectious diseases in pigs (including the viruses of the pestivirus group).

Sterility

The vaccine complies with the test for sterility prescribed in the monograph on *Vaccines for veterinary use (0062)*.

POTENCY

Vaccinate according to the recommended schedule not less than seven gilts, 5 to 6 months old, which do not have antibodies against porcine parvovirus or against a fraction of the virus. The interval between vaccination and service is that stated on the label. Mate the gilts on two consecutive days immediately following signs of oestrus. Keep not less than five unvaccinated mated gilts of the same age as controls. At about the 40th day of gestation, challenge all gilts using a suitable strain of porcine parvovirus. Slaughter the gilts at about the 90th day of gestation and examine their foetuses for infection with porcine parvovirus as demonstrated by the presence of either virus or antibodies. The vaccine complies with the test if not fewer than 80 per cent of the total number of piglets from vaccinated gilts are protected from infection. The test is not valid unless: not fewer than seven vaccinated gilts and five control gilts are challenged; not fewer than 90 per cent of piglets from the control gilts are infected; and the average number of piglets per litter for the vaccinated gilts is not less than six.

Ph Eur

Porcine Progressive Atrophic Rhinitis Vaccine, Inactivated

(Porcine Progressive Atrophic Rhinitis Vaccine (Inactivated), Ph Eur monograph 1361)

Ph Eur

DEFINITION

Porcine progressive atrophic rhinitis vaccine (inactivated) is a preparation containing either the dermonecrotic exotoxin of *Pasteurella multocida*, treated to render it harmless while maintaining adequate immunogenic activity, or a genetically modified form of the exotoxin which has adequate immunogenic activity and which is free from toxic properties; the vaccine may also contain cells and/or antigenic components of one or more suitable strains of *P. multocida* and/or *Bordetella bronchiseptica*. This monograph applies to vaccines administered to sows and gilts for protection of their progeny.

PRODUCTION

The bacterial strains used for production are cultured separately in suitable media. The toxins and/or cells are treated to render them safe.

Detoxification A test for detoxification of the dermonecrotic exotoxin of *P. multocida* is carried out immediately after detoxification. The concentration of detoxified exotoxin used in the test is not less than that in the vaccine. The suspension complies with the test if no toxic dermonecrotic exotoxin is detected. The test for detoxification is not required where the vaccine is prepared using a toxin-like protein free from toxic properties, produced by expression of a modified form of the corresponding gene.

Antigen content The content of the dermonecrotic exotoxin of *P. multocida* in the detoxified suspension or the toxin-like protein in the harvest is determined by a suitable immunochemical method *(2.7.1)*, such as an enzyme-linked immunosorbent assay and the value found is used in the

formulation of the vaccine. The content of other antigens stated on the label is also determined *(2.7.1)*.

The vaccine may contain a suitable adjuvant.

CHOICE OF VACCINE COMPOSITION

The strains used for the preparation of the vaccine are shown to be satisfactory with respect to the production of the dermonecrotic exotoxin and the other antigens claimed to be protective. The vaccine is shown to be satisfactory with respect to safety *(5.2.6)* and efficacy *(5.2.7)*.

Production of antigens The production of antigens claimed to be protective is verified by a suitable bioassay or immunochemical method *(2.7.1)*, carried out on the antigens obtained from each of the vaccine strains under the conditions used for the production of the vaccine.

The following tests may be used during demonstration of safety and immunogenicity.

Safety

A. Carry out the test for each route of administration stated on the label. Use pigs that do not have antibodies against the components of the vaccine, that are from a herd or herds where there are no signs of atrophic rhinitis and that have not been vaccinated against atrophic rhinitis. If the vaccine is intended for use in pregnant animals, carry out the test in pregnant sows or gilts, vaccinating them at the recommended stage of pregnancy. Administer a double dose of vaccine by a recommended route to each of not fewer than 10 sows or gilts. Administer a single dose of vaccine to each of the animals after the recommended interval. Observe the pigs until farrowing. Record body temperature the day before vaccination, at vaccination, 2 h, 4 h and 6 h later and then daily for 4 days; note the maximum temperature increase for each animal. Note any effects on gestation and the offspring. No abnormal local or systemic reaction occurs; the average temperature increase for all animals does not exceed 1.5 °C and no animal shows a rise greater than 2 °C.

B. The animals used for field trials are also used to evaluate safety. Use not fewer than 3 groups each of not fewer than 20 animals with corresponding groups of not fewer than 10 controls. Examine the injection site for local reactions after vaccination. Record body temperature the day before vaccination, at vaccination, at the time interval after which a rise in temperature, if any, was seen in test A, and daily during the 2 days following vaccination; note the maximum temperature increase for each animal. No abnormal local or systemic reaction occurs; the average temperature increase for all animals does not exceed 1.5 °C and no animal shows a rise greater than 2 °C.

Immunogenicity The test described under Potency is suitable for demonstration of immunogenicity.

BATCH TESTING
Batch potency test

The test described under Potency is not carried out for routine testing of batches of vaccine. It is carried out, for a given vaccine, on one or more occasions, as decided by or with the agreement of the competent authority; where the test is not carried out, a suitable validated test is carried out, the criteria for acceptance being set with reference to a batch of vaccine that has given satisfactory results in the test described under Potency. The following test may be used after a satisfactory correlation with the test described under Potency has been established.

Use not fewer than 5 pigs not less than 3 weeks old and that do not have antibodies against the components of the vaccine. Vaccinate each pig by a recommended route and according to the recommended schedule. Maintain not fewer than 2 pigs of the same origin as unvaccinated controls under the same conditions.

Alternatively, if the nature of the antigens allows reproducible results to be obtained, a test in susceptible laboratory animals may be carried out. To obtain a valid assay, it may be necessary to carry out a test using several groups of animals, each receiving a different quantity of vaccine. For each quantity of vaccine, carry out the test as follows: vaccinate not fewer than 5 animals with a suitable quantity of vaccine. Maintain not fewer than 2 animals of the same species and origin as unvaccinated controls. Where the schedule stated on the label requires a booster injection to be given, a booster vaccination may also be given in this test provided it has been demonstrated that this will still provide a suitably sensitive test system. At a given interval within the range of 14 to 21 days after the last administration, collect blood from each animal and prepare serum samples. Use a validated test such as an enzyme-linked immunosorbent assay to measure the antibody response to each of the antigens stated on the label. The test is not valid and must be repeated if there is a significant antibody titre in the controls. The vaccine complies with the test if the antibody responses of the vaccinated animals are not significantly less than those obtained with a batch of vaccine that has given satisfactory results in the test or tests (as applicable) described under Potency.

Where animals seronegative for the antigens stated on the label are not available, seropositive animals may be used in the above test. During the development of a test with seropositive animals, particular care will be required during the validation of the test system to establish that the test is suitably sensitive and to specify acceptable pass, fail and retest criteria. It will be necessary to take into account the range of prevaccination antibody titres and to establish the acceptable minimum antibody titre rise after vaccination in relation to these.

Bacterial endotoxins
A test for bacterial endotoxins (2.6.14) is carried out on the batch or, where the nature of the adjuvant prevents performance of a satisfactory test, on the bulk antigen or the mixture of bulk antigens immediately before addition of the adjuvant. The maximum acceptable amount of bacterial endotoxins is that found for a batch of vaccine shown satisfactory in safety test A given under Choice of vaccine composition or in the safety test described under Tests, carried out using 10 pigs. Where the latter test is used, note the maximum temperature increase for each animal; the average temperature increase for all animals does not exceed 1.5 °C. The method chosen for determining the amount of bacterial endotoxin present in the vaccine batch used in the safety test for determining the maximum acceptable level of endotoxin is used subsequently for testing of each batch.

IDENTIFICATION
In animals free from specific antibodies against the antigens stated on the label, the vaccine stimulates the production of antibodies against these antigens.

TESTS
Safety
Use not fewer than 2 pigs that do not have antibodies against P. multocida and that preferably do not have antibodies against B. bronchiseptica. Administer to each pig a double dose of vaccine by a recommended route. Observe the pigs for 14 days. Record body temperature the day before

vaccination, at vaccination, 2 h, 4 h and 6 h later and then daily for 2 days. No abnormal local or systemic reaction occurs; a transient temperature increase not exceeding 2 °C may occur.

Sterility (2.6.1)
The vaccine complies with the test for sterility prescribed in the monograph on Vaccines for veterinary use (0062).

POTENCY
Use pigs that do not have antibodies against the components of the vaccine, that are from a herd or herds where there are no signs of atrophic rhinitis and that have not been vaccinated against atrophic rhinitis.

A. Vaccines containing dermonecrotic exotoxin of P. multocida (with or without cells of P. multocida).

Use not fewer than 12 breeder pigs. Vaccinate not fewer than 6 randomly chosen pigs at the stage of pregnancy or non-pregnancy and by the route and schedule stated on the label. Maintain not fewer than 6 of the remaining pigs as unvaccinated controls under the same conditions. From birth allow all the piglets from the vaccinated and unvaccinated breeder pigs to feed from their own dam.

Constitute from the progeny 2 challenge groups each of not fewer than 30 piglets chosen randomly, taking not fewer than 3 piglets from each litter. On the 2 consecutive days preceding challenge, the mucosa of the nasal cavity of the piglets may be treated by instillation of 0.5 ml of a solution of acetic acid (10 g/l $C_2H_4O_2$) in isotonic buffered saline pH 7.2.

Challenge each piglet at 10 days of age by the intranasal route with a sufficient quantity of a toxigenic strain of P. multocida.

At the age of 42 days, kill the piglets of the 2 groups and dissect the nose of each of them transversally at premolar-1. Examine the ventral and dorsal turbinates and the nasal septum for evidence of atrophy or distortion and grade the observations on the following scales:

Turbinates
0 no atrophy
1 slight atrophy
2 moderate atrophy
3 severe atrophy
4 very severe atrophy with almost complete disappearance of the turbinate

The maximum score is 4 for each turbinate and 16 for the sum of the 2 dorsal and 2 ventral turbinates.

Nasal septum
0   no deviation
1   very slight deviation
2   deviation of the septum

The maximum total score for the turbinates and the nasal septum is 18.

The test is not valid and must be repeated if fewer than 80 per cent of the progeny of each litter of the unvaccinated breeder pigs have a total score of at least 10. The vaccine complies with the test if a significant reduction in the total score has been demonstrated in the group from the vaccinated breeder pigs compared to that from the unvaccinated breeder pigs.

B. Vaccines containing P. multocida dermonecrotic exotoxin (with or without cells of P. multocida) and cells and/or antigenic components of B. bronchiseptica.

Use not fewer than 24 breeder pigs. Vaccinate not fewer than 12 randomly chosen pigs at the stage of pregnancy or non-pregnancy and by the route and schedule stated on the label. Maintain not fewer than 12 of the remaining pigs as unvaccinated controls under the same conditions. From birth allow all the piglets from the vaccinated and unvaccinated breeder pigs to feed from their own dam.

Using groups of not fewer than 6 pigs, constitute from their progeny 2 challenge groups from vaccinated pigs and 2 groups from unvaccinated pigs each group consisting of not fewer than 30 piglets chosen randomly, taking not fewer than 3 piglets from each litter. On the 2 consecutive days preceding challenge, the mucosa of the nasal cavity of the piglets may be treated by instillation of 0.5 ml of a solution of acetic acid (10 g/l $C_2H_4O_2$) in isotonic buffered saline pH 7.2.

For a group of piglets from not fewer than 6 vaccinated pigs and a group from not fewer than 6 controls, challenge each piglet by the intranasal route at 10 days of age with a sufficient quantity of a toxigenic strain of *P. multocida*.

For the other group of piglets from not fewer than 6 vaccinated pigs and the other group from not fewer than 6 controls, challenge each piglet at 7 days of age by the intranasal route with a sufficient quantity of *B. bronchiseptica*. In addition, challenge each piglet at 10 days of age by the intranasal route with a sufficient quantity of a toxigenic strain of *P. multocida*.

At the age of 42 days, kill the piglets of the 4 groups and dissect the nose of each of them transversally at premolar-1. Examine the ventral and dorsal turbinates and the nasal septum for evidence of atrophy or distortion and grade the observations on the scale described above.

The test is not valid and must be repeated if fewer than 80 per cent of the progeny of each litter of the unvaccinated breeder pigs have a total score of at least 10. The vaccine complies with the test if a significant reduction in the total score has been demonstrated in the groups from the vaccinated breeder pigs compared to the corresponding group from the unvaccinated breeder pigs.

LABELLING

The label states the protective antigens present in the vaccine.

Ph Eur

Rabies Vaccine for Foxes, Living

(Rabies Vaccine (Live, Oral) for Foxes, Ph Eur monograph 0746)

Ph Eur

DEFINITION

Rabies vaccine (live, oral) for foxes is a preparation of an immunogenic strain of an attenuated rabies virus.
The vaccine is incorporated in a bait in such a manner as to enable the tests prescribed below to be performed aseptically.

PRODUCTION

The attenuated virus strain is grown in suitable cell cultures (5.2.4); if the cell cultures are of mammalian origin, they are shown to be free from rabies virus. The virus suspension is harvested on one or more occasions within 14 days of inoculation. Multiple harvests from a single cell lot may be pooled and considered as a single harvest. The viral suspension may be mixed with a suitable stabiliser. The vaccine may be freeze-dried or liquid. A freeze-dried vaccine has to be reconstituted before use.

CHOICE OF VACCINE STRAIN

Only a virus strain shown to be satisfactory with respect to immunogenicity (see Potency) and the following characteristics may be used in the preparation of the vaccine:
— when administered orally at the dose and by the method recommended for use to forty foxes, it causes no sign of rabies within 180 days of administration,
— when administered orally at ten times the recommended dose to each of ten foxes, it causes no sign of rabies within 180 days of administration,
— when administered orally at ten times the recommended dose to each of ten dogs, it causes no sign of rabies within 180 days of administration,
— when administered orally at ten times the recommended dose to each of ten cats, it causes no sign of rabies within 180 days of administration,
— in natural and experimental conditions, the virus strain does not spread from one animal to another in wild rodents,
— the virus strain has one or more stable genetic markers that may be used to discriminate the vaccine strain from other rabies virus strains.

BATCH TESTING

If the test for potency has been carried out with satisfactory results on a representative batch of vaccine, this test may be omitted as a routine control on other batches of vaccine prepared from the same seed lot.

IDENTIFICATION

A. When mixed with a monospecific rabies antiserum, the vaccine is no longer able to infect susceptible cell cultures into which it is inoculated.

B. A test is carried out to demonstrate the presence of the genetic marker.

TESTS

Extraneous viruses

(a) Mix the vaccine with a specific neutralising rabies virus antiserum. It no longer provokes cytopathic effects in susceptible cell cultures. It shows no evidence of haemagglutinating or haemadsorbing agents.

(b) Inoculate 1 in 10 and 1 in 1000 dilutions of the vaccine into susceptible cell cultures. Incubate at 37 °C. After 2, 4 and 6 days, stain the cells with a panel of monoclonal antibodies that do not react with the vaccine strain but that react with other strains of rabies virus (for example, street virus, Pasteur strain). The vaccine shows no evidence of contaminating rabies virus.

Bacterial and fungal contamination

The vaccine complies with the test for sterility prescribed in the monograph on *Vaccines for veterinary use (0062)*.

Mycoplasmas *(2.6.7)*

The vaccine complies with the test for mycoplasmas.

Virus titre

Titrate the vaccine in suitable cell cultures. One dose of the vaccine contains not less than the quantity of virus equivalent to the minimum titre stated on the label.

POTENCY

Use not fewer than thirty-five foxes, at least three months old, free from rabies-neutralising antibodies. Administer orally and with the bait stated on the label to each of not fewer than twenty-five animals a volume of the vaccine containing a quantity of virus equivalent to the minimum titre stated on the label. Keep not fewer than ten animals as controls. Observe all the animals for 180 days. No animal shows signs of rabies. The test is not valid if fewer than twenty-five vaccinated animals survive after this observation period. On the 180th day after vaccination, challenge all foxes by the intramuscular injection of virulent rabies virus of a strain approved by the competent authority. Observe the animals for 90 days. Animals that die from causes not attributable to rabies are eliminated. The test is not valid if the number of such deaths reduces the number of vaccinated animals in the test to fewer than twenty-five. The vaccine complies with the test if not more than two of twenty-five vaccinated animals (or a statistically equivalent number if more than twenty-five vaccinated animals are challenged) show signs of rabies. The test is not valid unless at least nine control animals (or a statistically equivalent number if more than ten control animals are challenged) show signs of rabies and the presence of rabies virus in their brain is demonstrated by the fluorescent-antibody test or some other reliable method.

LABELLING

The label states the nature of the genetic marker of the virus strain.

Ph Eur

Rabies Veterinary Vaccine, Inactivated

(_Rabies Vaccine (Inactivated) for Veterinary Use, Ph Eur monograph 0451_)

Ph Eur

DEFINITION

Rabies vaccine (inactivated) for veterinary use is a liquid or freeze-dried preparation of fixed rabies virus inactivated by a suitable method.

PRODUCTION

The vaccine is prepared from virus grown either in suitable cell lines or in primary cell cultures from healthy animals (_5.2.4_). The virus suspension is harvested on one or more occasions within 28 days of inoculation. Multiple harvests from a single production cell culture may be pooled and considered as a single harvest. The rabies virus is inactivated by a suitable method.

Inactivation The test for residual live rabies virus is carried out by inoculation of the inactivated virus into the same type of cell culture as that used in the production of the vaccine or a cell culture shown to be at least as sensitive; the quantity of inactivated virus used in the test is equivalent to not less than 25 doses of the vaccine. After incubation for 4 days, a subculture is made using trypsinised cells; after incubation for a further 4 days, the cultures are examined for residual live rabies virus by an immunofluorescence test. No live virus is detected.

Antigen content The content of rabies virus glycoprotein is determined by a suitable immunochemical method (_2.7.1_). The content is within the limits approved for the particular preparation.

The vaccine may contain one or more adjuvants.

CHOICE OF VACCINE COMPOSITION

The vaccine is shown to be satisfactory with respect to immunogenicity for each species for which it is recommended. The suitability of the vaccine with respect to immunogenicity for carnivores (cats and dogs) is demonstrated by direct challenge. For other species, if a

challenge test has been carried out for the vaccine in cats or dogs, an indirect test is carried out by determining the antibody level following vaccination of not fewer than twenty animals according to the recommended schedule; the vaccine is satisfactory if, after the period claimed for protection, the mean rabies virus antibody level in the serum of the animals is not less than 0.5 IU/ml and if not more than 10 per cent of the animals have an antibody level less than 0.1 IU/ml. The test described below may be used to demonstrate immunogenicity in cats and dogs.

Immunogenicity Use not fewer than 35 susceptible animals of the minimum age recommended for vaccination. Take a blood sample from each animal and test individually for antibodies against rabies virus to determine susceptibility. Administer by the recommended route to each of not fewer than 25 animals one dose of vaccine. Keep not fewer than 10 animals as controls. Observe all the animals for a period equal to the claimed duration of immunity. No animal shows signs of rabies. On the last day of the claimed period for duration of immunity or later, challenge all animals by intramuscular injection of virulent rabies virus of a strain approved by the competent authority. Observe the animals for 90 days. Animals that die from causes not attributable to rabies are eliminated. The test is not valid if the number of such deaths reduces the number of vaccinated animals in the test to fewer than 25. The test is not valid unless at least eight control animals (or a statistically equivalent number if more than 10 control animals are challenged) show signs of rabies and the presence of rabies virus in their brain is demonstrated by the fluorescent-antibody test or some other suitable method. The vaccine complies with the test if not more than 2 of the 25 vaccinated animals (or a statistically equivalent number if more than 25 vaccinated animals are challenged) show signs of rabies.

BATCH TESTING

The test described under Potency is not necessarily carried out for routine testing of batches of vaccine. It is carried out, for a given vaccine, on one or more occasions, as decided by or with the agreement of the competent authority; where the test is not carried out, a suitable validated alternative method is used, the criteria for acceptance being set with reference to a batch of vaccine that has given satisfactory results in the test described above for immunogenicity or in the test described under Potency. The following test may be used after a suitable correlation with the test described above for immunogenicity or the test described under Potency has been established.

Batch potency test

Use 5 mice each weighing 18 g to 20 g. Vaccinate each mouse subcutaneously or intramuscularly using one-fifth of the recommended dose volume. Take blood samples 14 days after the injection and test the sera individually for rabies antibody using the rapid fluorescent focus inhibition test described for _Human rabies immunoglobulin (0723)_.

The amount of antibody is not less than that produced by a vaccine that has been found satisfactory with respect to immunogenicity as described above or in the test described under Potency.

Antigen content

The quantity of rabies virus glycoprotein per dose, determined by a suitable immunochemical method (_2.7.1_), is not significantly lower than that of a batch that has been found satisfactory with respect to immunogenicity as described above or in the test described under Potency.

IDENTIFICATION

When injected into animals, the vaccine stimulates the production of specific neutralising antibodies.

TESTS

Safety

If the vaccine is intended for more than one species including one belonging to the order of Carnivora, carry out the test in dogs. Otherwise use one of the species for which the vaccine is intended. Administer, by a recommended route, a double dose of vaccine to each of 2 animals having no antibodies against rabies virus. Observe the animals for 14 days. No abnormal local or systemic reaction occurs.

Inactivation

Carry out the test using a pool of the contents of 5 containers.

For vaccines which do not contain an adjuvant, carry out a suitable amplification test for residual infectious rabies virus using the same type of cell culture as that used in the production of the vaccine or a cell culture shown to be at least as sensitive. No live virus is detected.

For vaccines that contain an adjuvant, inject intracerebrally into each of not fewer than 10 mice each weighing 11 g to 15 g 0.03 ml of a pool of at least 5 times the smallest stated dose. To avoid interference from any antimicrobial preservative or the adjuvant, the vaccine may be diluted not more than 10 times before injection. In this case or if the vaccine strain is pathogenic only for unweaned mice, carry out the test on mice 1 to 4 days old. Observe the animals for 21 days. If more than 2 animals die during the first 48 h, repeat the test. From the third to the twenty-first days following the injection, the animals show no signs of rabies and immunofluorescence tests carried out on the brains of the animals show no indication of the presence of rabies virus.

Sterility

The vaccine complies with the test for sterility prescribed in the monograph on *Vaccines for veterinary use (0062)*.

POTENCY

The potency of rabies vaccine is determined by comparing the dose necessary to protect mice against the clinical effects of the dose of rabies virus defined below, administered intracerebrally, with the quantity of a reference preparation, calibrated in International Units, necessary to provide the same protection.

The International Unit is the activity of a stated quantity of the International Standard. The equivalence in International Units of the International Standard is stated by the World Health Organisation.

Rabies vaccine (inactivated) for veterinary use BRP is calibrated in International Units against the International Standard.

The test described below uses a parallel-line model with at least 3 points for the vaccine to be examined and the reference preparation. Once the analyst has experience with the method for a given vaccine, it is possible to carry out a simplified test using one dilution of the vaccine to be examined. Such a test enables the analyst to determine that the vaccine has a potency significantly higher than the required minimum but will not give full information on the validity of each individual potency determination. It allows a considerable reduction in the number of animals required for the test and should be considered by each laboratory in accordance with the provisions of the European Convention for the Protection of Vertebrate Animals used for Experimental and other Scientific Purposes.

Selection and distribution of the test animals Use in the test healthy female mice about 4 weeks old and from the same stock. Distribute the mice into at least 10 groups of not fewer than 10 mice.

Preparation of the challenge suspension Inoculate a group of mice intracerebrally with the CVS strain of rabies virus and when the mice show signs of rabies, but before they die, kill the mice and remove the brains and prepare a homogenate of the brain tissue in a suitable diluent. Separate gross particulate matter by centrifugation and use the supernatant liquid as challenge suspension. Distribute the suspension in small volumes in ampoules, seal and store at a temperature below $-60\ °C$. Thaw one ampoule of the suspension and make serial dilutions in a suitable diluent. Allocate each dilution to a group of mice and inject intracerebrally into each mouse 0.03 ml of the dilution allocated to its group. Observe the animals for 14 days and record the number in each group that, between the fifth and the fourteenth days, develop signs of rabies. Calculate the ID_{50} of the undiluted suspension.

Determination of potency of the vaccine to be examined Prepare at least three serial dilutions of the vaccine to be examined and three similar dilutions of the reference preparation. Prepare the dilutions such that those containing the largest quantity of vaccine may be expected to protect more than 50 per cent of the animals into which they are injected and those containing the smallest quantities of vaccine may be expected to protect less than 50 per cent of the animals into which they are injected. Allocate each dilution to a different group of mice and inject intraperitoneally into each mouse 0.5 ml of the dilution allocated to its group. 14 days after the injection prepare a suspension of the challenge virus such that, on the basis of the preliminary titration, it contains about 50 ID_{50} in each 0.03 ml. Inject intracerebrally into each vaccinated mouse 0.03 ml of this suspension. Prepare 3 suitable serial dilutions of the challenge suspension. Allocate the challenge suspension and the 3 dilutions one to each of 4 groups of 10 unvaccinated mice and inject intracerebrally into each mouse 0.03 ml of the suspension or one of the dilutions allocated to its group. Observe the animals in each group for 14 days. The test is not valid if more than 2 mice of any group die within the first 4 days after challenge. Record the numbers in each group that show signs of rabies in the period 5 days to 14 days after challenge.

The test is not valid unless:

— for both the vaccine to be examined and the reference preparation the 50 per cent protective dose lies between the smallest and the largest dose given to the mice,

— the titration of the challenge suspension shows that 0.03 ml of the suspension contained at least 10 ID_{50},

— the confidence limits ($P = 0.95$) are not less than 25 per cent and not more than 400 per cent of the estimated potency,

— the statistical analysis shows a significant slope and no significant deviations from linearity or parallelism of the dose-response lines.

The vaccine complies with the test if the estimated potency is not less than 1 IU in the smallest prescribed dose.

LABELLING

The label states:

— the type of cell culture used to prepare the vaccine and the species of origin,

— the minimum number of International Units per dose,

— the minimum period for which the vaccine provides protection.

Ruminant E. Coli Vaccine, Inactivated

Ruminant Escherichia Coli Vaccine, Inactivated

(Neonatal Ruminant Colibacillosis Vaccine (Inactivated), Ph Eur monograph 0961)

Ph Eur _____

DEFINITION

Neonatal ruminant colibacillosis vaccine (inactivated) is prepared from cultures of one or more suitable strains of *Escherichia coli*, carrying one or more adhesin factors or enterotoxins. This monograph applies to vaccines administered by injection to dams for protection of newborn offspring against enteric forms of colibacillosis.

PRODUCTION

The *E. coli* strains used for production are cultured separately in a suitable medium. The cells or toxins are processed to render them safe and are blended.

The vaccine may contain one or more suitable adjuvants.

CHOICE OF VACCINE COMPOSITION

The *E. coli* strains used in the production of the vaccine are shown to be satisfactory with respect to expression of antigens and the vaccine is shown to be satisfactory with respect to safety and immunogenicity. The following tests may be used during demonstration of safety (*5.2.6*) and efficacy (*5.2.7*).

Expression of antigens The expression of antigens that stimulate a protective immune response is verified by a suitable immunochemical method (*2.7.1*) carried out on the antigen obtained from each of the vaccine strains under the conditions used for the production of the vaccine.

Safety

A. A double dose of vaccine is administered to each of 10 pregnant animals of each of the species for which the vaccine is intended and that have not been vaccinated against colibacillosis. 1 dose is administered to each animal after the interval stated on the label. The animals are observed until parturition has occurred. Record body temperature the day before vaccination, at vaccination, 2 h, 4 h and 6 h later and then daily for 4 days; note the maximum temperature increase for each animal. No abnormal local or systemic reaction occurs; the average temperature increase for all animals does not exceed 1.5 °C and no animal shows a rise greater than 2 °C. Any effects on gestation or the offspring are noted.

B. Safety is demonstrated in field trials for each species for which the vaccine is intended by administering the intended dose to at least 60 animals from 3 different stocks, by the route and according to the schedule stated on the label. At least 30 animals from the same stocks are assigned to control groups. The animals are observed for 14 days after the last dose. No abnormal local or systemic reaction is noted and, in particular, no rise in temperature of more than 1.5 °C occurs within 2 days of administration of each dose of vaccine.

Immunogenicity The suitability of the vaccine with respect to immunogenicity must be demonstrated for each species for which it is intended. This may be demonstrated by the test described under Potency.

BATCH TESTING

Batch potency test

The test described under Potency is not carried out for routine testing of batches of vaccine. It is carried out, for a given vaccine, on one or more occasions, as decided by or with the agreement of the competent authority; where the test is not carried out, a suitable validated test is carried out, the criteria for acceptance being set with reference to a batch of vaccine that has given satisfactory results in the test described under Potency.
The following test may be used after a suitable correlation with the test described under Potency has been established by a statistical evaluation.

To obtain a valid assay, it may be necessary to carry out a test using several groups of animals, each receiving a different dose. For each dose required, carry out the test as follows. Vaccinate not fewer than 5 animals (for example rabbits, guinea-pigs, rats or mice), free from specific antibodies against the antigens stated on the label, using one injection of a suitable dose. Maintain 2 animals as unvaccinated controls. Where the schedule stated on the label requires a booster injection to be given, a booster vaccination may also be given in this test provided it has been demonstrated that this will still provide a suitably sensitive test system. At a given interval within the range of 14 to 21 days after the last injection, collect blood from each animal and prepare serum samples. Use a suitable validated test such as an enzyme-linked immunosorbent assay (*2.7.1*) to measure the antibody response to each of the protective antigens stated on the label. The antibody levels are not significantly less than those obtained with a batch that has given satisfactory results in the test described under Potency and there is no significant increase in antibody titre in the controls.

Where seronegative animals are not available, seropositive animals may be used in the above test. During the development of a test with seropositive animals, particular care will be required during the validation of the test system to establish that the test is suitably sensitive and to specify acceptable pass, fail and retest criteria. It will be necessary to take into account the range of possible prevaccination titres and establish the acceptable minimum titre rise after vaccination in relation to these.

Bacterial endotoxins

A test for bacterial endotoxins (*2.6.14*) is carried out on the final lot or, where the nature of the adjuvant prevents performance of a satisfactory test, on the bulk antigen or the mixture of bulk antigens immediately before addition of the adjuvant. The maximum acceptable amount of bacterial endotoxins is that found for a batch of vaccine that has been shown satisfactory in safety test A given under Choice of vaccine composition or in the safety test described under Tests, carried out using 10 animals. Where the latter test is used, note the maximum temperature increase for each animal; the average temperature increase for all animals does not exceed 1.5 °C. The method chosen for determining the amount of bacterial endotoxin present in the vaccine batch used in the safety test for determining the maximum acceptable level of endotoxins is used subsequently for testing of each batch.

IDENTIFICATION

In animals free from specific antibodies against the antigens stated on the label, the vaccine stimulates the production of antibodies against these antigens.

TESTS

Safety

Use animals of one of the species for which the vaccine is recommended and preferably having no specific antibodies against the antigens stated on the label or, where justified, use animals with a low level of such antibodies as long as they have not been vaccinated against colibacillosis and administration of the vaccine does not cause an anamnestic response. Administer by a recommended route a double dose of vaccine to each of 2 animals. Observe the animals for 14 days. Record body temperature before vaccination, at vaccination, 2 h, 4 h and 6 h later and then daily for 2 days. No abnormal local or systemic reaction occurs; a transient temperature increase not exceeding 2 °C may occur.

Sterility

The vaccine complies with the test for sterility prescribed in the monograph on *Vaccines for veterinary use (0062)*.

POTENCY

Carry out the test with a challenge strain representing each type of antigen against which the vaccine is intended to protect: if a single strain with all the necessary antigens is not available, repeat the test using different challenge strains.

Use not fewer than 15 susceptible animals of one of the species for which the vaccine is recommended and which are free from specific antibodies against the antigens stated on the label. Take not fewer than 10 at random and vaccinate these at the recommended stage of pregnancy and according to the recommended schedule. Collect colostrum from all animals after parturition and store the samples individually in conditions that maintain antibody levels. Take not fewer than 15 newborn unsuckled animals and house them in an environment ensuring absence of enteric pathogens. Allocate a colostrum sample from not fewer than 10 vaccinated dams and not fewer than 5 controls to the offspring. After birth, feed the animals with the colostrum sample allocated to it. After feeding the colostrum and within 12 h of birth, challenge the animals orally with a pathogenic strain of *E. coli* and observe for 10 days. The strain must not be one used in the manufacture of the vaccine.

On each day, note clinical signs in each animal and score using the following scale:

0   no signs
1   slight diarrhoea
2   marked diarrhoea (watery faeces)
3   dead

Total scores for each animal over 10 days are calculated. The test is not valid unless 80 per cent of the offspring from the control animals die or show severe signs of disease. The vaccine complies with the test if there is a significant reduction in score in the group of animals from vaccinated dams compared with the group from the unvaccinated controls.

LABELLING

The label states the antigen or antigens contained in the vaccine that stimulate a protective immune response.

_____ *Ph Eur*

Salmonella Dublin Vaccine, Living

Calf Paratyphoid Vaccine, Living

DEFINITION

Salmonella Dublin Vaccine, Living is a suspension of a suitably modified rough strain of *Salmonella dublin*. The vaccine is prepared immediately before use by reconstitution from the dried vaccine with a suitable liquid.

PRODUCTION

The vaccine may be prepared using suitable cultures grown in solid or liquid media. The final product is freeze dried.

CAUTION *There is no evidence that the vaccine is harmful to man, but it is advisable to avoid undue exposure.*

The reconstituted vaccine complies with the requirements stated under Veterinary Vaccines, with the following modifications.

IDENTIFICATION

Consists of a suspension of Gram-negative bacilli having the morphological, cultural and serological characteristics of rough strains of *S. dublin*.

TESTS

Extraneous micro-organisms

Does not contain extraneous micro-organisms. Verify the absence of micro-organisms other than *Salmonella dublin* as described in the test for sterility under Veterinary Vaccines.

Safety

Complies with the test described under Veterinary Vaccines.

Viable count

No fewer than 2.5 x 10^9 *S. dublin* organisms in the dose stated on the label, determined by plate counts.

STORAGE

When stored under the prescribed conditions the dried vaccine may be expected to retain its potency for not less than 2 years. The reconstituted vaccine should be used immediately.

LABELLING

The label states the number of bacteria in the dose.

Salmonella Enteritidis Vaccine (Inactivated) for Chickens

(*Ph Eur monograph 1947*)

Ph Eur _____

1 DEFINITION

Salmonella Enteritidis vaccine (inactivated) for chickens is a preparation of a suitable strain or strains of *Salmonella enterica* Enteritidis, inactivated while maintaining adequate immunogenic properties. This monograph applies to vaccines intended for administration to chickens for reducing *S. enterica* Enteritidis colonisation and faecal excretion of *S. enterica* Enteritidis.

2 PRODUCTION

2-1 PREPARATION OF THE VACCINE

The seed material is cultured in a suitable medium; each strain is cultivated separately. During production, various parameters such as growth rate are monitored by suitable methods; the values are within the limits approved for the particular vaccine. Purity of the cultures and identity are verified on the harvest using suitable methods. After cultivation, the bacterial harvests are collected separately, inactivated by a suitable method, and blended. The vaccine may contain adjuvants.

2-2 CHOICE OF VACCINE COMPOSITION

The vaccine is shown to be satisfactory with respect to safety (*5.2.6*) and efficacy (*5.2.7*) for the birds for which it is intended. The following tests for safety (section 2-2-1) and immunogenicity (section 2-2-2) may be used during the demonstration of safety and efficacy.

2-2-1 Safety

Carry out the test for each route of administration to be recommended for vaccination, using in each case chickens not older than the minimum recommended age. Use a batch of vaccine containing not less than the maximum potency that may be expected in a batch of vaccine.

Use not fewer than 10 chickens from a flock free from specified pathogens (SPF) (5.2.2). Administer by a recommended route and method to each chicken a double dose of vaccine. If the recommended schedule requires a second dose, administer 1 additional dose to each chicken after at least 14 days. Observe the chickens at least daily until at least 21 days after the last administration of the vaccine.

The test is invalid if more than 10 per cent of the chickens show abnormal signs or die from causes not attributable to the vaccine. The vaccine complies with the test if no chicken shows abnormal local or systemic reactions or dies from causes attributable to the vaccine.

2-2-2 Immunogenicity
A test is carried out for each route and method of administration to be recommended. The vaccine administered to each animal is of minimum potency.

Use for the test not fewer than 60 SPF chickens (5.2.2) not older than the minimum age recommended for vaccination. Vaccinate not fewer than 30 chickens with no more than the minimum recommended number of doses of vaccine. Maintain not fewer than 30 chickens as controls for each group of vaccinates. Challenge both groups, 4 weeks after the last administration of vaccine, by oral administration to each chicken of a sufficient quantity of a strain of *S. enterica* Enteritidis that is able to colonise chickens. Take blood samples from control chickens on the day before challenge. Observe the chickens at least daily for 4 weeks. Take individual fresh faeces samples on day 1 after challenge and at least twice weekly (including day 7) until 14 days after challenge. Test the fresh faeces samples for the presence of *S. enterica* Enteritidis by direct plating. Euthanise all surviving chickens at the end of the observation period, take samples of liver and spleen and test for the presence of *S. enterica* Enteritidis by an appropriate method.

The test is invalid if antibodies against *S. enterica* Enteritidis are found in any control chicken before challenge.

The vaccine complies with the test if:
— the number of *S. enterica* Enteritidis in fresh faeces samples from vaccinated chickens after challenge at the different days of sampling is significantly lower in vaccinates than in controls and remains lower until the end of the test;
— the number of positive samples of liver and spleen is significantly lower in vaccinates than in controls.

2-3 MANUFACTURER'S TEST
2-3-1 Batch potency test
It is not necessary to carry out the Potency test (section 3-4) for each batch of the vaccine if it has been carried out using a batch of vaccine with a minimum potency. Where the test is not carried out, an alternative validated method is used, the criteria for acceptance being set with reference to a batch of vaccine that has given satisfactory results in the test described under Potency. The following test may be used.

Use not fewer than 15 SPF chickens (5.2.2). Maintain not fewer than 5 SPF chickens as controls. Administer to each of 10 chickens 1 dose of vaccine by a recommended route. Where the schedule stated on the label requires a booster injection to be given, a booster vaccination may also be given in this test provided it has been demonstrated that this will still provide a suitably sensitive test system. At a given interval after the last injection, collect blood from each vaccinated and control chicken and prepare serum samples. Measure the titre of antibodies against *S. enterica* Enteritidis

in each serum sample using a suitable validated serological method. Calculate the titre for the group of vaccinates.

The test is invalid if specific *S. enterica* Enteritidis antibodies are found in 1 or more sera from control chickens at a given interval after the time of administration of the vaccine in the vaccinated group.

The vaccine complies with the test if the antibody titres of the group of vaccinates at a given interval after each vaccination, where applicable, are not significantly lower than the value obtained with a batch that has given satisfactory results in the test described under Potency (section 3-4).

3 BATCH TESTS
3-1 Identification
In animals that do not have antibodies against *S. enterica* Enteritidis, the vaccine stimulates the production of such antibodies.

3-2 Bacteria and fungi
The vaccine and, where applicable, the liquid supplied with it comply with the test for sterility prescribed in the monograph *Vaccines for veterinary use (0062)*.

3-3 Safety
Use not fewer than 10 SPF chickens (5.2.2), not older than the minimum age recommended for vaccination. Administer a double dose of vaccine by a recommended route to each chicken. Observe the chickens at least daily for 21 days. The test is invalid if more than 20 per cent of the chickens show abnormal signs or die from causes not attributable to the vaccine. The vaccine complies with the test if no chicken shows notable signs of disease or dies from causes attributable to the vaccine.

3-4 Potency
The vaccine complies with the requirements of the test mentioned under Immunogenicity (section 2-2-2) when administered by a recommended route and method.

Ph Eur

Salmonella Typhimurium Vaccine (Inactivated) for Chickens

(*Ph Eur monograph 2361*)

Ph Eur

1 DEFINITION
Salmonella Typhimurium vaccine (inactivated) for chickens is a preparation of a suitable strain or strains of *Salmonella enterica* Typhimurium, inactivated while maintaining adequate immunogenic properties. This monograph applies to vaccines intended for administration to chickens for reducing *S. enterica* Typhimurium colonisation and faecal excretion of *S. enterica* Typhimurium.

2 PRODUCTION
2-1 PREPARATION OF THE VACCINE
The seed material is cultured in a suitable medium; each strain is cultivated separately. During production, various parameters such as growth rate are monitored by suitable methods; the values are within the limits approved for the particular vaccine. Purity of the cultures and identity are verified on the harvest using suitable methods. After cultivation, the bacterial harvests are collected separately, inactivated by a suitable method, and blended. The vaccine may contain adjuvants.

2-2 CHOICE OF VACCINE COMPOSITION

The vaccine is shown to be satisfactory with respect to safety (5.2.6) and efficacy (5.2.7) for the birds for which it is intended. The following tests for safety (section 2-2-1) and immunogenicity (section 2-2-2) may be used during the demonstration of safety and efficacy.

2-2-1 Safety

Carry out the test for each route of administration to be recommended for vaccination, using in each case chickens not older than the minimum recommended age. Use a batch of vaccine containing not less than the maximum potency that may be expected in a batch of vaccine.

Use not fewer than 10 chickens from a flock free from specified pathogens (SPF) (5.2.2). Administer by a recommended route and method to each chicken a double dose of vaccine. If the recommended schedule requires a second dose, administer 1 additional dose to each chicken after at least 14 days. Observe the chickens at least daily until at least 21 days after the last administration of the vaccine.

The test is invalid if more than 10 per cent of the chickens show abnormal signs or die from causes not attributable to the vaccine. The vaccine complies with the test if no chicken shows abnormal local or systemic reactions or dies from causes attributable to the vaccine.

2-2-2 Immunogenicity

A test is carried out for each route and method of administration to be recommended. The vaccine administered to each animal is of minimum potency.

Use for the test not fewer than 60 SPF chickens (5.2.2) not older than the minimum age recommended for vaccination. Vaccinate not fewer than 30 chickens with no more than the minimum recommended number of doses of vaccine. Maintain not fewer than 30 chickens as controls for each group of vaccinates. Challenge both groups, 4 weeks after the last administration of vaccine, by oral administration to each chicken of a sufficient quantity of a strain of S. enterica Typhimurium that is able to colonise chickens. Take blood samples from control chickens on the day before challenge. Observe the chickens at least daily for 4 weeks. Take individual fresh faeces samples on day 1 after challenge and at least twice weekly (including day 7) until 14 days after challenge. Test the fresh faeces samples for the presence of S. enterica Typhimurium by direct plating. Euthanise all surviving chickens at the end of the observation period, take samples of liver and spleen and test for the presence of S. enterica Typhimurium by an appropriate method.

The test is invalid if antibodies against S. enterica Typhimurium are found in any control chicken before challenge.

The vaccine complies with the test if:
— the number of S. enterica Typhimurium in fresh faeces samples from vaccinated chickens after challenge at the different days of sampling is significantly lower in vaccinates than in controls and remains lower until the end of the test;
— the number of positive samples of liver and spleen is significantly lower in vaccinates than in controls.

2-3 MANUFACTURER'S TEST
2-3-1 Batch potency test

It is not necessary to carry out the Potency test (section 3-4) for each batch of the vaccine if it has been carried out using a batch of vaccine with a minimum potency. Where the test is not carried out, an alternative validated method is used, the criteria for acceptance being set with reference to a batch

of vaccine that has given satisfactory results in the test described under Potency. The following test may be used.

Use not fewer than 15 SPF chickens (5.2.2). Maintain not fewer than 5 SPF chickens as controls. Administer to each of 10 chickens 1 dose of vaccine by a recommended route. Where the schedule stated on the label requires a booster injection to be given, a booster vaccination may also be given in this test provided it has been demonstrated that this will still provide a suitably sensitive test system. At a given interval after the last injection, collect blood from each vaccinated and control chicken and prepare serum samples. Measure the titre of antibodies against S. enterica Typhimurium in each serum sample using a suitable validated serological method. Calculate the titre for the group of vaccinates.

The test is invalid if specific S. enterica Typhimurium antibodies are found in 1 or more sera from control chickens at a given interval after the time of administration of the vaccine in the vaccinated group.

The vaccine complies with the test if the antibody titres of the group of vaccinates at a given interval after each vaccination, where applicable, are not significantly lower than the value obtained with a batch that has given satisfactory results in the test described under Potency (section 3-4).

3 BATCH TESTS
3-1 Identification

In animals that do not have antibodies against S. enterica Typhimurium, the vaccine stimulates the production of such antibodies.

3-2 Bacteria and fungi

The vaccine and, where applicable, the liquid supplied with it comply with the test for sterility prescribed in the monograph *Vaccines for veterinary use (0062)*.

3-3 Safety

Use not fewer than 10 SPF chickens (5.2.2), not older than the minimum age recommended for vaccination. Administer a double dose of vaccine by a recommended route to each chicken. Observe the chickens at least daily for 21 days. The test is invalid if more than 20 per cent of the chickens show abnormal signs or die from causes not attributable to the vaccine. The vaccine complies with the test if no chicken shows notable signs of disease or dies from causes attributable to the vaccine.

3-4 Potency

The vaccine complies with the requirements of the test mentioned under Immunogenicity (section 2-2-2) when administered by a recommended route and method.

Ph Eur

Swine Erysipelas Vaccine, Inactivated

(Swine Erysipelas Vaccine (Inactivated), Ph Eur monograph 0064)

Ph Eur

DEFINITION

Swine erysipelas vaccine (inactivated) is a preparation of one or more suitable strains of *Erysipelothrix rhusiopathiae* (*E. insidiosa*) inactivated by a suitable method. This monograph applies to vaccines intended to protect pigs against swine erysipelas.

PRODUCTION

The vaccine may contain an adjuvant.

CHOICE OF VACCINE COMPOSITION

The vaccine is shown to be satisfactory with respect to safety (5.2.6) and efficacy (5.2.7).

Immunogenicity

The test described under Potency is suitable to demonstrate immunogenicity of the vaccine with respect to *E. rhusiopathiae* serotypes 1 and 2. If claims are made concerning another serotype, then a further test to demonstrate immunogenicity against this serotype is necessary.

BATCH TESTING

Batch potency test

The test described under Potency is not carried out for routine testing of batches of vaccine. It is carried out, for a given vaccine, on one or more occasions, as decided by or with the agreement of the competent authority. Where the test is not carried out, a suitable validated alternative test is carried out, the criteria for acceptance being set with reference to a batch of vaccine that has given satisfactory results in the test described under Potency. The following test may be used after a satisfactory correlation with the test described under Potency has been established.

Use mice of a suitable strain (for example, NMRI) weighing 17-20 g, from a uniform stock and that do not have antibodies against swine erysipelas. Administer the vaccine to be examined to a group of 10 mice. Inject a suitable dose (usually 1/10 of the pig dose) subcutaneously into each mouse. At a given interval (for example, 21-28 days), depending on the vaccine to be examined, bleed the animals under anaesthesia. Pool the sera, using an equal volume from each mouse. Determine the level of antibodies by a suitable immunochemical method (2.7.1), for example, enzyme-linked immunosorbent assay with *erysipelas ELISA coating antigen BRP*. The antibody level is not significantly less than that obtained with a batch that has given satisfactory results in the test described under Potency.

IDENTIFICATION

Injected into animals that do not have antibodies against *E. rhusiopathiae*, it stimulates the production of such antibodies.

TESTS

Safety

Use pigs of the minimum age recommended for vaccination and preferably having no antibodies against swine erysipelas or, where justified, use pigs with a low level of such antibodies as long as they have not been vaccinated against Swine erysipelas and administration of the vaccine does not cause an anamnestic response. Administer a double dose of vaccine by a recommended route to each of 2 pigs. Observe the animals for 14 days. No abnormal local or systemic reaction occurs.

Sterility

It complies with the test for sterility prescribed in the monograph on *Vaccines for veterinary use (0062)*.

POTENCY

If the vaccine contains more than 1 serotype, a test for 2 serotypes may be carried out on a single group by injecting each challenge serotype on different flanks of the animals. Validation and acceptance criteria are applied separately to the respective injection sites. If the vaccine contains more than 1 serotype, the potency test may also be carried out using a separate group for each serotype.

Use not fewer than 15 pigs not less than 12 weeks old, weighing not less than 20 kg and that do not have antibodies against swine erysipelas. Divide the animals into 2 groups. Vaccinate a group of not fewer than 10 pigs according to the recommended schedule. Maintain a group of not fewer than 5 pigs as unvaccinated controls. 3 weeks after vaccination, challenge the vaccinated animals and the control group by separate intradermal injections of 0.1 ml of a virulent strain of each of serotype 1 and serotype 2 of *E. rhusiopathiae*. Observe the animals for 7 days. The vaccine complies with the test if not fewer than 90 per cent of the vaccinated animals remain free from diamond skin lesions at the injection site. The test is invalid if fewer than 80 per cent of control animals show typical signs of disease, i.e. diamond skin lesions at the injection sites.

Swine erysipelas bacteria serotype 1 BRP and *swine erysipelas bacteria serotype 2 BRP* are suitable for use as challenge strains.

LABELLING

The label states the serotypes of *E. rhusiopathiae* included in the vaccine.

Ph Eur

Swine Fever Vaccine, Living

(Swine-Fever Vaccine (Live), Classical, Freeze-dried, Ph Eur monograph 0065)

Ph Eur

DEFINITION

Freeze-dried classical swine-fever vaccine (live) is a preparation obtained from a strain of classical swine-fever virus which has lost its pathogenicity for the pig by adaptation either to cell cultures or to the rabbit.

PRODUCTION

For vaccine prepared in rabbits, the seed-lot (or the vaccine) is made from the homogenised organs and/or blood of rabbits from healthy colonies, sacrificed at the peak of the temperature rise following intravenous inoculation of the virus. The vaccine is freeze-dried.

CHOICE OF VACCINE STRAIN

Only a virus strain shown to be satisfactory with respect to the following characteristics may be used in the preparation of the vaccine: safety; non-transmissibility; irreversibility of attenuation; and immunogenic properties. The following tests may be used during demonstration of safety (5.2.6) and efficacy (5.2.7).

The dose of vaccine used throughout the following tests is determined by the manufacturer on the basis of prior experiments.

Tests in pigs

Selection of animals The piglets are 6 to 7 weeks old. The sows are primiparae. All animals are healthy and must have had no contact with swine-fever virus and serologically must be free from swine-fever and bovine viral diarrhoea antibodies. They must have a week in which to adapt themselves to the new quarters where the tests are to be carried out.

Safety

(a) Each of five piglets receives intramuscularly as a single injection ten doses of vaccine (group a).

(b) Five piglets are immunodepressed by the daily injection of 2 mg of prednisolone per kilogram of body mass for five consecutive days and on the third day they receive one dose of vaccine (group b).

The animals of groups (a) and (b) are observed for 21 days. They must remain in good health. The temperature curve and the weight curve must not differ significantly from those of control animals.

(c) Ten non-immune pregnant sows each receive two doses of vaccine intramuscularly as a single injection between the twenty-fifth and thirty-fifth days of gestation. Ten non-immune pregnant sows of the same age and of the same origin receive instead of the two doses of vaccine an equal volume of a 9 g/l solution of *sodium chloride R*. The vaccinal virus does not cause abnormalities in the gestation or in the piglets.

Non-transmissibility   Twelve piglets of the same origin are kept together. Six are vaccinated in the normal way and the six others are kept as contact controls. After 40 days, all the pigs are challenged by intramuscular inoculation of a sufficient quantity of the challenge virus (see Potency) to kill an unvaccinated piglet in 7 days. The vaccinated piglets resist challenge whereas the contact piglets must display the typical signs of swine fever.

Irreversibility of attenuation   Each of two piglets receives one dose of vaccine intramuscularly. Seven days later, 5 ml of blood is taken from each of the piglets and the samples are pooled. 5 ml of the pooled blood is injected intramuscularly into each of two other piglets. This operation is repeated six times. The animals must not display any sign of swine fever and must show normal growth.

Immunogenic properties   The immunogenic properties may be demonstrated by the method described for the determination of potency. The quantity of the vaccinal virus corresponding to one dose of vaccine contains at least 100 PD_{50}.

IDENTIFICATION

A. For vaccines prepared in rabbits and lapinised vaccines prepared in cell cultures, inject intravenously 0.5 ml of the vaccine reconstituted as stated on the label into one or more non-immunised rabbits and one or more rabbits immunised either with an identical dose of a vaccine of the same type injected by the same route at least 10 days and at most 2 months beforehand or with a sufficient dose of antiserum administered a few hours before the injection of the vaccine. Measure the temperature of the rabbits in the morning and the evening starting 24 h after the injection and continuing until the fifth day after the injection. The vaccine is identified by its specific pyrogenic character leading to a rise in temperature of at least 1.5 °C in the non-immunised rabbits only.

B. For non-lapinised vaccines prepared in cell cultures, the serum of pigs immunised with the vaccine neutralises the virus used in the preparation of the vaccine.

TESTS

Safety

Use three piglets complying with the requirements prescribed for the selection of animals under Choice of Vaccine Strain. Inject intramuscularly into each piglet ten doses of the reconstituted vaccine as a single injection. Observe the animals for 21 days. The temperature curve remains normal and the animals remain in apparent good health and display normal growth.

Extraneous viruses

Mix the vaccine with a monospecific antiserum and inoculate into susceptible cell cultures. No cytopathic effect is produced.

Carry out a haemagglutination test using chicken red blood cells and the supernatant liquid of the cell cultures. The test is negative. Carry out a haemadsorption test on the cell cultures. The test is negative.

Use ten mice each weighing 11 g to 15 g. Inject intracerebrally into each mouse 0.03 ml of the vaccine reconstituted so that 1 ml contains 1 dose. Observe the animals for 21 days. If more than two mice die within the first 48 h, repeat the test. From the third to the twenty-first day after the injection, the mice show no abnormalities attributable to the vaccine.

Bacterial and fungal contamination

The vaccine to be examined complies with the test for sterility prescribed in the monograph on *Vaccines for veterinary use (0062)*.

Mycoplasmas (2.6.7)

The vaccine complies with the test for mycoplasmas.

POTENCY

The potency is expressed as the number of 50 per cent protective doses (PD_{50}) for pigs contained in the dose indicated on the label. The vaccine contains at least 100 PD_{50} per dose.

Use piglets complying with the requirements for selection of animals described under Choice of Vaccine Strain. To two groups of five piglets inject intramuscularly:

— 1/40 of a dose of the vaccine to be examined into each piglet of the first group,
— 1/160 of a dose of the vaccine to be examined into each piglet of the second group.

Use two piglets as controls.

Prepare the dilutions using *buffered salt solution pH 7.2 R*. On the fourteenth day after the injection, inoculate intramuscularly into each vaccinated and control animal a sufficient quantity of challenge virus to kill an unvaccinated piglet in 7 days. The challenge virus preparation consists of blood of pigs infected experimentally by virus that has not been submitted to passage in cell cultures. The control animals die within the seven days of inoculation. Observe the vaccinated animals for 14 days. From the number of animals which survive without showing any sign of swine fever, calculate the number of PD_{50} contained in the vaccine using the usual statistical methods.

LABELLING

The label states that the vaccine has been prepared in cell cultures or in rabbits as appropriate.

_____ *Ph Eur*

Swine Influenza Vaccine, Inactivated

(Porcine Influenza Vaccine (Inactivated),
Ph Eur monograph 0963)

Ph Eur _____

DEFINITION

Porcine influenza vaccine (inactivated) is an aqueous suspension, an oily emulsion or a freeze-dried preparation of one or more inactivated strains of swine or human influenza virus. Suitable strains contain both haemagglutinin and neuraminidase.

PRODUCTION

The virus is propagated in the allantoic cavity of fertilised hen eggs from a healthy flock or in suitable cell cultures (5.2.4). Each virus strain is cultivated separately. After cultivation, the viral suspensions are collected separately and inactivated by a method that avoids destruction of the immunogenicity. If necessary, they may be purified.

An amplification test for residual infectious influenza virus is carried out on each batch of antigen immediately after inactivation by passage in the same type of substrate as that used for production (eggs or cell cultures) or a substrate shown to be at least as sensitive. The quantity of inactivated virus used in the test is equivalent to not less than 10 doses of the vaccine. No live virus is detected.

The vaccine may contain one or more suitable adjuvants; it may be freeze-dried.

CHOICE OF VACCINE COMPOSITION

The choice of strains is based on the antigenic types and sub-types observed in Europe. The vaccine is shown to be satisfactory with respect to safety and immunogenicity for pigs. The following tests may be used during demonstration of safety (5.2.6) and efficacy (5.2.7).

Safety

A. A test is carried out in each category of animal for which the vaccine is intended (sows, fattening pigs). The animals used do not have antibodies against swine influenza virus. 2 doses of vaccine are injected by the intended route into each of not fewer than 10 animals. After 14 days, 1 dose of vaccine is injected into each of the animals. The animals are observed for a further 14 days. During the 28 days of the test, no abnormal local or systemic reaction is produced.

B. The animals used in the test for immunogenicity are also used to evaluate safety. The rectal temperature of each vaccinated animal is measured at the time of vaccination and 24 h and 48 h later. No abnormal effect on rectal temperature is noted nor other systemic reactions (for example, anorexia). The injection site is examined for local reactions at slaughter. No abnormal local reaction occurs.

C. The animals used for field trials are also used to evaluate safety. A test is carried out in each category of animals for which the vaccine is intended (sows, fattening pigs). Not fewer than 3 groups each of not fewer than 20 animals in at least 2 locations are used with corresponding groups of not fewer than 10 controls. The rectal temperature of each animal is measured at the time of vaccination and 24 h and 48 h later. No abnormal effect on rectal temperature is noted. The injection site is examined for local reactions at slaughter. No abnormal local reaction occurs.

Immunogenicity The test described under Potency carried out using an epidemiologically relevant challenge strain or strains is suitable to demonstrate the immunogenicity of the vaccine.

IN-PROCESS TESTS

For vaccines produced in eggs, the content of bacterial endotoxins is determined on the virus harvest to monitor production.

BATCH POTENCY TEST

The test described below under Potency is not carried out for routine testing of batches of vaccine. It is carried out, for a given vaccine, on one or more occasions, as decided by or with the agreement of the competent authority; where the test is not carried out, a suitable validated test is carried out, the criteria for acceptance being set with reference to a batch of vaccine that has given satisfactory results in the test described under Potency.

The following test may be used after a satisfactory correlation with the test described under Potency has been established by a statistical evaluation.

Inject subcutaneously into each of 5 seronegative guinea-pigs, 5 to 7 weeks old, a quarter of the dose stated on the label. Collect blood samples before the vaccination and 21 days after vaccination. Determine for each sample the level of specific antibodies against each virus subtype in the vaccine by haemagglutination-inhibition or another suitable test. The vaccine complies with the test if the level of antibodies is not lower than that found for a batch of vaccine that gave satisfactory results in the potency test in pigs (see Potency).

IDENTIFICATION

When injected into healthy, susceptible animals, the vaccine stimulates the production of specific antibodies against the influenza virus subtypes included in the vaccine. The antibodies may be detected by a suitable immunochemical method (2.7.1).

TESTS
Safety

Use 2 pigs, free from antibodies against swine influenza virus and not older than the minimum age stated for vaccination. Inject into each pig a double dose of vaccine by the route stated on the label. Observe the animals for 14 days and then inject into each animal 1 dose of vaccine. Observe the animals for 14 days. No abnormal local or systemic reaction occurs during the 28 days of the test.

Inactivation

If the vaccine has been prepared in eggs, inoculate 0.2 ml into the allantoic cavity of each of 10 fertilised hen eggs, 9 to 11 days old. Incubate at a suitable temperature for 3 days. The death of any embryo within 24 h of inoculation is considered as non-specific mortality and the egg is discarded. The test is not valid unless at least 80 per cent of the eggs survive. Collect the allantoic fluid of each egg, pool equal quantities and carry out a second passage on fertilised eggs in the same manner. Incubate for 4 days; the allantoic fluid of these eggs shows no haemagglutinating activity.

If the vaccine has been prepared in cell cultures, carry out a suitable test for residual infectious influenza virus using 2 passages in the same type of cell culture as used in the production of vaccine. No live virus is detected. If the vaccine contains an oily adjuvant that interferes with this test, where possible separate the aqueous phase from the vaccine by means that do not diminish the capacity to detect residual infectious influenza virus.

Extraneous viruses

On the pigs used for the safety test, carry out tests for antibodies. The vaccine does not stimulate the formation of antibodies other than those against influenza virus. In particular, no antibodies against viruses pathogenic for pigs or against viruses which could interfere with the diagnosis of infectious diseases of pigs (including viruses of the pestivirus group) are detected.

Sterility

The vaccine complies with the test for sterility prescribed in the monograph on *Vaccines for veterinary use (0062)*.

POTENCY

Carry out a potency test for each subtype used in the preparation of the vaccine. Use not fewer than 20 pigs of the minimum age recommended for vaccination and that do not have antibodies against swine influenza virus. Vaccinate not fewer than 10 pigs as recommended on the label and keep not fewer than 10 pigs as unvaccinated controls. Take a blood sample from all control pigs immediately before challenge. 3 weeks after the last administration of vaccine, challenge all the pigs with a suitable quantity of a virulent influenza field virus by the intratracheal route. Kill half of the vaccinated and control pigs 24 h after challenge and the other half 72 h after challenge. For each pig, measure the quantity of influenza virus in 2 lung tissue homogenates, one from the left apical, cardiac and diaphragmatic lobes, and the other from the corresponding right lung lobes. Take equivalent samples from each animal. The test is invalid if antibodies against influenza virus are found in any control pig immediately before challenge. The vaccine complies with the test if, at both times of measurement, the mean virus titre in the pooled lung tissue samples of vaccinated pigs is significantly lower than that for control pigs, when analysed by a suitable statistical method such as the Wilcoxon Mann-Whitney test.

_____ Ph Eur

Cold-water Vibriosis Vaccine for Salmonids, Inactivated

(Vibriosis (Cold-water) Vaccine (Inactivated) for Salmonids, Ph Eur monograph 1580)

Ph Eur _____

DEFINITION
Cold-water vibriosis vaccine (inactivated) for salmonids is prepared from cultures of one or more suitable strains of *Vibrio salmonicida*.

PRODUCTION
The strains of *V. salmonicida* are cultured and harvested separately. The harvests are inactivated by a suitable method. They may be purified and concentrated. Whole or disrupted cells may be used and the vaccine may contain extracellular products of the bacterium released into the growth medium.

CHOICE OF VACCINE COMPOSITION
The strain or strains of *V. salmonicida* used are shown to be suitable with respect to production of antigens of assumed immunological importance. The vaccine is shown to be satisfactory with respect to safety (5.2.6) and immunogenicity (5.2.7) in the species of fish for which it is intended. The following tests may be used during demonstration of safety and immunogenicity.

Safety   Safety is tested in three different batches using test A, test B or both, depending on the recommendations for use.

A. *Vaccines intended for administration by injection.* A test is carried out in each species of fish for which the vaccine is intended. The fish used are from a population that does not have specific antibodies against *V. salmonicida* and which has not been vaccinated against nor exposed to cold-water vibriosis. The test is carried out in the conditions recommended for the use of the vaccine with a water temperature not less than 10 °C. An amount of vaccine corresponding to twice the recommended dose per mass unit for fish of the minimum body mass recommended for vaccination is administered intraperitoneally to each of not fewer than fifty fish of the minimum recommended body mass. The fish are observed for 21 days. No abnormal local or systemic reaction occurs. The test is invalid if more than 6 per cent of the fish die from causes not attributable to the vaccine.

B. *Vaccines intended for administration by immersion.* A test is carried out in each species of fish for which the vaccine is intended. The fish used are from a population that does not

have specific antibodies against *V. salmonicida* and which has not been vaccinated against nor exposed to cold-water vibriosis. The test is carried out in the conditions recommended for the use of the vaccine with a water temperature not less than 10 °C. Prepare an immersion bath at twice the recommended concentration. Not fewer than fifty fish, having not less than the minimum body mass recommended for vaccination are used. The fish are bathed for twice the recommended time. The fish are observed for 21 days. No abnormal local or systemic reaction occurs. The test is invalid if more than 6 per cent of the fish die from causes not attributable to the vaccine.

C. Safety is demonstrated in addition in field trials by administering the intended dose to a sufficient number of fish distributed in not fewer than two sets of premises. No abnormal reaction occurs.

Immunogenicity   The test described under Potency, carried out for each recommended route of administration, is suitable to demonstrate immunogenicity of the vaccine.

BATCH TESTING
Batch potency test   For routine testing of batches of vaccine, the test described under Potency may be carried out using groups of not fewer than thirty fish of one of the species for which the vaccine is intended; alternatively, a suitable validated test based on antibody response may be carried out, the criteria being set with reference to a batch of vaccine that has given satisfactory results in the test described under Potency. The following test may be used after a satisfactory correlation with the test described under Potency has been established.

Use fish from a population that does not have specific antibodies against *V. salmonicida* and that are within specified limits for body mass. Carry out the test at a defined temperature. Inject into each of not fewer than twenty-five fish one dose of vaccine, according to the instructions for use. Perform mock vaccination on a control group of not fewer than ten fish. Collect blood samples at a defined time after vaccination. Determine for each sample the level of specific antibodies against *V. salmonicida* by a suitable immunochemical method (2.7.1). The vaccine complies with the test if the mean level of antibodies is not significantly lower than that found for a batch that gave satisfactory results in the test described under Potency. The test is not valid if the control group shows antibodies against *V. salmonicida*.

IDENTIFICATION
When injected into fish that do not have specific antibodies against *V. salmonicida*, the vaccine stimulates the production of such antibodies.

TESTS
Safety
Use not fewer than ten fish of one of the species for which the vaccine is intended, having, where possible, the minimum body mass recommended for vaccination; if fish of the minimum body mass are not available, use fish not greater than twice this mass. Use fish from a population that does not have specific antibodies against *V. salmonicida* and that has not been vaccinated against nor exposed to cold-water vibriosis. Carry out the test in the conditions recommended for use of the vaccine with a water temperature not less than 10 °C. For vaccines administered by injection or immersion, inject intraperitoneally into each fish an amount of vaccine corresponding to twice the recommended dose per mass unit. For vaccines administered by immersion only, use a bath with double the recommended concentration and bathe the

fish for twice the recommended immersion time. Observe the animals for 21 days. No abnormal local or systemic reaction attributable to the vaccine occurs. The test is invalid if more than 10 per cent of the fish die from causes not attributable to the vaccine.

Sterility

The vaccine complies with the test for sterility prescribed in the monograph on *Vaccines for veterinary use (0062)*.

POTENCY

Carry out the test according to a protocol defining limits of body mass for the fish, water source, water flow and temperature limits, and preparation of a standardised challenge. Vaccinate not fewer than one hundred fish by a recommended route, according to the instructions for use. Perform mock vaccination on a control group of not fewer than one hundred fish; mark vaccinated and control fish for identification. Keep all the fish in the same tank or mix equal numbers of controls and vaccinates in each tank if more than one tank is used. Carry out challenge by injection at a fixed time interval after vaccination, defined according to the statement regarding development of immunity. Use for challenge a culture of *V. salmonicida* whose virulence has been verified. Observe the fish daily until at least 60 per cent specific mortality is reached in the control group. Plot for both vaccinates and controls a curve of specific mortality against time from challenge and determine by interpolation the time corresponding to 60 per cent specific mortality in controls. The test is invalid if the specific mortality is less than 60 per cent in the control group 21 days after the first death in the fish. Read from the curve for vaccinates the mortality (*M*) at the time corresponding to 60 per cent mortality in controls. Calculate the relative percentage survival (RPS) from the expression:

$$\left(1 - \frac{M}{60}\right) \times 100$$

The vaccine complies with the test if the RPS is not less than 60 per cent for vaccines administered by immersion and 90 per cent for vaccines administered by injection.

LABELLING

The label states information on the time needed for development of immunity after vaccination under the range of conditions corresponding to the recommended use.

Ph Eur

Vibriosis Vaccine for Salmonids, Inactivated

(Vibriosis Vaccine (Inactivated) for Salmonids, Ph Eur monograph 1581)

Ph Eur

DEFINITION

Vibriosis vaccine (inactivated) for salmonids is prepared from cultures of one or more suitable strains or serovars of *Vibrio anguillarum*; the vaccine may also include *Vibrio ordalii*.

PRODUCTION

The strains of *V. anguillarum* and *V. ordalii* are cultured and harvested separately. The harvests are inactivated by a suitable method. They may be purified and concentrated. Whole or disrupted cells may be used and the vaccine may contain extracellular products of the bacterium released into the growth medium.

CHOICE OF VACCINE COMPOSITION

The strains of *V. anguillarum* and *V. ordalii* used are shown to be suitable with respect to production of antigens of assumed immunological importance. The vaccine is shown to be satisfactory with respect to safety (5.2.6) and immunogenicity (5.2.7) in the species of fish for which it is intended. The following tests may be used during demonstration of safety and immunogenicity.

Safety Safety is tested in three different batches using test A, test B or both, depending on the recommendations for use.

A. *Vaccines intended for administration by injection.* A test is carried out in each species of fish for which the vaccine is intended. The fish used are from a population that does not have specific antibodies against the relevant serovars of *V. anguillarum* or where applicable *V. ordalii* and which has not been vaccinated against nor exposed to vibriosis. The test is carried out in the conditions recommended for the use of the vaccine with a water temperature not less than 10 °C. An amount of vaccine corresponding to twice the recommended dose per mass unit for fish of the minimum body mass recommended for vaccination is administered intraperitoneally to each of not fewer than fifty fish of the minimum recommended body mass. The fish are observed for 21 days. No abnormal local or systemic reaction occurs. The test is invalid if more than 6 per cent of the fish die from causes not attributable to the vaccine.

B. *Vaccines intended for administration by immersion.* A test is carried out in each species of fish for which the vaccine is intended. The fish used are from a population that does not have specific antibodies against the relevant serovars of *V. anguillarum* or where applicable *V. ordalii* and which has not been vaccinated against nor exposed to vibriosis. The test is carried out in the conditions recommended for the use of the vaccine with a water temperature not less than 10 °C. Prepare an immersion bath at twice the recommended concentration. Not fewer than fifty fish having the minimum body mass recommended for vaccination are used. The fish are bathed for twice the recommended time. The fish are observed for 21 days. No abnormal local or systemic reaction occurs. The test is invalid if more than 6 per cent of the fish die from causes not attributable to the vaccine.

C. Safety is also demonstrated in field trials by administering the intended dose to a sufficient number of fish distributed in not fewer than two sets of premises. No abnormal reaction occurs.

Immunogenicity The test described under Potency, carried out for each recommended route of administration is suitable to demonstrate immunogenicity of the vaccine.

BATCH TESTING

Batch potency test For routine testing of batches of vaccine, the test described under Potency may be carried out using groups of not fewer than thirty fish of one of the species for which the vaccine is intended; alternatively, a suitable validated test based on antibody response may be carried out, the criteria being set with reference to a batch of vaccine that has given satisfactory results in the test described under Potency. The following test may be used after a satisfactory correlation with the test described under Potency has been established.

Use fish from a population that does not have specific antibodies against the relevant serovars of *V. anguillarum* and where applicable *V. ordalii* and that are within specified limits for body mass. Carry out the test at a defined temperature. Inject into each of not fewer than twenty-five fish one dose of vaccine, according to the instructions for use. Perform mock vaccination on a control group of not fewer than ten fish. Collect blood samples at a defined time after vaccination. Determine for each sample the level of specific antibodies against the different serovars of *V. anguillarum* and against *V. ordalii* included in the vaccine by a suitable immunochemical method (*2.7.1*). The vaccine complies with the test if the mean levels of antibodies are not significantly lower than those found for a batch that gave satisfactory results in the test described under Potency. The test is not valid if the control group shows antibodies against the relevant serovars of *V. anguillarum* or, where applicable, against *V. ordalii*.

IDENTIFICATION

When injected into fish that do not have specific antibodies against *V. anguillarum* and, where applicable, *V. ordalii*, the vaccine stimulates the production of such antibodies.

TESTS

Safety

Use not fewer than ten fish of one of the species for which the vaccine is intended, having, where possible, the minimum body mass recommended for vaccination; if fish of the minimum body mass are not available, use fish not greater than twice this mass. Use fish from a population that does not have specific antibodies against the relevant serovars of *V. anguillarum* and, where applicable, *V. ordalii* and which has not been vaccinated against nor exposed to vibriosis. Carry out the test in the conditions recommended for the use of the vaccine with a water temperature not less than 10 °C. For vaccines administered by injection or immersion, inject intraperitoneally into each fish an amount of vaccine corresponding to twice the recommended dose per mass unit. For vaccines administered by immersion only, use a bath with double the recommended concentration and bathe the fish for twice the recommended immersion time. Observe the animals for 21 days. No abnormal local or systemic reaction attributable to the vaccine occurs. The test is invalid if more than 10 per cent of the fish die from causes not attributable to the vaccine.

Sterility

The vaccine complies with the test for sterility prescribed in the monograph on *Vaccines for veterinary use (0062)*.

POTENCY

Carry out a separate test for each species and each serovar included in the vaccine. Carry out the test according to a protocol defining limits of body mass for the fish, water source, water flow and temperature limits, and preparation of a standardised challenge. Vaccinate not fewer than one hundred fish by a recommended route, according to the instructions for use. Perform mock vaccination on a control group of not fewer than one hundred fish; mark vaccinated and control fish for identification. Keep all the fish in the same tank or mix equal numbers of controls and vaccinates in each tank if more than one tank is used. Carry out challenge by injection at a fixed time interval after vaccination, defined according to the statement regarding development of immunity. Use for challenge cultures of *V. anguillarum* or *V. ordalii* whose virulence has been verified. Observe the fish daily until at least 60 per cent specific mortality is reached in the control group. Plot for both vaccinates and controls a curve of specific mortality against time from challenge and determine by interpolation the time corresponding to 60 per cent specific mortality in controls.

The test is invalid if the specific mortality is less than 60 per cent in the control group 21 days after the first death in the fish. Read from the curve for vaccinates the mortality (*M*) at the time corresponding to 60 per cent mortality in controls. Calculate the relative percentage survival (RPS) from the expression:

$$\left(1 - \frac{M}{60}\right) \times 100$$

The vaccine complies with the test if the RPS is not less than 60 per cent for vaccines administered by immersion and 75 per cent for vaccines administered by injection.

LABELLING

The label states:
— the serovar or serovars of *V. anguillarum* included in the vaccine,
— where applicable, that the vaccine includes *V. ordalii*,
— information on the time needed for development of immunity after vaccination under the range of conditions corresponding to the recommended use.

Ph Eur

DIAGNOSTIC PREPARATIONS

Avian Tuberculin Purified Protein Derivative

Avian Tuberculin P.P.D.

(Ph Eur monograph 0535)

Ph Eur _____

DEFINITION

Avian tuberculin purified protein derivative (avian tuberculin PPD) is a preparation obtained from the heat-treated products of growth and lysis of *Mycobacterium avium* capable of revealing a delayed hypersensitivity in an animal sensitised to micro-organisms of the same species.

PRODUCTION

It is obtained from the water-soluble fractions prepared by heating in free-flowing steam and subsequently filtering cultures of *M. avium* grown in a liquid synthetic medium. The active fraction of the filtrate, consisting mainly of protein, is isolated by precipitation, washed and re-dissolved. An antimicrobial preservative that does not give rise to false positive reactions, such as phenol, may be added. The final sterile preparation, free from mycobacteria, is distributed aseptically into sterile tamper-proof glass containers, which are then closed so as to prevent contamination.
The preparation may be freeze-dried.

The identification, the tests and the determination of potency apply to the liquid form and to the freeze-dried form after reconstitution as stated on the label.

IDENTIFICATION

Inject a range of graded doses intradermally at different sites into suitably sensitised albino guinea-pigs, each weighing not less than 250 g. After 24-28 h, reactions appear in the form of oedematous swellings with erythema, with or without necrosis, at the points of injection. The size and severity of the reactions vary according to the dose. Unsensitised guinea-pigs show no reactions to similar injections.

TESTS

pH *(2.2.3)*
6.5 to 7.5.

Phenol *(2.5.15)*
Maximum 5 g/l, if the preparation to be examined contains phenol.

Sensitising effect
Use a group of 3 guinea-pigs that have not been treated with any material that will interfere with the test. On 3 occasions at intervals of 5 days, inject intradermally into each guinea-pig a dose of the preparation to be examined equivalent to 500 IU in 0.1 ml. 15-21 days after the 3rd injection, inject the same dose (500 IU) intradermally into these animals and into a control group of 3 guinea-pigs of the same mass, which have not previously received injections of tuberculin. 24-28 h after the last injections, the reactions of the 2 groups are not significantly different.

Toxicity
Use 2 guinea-pigs, each weighing not less than 250 g, that have not previously been treated with any material that will interfere with the test. Inject subcutaneously into each guinea-pig 0.5 ml of the preparation to be examined. Observe the animals for 7 days. No abnormal effects occur during the observation period.

Sterility
It complies with the test for sterility prescribed in the monograph *Vaccines for veterinary use (0062)*.

POTENCY

The potency of avian tuberculin purified protein derivative is determined by comparing the reactions produced in sensitised guinea-pigs by the intradermal injection of a series of dilutions of the preparation to be examined with those produced by known concentrations of a reference preparation calibrated in International Units.

The International Unit is the activity contained in a stated amount of the International Standard. The equivalence in International Units of the International Standard is stated by the World Health Organisation.

Sensitise not fewer than 8 albino guinea-pigs, each weighing 400-600 g, by the deep intramuscular injection of a suitable dose of inactivated or live *M. avium*. Not less than 4 weeks after the sensitisation of the guinea-pigs, shave their flanks to provide space for not more than 4 injection sites on each side. Prepare dilutions of the preparation to be examined and of the reference preparation using isotonic phosphate-buffered saline (pH 6.5-7.5) containing 0.005 g/l of *polysorbate 80 R*. Use not fewer than 3 doses of the reference preparation and not fewer than 3 doses of the preparation to be examined. Choose the doses such that the lesions produced have a diameter of not less than 8 mm and not more than 25 mm. Allocate the dilutions randomly to the sites, for example using a Latin square design. Inject each dose intradermally in a constant volume of 0.1 ml or 0.2 ml. Measure the diameters of the lesions after 24-28 h and calculate the results of the test using the usual statistical methods (for example, 5.3) and assuming that the diameters of the lesions are directly proportional to the logarithm of the concentration of the tuberculins.

The test is not valid unless the confidence limits ($P = 0.95$) are not less than 50 per cent and not more than 200 per cent of the estimated potency. The estimated potency is not less than 75 per cent and not more than 133 per cent of the stated potency. The stated potency is not less than 20 000 IU/ml.

STORAGE

Protected from light, at a temperature of 5 ± 3 °C.

LABELLING

The label states:
— the potency in International Units per millilitre;
— the name and quantity of any added substance;
— for freeze-dried preparations:
— the name and volume of the reconstituting liquid to be added;
— that the product is to be used immediately after reconstitution.

_____ *Ph Eur*

Bovine Tuberculin Purified Protein Derivative

Bovine Tuberculin P.P.D.

(*Ph Eur monograph 0536*)

Ph Eur

DEFINITION

Bovine tuberculin purified protein derivative (bovine tuberculin PPD) is a preparation obtained from the heat-treated products of growth and lysis of *Mycobacterium bovis* capable of revealing a delayed hypersensitivity in an animal sensitised to micro-organisms of the same species.

PRODUCTION

It is obtained from the water-soluble fractions prepared by heating in free-flowing steam and subsequently filtering cultures of *M. bovis* grown in a liquid synthetic medium. The active fraction of the filtrate, consisting mainly of protein, is isolated by precipitation, washed and re-dissolved. An antimicrobial preservative that does not give rise to false positive reactions, such as phenol, may be added. The final sterile preparation, free from mycobacteria, is distributed aseptically into sterile, tamper-proof glass containers, which are then closed so as to prevent contamination.
The preparation may be freeze-dried.

The identification, the tests and the determination of potency apply to the liquid form and to the freeze-dried form after reconstitution as stated on the label.

IDENTIFICATION

Inject a range of graded doses intradermally at different sites into suitably sensitised albino guinea-pigs, each weighing not less than 250 g. After 24-28 h, reactions appear in the form of oedematous swellings with erythema, with or without necrosis, at the points of injection. The size and severity of the reactions vary according to the dose. Unsensitised guinea-pigs show no reactions to similar injections.

TESTS

pH (*2.2.3*)
6.5 to 7.5.

Phenol (*2.5.15*)
Maximum 5 g/l, if the preparation to be examined contains phenol.

Sensitising effect
Use a group of 3 guinea-pigs that have not been treated with any material that will interfere with the test. On 3 occasions at intervals of 5 days, inject intradermally into each guinea-pig a dose of the preparation to be examined equivalent to 500 IU in 0.1 ml. 15-21 days after the 3rd injection, inject the same dose (500 IU) intradermally into these animals and into a control group of 3 guinea-pigs of the same mass, which have not previously received injections of tuberculin. 24-28 h after the last injections, the reactions of the 2 groups are not significantly different.

Toxicity
Use 2 guinea-pigs, each weighing not less than 250 g, that have not previously been treated with any material that will interfere with the test. Inject subcutaneously into each guinea-pig 0.5 ml of the preparation to be examined. Observe the animals for 7 days. No abnormal effects occur during the observation period.

Sterility
It complies with the test for sterility prescribed in the monograph *Vaccines for veterinary use (0062)*.

POTENCY

The potency of bovine tuberculin purified protein derivative is determined by comparing the reactions produced in sensitised guinea-pigs by the intradermal injection of a series of dilutions of the preparation to be examined with those produced by known concentrations of a reference preparation calibrated in International Units.

The International Unit is the activity contained in a stated amount of the International Standard. The equivalence in International Units of the International Standard is stated by the World Health Organisation.

Sensitise not fewer than 8 albino guinea-pigs, each weighing 400-600 g, by the deep intramuscular injection of 0.0001 mg of wet mass of living *M. bovis* of strain AN5 suspended in 0.5 ml of a 9 g/l solution of *sodium chloride R*. Not less than 4 weeks after the sensitisation of the guinea-pigs, shave their flanks to provide space for not more than 4 injection sites on each side. Prepare dilutions of the preparation to be examined and of the reference preparation using isotonic phosphate-buffered saline (pH 6.5-7.5) containing 0.005 g/l of *polysorbate 80 R*. Use not fewer than 3 doses of the reference preparation and not fewer than 3 doses of the preparation to be examined. Choose the doses such that the lesions produced have a diameter of not less than 8 mm and not more than 25 mm. Allocate the dilutions randomly to the sites, for example using a Latin square design. Inject each dose intradermally in a constant volume of 0.1 ml or 0.2 ml. Measure the diameters of the lesions after 24-28 h and calculate the results of the test using the usual statistical methods (for example, *5.3*) and assuming that the diameters of the lesions are directly proportional to the logarithm of the concentration of the tuberculins.

The test is not valid unless the confidence limits ($P = 0.95$) are not less than 50 per cent and not more than 200 per cent of the estimated potency. The estimated potency is not less than 66 per cent and not more than 150 per cent of the stated potency. The stated potency is not less than 20 000 IU/ml.

STORAGE

Protected from light, at a temperature of 5 ± 3 °C.

LABELLING

The label states:
— the potency in International Units per millilitre;
— the name and quantity of any added substance;
— for freeze-dried preparations:
  — the name and volume of the reconstituting liquid to be added;
  — that the product is to be used immediately after reconstitution.

Ph Eur

Mallein Purified Protein Derivative

Mallein P.P.D.

DEFINITION

Mallein Purified Protein Derivative is a preparation of the heat treated products of growth and lysis of *Pseudomonas mallei*. It contains not less than 0.95 mg per ml and not more than 1.05 mg per ml of purified protein derivative.

PRODUCTION

It is prepared from the water-soluble fractions obtained by heating in free-flowing steam and subsequently filtering cultures of the glanders bacillus grown in a liquid synthetic medium. The active fraction of the filtrate, which is predominantly protein, is isolated by precipitation, washed and redissolved in phosphate buffered saline at neutral pH. It is then distributed in sterile containers that are inert towards the contents and sealed so as to exclude micro-organisms. A suitable preservative may be added.

CAUTION *Mallein P.P.D. is not dangerous to man, but the organism from which it is prepared is pathogenic to man and may be fatal if an infection is untreated. If an infection is suspected treatment should begin without delay.*

IDENTIFICATION

Inject small doses intradermally into suitable guinea-pigs that have been sensitised with killed *P. mallei* in oily adjuvant. Oedematous swellings occur at the point of injection after 48 hours.

TESTS

Acidity or alkalinity
pH, 6.5 to 7.5, Appendix V L.

Phenol
For preparations containing phenol as a preservative, not more than 0.5% w/v, determined by the method described under Veterinary Antisera.

Sterility
Complies with the *test for sterility*, Appendix XVI A, using Method I: Membrane filtration, whenever possible and particularly when the volume in a container is greater than 100 ml, with the following modifications.

Incubate the media for not less than 14 days at 30° to 35° in the test intended to detect bacteria and at 20° to 25° in the test intended to detect fungi.

Use the quantities stated under Application of the test to injectable preparations except that when the quantity in each container[1] is 20 ml or more of a liquid, the minimum quantity to be used for each medium is 10% of the contents or 5 ml, whichever is the less.

Abnormal toxicity
Inject 0.5 ml subcutaneously into each of two guinea-pigs. Neither shows a significant local or systemic reaction within 7 days.

ASSAY

To 2.5 ml add 2.5 ml of *water* and 2.5 ml of a 40% w/v solution of *trichloroacetic acid*, mix, allow to stand for 30 minutes and centrifuge for 15 minutes. Discard the supernatant liquid and dissolve the residue in 0.5 ml of 5M *sodium hydroxide*. Transfer the solution to a Kjeldahl flask with the aid of 6 ml of *water* and add about 0.1 g of a mixture of 100 parts of *potassium sulphate*, 10 parts of *copper(II) sulphate* and 5 parts of *selenium dioxide* and 1 ml of *nitrogen-free sulphuric acid*. Evaporate the water and continue heating until a brown deposit appears. Dissolve the deposit by the addition of 0.5 ml of *hydrogen peroxide solution (100 vol)*, continue heating until white fumes of sulphur trioxide appear and boil rapidly for at least 10 minutes. (If while heating a brown deposit again appears, add a further 0.5 ml of *hydrogen peroxide solution (100 vol)*. Transfer to an ammonia distillation apparatus with the aid of 5 ml of *water* and add 5 ml of a 50% w/v solution of *sodium hydroxide* to form a lower layer. Distil for 3 minutes, collecting the distillate in a mixture of 5 ml of a 2% w/v solution of *boric acid* and 0.05 ml of a solution containing 0.066% w/v of *methyl red* and 0.033% w/v of *bromocresol green* in *ethanol (96%)* and titrate with 0.00447M *sulphuric acid VS* (prepared by diluting 89.3 ml of 0.05M *sulphuric acid VS* to 1000 ml

with *water*). Repeat the operation using 2.5 ml of *water* in place of the preparation being examined. The difference between the titrations represents the ammonia liberated by the substance being tested. Each ml of 0.00447M *sulphuric acid VS* is equivalent to 0.875 mg of purified protein derivative.

STORAGE

Mallein Purified Protein Derivative should be protected from light and stored at a temperature between 2° and 8°. Under these conditions it may be expected to retain its potency for not less than 6 months.

LABELLING

The label states (1) the volume of the contents; (2) the date after which the preparation is not intended to be used; (3) that the preparation is to be used for animals only; (4) the conditions under which it should be stored; (5) the name and percentage of any added preservative; (6) the dose.

ANNEX

Guidance to manufacturers performing the test for sterility in determining the number of containers to be tested, the manufacturer should have regard to the environmental conditions of manufacture, the volume of preparation per container and any other special considerations applying to the preparation concerned. With respect to diagnostic preparations for veterinary use, 1% of the containers in a batch, with a minimum of three and a maximum of 10 is considered a suitable number assuming that the preparation has been manufactured under appropriately validated conditions designed to exclude contamination.

---

[1] Guidance to manufacturers on the number of containers is provided in the Annex to this monograph.

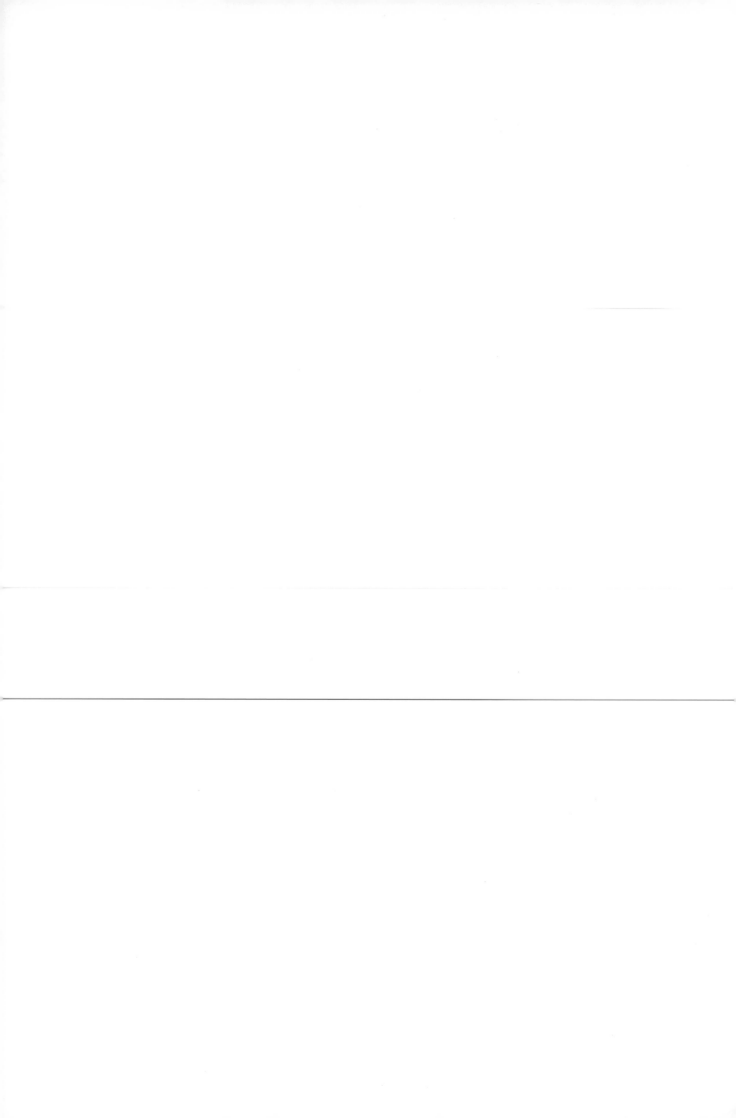

Monographs

Surgical Materials

SUTURES

Sterile Catgut in Distributor

*(Catgut, Sterile, in Distributor for Veterinary Use,
Ph Eur monograph 0660)*

Ph Eur

DEFINITION
Sterile catgut in distributor for veterinary use consists of strands prepared from collagen taken from the intestinal membranes of mammals. After cleaning, the membranes are split longitudinally into strips of varying width, which, when assembled in small numbers, according to the diameter required, are twisted under tension, dried, polished, selected and sterilised. The strands may be treated with chemical substances such as chromium salts to prolong absorption and glycerol to make them supple, provided such substances do not reduce tissue acceptability.

The strand is presented in a distributor that allows the withdrawal and use of all or part of it in aseptic conditions. The design of the distributor is such that with suitable handling the sterility of the content is maintained even when part of the strand has been withdrawn. It may be stored dry or in a preserving liquid to which an antimicrobial preservative but not an antibiotic may be added.

TESTS
If stored in a preserving liquid, remove the strand from the distributor and measure promptly and in succession the length, diameter and breaking load. If stored in the dry state, immerse the strand in alcohol R or a 90 per cent V/V solution of 2-propanol R for 24 h and proceed with the measurements as indicated above.

Length
Measure the length without applying to the strand more tension than is necessary to keep it straight. The length is not less than 95 per cent of the length stated on the label. If the strand consists of several sections joined by knots, the length of each section is not less than 2.5 m.

Diameter
Carry out the test using a suitable instrument capable of measuring with an accuracy of at least 0.002 mm and having a circular pressor foot 10 mm to 15 mm in diameter. The pressor foot and the moving parts attached to it are weighted so as to apply a total load of 100 ± 10 g to the strand being tested. When making the measurements, lower the pressor foot slowly to avoid crushing the strand. Make not fewer than one measurement per 2 m of length. If the strand consists of several sections joined by knots, make not fewer than three measurements per section. In any case make not fewer than twelve measurements. Make the measurements at points evenly spaced along the strand or along each section. The strand is not subjected to more tension than is necessary to keep it straight during measurement. The average of the measurements carried out on the strand being tested and not less than two-thirds of the individual measurements are within the limits given in the column under A in Table 0660.-1 for the gauge number concerned. None of the measurements is outside the limits given in the columns under B in Table 0660.-1 for the gauge number concerned.

Table 0660.-1. – *Diameters and breaking loads*

Gauge number	Diameter (millimetres)				Breaking load (newtons)	
	A		B		C	D
	min.	max.	min.	max.		
1	0.100	0.149	0.085	0.175	1.8	0.4
1.5	0.150	0.199	0.125	0.225	3.8	0.7
2	0.200	0.249	0.175	0.275	7.5	1.8
2.5	0.250	0.299	0.225	0.325	10	3.8
3	0.300	0.349	0.275	0.375	12.5	7.5
3.5	0.350	0.399	0.325	0.450	20	10
4	0.400	0.499	0.375	0.550	27.5	12.5
5	0.500	0.599	0.450	0.650	38.4	20.0
6	0.600	0.699	0.550	0.750	45.0	27.5
7	0.700	0.799	0.650	0.850	60.0	38.0
8	0.800	0.899	0.750	0.950	70.0	45.0

Minimum breaking load
The minimum breaking load is determined over a simple knot formed by placing one end of a strand held in the right hand over the other end held in the left hand, passing one end over the strand and through the loop so formed (see Figure 0660.-1) and pulling the knot tight.

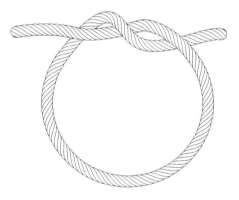

Figure 0660.-1. – *Simple knot*

Make not fewer than one measurement per 2 m of length. If the strand consists of several sections joined by knots, make not fewer than three measurements per section and, in any case, not fewer than one measurement per 2 m of length at points evenly spaced along the strand or along each section. Determine the breaking load using a suitable tensilometer. The apparatus has two clamps for holding the strand, one of which is mobile and is driven at a constant rate of 30 cm per minute. The clamps are designed so that the strand being tested can be attached without any possibility of slipping. At the beginning of the test the length of strand between the clamps is 12.5 cm to 20 cm and the knot is midway between the clamps. Set the mobile clamp in motion and note the force required to break the strand. If the strand breaks in a clamp or within 1 cm of it, the result is discarded and the test repeated on another part of the strand. The average of all the results, excluding those legitimately discarded, is equal to or greater than the value in column C and no value is less than that given in column D in Table 0660.-1 for the gauge number concerned.

Soluble chromium compounds

Place 0.25 g in a conical flask containing 1 ml of *water R* per 10 mg of catgut. Stopper the flask, allow to stand at 37 ± 0.5 °C for 24 h, cool and decant the liquid. Transfer 5 ml to a small test tube and add 2 ml of a 10 g/l solution of *diphenylcarbazide R* in *alcohol R* and 2 ml of *dilute sulphuric acid R*. The solution is not more intensely coloured than a standard prepared at the same time using 5 ml of a solution containing 2.83 μg of *potassium dichromate R* per millilitre, 2 ml of *dilute sulphuric acid R* and 2 ml of a 10 g/l solution of *diphenylcarbazide R* in *alcohol R* (1 ppm of Cr).

Sterility (*2.6.1*)

It complies with the test for sterility as applied to catgut and other surgical sutures. Carry out the test on three sections, each 30 cm long, cut off respectively from the beginning, the centre and the end of the strand.

STORAGE

Store protected from light and heat.

LABELLING

The label states:
— the gauge number,
— the length in centimetres or in metres.

Ph Eur

Sterile Non-absorbable Strands in Distributor

(Strands, Sterile Non-absorbable, in Distributor for Veterinary Use, Ph Eur monograph 0605)

Ph Eur

DEFINITION

The statements in this monograph are intended to be read in conjunction with the individual monographs on sterile non-absorbable strands in distributor for veterinary use in the Pharmacopoeia. The requirements do not necessarily apply to sterile non-absorbable strands which are not the subject of such monographs.

Sterile non-absorbable strands in distributor for veterinary use are strands which, when introduced into a living organism, are not metabolised by that organism. Sterile non- absorbable strands vary in origin, which may be animal, vegetable or synthetic. They occur as cylindrical monofilaments or as multifilament strands. Multifilament strands consist of elementary fibres which are assembled by twisting, cabling or braiding. Such strands may be sheathed. Sterile non- absorbable strands may be treated to render them non-capillary, and they may be coloured with colouring matter or pigments authorised by the competent authority. The strands are sterilised.

They are presented in a suitable distributor that allows the withdrawal and use of all or part of the strand in aseptic conditions. The design of the distributor is such that with suitable handling the sterility of the content is maintained even when part of the strand has been removed. They may be stored dry or in a preserving liquid to which an antimicrobial preservative but not an antibiotic may be added.

TESTS

Remove the strand from the distributor and measure promptly and in succession the length, diameter and minimum breaking load.

Length

Measure the length in the condition in which the strand is presented and without applying more tension than is necessary to keep it straight. The length of the strand is not less than 95 per cent of the length stated on the label.

Diameter

Unless otherwise prescribed, measure the diameter by the following method using the strand in the condition in which it is presented. Use a suitable instrument capable of measuring with an accuracy of at least 0.002 mm and having a circular pressor foot 10 mm to 15 mm in diameter. The pressor foot and the moving parts attached to it are weighted so as to apply a total load of 100 ± 10 g to the strand being tested. When making the measurements, lower the pressor foot slowly to avoid crushing the strand. Make not fewer than one measurement per 2 m of length and in any case not fewer than 12 measurements at points evenly spaced along the strand. During the measurement submit monofilament strands to a tension not greater than that required to keep them straight. Submit multifilament strands to a tension not greater than one-fifth of the minimum breaking load shown in column C of Table 0605.-1 appropriate to the gauge number and type of material concerned or 10 N whichever is less. For multifilament strands of gauge number above 1.5 make two measurements at each point, the second measurement being made after rotating the strand through 90°. The diameter of that point is the average of the two measurements. The average of the measurements carried out on the strand being tested and not less than two-thirds of the individual measurements are within the limits given in the columns under A in Table 0605.-1 for the gauge number concerned. None of the measurements is outside the limits given in the columns under B in Table 0605.-1 for the gauge number concerned.

Table 0605.-1. – *Diameters and minimum breaking loads*

Gauge number	Diameter (millimetres)				Minimum breaking load (newtons)			
	A		B		Linen thread		All other non-absorbable strands	
	min.	max.	min.	max.	C	D	C	D
0.5	0.050	0.069	0.045	0.085	-	-	1.0	0.35
0.7	0.070	0.099	0.060	0.125	1.0	0.3	1.5	0.60
1	0.100	0.149	0.085	0.175	2.5	0.6	3.0	1.0
1.5	0.150	0.199	0.125	0.225	5.0	1.0	5.0	1.5
2	0.200	0.249	0.175	0.275	8.0	2.5	9.0	3.0
2.5	0.250	0.299	0.225	0.325	9.0	5.0	13.0	5.0
3	0.300	0.349	0.275	0.375	11.0	8.0	15.0	9.0
3.5	0.350	0.399	0.325	0.450	15.0	9.0	22.0	13.0
4	0.400	0.499	0.375	0.550	18.0	11.0	27.0	15.0
5	0.500	0.599	0.450	0.650	26.0	15.0	35.0	22.0
6	0.600	0.699	0.550	0.750	37.0	18.0	50.0	27.0
7	0.700	0.799	0.650	0.850	50.0	26.0	62.0	35.0
8	0.800	0.899	0.750	0.950	65.0	37.0	73.0	50.0

Minimum breaking load

Unless otherwise prescribed, determine the minimum breaking load by the following method using the strand in the condition in which it is presented. The minimum breaking load is determined over a simple knot formed by placing one end of a strand held in the right hand over the other end held in the left hand, passing one end over the strand and through the loop so formed (see Figure 0605.-1) and pulling the knot tight.

Make not fewer than one measurement per 2 m of length at points evenly spaced along the strand. Determine the breaking load using a suitable tensilometer. The apparatus has two clamps for holding the strand, one of which is mobile and is driven at a constant rate of 30 cm per minute. The clamps are designed so that the strand being tested can be attached with-out any possibility of slipping. At the beginning of the test the length of strand between the clamps is 12.5 cm to 20 cm and the knot is midway between the clamps. Set the mobile clamp in motion and note the force required to break the strand. If the strand breaks in a clamp or within 1 cm of it, the result is discarded and the test repeated on another part of the strand. The average of all the results, excluding those legitimately discarded, is equal to or greater than the value in column C and no value is less than that given in column D in Table 0605.-1 for the gauge number and type of material concerned.

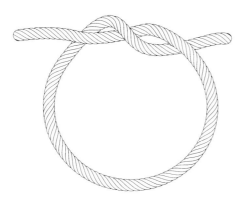

Figure 0605.-1. – *Simple knot*

Sterility (*2.6.1*)
They comply with the test for sterility as applied to catgut and other surgical sutures. Carry out the test on three sections each 30 cm long, cut off respectively from the beginning, the centre and the end of the strand.

Extractable colour
Strands that are dyed and intended to remain so during use comply with the test for extractable colour. Place 0.25 g of the strand to be examined in a conical flask, add 25.0 ml of *water R* and cover the mouth of the flask with a short-stemmed funnel. Boil for 15 min, cool and adjust to the original volume with *water R*. Depending on the colour of the strand, prepare the appropriate reference solution as described in Table 0605.-2 using the primary colour solutions (*2.2.2*).

Table 0605.-2. – *Colour reference solutions*

Colour of strand	Composition of reference solution (parts by volume)			
	Red primary solution	Yellow primary solution	Blue primary solution	Water
Yellow - brown	0.2	1.2	–	8.6
Pink - red	1.0	–	–	9.0
Green - blue	–	–	2.0	8.0
Violet	1.6	–	8.4	–

The test solution is not more intensely coloured than the appropriate reference solution.

STORAGE
Store protected from light and heat.

LABELLING
The label states:
— the gauge number,
— the length in centimetres or in metres,
— where appropriate, that the strand is coloured and intended to remain so during use.

Ph Eur

Sterile Linen Thread in Distributor

(*Linen Thread, Sterile, in Distributor for Veterinary Use, Ph Eur monograph 0608*)

Ph Eur

DEFINITION
Sterile linen thread in distributor for veterinary use consists of the pericyclic fibres of the stem of *Linum usitatissimum* L. The elementary fibres, 2.5 cm to 5 cm long, are assembled in bundles 30 cm to 80 cm long and spun into continuous lengths of suitable diameter. The thread may be creamy-white or may be coloured with colouring matter authorised by the competent authority. The thread is sterilised.

IDENTIFICATION
A. Dissect the end of a thread, using a needle or fine tweezers, to isolate a few individual fibres. Examined under a microscope, the fibres are seen to be 12 µm to 31 µm wide and, along the greater part of their length, have thick walls, sometimes marked with fine longitudinal striations, and a narrow lumen. The fibres gradually narrow to a long, fine point. Sometimes there are unilateral swellings with transverse lines.

B. Impregnate isolated fibres with *iodinated zinc chloride solution R*. The fibres are coloured violet-blue.

TESTS
It complies with the tests prescribed in the monograph on *Strands, sterile non-absorbable, in distributor for veterinary use (0605)*.

If stored in a dry state, expose to an atmosphere with a relative humidity of 65 ± 5 per cent at 20 ± 2 °C for 4 h immediately before measuring the diameter and for the determination of minimum breaking load immerse in water R at room temperature for 30 min immediately before carrying out the test.

STORAGE
See the monograph on *Strands, sterile non-absorbable, in distributor for veterinary use (0605)*.

LABELLING
See the monograph on *Strands, sterile non-absorbable, in distributor for veterinary use (0605)*.

Ph Eur

Sterile Poly(ethylene terephthalate) Suture in Distributor

(Poly(ethylene terephthalate) Suture, Sterile, in Distributor for Veterinary Use, Ph Eur monograph 0607)

Ph Eur _____

DEFINITION
Sterile poly(ethylene terephthalate) suture in distributor for veterinary use is obtained by drawing poly(ethylene terephthalate) through a suitable die. The suture is prepared by braiding very fine filaments in suitable numbers, depending on the gauge required. It may be whitish in colour, or may be coloured with authorised colouring matter or pigments authorised by the competent authority. The suture is sterilised.

CHARACTERS
It is practically insoluble in most of the usual organic solvents, but is attacked by strong alkaline solutions. It is incompatible with phenols.

IDENTIFICATION
A. It dissolves with difficulty when heated in *dimethylformamide R* and in *dichlorobenzene R*.

B. To about 50 mg add 10 ml of *hydrochloric acid R1*. The material remains intact even after immersion for 6 h.

TESTS
It complies with the tests prescribed in the monograph on *Strands, sterile non-absorbable, in distributor for veterinary use (0605)*.

STORAGE
See the monograph on *Strands, sterile non-absorbable, in distributor for veterinary use (0605)*.

LABELLING
See the monograph on *Strands, sterile non-absorbable, in distributor for veterinary use (0605)*.

_____ *Ph Eur*

Sterile Polyamide 6 Suture in Distributor

(Polyamide 6 Suture, Sterile, in Distributor for Veterinary Use, Ph Eur monograph 0609)

NOTE The name Nylon 6 as a synonym for Polyamide 6 may be used freely in many countries, including Great Britain and Northern Ireland, but exclusive proprietary rights in this name are claimed in certain other countries.

Ph Eur _____

DEFINITION
Sterile polyamide 6 suture in distributor for veterinary use is obtained by drawing through a suitable die a synthetic plastic material formed by the polymerisation of ε-caprolactam. It consists of smooth, cylindrical monofilaments or braided filaments, or lightly twisted strands sheathed with the same material. It may be coloured with colouring matter authorised by the competent authority. The suture is sterilised.

CHARACTERS
It is practically insoluble in the usual organic solvents; it is not attacked by dilute alkaline solutions (for example a

100 g/l solution of sodium hydroxide) but is attacked by dilute mineral acids (for example 20 g/l sulphuric acid), by hot glacial acetic acid and by 70 per cent *m/m* formic acid.

IDENTIFICATION
A. Heat about 50 mg with 0.5 ml of *hydrochloric acid R1* in a sealed glass tube at 110 °C for 18 h and allow to stand for 6 h. No crystals appear.

B. To about 50 mg add 10 ml of *hydrochloric acid R1*. The material disintegrates in the cold and dissolves completely within a few minutes.

C. It dissolves in a 70 per cent *m/m* solution of *anhydrous formic acid R*.

TESTS
It complies with the tests prescribed in the monograph on *Strands, sterile non-absorbable, in distributor for veterinary use (0605)* and with the following test:

Monomer and oligomers
In a continuous-extraction apparatus, treat 1.00 g with 30 ml of *methanol R* at a rate of at least three extractions per hour for 7 h. Evaporate the extract to dryness, dry the residue at 110 °C for 10 min, allow to cool in a desiccator and weigh. The residue weighs not more than 20 mg (2 per cent).

STORAGE
See the monograph on *Strands, sterile non-absorbable, in distributor for veterinary use (0605)*.

LABELLING
See the monograph on *Strands, sterile non-absorbable, in distributor for veterinary use (0605)*.

The label states whether the suture is braided, monofilament or sheathed.

_____ *Ph Eur*

Sterile Polyamide 6/6 Suture in Distributor

(Polyamide 6/6 Suture, Sterile, in Distributor for Veterinary Use, Ph Eur monograph 0610)

NOTE The name Nylon 6/6 as a synonym for Polyamide 6/6 may be used freely in many countries including Great Britain and Northern Ireland, but exclusive proprietary rights in this name are claimed in certain other countries.

Ph Eur _____

DEFINITION
Sterile polyamide 6/6 suture in distributor for veterinary use is obtained by drawing through a suitable die a synthetic plastic material formed by the polycondensation of hexamethylene-diamine and adipic acid. It consists of smooth, cylindrical monofilaments or braided filaments, or lightly twisted strands sheathed with the same material. It may be coloured with authorised colouring matter or pigments authorised by the competent authority. The suture is sterilised.

CHARACTERS
It is practically insoluble in the usual organic solvents; it is not attacked by dilute alkaline solutions (for example a 100 g/l solution of sodium hydroxide) but is attacked by dilute mineral acids (for example 20 g/l sulphuric acid), by hot glacial acetic acid and by 80 per cent *m/m* formic acid.

IDENTIFICATION

A. In contact with a flame it melts and burns, forming a hard globule of residue and gives off a characteristic odour resembling that of celery.

B. Place about 50 mg in an ignition tube held vertically and heat gently until thick fumes are evolved. When the fumes fill the tube, withdraw it from the flame and insert a strip of *nitrobenzaldehyde paper R*. A violet-brown colour slowly appears on the paper and fades slowly in air; it disappears immediately on washing with *dilute sulphuric acid R*.

C. To about 50 mg add 10 ml of *hydrochloric acid R1*. The material disintegrates in the cold and dissolves within a few minutes.

D. It does not dissolve in a 70 per cent *m/m* solution of *anhydrous formic acid R* but dissolves in an 80 per cent *m/m* solution of *anhydrous formic acid R*.

TESTS

It complies with the tests prescribed in the monograph on *Strands, sterile non-absorbable, in distributor for veterinary use (0605)*.

STORAGE

See the monograph on *Strands, sterile non-absorbable, in distributor for veterinary use (0605)*.

LABELLING

See the monograph on *Strands, sterile non-absorbable, in distributor for veterinary use (0605)*.

The label states whether the suture is braided, monofilament or sheathed.

Ph Eur

LABELLING

See the monograph on *Strands, sterile non-absorbable, in distributor for veterinary use (0605)*.

Ph Eur

Sterile Braided Silk Suture in Distributor

(Silk Suture, Sterile, Braided, in Distributor for Veterinary Use, Ph Eur monograph 0606)

Ph Eur

DEFINITION

Sterile braided silk suture in distributor for veterinary use is obtained by braiding a variable number of threads, according to the diameter required, of degummed silk obtained from the cocoons of the silkworm *Bombyx mori* L. It may be coloured with colouring matter authorised by the competent authority. The suture is sterilised.

IDENTIFICATION

A. Dissect the end of a strand, using a needle or fine tweezers, to isolate a few individual fibres. The fibres are sometimes marked with very fine longitudinal striations parallel to the axis of the strand. Examined under a microscope, a cross-section is more or less triangular or semi-circular, with rounded edges and without a lumen.

B. Impregnate isolated fibres with *iodinated potassium iodide solution R*. The fibres are coloured pale yellow.

TESTS

It complies with the tests prescribed in the monograph on *Strands, sterile non-absorbable, in distributor for veterinary use (0605)*.

STORAGE

See the monograph on *Strands, sterile non-absorbable, in distributor for veterinary use (0605)*.

Infrared Reference Spectra

Preparation of Infrared Reference Spectra

All spectra presented in this section were recorded using either a Perkin-Elmer model 682 dispersive infrared spectrophotometer or a Perkin Elmer model 16PC Fourier transform infrared spectrophotometer.

Pressed discs, 13 mm in diameter, were prepared using potassium bromide or potassium chloride. Liquid paraffin mulls and thin films were prepared between potassium bromide plates, and gas and solution spectra were prepared using cells with potassium bromide windows. Solution spectra were prepared against a solvent reference and all other spectra were recorded against air.

For solution spectra the regions of the spectrum within which the solvent shows strong absorption should be disregarded. Solvent 'cut-offs' in the reference spectra may be recorded as horizontal straight lines or may appear as blank regions on the spectrum.

Polystyrene

Instrument: Dispersive

Phase: Thin Film Thickness: 0.038mm

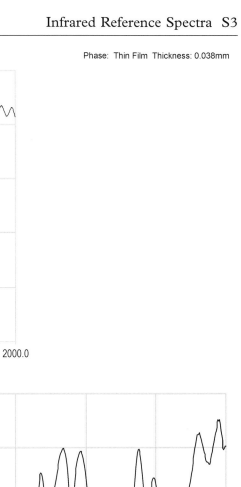

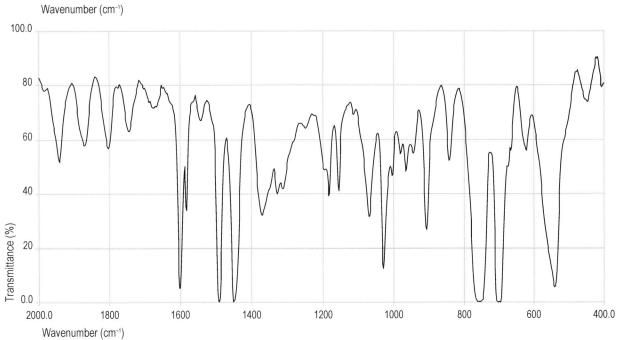

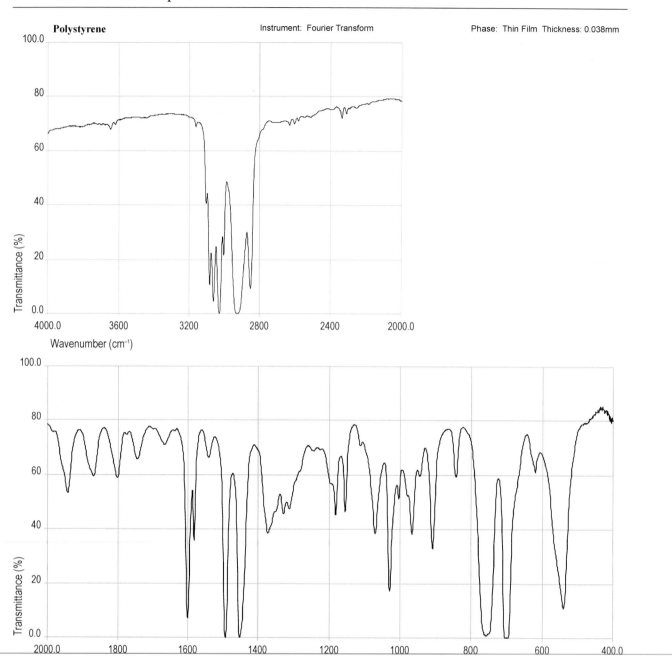

Polystyrene   Instrument: Fourier Transform   Phase: Thin Film Thickness: 0.038mm

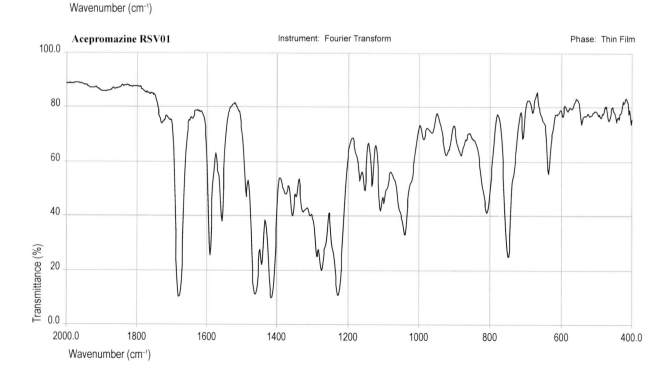

Acepromazine RSV01   Instrument: Fourier Transform   Phase: Thin Film

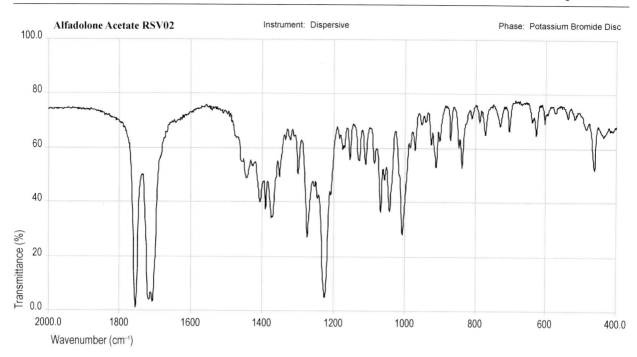

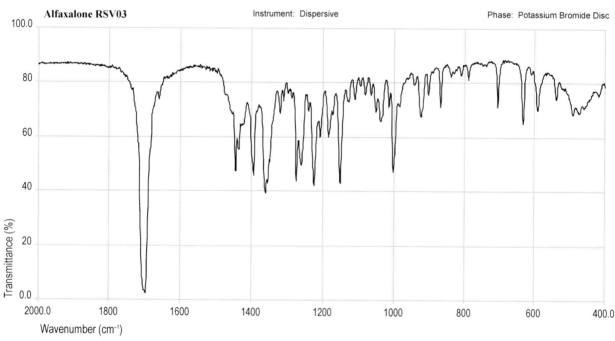

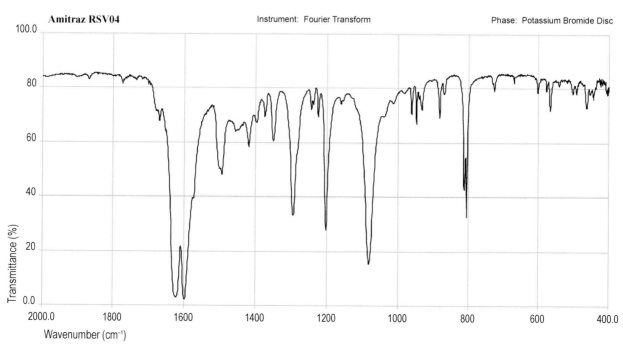

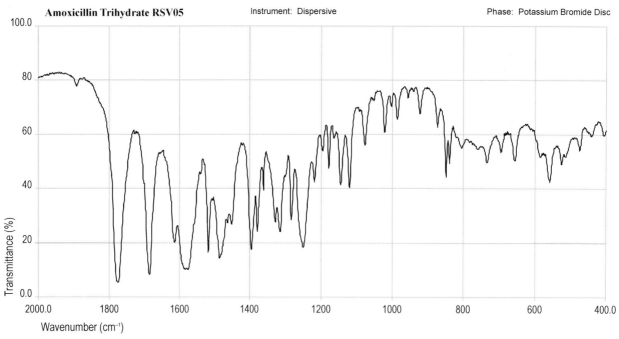

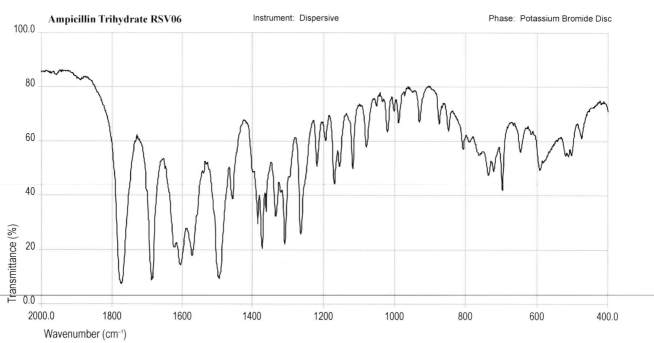

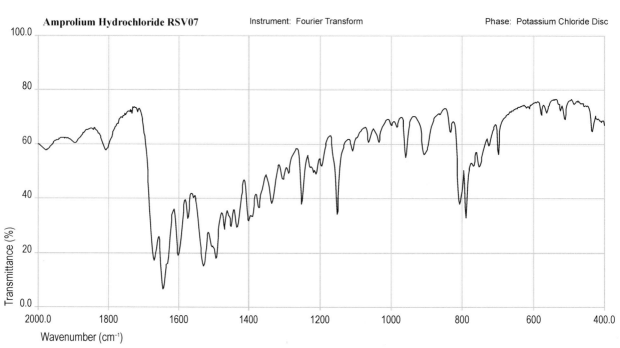

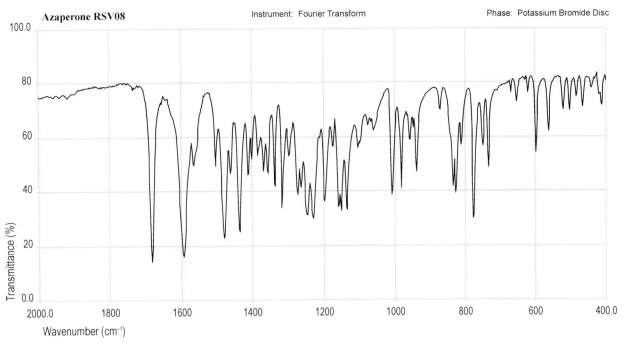

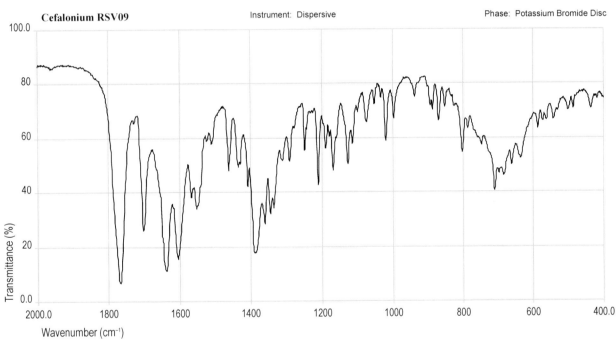

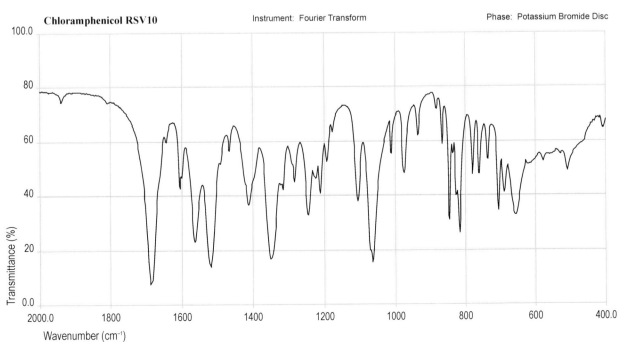

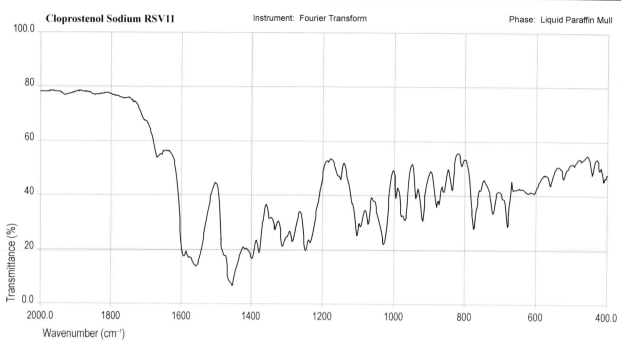

Cloprostenol Sodium RSV11 Instrument: Fourier Transform Phase: Liquid Paraffin Mull

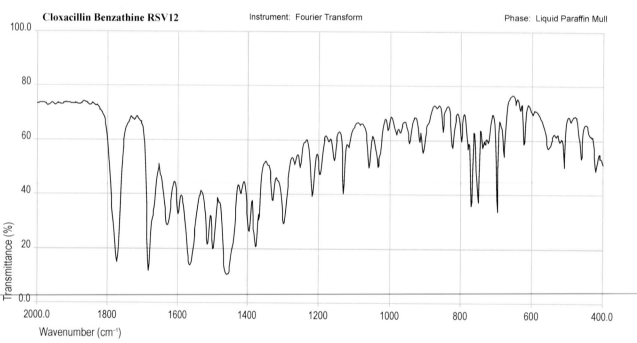

Cloxacillin Benzathine RSV12 Instrument: Fourier Transform Phase: Liquid Paraffin Mull

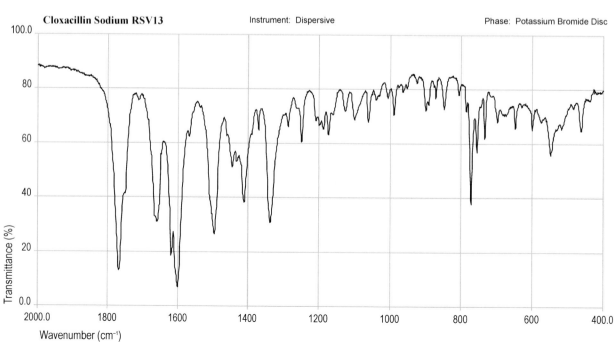

Cloxacillin Sodium RSV13 Instrument: Dispersive Phase: Potassium Bromide Disc

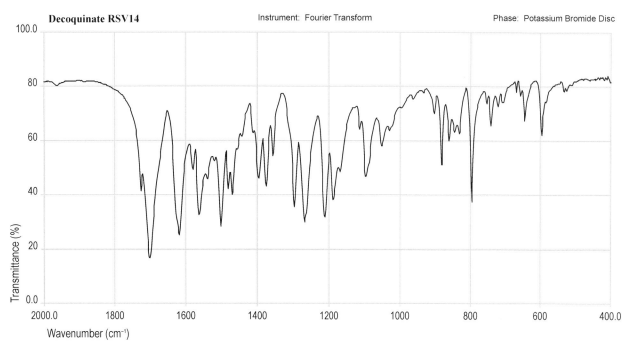

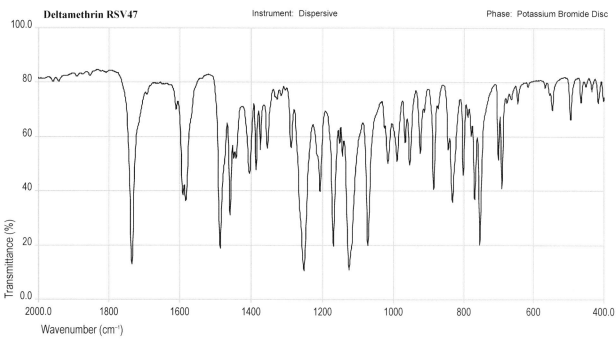

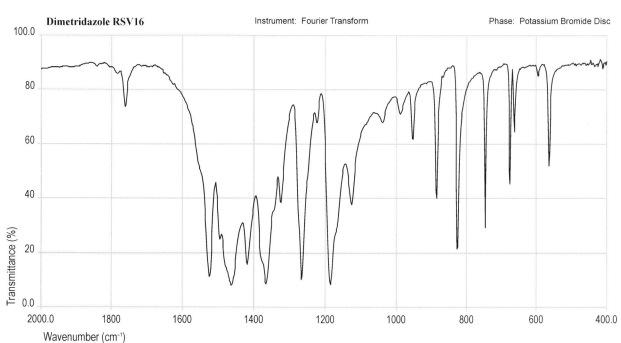

Dimpylate RSV49   Instrument: Fourier Transform   Phase: Thin Film

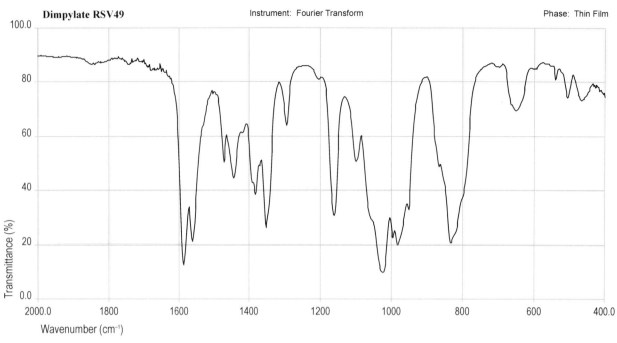

Dinitolmide RSV17   Instrument: Fourier Transform   Phase: Potassium Bromide Disc

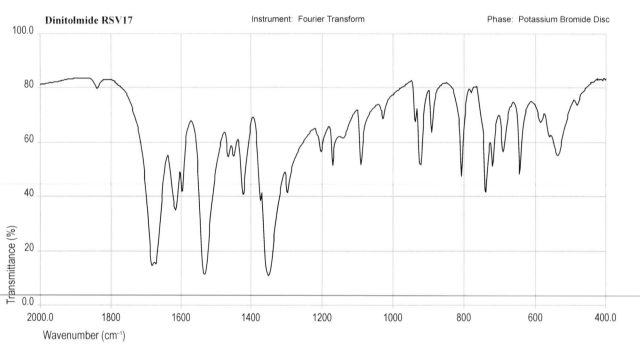

Diprenorphine Hydrochloride RSV18   Instrument: Fourier Transform   Phase: Potassium Chloride Disc

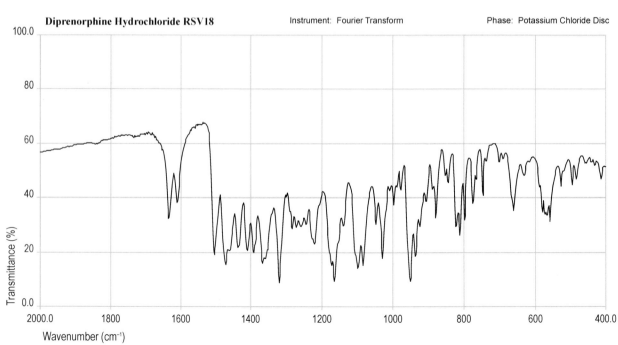

Etamiphylline RSV19 Instrument: Dispersive Phase: Liquid Paraffin Mull

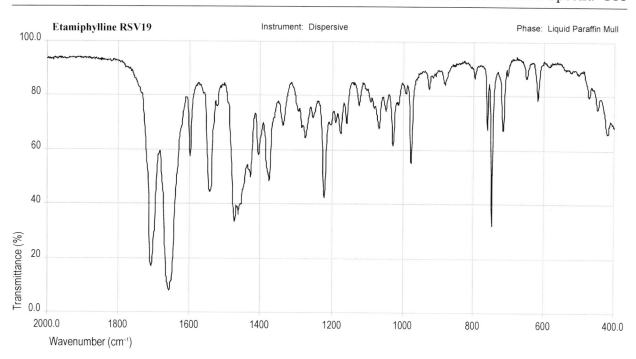

Etamiphylline Camsilate RSV51 Instrument: Dispersive Phase: Liquid Paraffin Mull

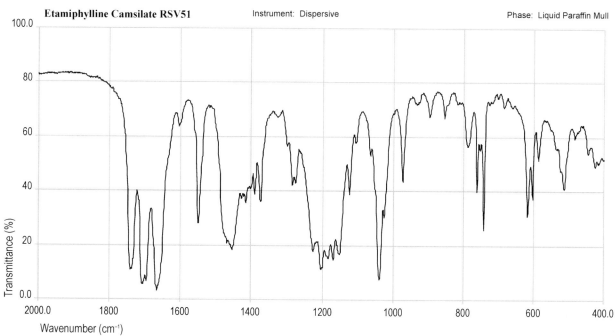

Ethopabate RSV20 Instrument: Fourier Transform Phase: Potassium Bromide Disc

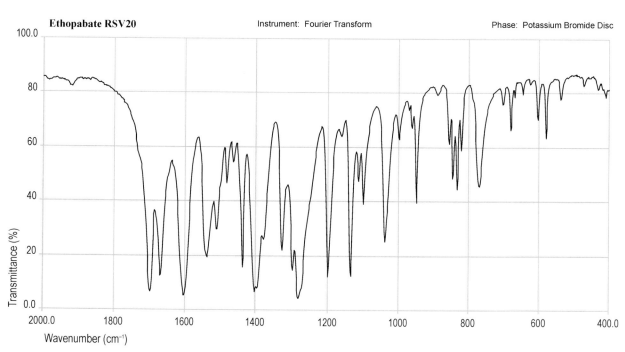

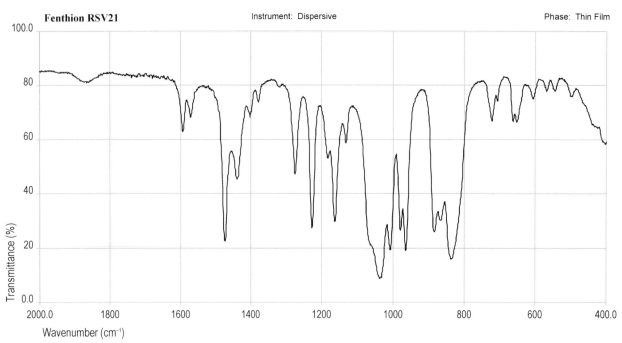

Fenthion RSV21 Instrument: Dispersive Phase: Thin Film

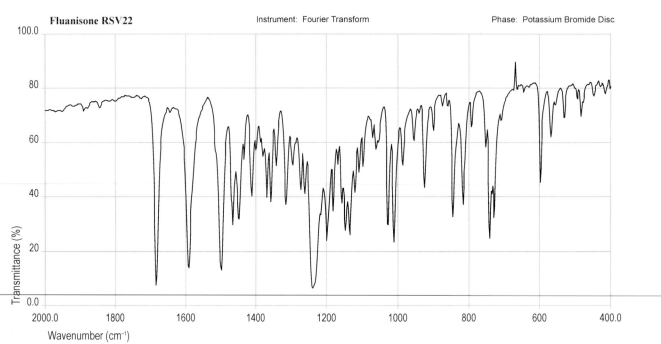

Fluanisone RSV22 Instrument: Fourier Transform Phase: Potassium Bromide Disc

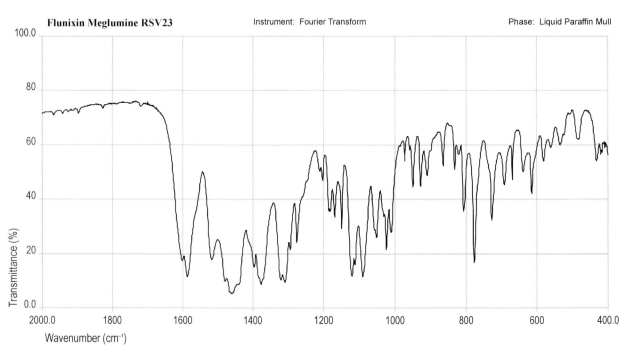

Flunixin Meglumine RSV23 Instrument: Fourier Transform Phase: Liquid Paraffin Mull

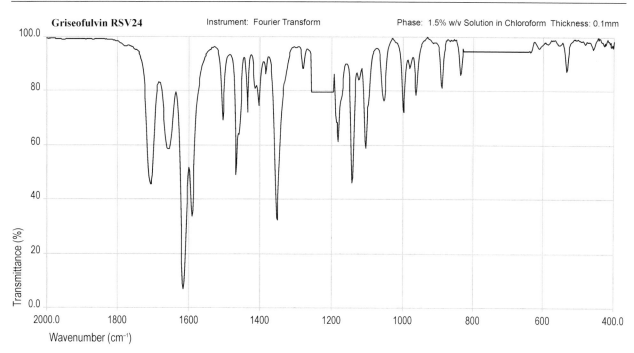

Griseofulvin RSV24   Instrument: Fourier Transform   Phase: 1.5% w/v Solution in Chloroform Thickness: 0.1mm

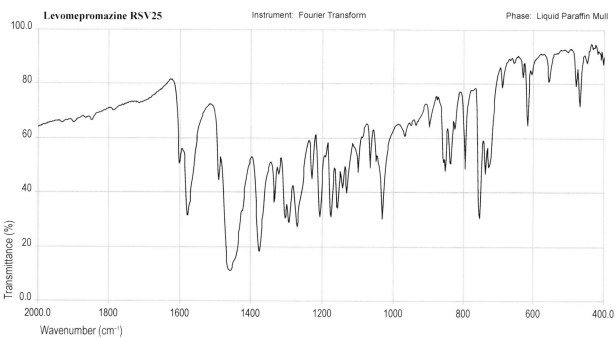

Levomepromazine RSV25   Instrument: Fourier Transform   Phase: Liquid Paraffin Mull

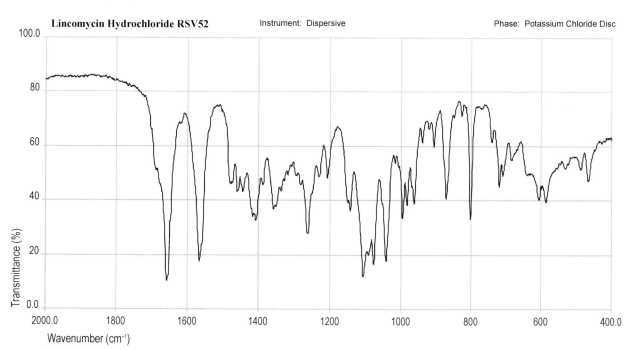

Lincomycin Hydrochloride RSV52   Instrument: Dispersive   Phase: Potassium Chloride Disc

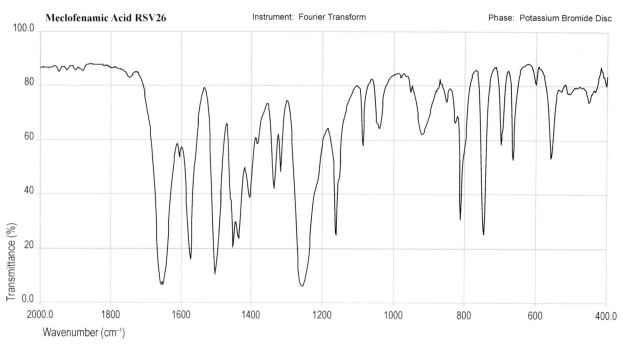

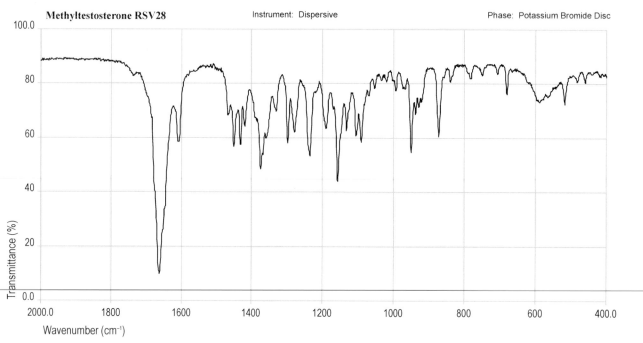

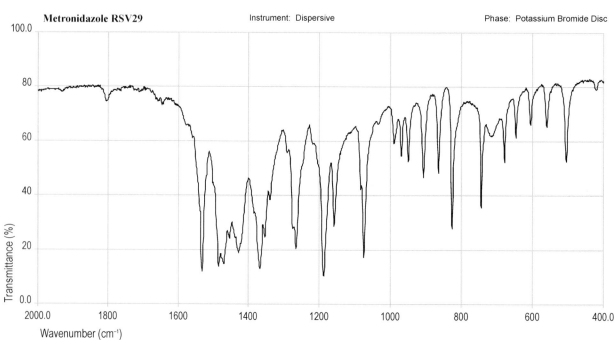

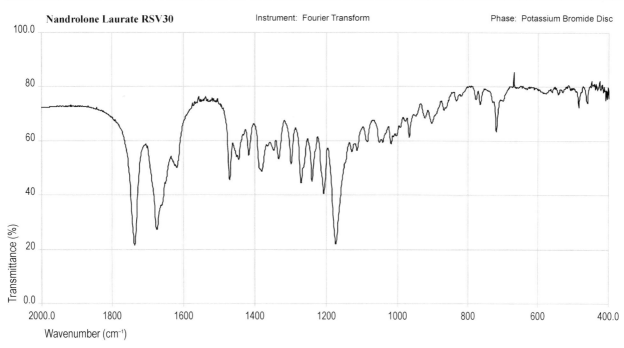

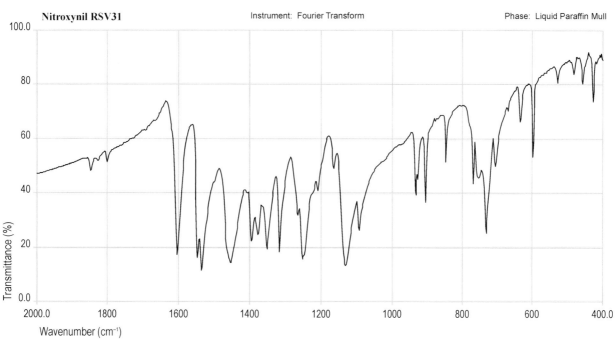

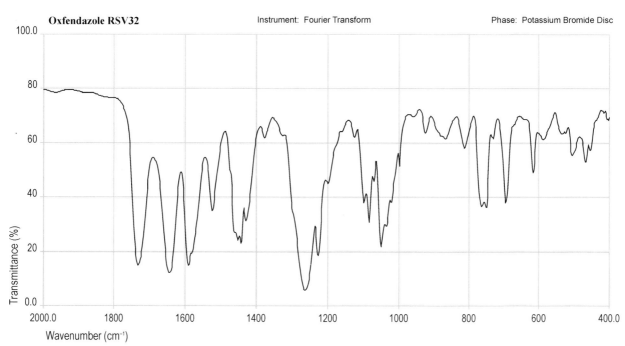

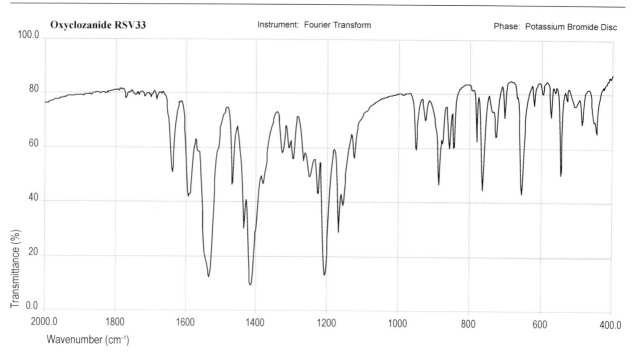

Oxyclozanide RSV33   Instrument: Fourier Transform   Phase: Potassium Bromide Disc

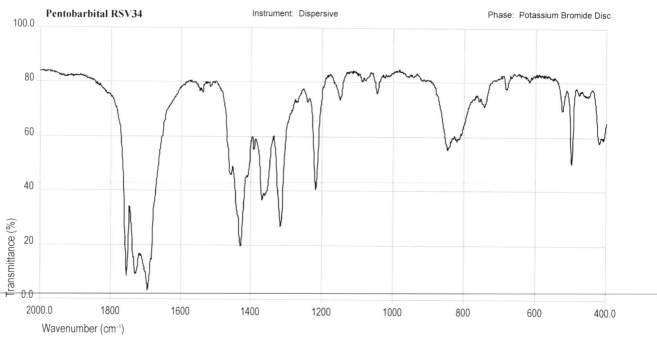

Pentobarbital RSV34   Instrument: Dispersive   Phase: Potassium Bromide Disc

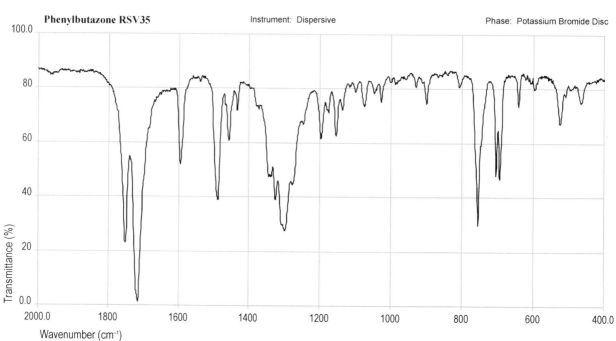

Phenylbutazone RSV35   Instrument: Dispersive   Phase: Potassium Bromide Disc

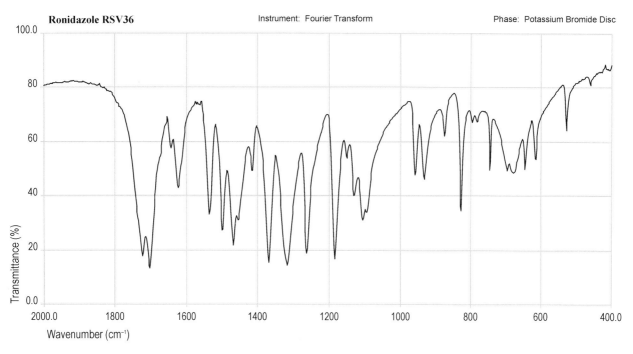

Ronidazole RSV36 Instrument: Fourier Transform Phase: Potassium Bromide Disc

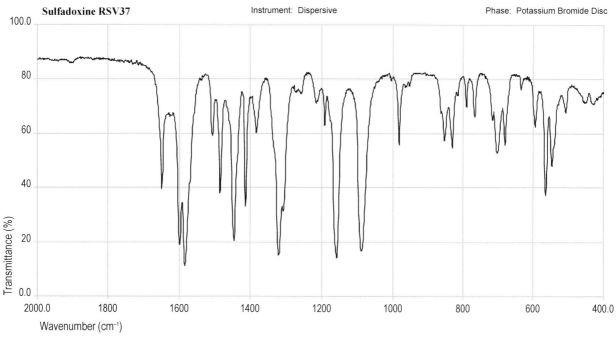

Sulfadoxine RSV37 Instrument: Dispersive Phase: Potassium Bromide Disc

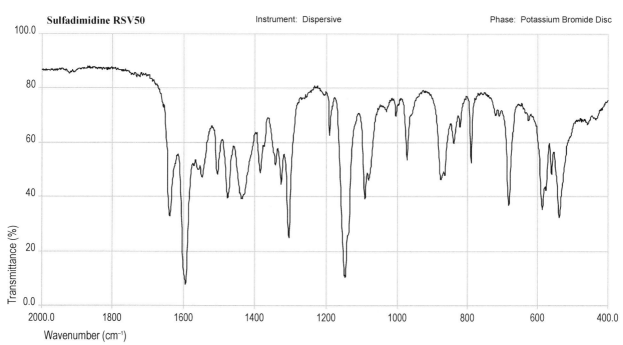

Sulfadimidine RSV50 Instrument: Dispersive Phase: Potassium Bromide Disc

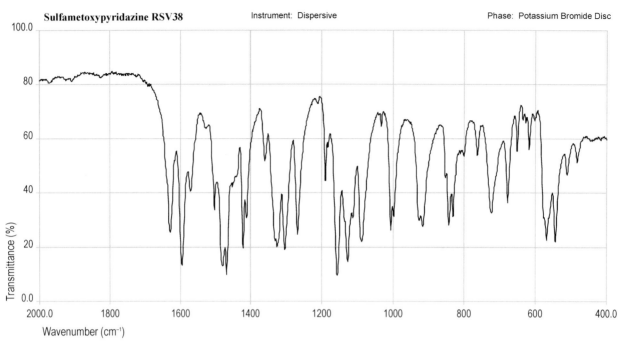

Sulfametoxypyridazine RSV38　　　Instrument: Dispersive　　　Phase: Potassium Bromide Disc

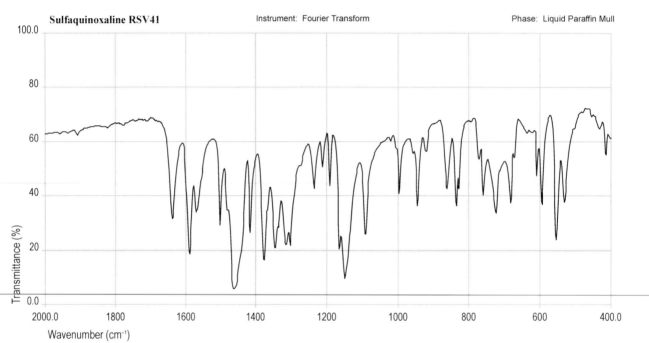

Sulfaquinoxaline RSV41　　　Instrument: Fourier Transform　　　Phase: Liquid Paraffin Mull

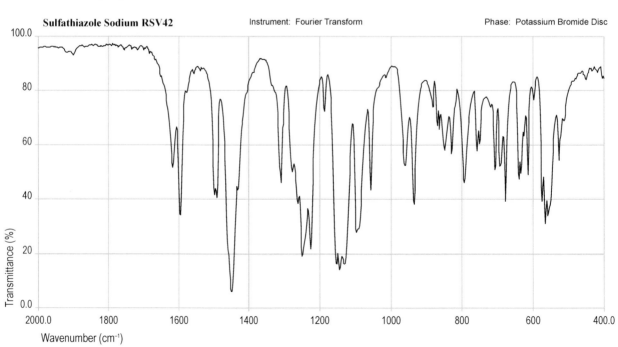

Sulfathiazole Sodium RSV42　　　Instrument: Fourier Transform　　　Phase: Potassium Bromide Disc

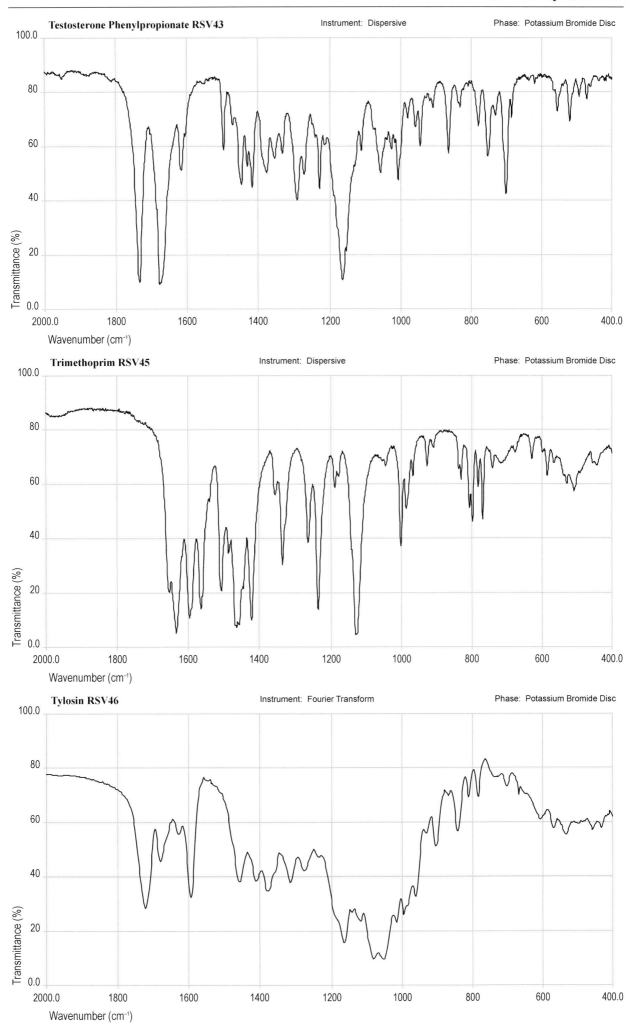

Appendices

When a method, test or other matter described in an appendix is invoked in a monograph reproduced from the European Pharmacopoeia, Part III of the general notices applies. When a method, test or other matter described in an appendix is invoked in any other monograph, Part II of general notices applies.

Any reference to an appendix that is not contained within this edition of the British Pharmacopoeia (Veterinary) is to be construed as a reference to the said appendix contained within the *British Pharmacopoeia 2004* modified as necessary by amendments.

The following appendices are included in this section of the British Pharmacopoeia (Veterinary).

European Pharmacopoeia Equivalent Texts

In monographs reproduced from the European Pharmacopoeia the analytical methods, tests and other supporting texts are invoked by means of the reference number of the text in the general Chapters of the European Pharmacopoeia. The table below lists the contents of the General Chapters of the European Pharmacopoeia and gives the British Pharmacopoeia or British Pharmacopoeia (Veterinary) equivalents. It is provided for information but it is emphasised that for texts of the European Pharmacopoeia, in cases of doubt or dispute the text published by the Council of Europe is authoritative. Appendices of the British Pharmacopoeia (Veterinary) are identified by inclusion of '(Vet)' after the Appendix letter, for example, Appendix XV J(Vet) 1.

Ph. Eur.	Subject of text	British Pharmacopoeia reference
1	General Notices	†
2.1.1	Droppers	Appendix I A
2.1.2	Sintered-glass filters	Appendix XVII B2
2.1.3	UV lamps	Appendix III A
2.1.4	Sieves	Appendix XVII B1
2.1.5	Tubes for comparative tests	Appendix VII
2.1.6	Gas detector tubes	Appendix IX K
2.2.1	Clarity and degree of opalescence of liquids	Appendix IV A
2.2.2	Degree of coloration of liquids	Appendix IV B
2.2.3	Potentiometric determination of pH	Appendix V L
2.2.4	Reaction of solution, pH and indicator colour	Appendix V K
2.2.5	Relative density	Appendix V G
2.2.6	Refractive index	Appendix V E
2.2.7	Optical rotation	Appendix V F
2.2.8	Viscosity	Appendix V H
2.2.9	Capillary viscometer method	Appendix V H, Method II
2.2.10	Rotating viscometer method	Appendix V H, Method III
2.2.11	Distillation range	Appendix V C
2.2.12	Boiling point	Appendix V D
2.2.13	Water by distillation range	Appendix IX C, Method II
2.2.14	Melting point: Capillary method	Appendix V A, Method I
2.2.15	Melting point: Open capillary method	Appendix V A, Method IV
2.2.16	Melting point: Instantaneous method	Appendix V A, Method V
2.2.17	Drop point	Appendix V A, Method III
2.2.18	Freezing point	Appendix V B
2.2.19	Amperometric titrations	Appendix VIII B
2.2.20	Potentiometric titrations	Appendix VIII B
2.2.21	Fluorimetry	Appendix II E
2.2.22	Atomic emission spectrometry	Appendix II D
2.2.23	Atomic absorption spectrometry	Appendix II D
2.2.24	Infrared spectrophotometry	Appendix II A
2.2.25	Visible and ultraviolet spectrophotometry	Appendix II B
2.2.26	Paper chromatography	Appendix III E
2.2.27	Thin-layer chromatography	Appendix III A
2.2.28	Gas chromatography	Appendix III B
2.2.29	Liquid chromatography	Appendix III D
2.2.30	Size-exclusion chromatography	Appendix III C
2.2.31	Electrophoresis	Appendix III F
2.2.32	Loss on drying	Appendix IX D
2.2.33	Nuclear magnetic resonance spectrometry	Appendix II C
2.2.34	Thermogravimetry	Appendix V M
2.2.35	Osmolality	Appendix V N
2.2.36	Ion-selective potentiometry	Appendix VIII E
2.2.37	X-ray fluorescent spectrophotometry	Appendix II F
2.2.38	Conductivity	Appendix V O
2.2.39	Molecular mass distribution in dextrans	Appendix III C
2.2.40	Near infrared spectrometry	Appendix II A

† *Reproduced in full as Part III of the General Notices of the British Pharmacopoeia and British Pharmacopoeia (Veterinary).*

2.2.41	Circular dichroism	Appendix V J
2.2.42	Density of solids	Appendix V Q
2.2.43	Mass spectrometry	Appendix II G
2.2.44	Total organic carbon in water	Appendix V P
2.2.45	Supercritical fluid chromatography	Appendix III H
2.2.46	Chromatographic separation techniques	Appendix III
2.2.47	Capillary electrophoresis	Appendix III G
2.2.48	Raman spectroscopy	Appendix II H
2.2.49	Falling ball viscometer method	Appendix V H, Method IV
2.2.54	Isoelectric focussing	Appendix III J
2.2.55	Peptide mapping	Appendix III K
2.2.56	Amino acid analysis	Appendix III L
2.3.1	Identification reactions	Appendix VI
2.3.2	Identification of fatty oils by TLC	Appendix X N
2.3.3	Identification of phenothiazines by TLC	Appendix III A
2.3.4	Odour	Appendix VI
	Limit test for:	
2.4.1	– ammonium	Appendix VII
2.4.2	– arsenic	Appendix VII
2.4.3	– calcium	Appendix VII
2.4.4	– chloride	Appendix VII
2.4.5	– fluorides	Appendix VII
2.4.6	– magnesium	Appendix VII
2.4.7	– magnesium and alkaline-earth metals	Appendix VII
2.4.8	– heavy metals	Appendix VII
2.4.9	– iron	Appendix VII
2.4.10	– lead in sugars	Appendix VII
2.4.11	– phosphates	Appendix VII
2.4.12	– potassium	Appendix VII
2.4.13	– sulphate	Appendix VII
2.4.14	Sulphated ash	Appendix IX A, Method II
2.4.15	Limit test for nickel in polyols	Appendix VII
2.4.16	Total ash	Appendix XI J, Method II
2.4.17	Limit test for aluminium	Appendix VII
2.4.18	Free formaldehyde	Appendix XV D
2.4.19	Alkaline impurities in fatty oils	Appendix X N
2.4.20	Antioxidants in fatty oils	*Suppressed 1/1/99*
2.4.21	Foreign oils in fatty oils by TLC	Appendix X N
2.4.22	Composition of fatty acids by gas chromatography	Appendix X N
2.4.23	Sterols in fatty oils	Appendix X Q
2.4.24	Residual solvents	Appendix VIII L
2.4.25	Residual ethylene oxide and dioxan	Appendix VIII M
2.4.26	N,N-Dimethylaniline	Appendix VIII N
2.4.27	Heavy metals in herbal drugs and fatty oils	Appendix VII
2.4.28	2-Ethylhexanoic acid	Appendix VIII O
2.4.29	Composition of fatty acids in oils rich in omega-3-acids	Appendix X P
2.4.30	Ethylene glycol and diethylene glycol in ethoxylated substances	Appendix VIII K
2.5.1	Acid value	Appendix X B
2.5.2	Ester value	Appendix X C
2.5.3	Hydroxyl value	Appendix X D
2.5.4	Iodine value	Appendix X E
2.5.5	Peroxide value	Appendix X F
2.5.6	Saponification value	Appendix X G, Method II
2.5.7	Unsaponifiable matter	Appendix X H, Method II
2.5.8	Assay of primary aromatic amino nitrogen	Appendix VIII B
2.5.9	Semi-micro determination of nitrogen by sulphuric acid digestion	Appendix VIII H
2.5.10	Oxygen-flask method	Appendix VIII C
2.5.11	Complexometric titrations	Appendix VIII D
2.5.12	Semi-micro determination of water	Appendix IX C, Method I
2.5.13	Aluminium in adsorbed vaccines	Appendix XV B
2.5.14	Calcium in adsorbed vaccines	Appendix XV C
2.5.15	Phenol in immunosera and vaccines	Appendix XV E
	Polysaccharide vaccines:	
2.5.16	– protein	Appendix XV G
2.5.17	– nucleic acids	Appendix XV G
2.5.18	– phosphorus	Appendix XV G

2.5.19	– *O*-acetyl	Appendix XV G
2.5.20	– hexosamines	Appendix XV G
2.5.21	– methylpentoses	Appendix XV G
2.5.22	– uronic acids	Appendix XV G
2.5.23	– sialic acid	Appendix XV G
2.5.24	Carbon dioxide in medicinal gases	Appendix IX F
2.5.25	Carbon monoxide in medicinal gases	Appendix IX E
2.5.26	Nitrogen monoxide and nitrogen dioxide in medicinal gases	Appendix IX G
2.5.27	Oxygen in medicinal gases	Appendix IX H
2.5.28	Water in medicinal gases	Appendix IX J
2.5.29	Sulphur dioxide	Appendix IX B Method II
2.5.30	Oxidising substances	Appendix X L
2.5.31	Ribose in polysaccharide vaccines	Appendix XV G
2.5.32	Micro determination of water	Appendix IX C, Method III
2.5.33	Total protein assay	Appendix VIII P
2.5.34	Acetic acid in synthetic peptides	Appendix VIII Q
2.5.35	Nitrous oxide in gases	Appendix IX L
2.5.36	Anisidine value	Appendix X O
2.6.1	Sterility	Appendix XVI A
2.6.2	Mycobacteria	Appendix XVI B4
2.6.3	Extraneous viruses using fertilised eggs	now Appendix XVI B (Vet) 4 *and* Appendix XVI B (Vet) 5
2.6.4	Leucosis virus	now Appendix XVI B (Vet) 4 *and* Appendix XVI B (Vet) 5
2.6.5	Extraneous viruses using cell cultures	now Appendix XVI B (Vet) 4 *and* Appendix XVI B (Vet) 5
2.6.6	Extraneous agents using chicks	now Appendix XVI B (Vet) 4 *and* Appendix XVI B (Vet) 5
2.6.7	Mycoplasmas	Appendix XVI B3 *and* Appendix XVI B(Vet) 3
2.6.8	Pyrogens	Appendix XIV D
2.6.9	Abnormal toxicity	Appendix XIV E
2.6.10	Histamine	Appendix XIV G
2.6.11	Depressor substances	Appendix XIV F
2.6.12	Total viable aerobic count	Appendix XVI B2
2.6.13	Specified micro-organisms	Appendix XVI B1
2.6.14	Bacterial endotoxins	Appendix XIV C
2.6.15	Prekallikrein activator	Appendix XIV J8
2.6.16	Extraneous agents in viral vaccines	Appendix XVI B5
2.6.17	Anticomplementary activity of immunoglobulins	Appendix XIV J9
2.6.18	Neurovirulence of live viral vaccines	Appendix XV F1
2.6.19	Neurovirulence of poliomyelitis vaccine (oral)	Appendix XV F2
2.6.20	Anti-A and anti-B haemagglutinins (indirect method)	Appendix XIV J7
2.6.21	Nucleic acid amplification	Appendix XIV L
2.6.22	Activated coagulation factors	Appendix XIV J11
2.6.24	Avian viral vaccines: tests for extraneous agents in seed lots	Appendix XVI B (Vet) 4
2.6.25	Avian live virus vaccines: tests for extraneous agents in batches of finished Product	Appendix XVI B (Vet) 5
2.7.1	Immunochemical methods	Appendix XIV B
2.7.2	Microbiological assay of antibiotics	Appendix XIV A
2.7.4	Assay of coagulation factor VIII	Appendix XIV J2
2.7.5	Assay of heparin	Appendix XIV J5
2.7.6	Assay of diphtheria vaccine (adsorbed)	Appendix XIV K1
2.7.7	Assay of pertussis vaccine	Appendix XIV K2
2.7.8	Assay of tetanus vaccine (adsorbed)	Appendix XIV K3
2.7.9	Fc function of immunoglobulins	Appendix XIV J6
2.7.10	Assay of coagulation factor VII	Appendix XIV J1
2.7.11	Assay of coagulation factor IX	Appendix XIV J3
2.7.12	Assay of heparin in coagulation factors	Appendix XIV J4
2.7.13	Assay of anti-D immunoglobulin	Appendix XIV J10
2.7.14	Assay of hepatitis A vaccine	Appendix XIV K4
2.7.15	Assay of hepatitis B (rDNA) vaccine	Appendix XIV K5
2.7.16	Assay of pertussis vaccine (acellular)	Appendix XIV K6
2.7.17	Assay of human antithrombin III	Appendix XIV J12

2.7.18	Assay of human coagulation factor II	Appendix XIV J13
2.7.19	Assay of human coagulation factor X	Appendix XIV J14
2.7.20	*In vivo* assay of poliomyelitis vaccine (inactivated)	Appendix XIV K7
2.7.22	Assay of human coagulation factor XI	Appendix XIV J15
2.8.1	Ash insoluble in hydrochloric acid	Appendix XI K, Method II
2.8.2	Foreign matter	Appendix XI D
2.8.3	Stomata and stomatal index	Appendix XI H
2.8.4	Swelling index	Appendix XI C
2.8.5	Water in essential oils	Appendix X M
2.8.6	Foreign esters	Appendix X M
2.8.7	Fatty oils and resinified volatile oils	Appendix X M
2.8.8	Odour and taste of volatile oils	Appendix X M
2.8.9	Residue on evaporation	Appendix X M
2.8.10	Solubility in ethanol (volatile oils)	Appendix X M
2.8.11	Determination of cineole	Appendix X J
2.8.12	Essential oil content of crude drugs	Appendix XI E
2.8.13	Pesticide residues	Appendix XI L
2.8.14	Determination of tannins in herbal drugs	Appendix XI M
2.8.15	Bitterness value	Appendix XI N
2.8.16	Dry residue of extracts	Appendix XI P
2.8.17	Loss on drying of extracts	Appendix XI Q
2.9.1	Disintegration: tablets and capsules	Appendix XII A
2.9.2	Disintegration: suppositories and pessaries	Appendix XII C
2.9.3	Dissolution: solid oral dosage forms	Appendix XII D
2.9.4	Dissolution: transdermal patches	Appendix XII E
2.9.5	Uniformity of mass	Appendix XII G
2.9.6	Uniformity of content	Appendix XII H
2.9.7	Friability of uncoated tablets	Appendix XVII G
2.9.8	Resistance to crushing of tablets	Appendix XVII H
2.9.9	Measurement of consistency by penetrometry	Appendix XVII F
2.9.10	Ethanol content and alcoholimetric tablets	Appendix VIII F, Method III
2.9.11	Methanol and 2-propanol	Appendix VIII G
2.9.12	Sieve test	Appendix XVII A1
2.9.13	Particle size by microscopy (limit test)	Appendix XVII A2
2.9.14	Specific surface area by gas permeability	Appendix XVII C
2.9.15	Apparent volume	Appendix XVII D
2.9.16	Flowability	Appendix XVII E
2.9.17	Extractable volume of parenteral preparations	Appendix XII J
2.9.18	Aerodynamic assessment of fine particles	Appendix XII F
2.9.19	Particulate contamination: sub-visible particles	Appendix XIII A
2.9.20	Particulate contamination: visible particles	Appendix XIII B
2.9.22	Softening time of lipophilic suppositories	Appendix XVII J
2.9.23	Pycnometric density of solids	Appendix XVII K
2.9.24	Resistance to rupture of suppositories and pessaries	Appendix XVII L
2.9.25	Drug release from medicated chewing gum	Appendix XII K
2.9.26	Specific surface area by gas adsorption	Appendix XVII M
2.9.27	Uniformity of mass of delivered doses from multidose containers	Appendix XII L
2.9.28	Test for deliverable mass or volume of liquid and semi-solid preparations	Appendix XII M
2.9.40	Uniformity of dosage units	Appendix XII N
3.1.1	Material used for containers for human blood and blood components	Appendix XX A
3.1.1.1	Materials based on PVC for blood and blood components	Appendix XX A1
3.1.1.2	Materials based on PVC for tubing used in sets for the transfusion of blood and blood components	Appendix XX A2
3.1.3	Polyolefines	Appendix XX B
3.1.4	Polyethylene - without additives	Appendix XX C1
3.1.5	Polyethylene - with additives	Appendix XX C2
3.1.6	Polypropylene	Appendix XX D
3.1.7	Poly(ethylene–vinyl acetate)	Appendix XX E
3.1.8	Silicone oil used as a lubricant	Appendix XX F1
3.1.9	Silicone elastomer for closures and tubing	Appendix XX F2
3.1.10	Materials based on non-plasticised PVC for containers for non-injectable, aqueous solutions	Appendix XX A3
3.1.11	Materials based on non-plasticised PVC for containers for dry dosage forms for oral administration	Appendix XX A4
3.1.12	*vacant*	

Appendix XV

A (Vet). Terminology used in monographs on vaccines and certain other products

(Ph. Eur. general text 5.2.1)
For some items, alternative terms commonly used in connection with vaccines for human use are shown in parentheses.

SEED-LOT SYSTEM

A seed-lot system is a system according to which successive batches of a product are derived from the same master seed lot. For routine production, a working seed lot may be prepared from the master seed lot. The origin and the passage history of the master seed lot and the working seed lot are recorded.

MASTER SEED LOT

A culture of a micro-organism distributed from a single bulk into containers and processed together in a single operation in such a manner as to ensure uniformity and stability and to prevent contamination. A master seed lot in liquid form is usually stored at or below –70°C. A freeze-dried master seed lot is stored at a temperature known to ensure stability.

WORKING SEED LOT

A culture of a micro-organism derived from the master seed lot and intended for use in production. Working seed lots are distributed into containers and stored as described above for master seed lots.

CELL-SEED SYSTEM (CELL-BANK SYSTEM)

A system whereby successive batches (final lots) of a product are manufactured by culture in cells derived from the same master cell seed (master cell bank). A number of containers from the master cell seed (master cell bank) are used to prepare a working cell seed (working cell bank). The cell-seed system (cell-bank system) is validated for the highest passage level achieved during routine production.

MASTER CELL SEED (MASTER CELL BANK)

A culture of cells distributed into containers in a single operation, processed together and stored in such a manner as to ensure uniformity and stability and to prevent contamination. A master cell seed (master cell bank) is usually stored at –70°C or lower.

WORKING CELL SEED (WORKING CELL BANK)

A culture of cells derived from the master cell seed (master cell bank) and intended for use in the preparation of production cell cultures. The working cell seed (working cell bank) is distributed into containers, processed and stored as described for the master cell seed (master cell bank).

PRIMARY CELL CULTURES

Cultures of cells obtained by trypsination of a suitable tissue or organ. The cells are essentially identical to those of the tissue of origin and are no more than five *in vitro* passages from the initial preparation from the animal tissue.

CELL LINES

Cultures of cells that have a high capacity for multiplication *in vitro*. In diploid cell lines, the cells have essentially the same characteristics as those of the tissue of origin. In continuous cell lines, the cells are able to multiply indefinitely in culture and may be obtained from healthy or tumoral tissue. Some continuous cell lines have oncogenic potential under certain conditions.

PRODUCTION CELL CULTURE

A culture of cells intended for use in production; it may be derived from one or more containers of the working cell seed (working cell bank) or it may be a primary cell culture.

CONTROL CELLS

A quantity of cells set aside, at the time of virus inoculation, as uninfected cell cultures. The uninfected cells are incubated under similar conditions to those used for the production cell cultures.

SINGLE HARVEST

Material derived on one or more occasions from a single production cell culture inoculated with the same working seed lot or a suspension derived from the working seed lot, incubated, and harvested in a single production run.

MONOVALENT POOLED HARVEST

Pooled material containing a single strain or type of micro-organism or antigen and derived from a number of eggs, cell culture containers etc. that are processed at the same time.

FINAL BULK VACCINE

Material that has undergone all the steps of production except for the final filling. It consists of one or more monovalent pooled harvests, from cultures of one or more species or types of micro-organism, after clarification, dilution or addition of any adjuvant or other auxiliary substance. It is treated to ensure its homogeneity and is used for filling the containers of one or more batches (final lots).

BATCH (FINAL LOT)

A collection of closed, final containers or other final dosage units that are expected to be homogeneous and equivalent with respect to risk of contamination during filling or preparation of the final product. The dosage units are filled, or otherwise prepared, from the same final bulk vaccine, freeze dried together (if applicable) and closed in one continuous working session. They bear a distinctive number or code identifying the batch (final lot). Where a final bulk vaccine is filled and/or freeze dried in several separate sessions, there results a related set of batches (final lots) that are usually identified by the use of a common part in the distinctive number or code; these related batches (final lots) are sometimes referred to as sub-batches, sub-lots or filling lots.

COMBINED VACCINE

A multicomponent preparation formulated so that different antigens are administered simultaneously. The different antigenic components are intended to protect against different strains or types of the same organism and/or different organisms. A combined vaccine may be supplied by the manufacturer either as a single liquid or freeze-dried preparation or as several constituents with directions for admixture before use.

H (Vet). Chicken flocks free from specified pathogens for the production and quality control of vaccines

(Ph. Eur. method 5.2.2)
Where specified, chickens, embryos or cell cultures used for the production or quality control of vaccines are derived from eggs produced by chicken flocks free from specified pathogens (SPF). The SPF status of a flock is ensured by means of the system described below. The list of micro-

organisms given is based on current knowledge and will be updated as necessary.

A flock is defined as a group of birds sharing a common environment and having their own caretakers who have no contact with non-SPF flocks. Once a flock is defined, no non-SPF birds are added to it.

Each flock is housed so as to minimise the risk of contamination. The facility in which the flock is housed must not be sited near to any non-SPF flocks of birds with the exception of flocks that are in the process of being established as SPF flocks and that are housed in facilities and conditions appropriate to SPF flocks. The SPF flock is housed within an isolator or in a building with filtered air under positive pressure. Appropriate measures are taken to prevent entry of rodents, wild birds, insects and unauthorised personnel.

Personnel authorised to enter the facility must have no contact with other birds or with agents potentially capable of infecting the flock. It is advisable for personnel to shower and change clothing or to wear protective clothing before entering the controlled facility.

Wherever possible, items taken into the facility are sterilised. In particular it is recommended that the feed is suitably treated to avoid introduction of undesirable micro-organisms and that water is at least of potable quality, for example from a chlorinated supply. No medication is administered to birds within the flock that might interfere with detection of any disease.

A permanent record is kept of the general health of the flock and any abnormality is investigated. Factors to be monitored include morbidity, mortality, general physical condition, feed consumption, daily egg production and egg quality, fertility and hatchability. Records are maintained for a period of at least 5 years. Details of any deviation from normal in these performance parameters or detection of any infection are notified to the users of the eggs as soon as practicable.

The tests or combination of tests described below must have suitable specificity and sensitivity with respect to relevant serotypes of the viruses. Samples for testing are taken at random.

A positive result for chicken anaemia virus (CAV) does not necessarily exclude use of material derived from the flock, but live vaccines for use in birds less than 7 days old shall be produced using material from CAV-negative flocks. Inactivated vaccines for use in birds less than 7 days old may be produced using material from flocks that have not been shown to be free from CAV, provided it has been demonstrated that the inactivation process inactivates CAV.

Establishment of an SPF flock

A designated SPF flock is derived from chickens shown to be free from vertically-transmissible agents listed in Table 5.2.2-1. This is achieved by testing of 2 generations prior to the designated SPF flock. A general scheme for the procedure to be followed in establishing and maintaining an SPF flock is shown diagrammatically in Table 5.2.2.-2.

In order to establish a new SPF flock, a series of tests must be conducted on 3 generations of birds. All birds in the first generation must be tested at least once before the age of 20 weeks for freedom from avian leucosis group-antigen and tested by an enzyme immunoassay (EIA) for freedom of antibodies to avian leucosis virus subtypes A, B and J. All birds must also be tested for freedom from antibodies to the vertically-transmissible agents listed in Table 5.2.2-1. From the age of 8 weeks the flock is tested for freedom from

Salmonella. Clinical examination is carried out on the flock from 8 weeks of age and the birds must not exhibit any signs of infectious disease. The test methods to be used for these tests are given in the table and further guidance is also given in the section below on routine testing of designated SPF flocks. From 20 weeks of age, the flock is tested as described under Routine testing of designated SPF flocks. All stages of this testing regime are also applied to the subsequent 2 generations, except the testing of every bird before lay for vertically-transmissible agents. All test results must indicate freedom from pathogens in all 3 generations for the flock consisting of the third generation to be designated as SPF.

SPF embryos derived from another designated SPF flock contained within a separate facility on the same site may be introduced. From 8 weeks of age, these replacement birds are regarded as a flock and are tested in accordance with test procedures described above.

Initial testing requirements for subsequent generations derived from a designated SPF flock

Where a replacement flock is derived exclusively from a fully established SPF flock the new generation is tested prior to being designated as SPF. In addition to the tests for *Salmonella* and monitoring of the general health and performance of the flock, further specific testing from the age of 8 weeks is required. Tests are performed on two 5 per cent samples of the flock (minimum 10, maximum 200 birds) taken with an interval of at least 4 weeks between the ages of 12-16 weeks and 16-20 weeks.

All samples are collected and tested individually. Blood samples for antibody tests and suitable samples for testing for leucosis antigen are collected. The test methods to be used are as described under Routine testing of designated SPF flocks. Only when all tests have confirmed the absence of infection may the new generation be designated as SPF.

Routine testing of designated SPF flocks

General examination and necropsy

Clinical examination is carried out at least once per week throughout the life of the flock in order to verify that the birds are free from fowl-pox virus and signs of any other infection. In the event of mortality exceeding 0.1 per cent per week, necropsy is performed on all available carcasses to verify that there is no sign of infection. Where appropriate, histopathological and/or microbiological/virological studies are performed to confirm diagnosis. Specific examination for tuberculosis lesions is carried out and histological samples from any suspected lesions are specifically stained to verify freedom from *Mycobacterium avium*. Caecal contents of all available carcasses are examined microbiologically for the presence of *Salmonella spp.* using the techniques described below. Where appropriate, caecal samples from up to 5 birds may be pooled.

Cultural testing for Salmonella spp

Cultural testing for *Salmonella* spp. is performed either by testing samples of droppings or cloacal swabs or by testing of drag swabs. Where droppings or cloacal swabs are tested, a total of 60 samples within each 4-week period is tested throughout the entire life of the flock. Tests may be performed on pools of up to 10 samples. Where drag swabs are tested, a minimum of 2 drag swabs are tested during each 4-week period throughout the entire life of the flock. Detection of *Salmonella spp.* in these samples is performed by pre-enrichment of the samples followed by culture using *Salmonella*-selective media.

Table 5.2.2.-1

Agent	Test to be used**	Vertical transmission	Rapid/slow spread
Avian adenoviruses, group 1	AGP, EIA	yes	slow
Avian encephalomyelitis virus	AGP, EIA	yes	rapid
Avian infectious bronchitis virus	HI, EIA	no	rapid
Avian infectious laryngotracheitis virus	VN, EIA	no	slow
Avian leucosis viruses	EIA for virus, VN for antibody	yes	slow
Avian nephritis virus	IS	no	slow
Avian orthoreoviruses	IS, EIA	yes	slow
Avian reticuloendotheliosis virus	AGP, IS, EIA	yes	slow
Chicken anaemia virus	IS, EIA, VN	yes	slow
Egg drop syndrome virus	HI, EIA	yes	slow
Infectious bursal disease virus	Serotype 1: AGP, EIA, VN Serotype 2: VN	no	rapid
Influenza A virus	AGP, EIA, HI	no	rapid
Marek's disease virus	AGP	no	rapid
Newcastle disease virus	HI, EIA	no	rapid
Turkey rhinotracheitis virus	EIA	no	slow
Mycoplasma gallisepticum	Agg and HI to confirm a positive test, EIA, HI	yes	slow
Mycoplasma synoviae	Agg and HI to confirm a positive test, EIA, HI	yes	rapid
Salmonella pullorum	Agg	yes	slow

Agg: agglutination
AGP: agar gel precipitation; the technique is suitable where testing is carried out weekly
EIA: enzyme immunoassay

HI: haemagglutination inhibition
IS: immunostaining
VN: virus neutralisation

**Subject to agreement by the competent authority, other types of test may be used provided they are at least as sensitive as those indicated and of appropriate specificity.

Tests for avian leucosis antigen
Prior to the commencement of laying, cloacal swabs or blood samples (using buffy coat cultivation) are tested for the presence of group-specific leucosis antigen. A total of 5 per cent (minimum 10, maximum 200) of the flock is sampled during each 4-week period. During lay, albumen samples from 5 per cent (minimum 10, maximum 200) of the eggs are tested in each 4-week period. Tests are performed by EIA for group-specific antigen using methods that are capable of detecting antigen from subgroups A, B and J.

Test for antibodies to other agents
Tests for antibodies to all agents listed in Table 5.2.2.-1 are performed throughout the laying period of the flock. In each 4-week period, samples are taken from 5 per cent (minimum 10, maximum 200) of the flock. It is recommended that 1.25 per cent of the flock is sampled each week since some test methods for some agents must be conducted on a weekly basis. Table 5.2.2.-1 classifies the agents into those that spread rapidly through the flock and those that spread slowly or may not infect the entire flock. For those agents listed as slowly spreading, each sample is tested individually.
For those agents listed as rapidly spreading, at least 20 per cent of the samples collected in each 4-week period are tested individually or, where serum neutralisation or

ELISA tests are employed, all of the samples may be tested individually or by preparing pools of 5 samples, collected at the same time.

Suitable methods to be used for detection of the agents are shown in Table 5.2.2.-1. Subject to agreement by the competent authority, other test methods may be used provided they are shown to be at least as sensitive as those indicated and of appropriate specificity.

Tests to be conducted at the end of the laying period

Following the last egg collection, final testing to confirm the absence of vertically-transmissible agents indicated in Table 5.2.2.-1 is performed. After the last egg collection, a minimum of 5 per cent of the flock (minimum 10, maximum 200) is retained for at least 4 weeks. Blood samples are collected from every bird in the group during the 4-week period with at least 1.25 per cent of the birds (25 per cent of the sample) being bled not earlier than 4 weeks after the final egg collection. Serum samples are tested for vertically-transmissible agents (as defined by Table 5.2.2.-1) using the methods indicated. Where sampling is performed on a weekly basis, at least 1.25 per cent of the birds (25 per cent of the sample) are tested each week during this period.
Alternatively, within 4 weeks of the final egg collection blood and/or other suitable sample materials are collected from at

Table 5.2.2-2. – *Schematic description of the establishment and maintenance of SPF flocks*

NEW STOCK	Establish freedom from vertically-transmissible agents
	Test all birds for avian leucosis antigen and antibodies prior to 20 weeks of age
	Test for *Salmonella* spp. and perform general clinical observation from 8 weeks of age
	Carry out routine testing for specified agents from 20 weeks of age
2nd GENERATION	Test all birds for avian leucosis antigen and antibodies prior to 20 weeks of age
	Test for *Salmonella* spp. and perform general clinical observation from 8 weeks of age
	Carry out routine testing for specified agents from 20 weeks of age
3rd GENERATION	Test all birds for avian leucosis antigen and antibodies prior to 20 weeks of age
	Test for *Salmonella* spp. and perform general clinical observation from 8 weeks of age
DESIGNATE FLOCK AS SPF IF ALL TESTS ARE SATISFACTORY	
3rd GENERATION	Carry out routine testing for specified agents from 20 weeks of age
	Carry out post-lay testing for vertically-transmissible agents
SUBSEQUENT GENERATIONS	Test two 5 per cent samples for avian leucosis antigen and for antibodies against specified agents between 12 and 20 weeks of age
	Test for *Salmonella* spp. and perform general clinical observation from 8 weeks of age
	Carry out routine testing for specified agents from 20 weeks of age
	Carry out post-lay testing for vertically-transmissible agents

least 5 per cent of the flock and tested for the presence of vertically-transmissible agents using validated nucleic acid amplification techniques *(2.6.21)*.

Action to be taken in the event of detection of a specified agent

If evidence is found of contamination of the flock by an agent listed as slowly spreading in Table 5.2.2.-1, all materials derived from the flock during the 4-week period immediately preceding the date on which the positive sample was collected are considered unsatisfactory. Similarly, if evidence is found of contamination of the flock by an agent listed as rapidly spreading in Table 5.2.2.-1, all materials derived from the flock during the 2-week period immediately preceding the date on which the positive sample was collected are considered unsatisfactory. Any product manufactured with such materials, and for which the use of SPF materials is required, is considered unsatisfactory and must be discarded; any quality control tests conducted using the materials are invalid.

Producers must notify users of all eggs of the evidence of contamination as soon as possible following the outbreak.

Any flock in which an outbreak of any specified agent is confirmed may not be redesignated as an SPF flock. Any progeny derived from that flock during or after the 4-week period prior to the last negative sample being collected may not be designated as SPF.

J (Vet) 1. Cell Cultures for the Production of Veterinary Vaccines

(Ph. Eur. method 5.2.4)
Cell cultures for the production of vaccines for veterinary use comply with the requirements of this section. It may also be necessary that cell cultures used for testing of vaccines for veterinary use also comply with some or all of these requirements.

For most mammalian viruses, propagation in cell lines is possible and the use of primary cells is then not acceptable.

Permanently infected cells used for production of veterinary vaccines comply with the appropriate requirements described below. The cells shall be shown to be infected only with the agent stated.

Cell lines

Cell lines are normally handled according to a cell-seed system. Each master cell seed is assigned a specific code for identification purposes. The master cell seed is stored in aliquots at – 70 °C or lower. Production of vaccine is not normally undertaken on cells more than twenty passages from the master cell seed. Where suspension cultures are used, an increase in cell numbers equivalent to approximately three population doublings is considered equivalent to one passage. If cells beyond twenty passage levels are to be used for production, it shall be demonstrated, by validation or further testing, that the production cell cultures are essentially similar to the master cell seed with regard to their biological characteristics and purity and that the use of such cells has no deleterious effect on vaccine production.

The history of the cell line shall be known and recorded in detail (for example, origin, number of passages and media used for multiplication, storage conditions).

The method of storing and using the cells, including details of how it is ensured that the maximum number of passages permitted is not exceeded during product manufacture, are recorded. A sufficient quantity of the master cell seed and each working cell seed are kept for analytical purposes.

The tests described below are carried out (as prescribed in Table 5.2.4.-1) on a culture of the master cell seed and the working cell seed or on cell cultures from the working cell seed at the highest passage level used for production and derived from a homogeneous sample demonstrated to be representative.

Characteristics of Culture The appearance of cell monolayers, before and after histological staining, is described. Information, if possible numerical data, is provided especially on the speed and rate of growth. Similarly, the presence or absence of contact inhibition, polynucleated cells and any other cellular abnormalities are specified.

Karyotype   A chromosomal examination is made of not fewer than fifty cells undergoing mitosis in the master cell seed and at a passage level at least as high as that to be used in production. Any chromosomal marker present in the master cell seed must also be found in the high passage cells and the modal number of chromosomes in these cells must not be more than 15 per cent higher than of cells of the master cell seed. The karyotypes must be identical. If the modal number exceeds the level stated, if the chromosomal markers are not found in the working cell seed at the highest level used for production or if the karyotype differs, the cell line shall not be used for manufacture.

Table 5.2.4.-1. – *Cell culture stage at which tests are carried out*

	Master cell seed	Working cell seed	Cell from working cell seed at highest passage level
General microscopy	+	+	+
Bacteria and fungi	+	+	–
Mycoplasmas	+	+	–
Viruses	+	+	–
Identification of species	+	–	+
Karyotype	+	–	+
Tumorigenicity	+	–	–

Identification of the Species   It shall be shown, by one validated method, that the master cell seed and the cells from the working cell seed at the highest passage level used for production come from the species of origin specified. When a fluorescence test is carried out and the corresponding serum to the species of origin of cells is used and shows that all the tested cells are fluorescent, it is not necessary to carry out other tests with reagents able to detect contamination by cells of other species.

Bacterial and Fungal Contamination   The cells comply with the test for sterility (2.6.1). The sample of cells to be examined consists of not less than the number of cells in a monolayer with an area of 70 cm² or, for cells grown in suspension, an approximately equivalent number of cells. The cells are maintained in culture for at least 15 days without antibiotics before carrying out the test.

Mycoplasmas (Appendix XVI B (Vet) 3)   The cells comply with the test for mycoplasmas. The cells are maintained in culture for at least 15 days without antibiotics before carrying out the test.

Absence of Contaminating Viruses   The cells must not be contaminated by viruses; suitably sensitive tests, including those prescribed below, are carried out.

The monolayers tested shall have an area of at least 70 cm², and shall be prepared and maintained using medium and additives, and grown under similar conditions to those used for the preparation of the vaccine. The monolayers are maintained in culture for a total of at least 28 days. Subcultures are made at 7-day intervals, unless the cells do not survive for this length of time, when the subcultures are made on the latest day possible. Sufficient cells, in suitable containers, are produced for the final subculture to carry out the tests specified below.

The monolayers are examined regularly throughout the incubation period for the possible presence of cytopathic effects and at the end of the observation period for cytopathic effects, haemadsorbent viruses and specific viruses by immuno-fluorescence and other suitable tests as indicated below.

Detection of Cytopathic Viruses   Two monolayers of at least 6 cm² each are stained with an appropriate cytological stain. The entire area of each stained monolayer is examined for any inclusion bodies, abnormal numbers of giant cells or any other lesion indicative of a cellular abnormality which might be attributable to a contaminant.

Detection of Haemadsorbent Viruses   Monolayers totalling at least 70 cm² are washed several times with an appropriate buffer and a sufficient volume of a suspension of suitable red blood cells added to cover the surface of the monolayer evenly. After different incubation times cells are examined for the presence of haemadsorption.

Detection of Specified Viruses   Tests are carried out for freedom from contaminants specific for the species of origin of the cell line and for the species for which the product is intended. Sufficient cells on suitable supports are prepared to carry out tests for the agents specified. Suitable positive controls are included in each test. The cells are subjected to suitable tests, for example using fluorescein-conjugated antibodies or similar reagents.

Tests in Other Cell Cultures   Monolayers totalling at least 140 cm² are required. The cells are frozen and thawed at least three times and then centrifuged to remove cellular debris. Inoculate aliquots onto the following cells at any time up to 70 per cent confluency:

— primary cells of the source species;

— cells sensitive to viruses pathogenic for the species for which the vaccine is intended;

— cells sensitive to pestiviruses.

The inoculated cells are maintained in culture for at least 7 days, after which freeze-thawed extracts are prepared as above and inoculated onto sufficient fresh cultures of the same cell types to allow for the testing as described below. The cells are incubated for at least a further 7 days. The cultures are examined regularly for the presence of any cytopathic changes indicative of living organisms.

At the end of this period of 14 days, the inoculated cells are subjected to the following checks:

— freedom from cytopathic and haemadsorbent organisms, using the methods specified in the relevant paragraphs above,

— absence of pestiviruses and other specific contaminants by immunofluorescence or other validated methods as indicated in the paragraph above on Detection of Specified Viruses.

Tumorigenicity   The risk of a cell line for the target species must be evaluated and, if necessary, tests are carried out.

Primary Cells

For most mammalian vaccines, the use of primary cells is not acceptable for the manufacture of vaccines since cell lines can be used. If there is no alternative to the use of primary cells, the cells are obtained from a herd or flock free from specified pathogens, with complete protection from introduction of diseases (for example, disease barriers, filters on air inlets, suitable quarantine before introduction of animals). Chicken flocks comply with the requirements prescribed under *Chicken Flocks Free from Specified Pathogens for the Production and Quality Control of Vaccines (5.2.2)*. For all other species, the herd or flock is shown to be free from relevant specified pathogens. All the breeding stock in the herd or flock intended to be used to produce primary cells for vaccine manufacture is subject to a suitable monitoring procedure including regular serological checks carried out at least twice a year and two supplementary serological examinations performed in 15 per cent of the breeding stock in the herd between the two checks mentioned above.

Wherever possible, particularly for mammalian cells, a seed-lot system is used with, for example, a master cell seed formed after less than five passages, the working cell seed being no more than five passages from the initial preparation of the cell suspension from the animal tissues.

Each master cell seed, working cell seed and cells of the highest passage of primary cells are checked in accordance with Table 5.2.4.-2 and the procedure described below. The sample tested shall cover all the sources of cells used for the manufacture of the batch. No batches of vaccine manufactured using the cells may be released if any one of the checks performed produces unsatisfactory results.

Table 5.2.4.-2. – *Cell culture stage at which tests are carried out*

	Master cell seed	Working cell seed	Highest passage level
General microscopy	+	+	+
Bacteria and fungi	+	+	–
Mycoplasmas	+	+	–
Viruses	+	+	–
Identification of species	+	–	–

Characteristics of Cultures   The appearance of cell monolayers, before and after histological staining, is described. Information, if possible numerical data, is recorded, especially on the speed and rate of growth. Similarly, the presence or absence of contact inhibition, polynucleated cells and any other cellular abnormalities are specified.

Identification of Species   It shall be demonstrated by one validated test that the master cell seed comes from the specified species of origin.

When a fluorescence test is carried out and the corresponding serum to the species of origin of cells is used and shows that all the tested cells are fluorescent, it is not necessary to carry out other tests with reagents able to detect contamination by cells of other species.

Bacterial and Fungal Sterility   The cells comply with the test for sterility (*2.6.1*). The sample of cells to be examined consists of not less than the number of cells in a monolayer with an area of 70 cm^2 or for cells grown in suspension an approximately equivalent number of cells. The cells are maintained in culture for at least 15 days without antibiotics before carrying out the test.

Mycoplasmas (Appendix XVI B (Vet) 3)   The cells comply with the test for mycoplasmas. The cells are maintained in culture for at least 15 days without antibiotics before carrying out the test.

Absence of Contaminating Viruses   The cells must not be contaminated by viruses; suitably sensitive tests, including those prescribed below are carried out.

The monolayers tested shall be at least 70 cm^2, and shall be prepared and maintained in culture using the same medium and additives, and under similar conditions to those used for the preparation of the vaccine.

The monolayers are maintained in culture for a total of at least 28 days or for the longest period possible if culture for 28 days is impossible. Subcultures are made at 7-day intervals, unless the cells do not survive for this length of time when the subcultures are made on the latest day possible. Sufficient cells, in suitable containers are produced for the final subculture to carry out the tests specified below.

The monolayers are examined regularly throughout the incubation period for the possible presence of cytopathic effects and at the end of the observation period for cytopathic effects, haemadsorbent viruses and specific viruses by immunofluorescence and other suitable tests as indicated below.

Detection of Cytopathic Viruses   Two monolayers of at least 6 cm^2 each are stained with an appropriate cytological stain. Examine the entire area of each stained monolayer for any inclusion bodies, abnormal numbers of giant cells or any other lesion indicative of a cellular abnormality that might be attributable to a contaminant.

Detection of Haemadsorbent Viruses   Monolayers totalling at least 70 cm^2 are washed several times with a suitable buffer solution and a sufficient volume of a suspension of suitable red blood cells added to cover the surface of the monolayer evenly. After different incubation times, examine cells for the presence of haemadsorption.

Detection of Specified Viruses   Tests are be carried out for freedom of contaminants specific for the species of origin of the cells and for the species for which the product is intended.

Sufficient cells on suitable supports are prepared to carry out tests for the agents specified. Suitable positive controls are included in each test. The cells are subjected to suitable tests using fluorescein-conjugated antibodies or similar reagents.

Tests in Other Cell Cultures   Monolayers totalling at least 140 cm^2 are required. The cells are frozen and thawed at least three times and then centrifuged to remove cellular debris. Aliquots are inoculated onto the following cells at any time up to 70 per cent confluency:

— primary cells of the source species;

— cells sensitive to viruses pathogenic for the species for which the vaccine is intended;

— cells sensitive to pestiviruses.

The inoculated cells are maintained in culture for at least 7 days, after which freeze-thawed extracts are prepared as above, and inoculated onto sufficient fresh cultures of the same cell types to allow for the testing as described below. The cells are incubated for at least a further 7 days.

All cultures are regularly examined for the presence of any cytopathic changes indicative of living organisms.

At the end of this period of 14 days, the inoculated cells are subjected to the following checks:

— freedom from cytopathic and haemadsorbent organisms is demonstrated using the methods specified in the relevant paragraphs above;

— relevant substrates are tested for the absence of pestiviruses and other specific contaminants by immunofluorescence or other validated methods as indicated in the paragraph above on Detection of Specified Viruses.

J (Vet) 2. Substances of Animal Origin for the Production of Veterinary Vaccines

(Ph. Eur. method 5.2.5)

Substances of animal origin (for example, serum, trypsin and serum albumin) may be used during the manufacture of veterinary immunological products, as ingredients of culture media etc. or as added constituents of vaccines or diluents. It is recommended to reduce, wherever practicable, the use of such substances.

Certain restrictions are placed upon the use of such substances to minimise the risk associated with pathogens that may be present in them:

— The use of substances of animal origin as constituents of vaccines or diluents is not generally acceptable except where such substances are sterilised by a suitable, validated method. Where the use of such substances has been shown to be essential and sterilisation is not possible, the criteria described under Requirements apply.

— Substances of animal origin used during production are either subjected to a suitable, validated sterilisation or inactivation procedure or the substance is tested for the absence of extraneous organisms in accordance with the Requirements below. For inactivated vaccines, the method used for inactivation of the vaccine strain may also be validated for inactivation of possible contaminants from substances of animal origin.

In addition to the restrictions described below, manufacturers must consider restrictions on the handling of substances of animal origin in the vaccine manufacturing premises.

The restrictions imposed by these sections may need to be varied in accordance with changes in the incidence of disease in the country of origin and in Europe.

Requirements

Substances of animal origin comply with the requirements of the Pharmacopoeia (where a relevant monograph exists).

Source The risk related to the animal diseases occurring in the country of origin of the substance and to the potential infectious diseases occurring in the source species, in relation to the proposed recipient species must be carefully evaluated. The strictest possible selection criteria must be applied, in particular for substances for use in products intended for the same species and for substances of bovine, caprine, ovine and porcine origin.

Preparation Substances of animal origin are prepared from a homogeneous bulk designated with a batch number. A batch may contain substances derived from as many animals as desired but once defined and given a batch number, the batch is not added to or contaminated in any way.

All batches of substances shall be shown to be free from contaminants as described below and/or are subject to a validated inactivation procedure.

Inactivation The inactivation procedure chosen shall have been shown to be capable of reducing the titre of certain potential contaminants in the substance concerned by at least 10^6. If this reduction in titre cannot be shown experimentally, kinetic studies for the inactivation procedure must be carried out and shown to be satisfactory, taking into account the possible level of contamination.

The list of potential contaminating organisms that the procedure must be shown to be capable of inactivating must

be appropriate to the particular species of origin of the substance. The evidence for the efficacy of the procedure, which must relate to the current circumstances, may take the form of references to published literature or experimental data generated by the manufacturer.

Tests For examination of the substance for freedom from contaminants, any solids are dissolved or suspended in a suitable medium in such a way as to create a solution or suspension containing at least 300 g/l of the substance to be examined. If the substance is not soluble or where cytotoxic reactions occur, a lower concentration may be used.

Any batch of substance found to contain living organisms of any kind is unsatisfactory and is either discarded or reprocessed and shown to be satisfactory.

Freedom from extraneous viruses The solution or suspension of the solid substance or the undiluted liquid substance is tested for contaminants by suitably sensitive methods. These methods shall include tests in suitably sensitive cell cultures, including primary cells from the same species as the substances to be examined. A proportion of the cells is passaged at least twice.

The cells are observed regularly for 21 days for cytopathic effects. At the end of each 7 day period, a proportion of the original cultures is fixed, stained and examined for cytopathic effects; a proportion is tested for haemadsorbing agents; and a proportion is tested for specific agents by appropriate serodiagnostic tests.

Bacterial and fungal contamination Before use, substances are tested for sterility *(2.6.1)* and freedom from mycoplasmas, Appendix XVI B (Vet) 3, or sterilised to inactivate any bacterial, fungal or mycoplasmal contaminants.

K (Vet) 1. Evaluation of safety of veterinary vaccines and immunosera

(Ph. Eur. method 5.2.6)

The term "product" means either a vaccine or an immunoserum throughout the text.

During development, safety tests are carried out in the target species to show the risks from use of the product.

Vaccines

In laboratory tests, "dose" means that quantity of the product to be recommended for use and containing the maximum titre or potency likely to be contained in production batches. Live vaccines are prepared only from strains of organisms that have been shown to be safe. For live vaccines, use a batch or batches of vaccine containing virus/bacteria at the least attenuated passage level that will be present in a batch of vaccine.

For combined vaccines, the safety shall be demonstrated; for live components of combined vaccines, compliance with the special requirements for live vaccines stated below shall be demonstrated separately for each vaccine strain.

For inactivated vaccines, safety tests carried out on the combined vaccine may be regarded as sufficient to demonstrate the safety of the individual components.

Immunosera

In the tests, "dose" means the maximum quantity of the product to be recommended for use and containing the maximum potency and maximum total protein likely to be contained in production batches. In addition, if appropriate, the dose tested also contains maximum quantities of immunoglobulin or gammaglobulin.

The tests described below, modified or supplemented by tests described in the Production section of a monograph, may be carried out as part of the tests necessary during development to demonstrate the safety of the product.

LABORATORY TESTS

Safety of the administration of 1 dose For each of the recommended routes of administration, administer 1 dose of product to animals of each species and category for which use of the product is to be recommended. This must include animals of the youngest recommended age and pregnant animals, if appropriate. The animals are observed and examined at least daily for signs of abnormal local and systemic reactions. Where appropriate, these studies shall include detailed post-mortem macroscopic and microscopic examinations of the injection site. Other objective criteria are recorded, such as body temperature (for mammals) and performance measurements. The body temperatures are recorded on at least the day before and at the time of administration of the product, 4 h later and on the following 4 days. The animals are observed and examined until reactions may no longer be expected but, in all cases, the observation and examination period extends at least until 14 days after administration.

Examination of reproductive performance As part of the studies, examination of reproductive performance must also be considered when data suggest that the starting material from which the product is derived may be a risk factor. Where prescribed in a monograph, reproductive performance of males and non-pregnant and pregnant females and harmful effects on the progeny, including teratogenic and abortifacient effects, are investigated by each of the recommended routes of administration.

Safety of 1 administration of an overdose An overdose of the product is administered by each recommended route of administration to animals of the categories of the target species which are expected to be the most sensitive, such as animals of the youngest age and pregnant animals, if appropriate. The overdose normally consists of 10 doses of a live vaccine or 2 doses of an inactivated product or an immunoserum. For freeze-dried live vaccines, the 10 doses shall be reconstituted in a suitable volume of diluent for the test. The animals are observed and examined at least daily for signs of local and systemic reactions. Other objective criteria are recorded, such as body temperature (for mammals) and performance measurements. The animals are observed and examined for at least 14 days after administration. If the vaccine is intended for use in pregnant animals, carry out the test in these animals at the time for which use is not contra-indicated, and extend the observation period at least until parturtition. The animals are observed and effects on gestation or the offspring are recorded. In exceptional circumstances, notably for immunosera, where there is evidence that an overdose is not appropriate and an overdose test is not performed, a clear warning of the potential dangers of overdosing must be contained in the product literature.

Safety of the repeated administration of 1 dose
Repeated administration of 1 dose may be required to reveal any adverse effects induced by such administration. These tests are particularly important where the product, notably an immunoserum, may be administered on several occasions over a relatively short space of time. These tests are carried out on the most sensitive categories of the target species, using each recommended route of administration.
The number of administrations must be not less than the maximum number recommended; for vaccines, this shall take account of the number of administrations for primary vaccination and the 1st re-vaccination; for immunosera, it shall take account of the number of administrations required for treatment. The interval between administrations shall be suitable (e.g. period of risk or required for treatment) and appropriate to the recommendations of use. Although, for convenience, as far as vaccines are concerned, a shorter interval may be used in the study than that recommended in the field, an interval of at least 14 days must be allowed between administrations for the development of any hypersensitivity reaction. For immunosera, however, administration shall follow the recommended schedule. The animals are observed and examined at least daily for at least 14 days after the last administration for signs of systemic and local reactions. Other objective criteria are recorded, such as body temperature and performance measurements.

Residues In the case of live vaccines for well-established zoonotic diseases, the determination of residual vaccine organisms at the injection site may be required, in addition to the studies of dissemination described below.

Adverse effects on immunological functions Where the product might adversely affect the immune response of the animal to which the product is administered or of its progeny, suitable tests on the immunological functions are carried out.

Adverse effects from interactions Studies are undertaken to show a lack of adverse effect on the safety of the product when simultaneous administration is recommended or where administration of the product is recommended as part of a schedule of administration of products within a short period of time.

Special requirements for live vaccines The following laboratory tests must also be carried out with live vaccines.

a) Spread of the vaccine strain Spread of the vaccine strain from vaccinated to unvaccinated target animals is investigated using the recommended route of administration most likely to result in spread. Moreover, it may be necessary to investigate the safety of spread to non-target species that could be highly susceptible to a live vaccine strain. An assessment must be made of how many animal-to-animal passages are likely to be sustainable under normal circumstances together with an assessment of the likely consequences.

b) Dissemination in vaccinated animal Faeces, urine, milk, eggs, oral, nasal and other secretions shall be tested for the presence of the organism. Moreover, studies may be required of the dissemination of the vaccine strain in the body, with particular attention being paid to the predilection sites for replication of the organism. In the case of live vaccines for well-established zoonotic diseases for food-producing animals, these studies are obligatory.

c) Increase in virulence Use material from the passage level that is likely to be most virulent for the target species between the master seed lot and the final product.
The animals used are of an age suitable for recovery of the virus and the animals in all groups are of this age at the time of inoculation. The initial vaccination is carried out using the recommended route of administration most likely to lead to reversion to virulence. After this, not fewer than 5 further serial passages through animals of the target species are undertaken. The passages are undertaken by the route of administration most likely to lead to reversion to virulence. If the properties of the virus allow sequential passage to

5 groups via natural spreading, this method may be used, otherwise passage as described in each monograph is carried out and the maximally passaged virus that has been recovered is tested for increase in virulence. Not fewer than 2 animals are used for each passage. At each passage, the presence of living vaccine-derived organisms in the material used for passage is demonstrated. The safety of material from the highest successful passage is compared with that of unpassaged material.

For particular viruses, a monograph may require more passages in more animals if there is an indication from available data that this is relevant. At least the final passage is carried out using animals most appropriate to the potential risk being assessed.

d) Biological properties of the vaccine strain Other tests may be necessary to determine as precisely as possible the intrinsic biological properties of the vaccine strain (for example, neurotropism). For vector vaccines, evaluation is made of the risk of changing the tropism or virulence of the strain and where necessary specific tests are carried out. Such tests are systematically carried out where the product of a foreign gene is incorporated into the strain as a structural protein.

e) Recombination or genomic reassortment of strain The probability of recombination or genomic reassortment with field or other strains shall be considered.

B. Field Studies

Results from laboratory studies shall normally be supplemented with supportive data from field studies. Provided that laboratory tests have adequately assessed the safety and efficacy of a product under experimental conditions using vaccines of maximum and minimum titre or potency respectively, a single batch of product may be used to assess both safety and efficacy under field conditions. In these cases, a typical routine batch of intermediate titre or potency may be used.

For food-producing mammals, the studies include measurement of the body temperatures of a sufficient number of animals, before and after administration of the product; for other mammals, such measurements are carried out if the laboratory studies indicate that there might be a problem. The size and persistence of any local reaction and the proportion of animals showing local or systemic reactions are recorded. Performance measurements are made, where appropriate.

Performance measures for broilers include weekly mortality, feed conversion ratios, age at slaughter and weight, down grading and rejects at the processing plant. For vaccines for use in laying birds or in birds which may be maintained to lay, the effect of the vaccine on laying performance and hatchability is investigated, as appropriate.

C. Ecotoxicity

An assessment is made of the potential harmful effects of the product for the environment and any necessary precautionary measures to reduce such risks are identified. The likely degree of exposure of the environment to the product is assessed taking into account: the target species and mode of administration; excretion of the product; disposal of unused product. If these factors indicate that there will be significant exposure of the environment to the product, the potential ecotoxicity is evaluated taking into account the properties of the product.

K (Vet) 2. Evaluation of efficacy of veterinary vaccines and immunosera

(Ph. Eur. general text 5.2.7)
The term "product" means either a vaccine or an immunoserum throughout the text.

During development of the product, tests are carried out to demonstrate that the product is efficacious when administered by each of the recommended routes and methods of administration and using the recommended schedule to animals of each species and category for which use of the product is to be recommended. The type of efficacy testing to be carried out varies considerably depending on the particular type of product.

As part of tests carried out during development to establish efficacy, the tests described in the Production section of a monograph may be carried out; the following must be taken into account.

The dose to be used is that quantity of the product to be recommended for use and containing the minimum titre or potency expected at the end of the period of validity.

For live vaccines, use vaccine containing virus/bacteria at the most attenuated passage level that will be present in a batch of vaccine.

For immunosera, if appropriate, the dose tested also contains minimum quantities of immunoglobulin or gammaglobulin and/or total protein.

The efficacy evidence must support all the claims being made. For example, claims for protection against respiratory disease must be supported by at least evidence of protection from clinical signs of respiratory disease. Where it is claimed that there is protection from infection this must be demonstrated using re-isolation techniques. If more than one claim is made, supporting evidence for each claim is required.

Vaccines The influence of passively acquired and maternally derived antibodies on the efficacy of a vaccine is adequately evaluated. Any claims, stated or implied, regarding onset and duration of protection shall be supported by data from trials.

The efficacy of each of the components of multivalent and combined vaccines shall be demonstrated using the combined vaccine.

Immunosera Particular attention must be paid to providing supporting data for the efficacy of the regime that is to be recommended. For example, if it is recommended that the immunoserum needs only to be administered once to achieve a prophylactic or therapeutic effect then this must be demonstrated. Any claims, stated or implied, regarding onset and duration of protection or therapeutic effect must be supported by data from trials. For example, the duration of the protection afforded by a prophylactic dose of an antiserum must be studied so that appropriate guidance for the user can be given on the label.

Studies of immunological compatibility are undertaken when simultaneous administration is recommended or where it is a part of a usual administration schedule. Wherever a product is recommended as part of an administration scheme, the priming or booster effect or the contribution of the product to the efficacy of the scheme as a whole is demonstrated.

LABORATORY TESTS
In principle, demonstration of efficacy is undertaken under well-controlled laboratory conditions by challenge of the target animal under the recommended conditions of use.

In so far as possible, the conditions under which the challenge is carried out shall mimic the natural conditions for infection, for example with regard to the amount of challenge organism and the route of administration of the challenge.

Vaccines Unless otherwise justified, challenge is carried out using a strain different from the one used in the production of the vaccine.

If possible, the immune mechanism (cell-mediated/humoral, local/general, classes of immunoglobulin) that is initiated after the administration of the vaccine to target animals shall be determined.

Immunosera Data are provided from measurements of the antibody levels achieved in the target species after administration of the product, as recommended. Where suitable published data exist, references are provided to relevant published literature on protective antibody levels and challenge studies are avoided.

Where challenges are required, these can be given before or after administration of the product, in accordance with the indications and specific claims to be made.

FIELD TRIALS

In general, results from laboratory tests are supplemented with data from field trials, carried out, unless otherwise justified, with untreated control animals. Provided that laboratory tests have adequately assessed the safety and efficacy of a product under experimental conditions using vaccines of maximum and minimum titre or potency respectively, a single batch of product could be used to assess both safety and efficacy under field conditions. In these cases, a typical routine batch of intermediate titre or potency may be used. Where laboratory trials cannot be supportive of efficacy, the performance of field trials alone may be acceptable.

K (Vet) 3. Evaluation of safety of each batch of veterinary vaccines and immunosera

(Ph. Eur. general text 5.2.9)
The term "product" means either a vaccine or an immunoserum throughout the text.

Definition of abnormal reactions

During development studies, the type and degree of reactions expected after administration of the product are defined in the light of safety testing. This definition of normal or abnormal local and systemic reactions is then used as part of the operation procedure for the batch safety test to evaluate acceptable and unacceptable reactions.

Amount to be administered in the test

In the tests, "dose" means the quantity of the product to be recommended for use and containing the titre or potency within the limits specified for production batches.
The amount to be administered in the test is usually defined in a number of doses. For freeze-dried vaccines, the 10 doses are reconstituted in a suitable volume for the test.
For products consisting of a container of freeze-dried live component(s) and a container of inactivated component(s) to be used as a diluent, it may be necessary to use further liquid for the reconstitution of the freeze-dried component(s).
The contents of 2 containers of inactivated component mixed with the contents of a maximum number of freeze-dried live containers are to be injected in one site and the other live

freeze dried components reconstituted using a suitable solvent may be given at a separate site, if necessary and justified. For combined vaccines, safety tests carried out on the combined vaccine may be regarded as sufficient to demonstrate the safety of the individual components.

Route of administration

The product is administered by a recommended route. In principle, preference should be given to the application route with the higher possibility to detect reactions.
Where it is known, for example from development studies, that there is a particular risk, a 2nd administration is performed using a suitable dose and time interval as determined during development.

Target animal species and category of animals

Use animals of the minimum age recommended for vaccination or administration of the product and of the most sensitive species, unless otherwise justified and authorised.

Animal numbers

The number of animals to be used for the test is prescribed in the monographs. Generally 2 animals are used for a mammalian species and 10 for birds and fish.

Identification of animals

Unless otherwise justified, all animals are marked in a suitable way to ensure individual documentation of data for the whole observation period.

Observation period

Where objective criteria such as body temperature are to be recorded as described below, the animals are examined and observed for at least 3 days prior to administration of the product. After administration of the product, the animals are observed and examined at least once every day for a period of at least 14 days for signs of local and systemic reactions. On the day of administration of the product, at least one additional inspection is necessary after 4 h or at intervals as specified in the monograph. Where there is a 2nd administration of the product the period usually ends 14 days after the 2nd administration.

Local and systemic reactions

Animals showing severe abnormal local or systemic reactions are killed. All dead animals undergo a post-mortem with macroscopic examination. Additional microscopic and microbiological investigations may be indicated.

The animals are observed and examined for signs of local and systemic reactions. Where it is known to be a useful indicator, other criteria are recorded, such as body temperature, body mass, other performance measurements and food intake.

Local reactions As far as appropriate and possible, the size and persistence of any local reaction (including incidence of painful reactions) and the proportion of animals showing local reactions are recorded.

Systemic reactions Body temperature and if appropriate, body mass are documented as general indicators of systemic effects of administration of the product. In addition, all clinical signs are recorded.

Body temperature For mammals, the studies include measurement of body temperature during the observation period. The body temperatures are recorded beginning at least 3 days before administration of the product, at the time of administration, 4 h after and at suitable intervals.
The body temperature before administration of the product has to be within the physiological range. At least for

products where a significant increase in body temperature may be expected (e.g. endotoxin containing products or several live viral vaccines) or is specified in an individual monograph (e.g. not more than 2 °C for porcine actinobacillosis vaccine) it is recommended to use the mean temperature of the days before administration of the product (e.g. day − 3 to day 0) as the base line temperature to have clear guidance for evaluation of the test.

Body mass and food intake   Where it is known to be a reliable and useful indicator of safety, for example in young growing animals or in fish, the body mass is measured and documented shortly before administration and during the observation period. The food intake is monitored and documented as an indicator of the effect of administering the product. In most cases, it will be sufficient to record the daily ration has been consumed or partly or wholly rejected but, in some cases it may be necessary to record the actual weight of food consumed, if this is a relevant indicator of the safety of the product.

Clinical signs   All expected and unexpected clinical signs of a general nature are recorded, including changes in health status and behaviour changes.

Score sheets   The score sheets are prepared for each product in the light of expected signs. All parameters and data are recorded in score sheets. The score sheets contain general parameters but are also adapted for each kind of product to list clinical signs which might be more evident for a given product.

Criteria for repeating the test

If an abnormal sign occurs, the responsible veterinarian determines, based on post-mortem examination if necessary, whether this was due to the product or not. If it is not clear what caused the abnormal sign or where an animal is withdrawn for reasons unrelated to the product, the test may be repeated. If in the 2nd test, there is the same abnormal sign as in the 1st test, the product does not comply with the test. Any treatment administered to an animal during the observation period is recorded. If the treatment may interfere with the test, the test is not valid.

Appendix XVI

B (Vet) 3. Test for Absence of Mycoplasmas

(Ph. Eur. method 2.6.7 as applied to veterinary vaccines)
Where the test for mycoplasmas is prescribed for a master cell bank, for a working cell bank, for a virus seed lot or for control cells, both the culture method and the indicator cell culture method are used. Where the test for mycoplasmas is prescribed for a virus harvest, for a bulk vaccine or for the final lot (batch), the culture method is used. The indicator cell culture method may also be used, where necessary, for screening of media.

Culture method

Choice of culture media

The test is carried out using a sufficient number of both solid and liquid media to ensure growth in the chosen incubation conditions of small numbers of mycoplasmas that may be present in the product to be examined. Liquid media must contain phenol red. The range of media chosen is shown to have satisfactory nutritive properties for at least the organisms shown below. The nutritive properties of each new batch of medium are verified for the appropriate organisms in the list.

Acholeplasma laidlawii (vaccines for human and veterinary use where an antibiotic has been used during production)

Mycoplasma gallisepticum (where avian material has been used during production or where the vaccine is intended for use in poultry)

Mycoplasma hyorhinis (non-avian veterinary vaccines)

Mycoplasma orale (vaccines for human and veterinary use)

Mycoplasma pneumoniae (vaccines for human use) or other suitable species of D-glucose fermenter

Mycoplasma synoviae (where avian material has been used during production or where the vaccine is intended for use in poultry).

The test strains are field isolates having undergone not more than fifteen subcultures and are stored frozen or freeze-dried. After cloning the strains are identified as being of the required species by a suitable method, by comparison with type cultures, for example:

A. laidlawii	NCTC 10116	CIP 75.27	ATCC 23206
M. gallisepticum	NCTC 10115	CIP 104967	ATCC 19610
M. hyorhinis	NCTC 10130	CIP 104968	ATCC 17981
M. orale	NCTC 10112	CIP 104969	ATCC 23714
M. pneumoniae	NCTC 10119	CIP 103766	ATCC 15531
M. synoviae	NCTC 10124	CIP 104970	ATCC 25204

Incubation conditions

Divide inoculated media into two equal parts and incubate one in aerobic conditions and the other in microaerophilic conditions; for solid media maintain an atmosphere of adequate humidity to prevent desiccation of the surface. For aerobic conditions, incubate in an atmosphere of air containing, for solid media, 5 to 10 per cent of carbon dioxide. For microaerophilic conditions, incubate in an atmosphere of nitrogen containing, for solid media, 5 to 10 per cent of carbon dioxide.

Nutritive properties

Carry out the test for nutritive properties for each new batch of medium. Inoculate the chosen media with the appropriate test organisms; use not more than 100 CFU (colony-forming units) per 60 mm plate containing 9 ml of solid medium and not more than 40 CFU per 100 ml container of the corresponding liquid medium; use a separate plate and container for each species of organism. Incubate the media in the conditions that will be used for the test of the product to be examined (aerobically, microaerophilically or both, depending on the requirements of the test organism). The media comply with the test for nutritive properties if there is adequate growth of the test organisms accompanied by an appropriate colour change in liquid media.

Inhibitory substances

Carry out the test for nutritive properties in the presence of the product to be examined. If growth of the test organisms is notably less than that found in the absence of the product to be examined, the latter contains inhibitory substances that must be neutralised (or their effect otherwise countered, for example, by dilution) before the test for mycoplasmas is carried out. The effectiveness of the neutralisation or other process is checked by repeating the test for inhibitory substances after neutralisation.

Test for mycoplasmas in the product to be examined

For solid media, use plates 60 mm in diameter and containing 9 ml of medium. Inoculate each of not fewer than two plates of each solid medium with 0.2 ml of the product to be examined and inoculate 10 ml per 100 ml of each liquid medium. Incubate at 35 °C to 38 °C, aerobically and microaerophilically, for 21 days and at the same time incubate an uninoculated 100 ml portion of each liquid medium for use as a control. If any significant pH change occurs on addition of the product to be examined, restore the liquid medium to its original pH value by the addition of a solution of either sodium hydroxide or hydrochloric acid. On the first, second or third day after inoculation subculture each liquid culture by inoculating each of two plates of each solid medium with 0.2 ml and incubating at 35 °C to 38 °C aerobically and microaerophilically for not less than 21 days. Repeat the procedure on the sixth, seventh or eighth day and again on the thirteenth or fourteenth day of the test. Observe the liquid media every 2 or 3 days and if any colour change occurs subculture immediately. Observe solid media once per week.

If the liquid media show bacterial or fungal contamination, repeat the test. If, not earlier than 7 days after inoculation, not more than one plate at each stage of the test is accidentally contaminated with bacteria or fungi, or broken, that plate may be ignored provided that on immediate examination it shows no evidence of mycoplasmal growth. If, at any stage of the test, more than one plate is accidentally contaminated with bacteria or fungi, or broken, the test is invalid and must be repeated.

Include in the test positive controls prepared by inoculating not more than 100 CFU of suitable species such as *M. orale* and *M. pneumoniae*.

At the end of the incubation periods, examine all the inoculated solid media microscopically for the presence of mycoplasmas. The product passes the test if growth of mycoplasmas has not occurred in any of the inoculated media. If growth of mycoplasmas has occurred, the test may be repeated once using twice the amount of inoculum, media and plates; if growth of mycoplasmas does not occur, the product complies with the test. The test is invalid if the positive controls do not show growth of the relevant test organism.

Indicator cell culture method

Cell cultures are stained with a fluorescent dye that binds to DNA. Mycoplasmas are detected by their characteristic particulate or filamentous pattern of fluorescence on the cell surface and, if contamination is heavy, in surrounding areas.

Verification of the substrate

Using a Vero cell culture substrate, pretest the procedure using an inoculum of not more than 100 CFU (colony-forming units) of a strain growing readily in liquid or solid medium and demonstrate its ability to detect potential mycoplasma contaminants such as suitable strains of Mycoplasma hyorhinis and Mycoplasma orale. A different cell substrate may be used, for example the production cell line, if it has been demonstrated that it will provide at least equal sensitivity for the detection of potential mycoplasma contaminants.

TEST METHOD

Take not less than 1 ml of the product to be examined and use it to inoculate in duplicate, as described under Procedure, indicator cell cultures representing not less than 25 cm^2 of cell culture area at confluence.

Include in the test a negative (non-infected) control and two positive mycoplasma controls, such as M. hyorhinis and M. orale. Use an inoculum of not more than 100 CFU for the positive controls.

If for viral suspensions the interpretation of results is affected by marked cytopathic effects, the virus may be neutralised using a specific antiserum that has no inhibitory effects on mycoplasmas or a cell culture substrate that does not allow growth of the virus may be used. To demonstrate the absence of inhibitory effects of serum, carry out the positive control tests in the presence and absence of the antiserum.

PROCEDURE

1. Seed culture at a regular density (2×10^4 to 2×10^5 cells/ml, 4×10^3 to 2.5×10^4 cells/cm^2) and incubate at 36 ± 1 °C for at least 2 days. Inoculate the product to be examined and incubate for at least 2 days; make not fewer than one subculture. Grow the last subculture on coverslips in suitable containers or on some other surface suitable for the test procedure. Do not allow the last subculture to reach confluence since this would inhibit staining and impair visualisation of mycoplasmas.

2. Remove and discard the medium.

3. Rinse the monolayer with phosphate buffered saline pH 7.4 R, then with a mixture of equal volumes of phosphate buffered saline pH 7.4 R and a suitable fixing solution and finally with the fixing solution; when bisbenzimide R is used for staining, a freshly prepared mixture of 1 volume of glacial acetic acid R and 3 volumes of methanol R is a suitable fixing solution.

4. Add the fixing solution and allow to stand for 10 min.

5. Remove the fixing solution and discard.

6. If the monolayer is to be stained later, dry it completely. (Particular care is needed for staining of the slides after drying because of artefacts that may be produced.)

7. If the monolayer is to be stained directly, wash off the fixing solution twice with sterile water and discard the wash.

8. Add bisbenzimide working solution R or some other suitable DNA staining agent and allow to stand for 10 min.

9. Remove the stain and rinse the monolayer with water.

10. Mount each coverslip, where applicable, with a drop of a mixture of equal volumes of glycerol R and phosphate-citrate buffer solution pH 5.5 R; blot off surplus mountant from the edge of the coverslip.

11. Examine by epifluorescence (330 nm/380 nm excitation filter, LP 440 nm barrier filter) at 100-400 × magnification or greater.

12. Compare the microscopic appearance of the test cultures with that of the negative and positive controls, examining for extranuclear fluorescence. Mycoplasmas give pinpoints or filaments over the cytoplasm and sometimes in intercellular spaces.

The product to be examined complies with the test if there is no evidence of the presence of mycoplasmas in the test cultures inoculated with it. The test is invalid if the positive controls do not show the presence of the appropriate test organisms.

The following section is published for information.

Recommended media for the culture method

The following media are recommended. Other media may be used providing their ability to sustain the growth of mycoplasmas has been demonstrated on each batch in the presence and absence of the product to be examined.

Recommended media for the detection of Mycoplasma gallisepticum

(A) LIQUID MEDIUM

Beef heart infusion broth (1)	90.0 ml
Horse serum (unheated)	20.0 ml
Yeast extract (250 g/l)	10.0 ml
Thallium acetate (10 g/l solution)	1.0 ml
Phenol red (0.6 g/l solution)	5.0 ml
Penicillin (20 000 IU/ml)	0.25 ml
Deoxyribonucleic acid (2 g/l solution)	1.2 ml

Adjust to pH 7.8.

(B) SOLID MEDIUM

Prepare as described above replacing beef heart infusion broth by beef heart infusion agar containing 15 g/l of agar.

Recommended media for the detection of Mycoplasma synoviae

(A) LIQUID MEDIUM

Beef heart infusion broth (1)	90.0 ml
Essential vitamins (2)	0.025 ml
Glucose monohydrate (500 g/l solution)	2.0 ml
Swine serum (inactivated at 56 °C for 30 min)	12.0 ml
β-Nicotinamide adenine dinucleotide (10 g/l solution)	1.0 ml
Cysteine hydrochloride (10 g/l solution)	1.0 ml
Phenol red (0.6 g/l solution)	5.0 ml
Penicillin (20 000 IU/ml)	0.25 ml

Mix the solutions of β-nicotinamide adenine dinucleotide and cysteine hydrochloride and after 10 min add to the other ingredients. Adjust to pH 7.8.

(B) SOLID MEDIUM

Beef heart infusion broth (1)	90.0 ml
Ionagar (3)	1.4 g

Adjust to pH 7.8, sterilise by autoclaving then add:

Essential vitamins (2)	0.025 ml
Glucose monohydrate (500 g/l solution)	2.0 ml
Swine serum (unheated)	12.0 ml
β-Nicotinamide adenine dinucleotide (10 g/l solution)	1.0 ml
Cysteine hydrochloride (10 g/l solution)	1.0 ml
Phenol red (0.6 g/l solution)	5.0 ml
Penicillin (20 000 IU/ml)	0.25 ml

Recommended media for the detection of non-avian mycoplasmas

(A) LIQUID MEDIUM

Hanks' balanced salt solution (modified) (4)	800 ml
Distilled water	67 ml
Brain heart infusion (5)	135 ml
PPLO Broth (6)	248 ml
Yeast extract (170 g/l)	60 ml
Bacitracin	250 mg
Meticillin	250 mg
Phenol red (5 g/l)	4.5 ml
Thallium acetate (56 g/l)	3 ml
Horse serum	165 ml
Swine serum	165 ml

Adjust to pH 7.4 - 7.45.

(B) SOLID MEDIUM

Hanks' balanced salt solution (modified) (4)	200 ml
DEAE-dextran	200 mg
Ionagar (3)	15.65 mg

Mix well and sterilise by autoclaving. Cool to 100 °C. Add to 1740 ml of liquid medium as described above.

(1) Beef heart infusion broth

Beef heart (for preparation of the infusion)	500 g
Peptone	10 g
Sodium chloride	5 g
Distilled water to	1000 ml

Sterilise by autoclaving.

(2) Essential vitamins

Biotin	100 mg
Calcium pantothenate	100 mg
Choline chloride	100 mg
Folic acid	100 mg
i-Inositol	200 mg
Nicotinamide	100 mg
Pyridoxal hydrochloride	100 mg
Riboflavine	10 mg
Thiamine hydrochloride	100 mg
Distilled water to	1000 ml

(3) Ionagar

A highly refined agar for use in microbiology and immunology prepared by an ion-exchange procedure which results in a product having superior purity, clarity and gel strength.

It contains about:

Water	12.2 per cent
Ash	1.5 per cent
Acid-insoluble ash	0.2 per cent
Chlorine	0
Phosphate (calculated as P_2O_5)	0.3 per cent
Total nitrogen	0.3 per cent
Copper	8 ppm
Iron	170 ppm
Calcium	0.28 per cent
Magnesium	0.32 per cent

(4) Hanks' balanced salt solution (modified)

Sodium chloride	6.4 g
Potassium chloride	0.32 g
Magnesium sulphate heptahydrate	0.08 g
Magnesium chloride hexahydrate	0.08 g
Calcium chloride, anhydrous	0.112 g
Disodium hydrogen phosphate dihydrate	0.0596 g
Potassium dihydrogen phosphate, anhydrous	0.048 g
Distilled water to	800 ml

(5) Brain heart infusion

Calf-brain infusion	200 g
Beef-heart infusion	250 g
Proteose peptone	10 g
Glucose monohydrate	2 g
Sodium chloride	5 g
Disodium hydrogen phosphate, anhydrous	25 g
Distilled water to	1000 ml

(6) PPLO broth

Beef-heart infusion	50 g
Peptone	10 g
Sodium chloride	5 g
Distilled water to	1000 ml

B (Vet) 4. Avian Viral Vaccines: Tests for Extraneous Agents in Seed Lots

(Ph. Eur. method 2.6.24)

General provisions

a) In the following tests, chickens and/or chicken material such as eggs and cell cultures shall be derived from chicken flocks free from specified pathogens (SPF) *(5.2.2)*.

b) Cell cultures for the testing of extraneous agents comply with the requirements for the master cell seed of chapter *5.2.4. Cell cultures for the production of veterinary vaccines*, with the exception of the karyotype test and the tumorigenicity test, which do not have to be carried out.

c) In tests using cell cultures, precise specifications are given for the number of replicates, monolayer surface areas and minimum survival rate of the cultures. Alternative numbers of replicates and cell surface areas are possible as well, provided that a minimum of 2 replicates are used, the total surface area and the total volume of test substance applied are not less than that prescribed here and the survival rate requirements are adapted accordingly.

d) For a freeze-dried preparation, reconstitute using a suitable liquid. Unless otherwise stated or justified, the test substance must contain a quantity of virus equivalent to at least 10 doses of vaccine in 0.1 ml of inoculum.

e) If the virus of the seed lot would interfere with the conduct and sensitivity of the test, neutralise the virus in the preparation with a monospecific antiserum.

f) Monospecific antiserum and serum of avian origin used for cell culture or any other purpose, in any of these tests, shall be free of antibodies against and free from inhibitory effects on the organisms listed hereafter under 7 Antibody specifications for sera used in extraneous agents testing.

g) Where specified in a monograph or otherwise justified, if neutralisation of the virus of the seed lot is required but difficult to achieve, the *in vitro* tests described below are adapted, as required, to provide the necessary guarantees of freedom from contamination with an extraneous agent.

h) Other types of tests than those indicated may be used provided they are at least as sensitive as those indicated and of appropriate specificity. Nucleic acid amplification techniques (*2.6.21*) give specific detection for many agents and can be used after validation for sensitivity and specificity.

1. Test for extraneous agents using embryonated hens' eggs

Use a test substance, diluted if necessary, containing a quantity of neutralised virus equivalent to at least 10 doses of vaccine in 0.2 ml of inoculum. Suitable antibiotics may be added. Inoculate the test substance into 3 groups of 10 embryonated hens' eggs as follows:

— group 1: 0.2 ml into the allantoic cavity of each 9- to 11-day-old embryonated egg,

— group 2: 0.2 ml onto the chorio-allantoic membrane of each 9- to 11-day-old embryonated egg,

— group 3: 0.2 ml into the yolk sac of each 5- to 6-day-old embryonated egg.

Candle the eggs in groups 1 and 2 daily for 7 days and the eggs in group 3 for 12 days. Discard embryos that die during the first 24 h as non-specific deaths; the test is not valid unless at least 6 embryos in each group survive beyond the first 24 h after inoculation. Examine macroscopically for abnormalities all embryos which die more than 24 h after inoculation, or which survive the incubation period. Examine also the chorio-allantoic membranes of these eggs for any abnormality and test the allantoic fluids for the presence of haemagglutinating agents.

Carry out a further embryo passage. Pool separately material from live and from the dead and abnormal embryos. Inoculate each pool into 10 eggs for each route as described above, chorio-allantoic membrane material being inoculated onto chorio-allantoic membranes, allantoic fluids into the allantoic cavity and embryo material into the yolk sac. For eggs inoculated by the allantoic and chorio-allantoic routes, candle the eggs daily for 7 days, proceeding and examining the material as described above. For eggs inoculated by the yolk sac route, candle the eggs daily for 12 days, proceeding and examining the material as described above.

The seed lot complies with the test if no test embryo shows macroscopic abnormalities or dies from causes attributable to the seed lot and if examination of the chorio-allantoic membranes and testing of the allantoic fluids show no evidence of the presence of any extraneous agent.

2. Test in chicken kidney cells

Prepare 7 monolayers of chicken kidney cells, each monolayer having an area of about 25 cm^2. Maintain 2 monolayers as negative controls and treat these in the same way as the 5 monolayers inoculated with the test substance, as described below. Remove the culture medium when the cells reach confluence. Inoculate 0.1 ml of test substance onto each of the 5 monolayers. Allow adsorption for 1 h, add culture medium and incubate the cultures for a total of at least 21 days, subculturing at 4- to 7-day intervals. Each passage is made with pooled cells and fluids from all 5 monolayers after carrying out a freeze-thaw cycle. Inoculate 0.1 ml of pooled material onto each of 5 recently prepared monolayers of about 25 cm^2 each, at each passage. For the last passage, grow the cells also on a suitable substrate so as to obtain an area of about 10 cm^2 of cells from each of the monolayers for test A. The test is not valid if less than 80 per cent of the monolayers survive after any passage.

Examine microscopically all the cell cultures frequently throughout the entire incubation period for any signs of cytopathic effect or other evidence of the presence of contaminating agents in the test substance. At the end of the total incubation period, carry out the following procedures.

A. Fix and stain (with Giemsa or haematoxylin and eosin) about 10 cm^2 of confluent cells from each of the 5 monolayers. Examine the cells microscopically for any cytopathic effect, inclusion bodies, syncytial formation, or any other evidence of the presence of contaminating agents from the test substance.

B. Drain and wash about 25 cm^2 of cells from each of the 5 monolayers. Cover these cells with a 0.5 per cent suspension of washed chicken erythrocytes (using at least 1 ml of suspension for each 5 cm^2 of cells). Incubate the cells at 4 °C for 20 min and then wash gently in phosphate buffered saline pH 7.4. Examine the cells microscopically for haemadsorption attributable to the presence of a haemadsorbing agent in the test substance.

C. Test individual samples of the fluids from each cell culture using chicken erythrocytes for haemagglutination attributable to the presence of a haemagglutinating agent in the test substance.

The test is not valid if there are any signs of extraneous agents in the negative control cultures. The seed lot complies with the test if there is no evidence of the presence of any extraneous agent.

3. Test for avian leucosis viruses

Prepare at least 13 replicate monolayers of primary or secondary chick embryo fibroblasts from the tissues of 9- to 11-day-old embryos that are known to be genetically susceptible to subgroups A, B and J of avian leucosis viruses and that support the growth of exogenous but not endogenous avian leucosis viruses (cells from C/E strain chickens are suitable). Each replicate shall have an area of about 50 cm^2.

Remove the culture medium when the cells reach confluence. Inoculate 0.1 ml of the test substance onto each of 5 of the replicate monolayers. Allow adsorption for 1 h, and add culture medium. Inoculate 2 of the replicate monolayers with subgroup A avian leucosis virus (not more than 10 CCID$_{50}$ in 0.1 ml), 2 with subgroup B avian leucosis virus (not more than 10 CCID$_{50}$ in 0.1 ml) and 2 with subgroup J avian leucosis virus (not more than 10 $CCID_{50}$ in 0.1 ml) as positive controls. Maintain not fewer than 2 non-inoculated replicate monolayers as negative controls.

Incubate the cells for a total of at least 9 days, subculturing at 3- to 4-day intervals. Retain cells from each passage level and harvest the cells at the end of the total incubation period. Wash cells from each passage level from each replicate and resuspend the cells at 10^7 cells per millilitre in barbital-buffered saline for subsequent testing by a Complement Fixation for Avian Leucosis (COFAL) test or in phosphate buffered saline for testing by Enzyme-Linked Immunosorbent Assay (ELISA). Then, carry out 3 cycles of freezing and thawing to release any group-specific antigen and perform a COFAL test or an ELISA test on each extract to detect group-specific avian leucosis antigen if present.

The test is not valid if group-specific antigen is detected in fewer than 5 of the 6 positive control replicate monolayers or if a positive result is obtained in any of the negative control monolayers, or if the results for both of the 2 negative control monolayers are inconclusive. If the results for more than 1 of the test replicate monolayers are inconclusive, then further subcultures of reserved portions of the fibroblast monolayers shall be made and tested until an unequivocal result is obtained. If a positive result is obtained for any of the test monolayers, then the presence of avian leucosis virus in the test substance has been detected.

The seed lot complies with the test if there is no evidence of the presence of any avian leucosis virus.

4. Test for avian reticuloendotheliosis virus

Prepare 11 monolayers of primary or secondary chick embryo fibroblasts from the tissues of 9- to 11-day old chick embryos or duck embryo fibroblasts from the tissues of 13- to 14-day-old embryos, each monolayer having an area of about 25 cm^2.

Remove the culture medium when the cells reach confluence. Inoculate 0.1 ml of the test substance onto each of 5 of the monolayers. Allow adsorption for 1 h, and add culture medium. Inoculate 4 of the monolayers with avian reticuloendotheliosis virus as positive controls (not more than 10 $CCID_{50}$ in 0.1 ml). Maintain 2 non-inoculated monolayers as negative controls.

Incubate the cells for a total of at least 10 days, subculturing twice at 3- to 4-day intervals. The test is not valid if fewer than 3 of the 4 positive controls or fewer than 4 of the 5 test monolayers or neither of the 2 negative controls survive after any passage.

For the last subculture, grow the fibroblasts on a suitable substrate so as to obtain an area of about 10 cm^2 of confluent fibroblasts from each of the original 11 monolayers for the subsequent test: test about 10 cm^2 of confluent fibroblasts derived from each of the original 11 monolayers by immunostaining for the presence of avian reticuloendotheliosis virus. The test is not valid if avian reticuloendotheliosis virus is detected in fewer than 3 of the 4 positive control monolayers or in any of the negative control monolayers, or if the results for both of the 2 negative control monolayers are inconclusive. If the results for more than 1 of the test monolayers are inconclusive then further subcultures of reserved portions of the fibroblast monolayers shall be made and tested until an unequivocal result is obtained.

The seed lot complies with the test if there is no evidence of the presence of avian reticuloendotheliosis virus.

5. Test for chicken anaemia virus

Prepare eleven 20 ml suspensions of the MDCC-MSBI cell line or another cell line of equivalent sensitivity in 25 cm^2 cell culture flasks containing about 5×10^5 cells/ml. Inoculate 0.1 ml of test substance into each of 5 flasks. Inoculate 4 of the suspensions with 10 $CCID_{50}$ chicken anaemia virus as positive controls. Maintain not fewer than 2 non-inoculated suspensions. Maintain all the cell cultures for a total of at least 24 days, subculturing 8 times at 3- to 4-day intervals. During the subculturing the presence of chicken anaemia virus may be indicated by a metabolic colour change in the infected cultures, the culture fluids become red in comparison with the control cultures. Examine the cells microscopically for cytopathic effect. At this time or at the end of the incubation period, centrifuge the cells from each flask at low speed and resuspend at about 106 cells/ml and place 25 µl in each of 10 wells of a multi-well slide. Examine the cells by immunostaining.

The test is not valid if chicken anaemia virus is detected in fewer than 3 of the 4 positive controls or in any of the non-inoculated controls. If the results for more than 1 of the test suspensions are inconclusive, then further subcultures of reserved portions of the test suspensions shall be made and tested until an unequivocal result is obtained.

The seed lot complies with the test if there is no evidence of the presence of chicken anaemia virus.

6. Test for extraneous agents using chicks

Inoculate each of at least 10 chicks, with the equivalent of 100 doses of vaccine by the intramuscular route and with the equivalent of 10 doses by eye-drop. Chicks that are 2 weeks of age are used in the test except that if the seed virus is pathogenic for birds of this age, older birds may be used, if required and justified. In exceptional cases, for inactivated vaccines, the virus may be neutralised by specific antiserum if the seed virus is pathogenic for birds at the age of administration. Repeat these inoculations 2 weeks later. Observe the chicks for a period of 5 weeks from the day of the first inoculation. No antimicrobial agents shall be administered to the chicks during the test period. The test is not valid if fewer than 80 per cent of the chicks survive to the end of the test period.

Collect serum from each chick at the end of the test period. Test each serum sample for antibodies against each of the agents listed below (with the exception of the virus type of the seed lot) using one of the methods indicated for testing for the agent.

Clinical signs of disease in the chicks during the test period (other than signs attributable to the virus of the seed lot) and the detection of antibodies in the chicks after inoculation, (with the exception of antibodies to the virus of the seed lot) are classed as evidence of the presence of an extraneous agent in the seed lot.

It is recommended that sera from these birds is retained so that additional testing may be carried out if requirements change.

A. Standard tests

Agent	Type of test
Avian adenoviruses, group 1	SN, EIA, AGP
Avian encephalomyelitis virus	AGP, EIA
Avian infectious bronchitis virus	EIA, HI
Avian infectious laryngotracheitis virus	SN, EIA, IS
Avian leucosis viruses	SN, EIA
Avian nephritis virus	IS
Avian orthoreoviruses	IS, EIA
Avian reticuloendotheliosis virus	AGP, IS, EIA
Chicken anaemia virus	IS, EIA, SN
Egg drop syndrome virus	HI, EIA
Avian infectious bursal disease virus	Serotype 1: AGP, EIA, SN Serotype 2: SN
Influenza A virus	AGP, EIA, HI
Marek's disease virus	AGP
Newcastle disease virus	HI, EIA
Turkey rhinotracheitis virus	EIA
Salmonella pullorum	Agg

Agg: agglutination
AGP: agar gel precipitation
EIA: enzyme immunoassay (e.g. ELISA)
IS: immunostaining (e.g. fluorescent antibody)
HI: haemagglutination inhibition
SN: serum neutralisation

B. Additional tests for turkey extraneous agents

If the seed virus is of turkey origin or was propagated in turkey substrates, tests for antibodies against the following agents are also carried out.

Agent	Type of test
Chlamydia spp.	EIA
Avian infectious haemorrhagic enteritis virus	AGP
Avian paramyxovirus 3	HI
Avian infectious bursal disease virus type 2	SN

A test for freedom from turkey lympho-proliferative disease virus is carried out by intraperitoneal inoculation of twenty 4-week-old turkey poults. Observe the poults for 40 days. The test is not valid if more than 20 per cent of the poults die from non-specific causes. The seed lot complies with the test if sections of spleen and thymus taken from 10 poults 2 weeks after inoculation show no macroscopic or microscopic lesions (other than those attributable to the seed lot virus) and no poult dies from causes attributable to the seed lot.

C. Additional tests for duck extraneous agents

If the seed virus is of duck origin or was propagated in duck substrates, tests for antibodies against the following agents are also carried out.

Agent	Type of test
Chlamydia spp.	EIA
Duck and goose parvoviruses	SN, EIA
Duck enteritis virus	SN
Duck hepatitis virus type I	SN

The seed lot complies with the test if there is no evidence of the presence of any extraneous agent.

D. Additional tests for goose extraneous agents

If the seed virus is of goose origin or was prepared in goose substrates, tests for the following agents are also carried out.

Agent	Type of test
Duck and goose parvovirus	SN, EIA
Duck enteritis virus	SN
Goose haemorrhagic polyomavirus	test in goslings shown below or another suitable test

Inoculate subcutaneously the equivalent of at least 10 doses to each of ten 1-day-old susceptible goslings. Observe the goslings for 28 days. The test is not valid if more than 20 per cent of the goslings die from non-specific causes. The seed virus complies with the test if no gosling dies from causes attributable to the seed lot.

7. Antibody specifications for sera used in extraneous agents testing

All batches of serum to be used in extraneous agents testing either to neutralise the vaccine virus (seed lot or batch of finished product) and all batches of avian serum used as a supplement for culture media used for tissue culture propagation, shall be shown to be free of antibodies against and free from inhibitory effects on the following micro-organisms by suitably sensitive tests:

Avian adenoviruses
Avian encephalomyelitis virus
~~Avian infectious bronchitis viruses~~
Avian infectious bursal disease virus types 1 and 2
Avian infectious haemorrhagic enteritis virus
Avian infectious laryngotracheitis virus
Avian leucosis viruses
Avian nephritis virus
Avian paramyxoviruses 1 to 9
Avian orthoreoviruses
Avian reticuloendotheliosis virus
Chicken anaemia virus
Duck enteritis virus
Duck hepatitis virus type I
Egg drop syndrome virus
Fowl pox virus
Influenza viruses
Marek's disease virus
Turkey herpesvirus
Turkey rhinotracheitis virus

Non-immune serum for addition to culture media can be assumed to be free of antibodies against any of these viruses if the agent is known not to infect the species of origin of the serum and it is not necessary to test the serum for such antibodies. Monospecific antisera for virus neutralisation can be assumed to be free of the antibodies against any of these viruses if it can be shown that the immunising antigen could not have been contaminated with antigens derived from that virus and if the virus is known not to infect the species of origin of the serum; it is not necessary to test the serum for such antibodies. It is not necessary to retest sera obtained from birds from SPF chicken flocks (5.2.2).

Batches of sera prepared for neutralising the vaccine virus must not be prepared from any passage level derived from the virus isolate used to prepare the master seed lot or from an isolate cultured in the same cell line.

B (Vet) 5. Avian Live Virus Vaccines: Tests for Extraneous Agents in Batches of Finished Product

(Ph. Eur. method 2.6.25)

General provisions

a) In the following tests, chickens and/or chicken material such as eggs and cell cultures shall be derived from chicken flocks free from specified pathogens (SPF) *(5.2.2)*.

b) Cell cultures for the testing of extraneous agents comply with the requirements for the master cell seed of chapter *5.2.4. Cell cultures for the production of veterinary vaccines*, with the exception of the karyotype test and the tumorigenicity test, which do not have to be carried out.

c) In tests using cell cultures, precise specifications are given for the number of replicates, monolayer surface areas and minimum survival rate of the cultures. Alternative numbers of replicates and cell surface areas are possible as well, provided that a minimum of 2 replicates are used, the total surface area and the total volume of vaccine test applied are not less than that prescribed here and the survival rate requirements are adapted accordingly.

d) In these tests, use the liquid vaccine or reconstitute a quantity of the freeze-dried preparation to be tested with the liquid stated on the label or another suitable diluent such as water for injections. Unless otherwise stated or justified, the test substance contains the equivalent of 10 doses in 0.1 ml of inoculum.

e) If the vaccine virus would interfere with the conduct and sensitivity of the test, neutralise the virus in the preparation with a monospecific antiserum.

f) Where specified in a monograph or otherwise justified, if neutralisation of the vaccine virus is required but difficult to achieve, the *in vitro* tests described below are adapted, as required, to provide the necessary guarantees of freedom from contamination with an extraneous agent. Alternatively, or in addition to *in vitro* tests conducted on the batch, a test for extraneous agents may be conducted on chick sera obtained from testing the batch of vaccine, as decribed under 6 Test for extraneous agents using chicks of chapter *2.6.24. Test for extraneous agents in seed lots.*

g) Monospecific antiserum and serum of avian origin used for cell culture and any other purpose, in any of these tests, shall be free of antibodies against and free from

inhibitory effects on the organisms listed under 7 Antibody specifications for sera used in extraneous agents testing *(2.6.24)*.

h) Other types of tests than those indicated may be used provided they are at least as sensitive as those indicated and of appropriate specificity. Nucleic acid amplification techniques *(2.6.21)* give specific detection for many agents and can be used after validation for sensitivity and specificity.

1. Test for extraneous agents using embryonated hens' eggs

Prepare the test vaccine, diluted if necessary, to contain neutralised virus equivalent to 10 doses of vaccine in 0.2 ml of inoculum. Suitable antibiotics may be added. Inoculate the test vaccine into 3 groups of 10 embryonated hens' eggs as follows:

— group 1: 0.2 ml into the allantoic cavity of each 9- to 11-day-old embryonated egg,

— group 2: 0.2 ml onto the chorio-allantoic membrane of each 9- to 11-day-old embryonated egg,

— group 3: 0.2 ml into the yolk sac of each 5- to 6-day-old embryonated egg.

Candle the eggs in groups 1 and 2 daily for 7 days and the eggs in group 3 for 12 days. Discard embryos that die during the first 24 h as non-specific deaths; the test is not valid unless at least 6 embryos in each group survive beyond the first 24 h after inoculation. Examine macroscopically for abnormalities all embryos which die more than 24 h after inoculation, or which survive the incubation period. Examine also the chorio-allantoic membranes of these eggs for any abnormality and test the allantoic fluids for the presence of haemagglutinating agents.

Carry out a further embryo passage. Pool separately material from live and from the dead and abnormal embryos. Inoculate each pool into 10 eggs for each route as described above, chorio-allantoic membrane material being inoculated onto chorio-allantoic membranes, allantoic fluids into the allantoic cavity and embryo material into the yolk sac. For eggs inoculated by the allantoic and chorio-allantoic routes, candle the eggs daily for 7 days, proceeding and examining the material as described above. For eggs inoculated by the yolk sac route, candle the eggs daily for 12 days, proceeding and examining the material as described above.

The batch of vaccine complies with the test if no test embryo shows macroscopic abnormalities or dies from causes attributable to the vaccine and if examination of the chorio-allantoic membranes and testing of the allantoic fluids show no evidence of the presence of extraneous agents.

2. Test in chicken embryo fibroblast cells

Prepare 7 monolayers of primary or secondary chicken embryo fibroblasts, from the tissues of 9- to 11-day-old embryos, each monolayer having an area of about 25 cm^2. Maintain 2 monolayers as negative controls and treat these in the same way as the 5 monolayers inoculated with the test vaccine, as described below. Remove the culture medium when the cells reach confluence. Inoculate 0.1 ml of test vaccine onto each of 5 of the monolayers. Allow adsorption for 1 h and add culture medium. Incubate the cultures for a total of at least 21 days, subculturing at 4- to 5-day intervals. Each passage is made with pooled cells and fluids from all 5 monolayers after carrying out a freeze-thaw cycle. Inoculate 0.1 ml of pooled material onto each of 5 recently prepared monolayers of chicken embryo fibroblast cells, each monolayer having an area of about 25 cm² each as before. For the last passage, grow the cells also on a suitable substrate so as to obtain an area of about 10 cm² of cells from each of the monolayers, for test A. The test is not valid if less than 80 per cent of the test monolayers, or neither of the 2 negative control monolayers survive after any passage.

Examine microscopically all the cell cultures frequently throughout the entire incubation period for any signs of cytopathic effect or other evidence of the presence of contaminating agents in the test vaccine. At the end of the total incubation period, carry out the following procedures.

A. Fix and stain (with Giemsa or haematoxylin and eosin) about 10 cm² of confluent cells from each of the 5 original monolayers. Examine the cells microscopically for any cytopathic effect, inclusion bodies, syncytial formation, or any other evidence of the presence of a contaminating agent from the test vaccine.

B. Drain and wash about 25 cm² of cells from each of the 5 monolayers. Cover these cells with a 0.5 per cent suspension of washed chicken red blood cells (using at least 1 ml of suspension for each 5 cm² of cells). Incubate the cells at 4 °C for 20 min and then wash gently in phosphate buffered saline pH 7.4. Examine the cells microscopically for haemadsorption attributable to the presence of a haemadsorbing agent in the test vaccine.

C. Test individually samples of the fluid from each cell culture using chicken red blood cells for haemagglutination attributable to the presence of a haemagglutinating agent in the test vaccine.

The test is not valid if there are any signs of extraneous agents in the negative control cultures. The batch of vaccine complies with the test if there is no evidence of the presence of any extraneous agent.

3. Test for egg drop syndrome virus

Prepare 11 monolayers of chicken embryo liver cells, from the tissues of 14- to 16-day-old embryos, each monolayer having an area of about 25 cm². Remove the culture medium when the cells reach confluence. Inoculate 0.1 ml of test vaccine onto each of 5 of the monolayers (test monolayers). Allow adsorption for 1 h, add culture medium. Inoculate 4 of the monolayers with a suitable strain of egg drop syndrome virus (not more than 10 $CCID_{50}$ in 0.1 ml) to serve as positive control monolayers. Maintain 2 non-inoculated monolayers as negative control monolayers.

Incubate the cells for a total of at least 21 days, subculturing every 4-5 days. Each passage is made as follows: carry out a freeze-thaw cycle; prepare separate pools of the cells plus fluid from the test monolayers, from the positive control monolayers and from the negative control monolayers; inoculate 0.1 ml of the pooled material onto each of 5, 4 and 2 recently prepared monolayers of chicken embryo liver cells, each monolayer having an area of about 25 cm² as before. The test is not valid if fewer than 4 of the 5 test monolayers or fewer than 3 of the 4 positive controls or neither of the 2 negative control monolayers survive after any passage.

Examine microscopically all the cell cultures at frequent intervals throughout the entire incubation period for any signs of cytopathic effect or other evidence of the presence of a contaminating agent in the test vaccine. At the end of the total incubation period, carry out the following procedure: test separately, cell culture fluid from the test monolayers, positive control monolayers and negative control monolayers,

using chicken red blood cells, for haemagglutination attributable to the presence of haemagglutinating agents.

The test is not valid if egg drop syndrome virus is detected in fewer than 3 of the 4 positive control monolayers or in any of the negative control monolayers, or if the results for both of the 2 negative control monolayers are inconclusive. If the results for more than 1 of the test monolayers are inconclusive then further subcultures of reserved portions of the monolayers shall be made and tested until an unequivocal result is obtained.

The batch of vaccine complies with the test if there is no evidence of the presence of egg drop syndrome virus or any other extraneous agent.

4. Test for Marek's disease virus

Prepare 11 monolayers of primary or secondary chick embryo fibroblasts from the tissues of 9- to 11-day-old embryos, each monolayer having an area of about 25 cm². Remove the culture medium when the cells reach confluence. Inoculate 0.1 ml of test vaccine onto each of 5 of the monolayers (test monolayers). Allow adsorption for 1 h, and add culture medium. Inoculate 4 of the monolayers with a suitable strain of Marek's disease virus (not more than 10 $CCID_{50}$ in 0.1 ml) to serve as positive controls. Maintain 2 non-inoculated monolayers as negative controls.

Incubate the cultures for a total of at least 21 days, subculturing at 4- to 5-day intervals. Each passage is made as follows: trypsinise the cells, prepare separate pools of the cells from the test monolayers, from the positive control monolayers and from the negative control monolayers. Mix an appropriate quantity of each with a suspension of freshly prepared primary or secondary chick embryo fibroblasts and prepare 5, 4 and 2 monolayers, as before. The test is not valid if fewer than 4 of the 5 test monolayers or fewer than 3 of the 4 positive controls or neither of the 2 negative control monolayers survive after any passage.

Examine microscopically all the cell cultures frequently throughout the entire incubation period for any signs of cytopathic effect or other evidence of the presence of a contaminating agent in the test vaccine.

For the last subculture, grow the cells on a suitable substrate so as to obtain an area of about 10 cm² of confluent cells from each of the original 11 monolayers for the subsequent test: test about 10 cm² of confluent cells derived from each of the original 11 monolayers by immunostaining for the presence of Marek's disease virus. The test is not valid if Marek's disease virus is detected in fewer than 3 of the 4 positive control monolayers or in any of the negative control monolayers, or if the results for both of the 2 negative control monolayers are inconclusive.

The batch of vaccine complies with the test if there is no evidence of the presence of Marek's disease virus or any other extraneous agent.

5. Tests for turkey rhinotracheitis virus

A. In chicken embryo fibroblasts

NOTE: this test can be combined with Test 2 by using the same test monolayers and negative controls, for all stages up to the final specific test for turkey rhinotracheitis virus on cells prepared from the last subculture.

Prepare 11 monolayers of primary or secondary chick embryo fibroblasts from the tissues of 9- to 11-day-old embryos, each monolayer having an area of about 25 cm². Remove the culture medium when the cells reach confluence. Inoculate 0.1 ml of test vaccine onto each of 5 of the monolayers (test monolayers). Allow adsorption for 1 h, and add culture medium. Inoculate 4 of the monolayers with a suitable strain of turkey rhinotracheitis virus as positive controls (not more than 10 $CCID_{50}$ in 0.1 ml). Maintain 2 non-inoculated monolayers as negative controls.

Incubate the cultures for a total of at least 21 days, subculturing at 4- to 5-day intervals. Each passage is made as follows: carry out a freeze-thaw cycle; prepare separate pools of the cells plus fluid from the test monolayers, from the positive control monolayers and from the negative control monolayers; inoculate 0.1 ml of the pooled material onto each of 5, 4 and 2 recently prepared monolayers of chicken embryo fibroblasts cells, each monolayer having an area of about 25 cm^2 as before. The test is not valid if fewer than 4 of the 5 test monolayers or fewer than 3 of the 4 positive controls or neither of the 2 negative control monolayers survive after any passage.

For the last subculture, grow the cells on a suitable substrate so as to obtain an area of about 10 cm^2 of confluent cells from each of the original 11 monolayers for the subsequent test: test about 10 cm^2 of confluent cells derived from each of the original 11 monolayers by immunostaining for the presence of turkey rhinotracheitis virus. The test is not valid if turkey rhinotracheitis virus is detected in fewer than 3 of the 4 positive control monolayers or in any of the negative control monolayers, or if the results for both of the 2 negative control monolayers are inconclusive. If the results for both of the 2 test monolayers are inconclusive then further subcultures of reserved portions of the fibroblasts shall be made and tested until an unequivocal result is obtained.

The batch of vaccine complies with the test if there is no evidence of the presence of turkey rhinotracheitis virus or any other extraneous agent.

B. In Vero cells

Prepare 11 monolayers of Vero cells, each monolayer having an area of about 25 cm^2. Remove the culture medium when the cells reach confluence. Inoculate 0.1 ml of test vaccine onto each of 5 of the monolayers (test monolayers). Allow adsorption for 1 h, and add culture medium. Inoculate 4 of the monolayers with a suitable strain of turkey rhinotracheitis virus (not more than 10 $CCID_{50}$ in 0.1 ml) to serve as positive controls. Maintain 2 non-inoculated monolayers as negative controls.

Incubate the cultures for a total of at least 21 days, subculturing at 4- to 5-day intervals. Each passage is made as follows: carry out a freeze-thaw cycle. Prepare separate pools of the cells plus fluid from the test monolayers, from the positive control monolayers and from the negative control monolayers. Inoculate 0.1 ml of the pooled material onto each of 5, 4 and 2 recently prepared monolayers of Vero cells, each monolayer having an area of about 25 cm^2 as before. The test is not valid if fewer than 4 of the 5 test monolayers or fewer than 3 of the 4 positive controls or neither of the 2 negative controls survive after any passage.

For the last subculture, grow the cells on a suitable substrate so as to obtain an area of about 10 cm^2 of confluent cells from each of the original 11 monolayers for the subsequent test: test about 10 cm^2 of confluent cells derived from each of the original 11 monolayers by immunostaining for the presence of turkey rhinotracheitis virus. The test is not valid if turkey rhinotracheitis virus is detected in fewer than 3 of the 4 positive control monolayers or in any of the negative control monolayers, or if the results for both of the 2 negative control monolayers are inconclusive. If the results for more than 1 of the test monolayers are inconclusive then further subcultures of reserved portions of the monolayers shall be made and tested until an unequivocal result is obtained.

The batch of vaccine complies with the test if there is no evidence of the presence of turkey rhinotracheitis virus or any other extraneous agent.

6. Test for chicken anaemia virus

Prepare eleven 20 ml suspensions of the MDCC-MSBI cell line or another cell line of equivalent sensitivity in 25 cm^2 flasks containing about 5×10^5 cells/ml. Inoculate 0.1 ml of test vaccine into each of 5 of these flasks. Inoculate 4 other suspensions with 10 $CCID_{50}$ chicken anaemia virus as positive controls. Maintain not fewer than 2 non-inoculated suspensions. Maintain all the cell cultures for a total of at least 24 days, subculturing 8 times at 3- to 4-day intervals. During the subculturing the presence of chicken anaemia virus may be indicated by a metabolic colour change in the infected cultures, the culture fluids becoming red in comparison with the control cultures. Examine the cells microscopically for cytopathic effect. At this time or at the end of the incubation period, centrifuge the cells from each flask at low speed, resuspend at about 10^6 cells per millilitre and place 25 µl in each of 10 wells of a multi-well slide. Examine the cells by immunostaining.

The test is not valid if chicken anaemia virus is detected in fewer than 3 of the 4 positive controls or in any of the non-inoculated controls. If the results for more than 1 of the test suspensions are inconclusive then further subcultures of reserved portions of the test suspensions shall be made and tested until an unequivocal result is obtained.

The batch of vaccine complies with the test if there is no evidence of the presence of chicken anaemia virus.

7. Test for duck enteritis virus

This test is carried out for vaccines prepared on duck or goose substrates.

Prepare 11 monolayers of primary or secondary Muscovy duck embryo liver cells, from the tissues of 21- or 22-day-old embryos, each monolayer having an area of about 25 cm^2. Remove the culture medium when the cells reach confluence. Inoculate 0.1 ml of test vaccine onto each of 5 of the monolayers (test monolayers). Allow adsorption for 1 h and add culture medium. Inoculate 4 of the monolayers with a suitable strain of duck enteritis virus (not more than 10 $CCID_{50}$ in 0.1 ml) to serve as positive controls. Maintain 2 non-inoculated monolayers as negative controls.

Incubate the cultures for a total of at least 21 days, subculturing at 4- to 5-day intervals. Each passage is made as follows: trypsinise the cells and prepare separate pools of the cells from the test monolayers, from the positive control monolayers and from the negative control monolayers. Mix a portion of each with a suspension of freshly prepared primary or secondary Muscovy duck embryo liver cells to prepare 5, 4 and 2 monolayers, as before. The test is not valid if fewer than 4 of the 5 test monolayers or fewer than 3 of the 4 positive controls or neither of the 2 negative controls survive after any passage.

For the last subculture, grow the cells on a suitable substrate so as to obtain an area of about 10 cm^2 of confluent cells from each of the original 11 monolayers for the subsequent test: test about 10 cm^2 of confluent cells derived from each of the original 11 monolayers by immunostaining for the presence of duck enteritis virus. The test is not valid if duck enteritis virus is detected in fewer than 3 of the 4 positive control monolayers or in any of the negative control monolayers, or if the results for both of the 2 negative control monolayers are inconclusive. If the results for more than 1 of the test monolayers are inconclusive then further subcultures of reserved portions of the monolayers shall be made and tested until an unequivocal result is obtained.

The batch of vaccine complies with the test if there is no evidence of the presence of duck enteritis virus or any other extraneous agent.

8. Test for duck and goose parvoviruses

This test is carried out for vaccines prepared on duck or goose substrates.

Prepare a suspension of sufficient primary or secondary Muscovy duck embryo fibroblasts from the tissues of 16- to 18-day-old embryos, to obtain not fewer than 11 monolayers, each having an area of about 25 cm^2. Inoculate 0.5 ml of test vaccine into an aliquot of cells for 5 monolayers and seed into 5 replicate containers to form 5 test monolayers. Inoculate 0.4 ml of a suitable strain of duck parvovirus (not more than 10 CCID$_{50}$ in 0.1 ml) into an aliquot of cells for 4 monolayers and seed into 4 replicate containers to form 4 positive control monolayers. Prepare 2 non-inoculated monolayers as negative controls.

Incubate the cultures for a total of at least 21 days, subculturing at 4- to 5-day intervals. Each passage is made as follows: carry out a freeze-thaw cycle. Prepare separate pools of the cells plus fluid from the test monolayers, from the positive control monolayers and from the negative control monolayers. Inoculate 0.5 ml, 0.4 ml and 0.2 ml of the pooled materials into aliquots of a fresh suspension of sufficient primary or secondary Muscovy duck embryo fibroblast cells to prepare 5, 4 and 2 monolayers, as before. The test is not valid if fewer than 4 of the 5 test monolayers or fewer than 3 of the 4 positive controls or neither of the 2 negative controls survive after any passage.

For the last subculture, grow the cells on a suitable substrate so as to obtain an area of about 10 cm^2 of confluent cells from each of the original 11 monolayers for the subsequent test: test about 10 cm^2 of confluent cells derived from each of the original 11 monolayers by immunostaining for the presence of duck or goose parvovirus. The test is not valid if duck parvovirus is detected in fewer than 3 of the 4 positive control monolayers or in any of the negative control monolayers, or if the results for both of the 2 negative control monolayers are inconclusive.

The batch of vaccine complies with the test if there is no evidence of the presence of duck (or goose) parvovirus or any other extraneous agent.

Appendix XXI

B (Vet). Approved Synonyms

Where the English title at the head of a monograph in the European Pharmacopoeia is different from that at the head of the text incorporated into the British Pharmacopoeia or the British Pharmacopoeia (Veterinary), an Approved Synonym (or Approved Synonyms) is declared in accordance with section 65(8) of the Medicines Act 1968.

In accordance with the General Notice on Titles, the name or names given in the right-hand column of the list below are Approved Synonyms for the name at the head of the monograph of the European Pharmacopoeia given in the left-hand column. Where there is more than one entry in the right-hand column, the first entry is used as the title of the monograph in the British Pharmacopoeia or the British Pharmacopoeia (Veterinary) and the remaining entries are included as subsidiary titles.

Approved Synonyms and subsidiary titles have the same significance as the main title and are thus official titles.

Names made by changing the order of the words in an Approved Synonym, with the addition of a preposition when necessary, are also Approved Synonyms.

Where square brackets are used in a title these may be replaced by round brackets, and *vice versa*. The words 'per cent' may be replaced by the symbol '%'.

Where the word 'Injection' appears in the title or synonym of a monograph in the European Pharmacopoeia, the abbreviation 'Inj.' is declared to be an Approved Synonym for that part of the title.

A consolidated list of all Approved Synonyms is included in Appendix XXI B of the *British Pharmacopoeia*.

EUROPEAN PHARMACOPOEIA TITLE	APPROVED SYNONYM
Medicinal Substances and Formulated Preparations	
Azaperone for Veterinary Use	Azaperone
Clazuril for Veterinary Use	Clazuril
Closantel Sodium Dihydrate for Veterinary Use	Closantel Sodium Dihydrate
Dembrexine Hydrochloride Monohydrate for Veterinary Use	Dembrexine Hydrochloride Monohydrate
Detomidine Hydrochloride for Veterinary Use	Detomidine Hydrochloride
Diclazuril for Veterinary Use	Diclazuril
Dihydrostreptomycin Sulphate for Veterinary Use	Dihydrostreptomycin Sulphate
Enilconazole for Veterinary Use	Enilconazole
Equine Serum Gonadotrophin for Veterinary Use	Serum Gonadotrophin
Febantel for Veterinary Use	Febantel
Flunixin Meglumine for Veterinary Use	Flunixin Meglumine
Levamisole for Veterinary Use	Levamisole
Morantel Hydrogen Tartrate for Veterinary Use	Morantel Tartrate
Oxfendazole for Veterinary Use	Oxfendazole
Spectinomycin Sulphate Tetrahydrate for Veterinary Use	Spectinomycin Sulphate Tetrahydrate
Tiamulin for Veterinary Use	Tiamulin
Tiamulin Hydrogen Fumarate for Veterinary Use	Tiamulin Hydrogen Fumarate
Tylosin For Veterinary Use	Tylosin
Tylosin Phosphate Bulk Solution for Veterinary Use	Tylosin Phosphate
Tylosin Tartrate For Veterinary Use	Tylosin Tartrate
Valnemulin Hydrochloride for Veterinary Use	Valnemulin Hydrochloride

EUROPEAN PHARMACOPOEIA TITLE	APPROVED SYNONYM
Immunological Products (Veterinary)	
Anthrax Spore Vaccine (Live) for Veterinary Use	Anthrax Vaccine, Living
Aujeszky's Disease Vaccine (Inactivated) for Pigs	Aujeszky's Disease Vaccine, Inactivated
Aujeszky's Disease Vaccine (Live) for Pigs for Parenteral Administration, Freeze-dried	Aujeszky's Disease Vaccine, Living
Avian Infectious Bronchitis Vaccine (Live)	Avian Infectious Bronchitis Vaccine, Living
Avian Infectious Bursal Disease Vaccine (Inactivated)	Infectious Bursal Disease Vaccine, Inactivated Gumboro Disease Vaccine, Inactivated
Avian Infectious Bursal Disease Vaccine (Live)	Infectious Bursal Disease Vaccine, Living Gumboro Disease Vaccine, Living
Avian Infectious Encephalomyelitis Vaccine (Live)	Infectious Avian Encephalomyelitis Vaccine, Living Epidemic Tremor Vaccine, Living
Avian Infectious Laryngotracheitis Vaccine (Live)	Laryngotracheitis Vaccine, Living
Avian Paramyxovirus 3 Vaccine (Inactivated)	Avian Paramyxovirus 3 Vaccine, Inactivated
Bovine Parainfluenza Virus Vaccine (Live), Freeze-dried	Bovine Parainfluenza Virus Vaccine, Living
Bovine Respiratory Syncytial Virus Vaccine (Live), Freeze-dried	Bovine Respiratory Syncytial Virus Vaccine, Living
Brucellosis Vaccine (Live) (Brucella Melitensis Rev. 1 Strain) Freeze-dried, for Veterinary Use	Brucella Melitensis (Strain Rev. 1) Vaccine, Living
Canine Adenovirus Vaccine (Inactivated)	Canine Adenovirus Vaccine, Inactivated
Canine Adenovirus Vaccine (Live)	Canine Adenovirus Vaccine, Living
Canine Distemper Vaccine (Live), Freeze-dried	Canine Distemper Vaccine, Living
Canine Parvovirosis Vaccine (Inactivated)	Canine Parvovirus Vaccine, Inactivated
Canine Parvovirosis Vaccine (Live)	Canine Parvovirus Vaccine, Living
Clostridium Botulinum Vaccine for Veterinary Use	Clostridium Botulinum Vaccine Botulinum Vaccine
Clostridium Chauvoei Vaccine for Veterinary Use	Clostridium Chauvoei Vaccine Blackleg Vaccine
Clostridium Novyi (Type B) Vaccine for Veterinary Use	Clostridium Novyi Type B Vaccine Black Disease Vaccine
Clostridium Novyi Alpha Antitoxin for Veterinary Use	Clostridium Novyi Alpha Antitoxin
Clostridium Perfringens Beta Antitoxin for Veterinary Use	Clostridium Perfringens Beta Antitoxin
Clostridium Perfringens Epsilon Antitoxin for Veterinary Use	Clostridium Perfringens Epsilon Antitoxin Clostridium Perfringens Type D Antitoxin

EUROPEAN PHARMACOPOEIA TITLE	APPROVED SYNONYM
Clostridium Perfringens Vaccine for Veterinary Use Type B Type C Type D	Clostridium Perfringens Vaccines Clostridium Perfringens Type B Vaccine Lamb Dysentery Vaccine Clostridium Perfringens Type C Vaccine Struck Vaccine Clostridium Perfringens Type D Vaccine Pulpy Kidney Vaccine
Clostridium Septicum Vaccine for Veterinary Use	Clostridium Septicum VaccineBraxy Vaccine
Distemper Vaccine (Live) for Mustelids, Freeze-dried	Ferret and Mink Distemper Vaccine, Living
Egg Drop Syndrome '76 Vaccine (Inactivated)	Egg Drop Syndrome '76 (Adenovirus) Vaccine
Equine Herpesvirus Vaccine (Inactivated)	Equine Herpesvirus Vaccine, Inactivated
Equine Influenza Vaccine (Inactivated)	Equine Influenza Vaccine, Inactivated
Feline Calicivirosis Vaccine (Inactivated)	Feline Calicivirus Vaccine, Inactivated
Feline Calicivirosis Vaccine (Live), Freeze-dried	Feline Calicivirus Vaccine, Living
Feline Infectious Enteritis (Feline Panleucopenia) Vaccine (Inactivated)	Feline Infectious Enteritis Vaccine, Inactivated Feline Panleucopenia Vaccine, Inactivated
Feline Infectious Enteritis (Feline Panleucopenia) Vaccine (Live)	Feline Infectious Enteritis Vaccine, Living Feline Panleucopenia Vaccine, Living
Feline Leukaemia Vaccine (Inactivated)	Feline Leukaemia Vaccine, Inactivated
Feline Viral Rhinotracheitis Vaccine (Inactivated)	Feline Viral Rhinotracheitis Vaccine, Inactivated
Feline Viral Rhinotracheitis Vaccine (Live)	Feline Viral Rhinotracheitis Vaccine, Living
Foot-and-mouth Disease (Ruminants) Vaccine (Inactivated)	Foot and Mouth Disease (Ruminants) Vaccine
Fowl-pox Vaccine (Live)	Fowl Pox Vaccine, Living
Furunculosis Vaccine (Inactivated, oil-adjuvanted, Injectable) for Salmonids	Furunculosis Vaccine for Salmonids, Inactivated
Infectious Bovine Rhinotracheitis Vaccine (Live), Freeze-dried	Infectious Bovine Rhinotracheitis Vaccine, Living
Marek's Disease Vaccine (Live)	Marek's Disease Vaccine, Living Marek's Disease Vaccine (Turkey Herpes Virus) Marek's Disease Vaccine, Living (HVT)
Neonatal Piglet Colibacillosis Vaccine (Inactivated)	Porcine E. Coli Vaccine, Inactivated Porcine Escherichia Coli Vaccine, Inactivated
Neonatal Ruminant Colibacillosis Vaccine (Inactivated)	Ruminant E. Coli Vaccine, Inactivated Ruminant Escherichia Coli Vaccine, Inactivated
Newcastle Disease Vaccine (Inactivated)	Newcastle Disease Vaccine, Inactivated
Newcastle Disease Vaccine (Live)	Newcastle Disease Vaccine, Living

EUROPEAN PHARMACOPOEIA TITLE	APPROVED SYNONYM
Porcine Actinobacillosis Vaccine (Inactivated)	Porcine Actinobacillosis Vaccine, Inactivated
Porcine Influenza Vaccine (Inactivated)	Swine Influenza Vaccine, Inactivated
Porcine Parvovirosis Vaccine (Inactivated)	Porcine Parvovirus Vaccine, Inactivated
Porcine Progressive Atrophic Rhinitis Vaccine (Inactivated)	Porcine Progressive Atrophic Rhinitis Vaccine, Inactivated
Rabies Vaccine (Inactivated) for Veterinary Use	Rabies Veterinary Vaccine, Inactivated
Rabies Vaccine (Live, Oral) for Foxes	Rabies Vaccine for Foxes, Living
Swine Erysipelas Vaccine (Inactivated)	Swine Erysipelas Vaccine, Inactivated
Swine-fever Vaccine (Live), Classical, Freeze-dried	Swine Fever Vaccine, Living
Tetanus Antitoxin for Veterinary Use	Clostridium Tetani Antitoxin Tetanus Antitoxin (Veterinary)
Tetanus Vaccine for Veterinary Use	Clostridium Tetani Vaccines Clostridium Tetani Vaccine for Equidae *(for vaccines with an appropriate potency)* Tetanus Toxoids (Veterinary) Tetanus Toxoid for Equidae *(for vaccines with an appropriate potency)*
Tuberculin Purified Protein Derivative, Avian	Avian Tuberculin Purified Protein Derivative Avian Tuberculin P.P.D.
Tuberculin Purified Protein Derivative, Bovine	Bovine Tuberculin Purified Protein Derivative Bovine Tuberculin P.P.D.
Vibriosis (Cold-water) Vaccine (Inactivated) for Salmonids	Vibriosis Vaccine for Salmonids, Inactivated, Cold-water
Vibriosis Vaccine (Inactivated) for Salmonids	Vibriosis Vaccine for Salmonids, Inactivated

Index

Page numbers in **bold type** relate to monograph titles.